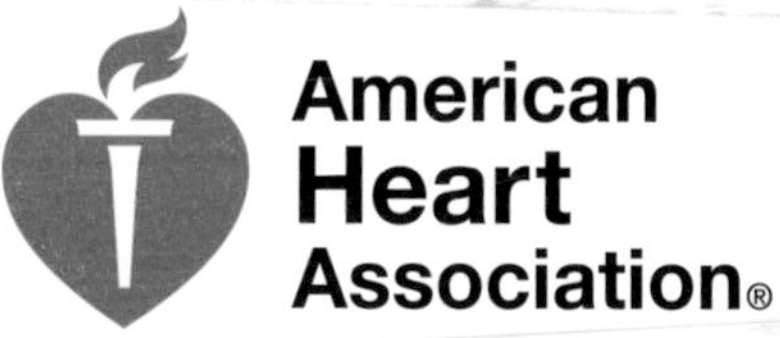

ACLS for Experienced Providers

MANUAL AND RESOURCE TEXT

Editors

Elizabeth Sinz, MD, *Senior Science Editor*
Kenneth Navarro, *Content Consultant*

Senior Managing Editor

Erik S. Soderberg, MS

Special Contributors

Benjamin S. Abella, MD, MPhil
Clifton W. Callaway, MD, PhD
Heba Costandy, MD, MS
Julie Crider, PhD
Michael Donnino, MD
David Gilmore, MD
Saket Girotra, MD
Farida Jeejeebhoy, MD
Richard Kerber, MD
Peter J. Kudenchuk, MD
Allen McCullough, PhD
Jeff Messerole, PS
Robert W. Neumar, MD, PhD
Brian O'Neil, MD
Peter D. Panagos, MD
Sallie Young, PharmD, BCPS, *Pharmacotherapy Editor*

ISBN 978-1-61669-313-8
Printed in the United States of America
First American Heart Association Printing April 2013
10 9 8 7 6 5 4 3 2 1

ACLS Subcommittee 2012-2013

Brian O'Neil, MD, *Chair*
Clifton W. Callaway, MD, PhD, *Immediate Past Chair, 2010-2012*
Michael Donnino, MD
Andrea Gabrielli, MD
Raúl J. Gazmuri, MD, PhD
Romergryko Geocadin, MD
Erik Hess, MD, MSc
Edward C. Jauch, MD, MS
Richard Kerber, MD
Peter J. Kudenchuk, MD
Eric Lavonas, MD
Ronald M. Lazar, PhD
Venu Menon, MD
Laurie J. Morrison, MD, MSc
Robert W. Neumar, MD, PhD
Graham Nichol, MD, MPH
Joseph P. Ornato, MD
Mary Ann Peberdy, MD
Scott M. Silvers, MD
Kimberly S. Staffey, MD
Mintu Turakhia, MD, MS
Terry L. Vanden Hoek, MD
Janice L. Zimmerman, MD

ACLS Subcommittee 2011-2012

Clifton W. Callaway, MD, PhD, *Chair*
Robert W. Neumar, MD, PhD, *Immediate Past Chair, 2008-2010*
Michael Donnino, MD
Andrea Gabrielli, MD
Raúl J. Gazmuri, MD, PhD
Romergryko Geocadin, MD
Erik Hess, MD, MSc
Edward C. Jauch, MD, MS
Richard Kerber, MD
Peter J. Kudenchuk, MD
Eric Lavonas, MD
Ronald M. Lazar, PhD
Venu Menon, MD
Laurie J. Morrison, MD, MSc
Graham Nichol, MD, MPH
Brian O'Neil, MD
Joseph P. Ornato, MD
Mary Ann Peberdy, MD
Scott M. Silvers, MD
Kimberly S. Staffey, MD
Mintu Turakhia, MD, MS
Terry L. Vanden Hoek, MD
Demetris Yannopoulos, MD
Janice L. Zimmerman, MD

Acknowledgments

Darren Hamilton, BA, MLIS
Moshe Levi, MD

References

The *ACLS for Experienced Providers Manual and Resource Text* is referenced with suggested reading, key references, landmark trials, and important meta-analyses. For more detailed references, refer to the *2010 AHA Guidelines for CPR and ECC.*

Note on Medication Doses

Emergency cardiovascular care is a dynamic science. Advances in treatment and drug therapies occur rapidly. Readers should use the following sources to check for changes in recommended doses, indications, and contraindications: the ECC Handbook, available as optional supplementary material, and the package insert product information sheet for each drug and medical device.

To find out about any updates or corrections to this text, visit **www.heart.org/cpr**, navigate to the page for this course, and click on "Updates."

To access the Student Website for this course, go to **www.heart.org/eccstudent** and enter this code: aclsresource

Contents

Contents

Chapter 1

Introduction

This Chapter

- Sudden Cardiac Death
- Chain of Survival
- Closing the Gaps
- Science Behind the Guidelines

Is There Incremental Benefit With ACLS?

Advanced cardiovascular life support (ACLS) providers face an important challenge—functioning as a team that implements and integrates both basic and advanced life support to save a person's life. The *2010 American Heart Association Guidelines for Cardiopulmonary Resuscitation and Emergency Cardiovascular Care (2010 AHA Guidelines for CPR and ECC)* reviewed evidence that showed that in both the in-hospital and out-of-hospital settings, many cardiac arrest patients do not receive high-quality cardiopulmonary resuscitation (CPR), and the majority do not survive. One study of in-hospital cardiac arrest showed that the quality of CPR was inconsistent and did not always meet guidelines recommendations.[1] Another study that evaluated the benefit of out-of-hospital ACLS found no additional advantage with ACLS, raising questions about current-day quality and benefit of ACLS interventions.[2] Over the years, however, patient outcomes after cardiac arrest have improved. In 2005, rates of survival to hospital discharge from witnessed out-of-hospital sudden cardiac arrest due to ventricular fibrillation (VF) were low, averaging 6% worldwide with little change before the 2005 conference. The 2012 Update of AHA's Heart Disease and Stroke Statistics showed that in the United States, the rate of survival to hospital discharge from emergency medical services (EMS)–treated non-traumatic out-of-hospital cardiac arrest had increased to 11.4%, and that of bystander-witnessed VF was 32.0%.[3] In the 2013 Update, these survival rates dropped to 9.5% and 28.4%, respectively.[4] Of adults who experienced in-hospital cardiac arrest, 24.2% survived to discharge. VF or pulseless ventricular tachycardia (VT) was the first recorded rhythm in 17.6%; and of these, 43.0% survived to discharge.[4]

To analyze these findings, a "back-to-basics" evidence review refocused on the essentials of CPR, the links in the Chain of Survival, and the integration of basic life support (BLS) with ACLS. Minimizing the interval between stopping chest compressions and delivering a shock (ie, minimizing the preshock pause) improves the chances of shock success[6] and patient survival.[7] The changes in the compression-ventilation ratio to 30:2 and in using 1 shock instead of 3 followed by immediate CPR were recommended to minimize interruptions in chest compressions.[8] Experts believe that high survival rates from both out-of-hospital and in-hospital sudden cardiac death are possible with strong systems of care.

High survival rates in studies are associated with several common elements:

- Training of knowledgeable healthcare providers
- Planned and practiced response
- Rapid recognition of sudden cardiac arrest
- Prompt provision of CPR
- Defibrillation within about 3 to 5 minutes of collapse
- Organized post–cardiac arrest care, which may improve survival for patients who achieve return of spontaneous circulation (ROSC) after cardiac arrest

Critical Concept	ACLS is optimized when a team leader effectively integrates high-quality CPR, including minimal interruption of high-quality chest compressions, with advanced life support strategies.

Critical Concept	Studies have shown that a reduction in the interval between compression and shock delivery can increase the predicted shock success. Interruptions in compressions should be minimized to 10 seconds or less.

When trained persons implement these elements early, ACLS has the best chance of producing a successful outcome. If the patient remains in cardiac arrest despite early interventions, 3 key elements of ACLS are now thought to provide optimal outcome and serve as a matrix for survival:

- **High-quality chest compressions delivered with minimal interruption**
- A team approach that integrates BLS and ACLS seamlessly
- Critical thinking and decision making by the team leader, who is responsible for organizing the team

Vasopressors, Antiarrhythmics, and Sequence of Actions During Treatment of Cardiac Arrest

At the time of the 2010 International Consensus Conference there were **no placebo-controlled human trials showing that any medication—vasopressor or antiarrhythmic drug—given routinely at any stage during cardiac arrest increases the rate of neurologically intact survival to hospital discharge.** Given this lack of documented effect of drug therapy in improving long-term outcome from cardiac arrest, the sequence for CPR deemphasizes drug administration and reemphasizes basic life support.

Coordination of Shock-Drug Sequence

To minimize interruptions in chest compressions for administration of drugs, the *2010 AHA Guidelines for CPR and ECC* recommend that healthcare providers resume CPR beginning with chest compressions *immediately* after a shock, without an intervening rhythm (or pulse) check.[9] Administer vasopressors or antiarrhythmics anytime during the 2-minute cycle as long as administration does not interrupt compressions or interfere with the next rhythm check. It will take time for the drug to be circulated by compressions and for the drug to take effect.

Healthcare providers should coordinate CPR and shock delivery so that, when a shock is indicated, it can be delivered as soon as possible after everyone is "cleared" from contact with the patient.

Sudden Cardiac Death

Sudden cardiac death (SCD) is the most dramatic presentation of acute coronary ischemia and a major public health problem in most developed countries today. Cardiovascular disease accounts for approximately one third of overall deaths. One third to one half of these are sudden and occur in the community. In 20%, SCD is the first, last, and only symptom. Trends in the incidence of SCD parallel coronary artery disease and atherogenic risk factors, particularly cigarette smoking. Accordingly, the incidence of sudden death has been declining in countries with decreasing rates of coronary artery disease. From 1950 to 1999, nonsudden coronary heart disease deaths in the United States decreased by 64% and SCD fell by 49%.[10] This decrease, the complexity of the problem, and recent therapeutic innovations have led to a false sense of security and progress.[1,8]

Who Dies Suddenly?

Definition

Previous studies and reviews of sudden death and cardiac arrest have been limited by the lack of uniform definitions. To address problems of definition, a panel of international experts developed consensus guidelines for the classification, definition, and reporting of sudden death and cardiac arrest.[11] In general, sudden death is used to describe collapse that occurs with minimal or no premonitory symptoms and death occurs less than 1 hour from onset of symptoms. Cardiac arrest is defined as a sudden cessation of cardiac mechanical activity, confirmed by unresponsiveness; apnea or agonal, gasping respirations; and the absence of a detectable pulse. SCD is often described as an unexpected death due to cardiac causes occurring within 1 hour of symptom onset whether the person has known or unknown cardiac disease. SCD is often related to cardiac arrhythmias.

Etiology

The underlying etiologies of atraumatic sudden death and its associated conditions are numerous and diverse. In general they can be separated into coronary (atherosclerotic and nonatherosclerotic) causes, noncoronary cardiac disease, and noncardiac events (Figure 1). Although coronary causes account for the majority of cases of sudden death, pulmonary, vascular, and central nervous system events occur in 15% to 30% of cases and are often undiagnosed. An underlying condition may be the cause of the cardiac arrest and serve as a trigger for sudden death. For example, hypoxia from any cause may exacerbate or cause coronary ischemia, resulting in cardiac arrest. The success of resuscitation and patient survival often depends on rapid identification and treatment of an underlying condition.

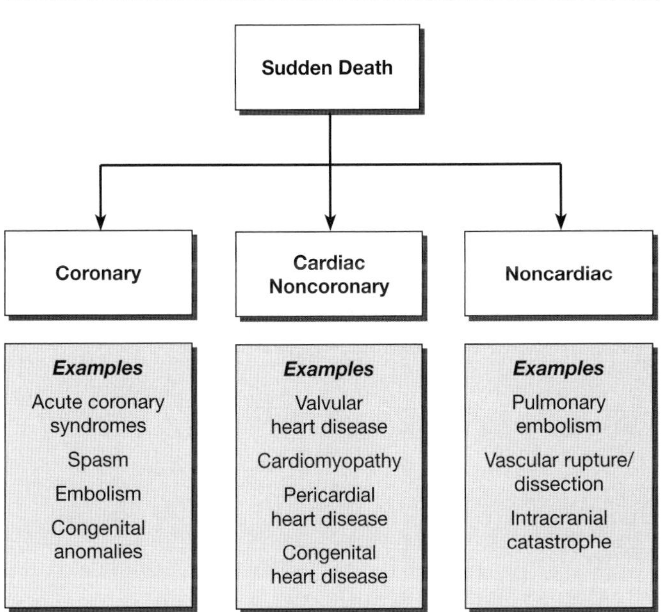

Figure 1. Three general classes of atraumatic sudden death. Deaths due to coronary heart disease are attributable largely to acute coronary syndromes. Hypertrophic obstructive cardiomyopathy is the most common cardiac noncoronary cause of sudden death in young adults.

Sudden Deaths Due to Cardiac Disease

It is difficult to estimate accurately the percentage of sudden deaths due to cardiac causes because many studies use the term *presumed cardiac etiology* in the absence of autopsy confirmation. Atherosclerotic coronary artery disease is by far the most common condition associated with SCD.[12] In one postmortem study of men with coronary artery disease, approximately 50% had an acute coronary thrombus and the rest had severe narrowing of their coronary arteries.[13] Most adult patients with sudden death have multivessel coronary disease, and they often have previous infarction as an associated finding even in the absence of prior known history of myocardial infarction. Fifty percent of men and 64% of women who die suddenly of coronary artery disease have no previous symptoms of this disease.[14] Autopsy studies have shown that 60% to 75% of SCDs are due to coronary artery disease (Figure 2) and acute coronary syndromes; the remainder are largely due to cardiomyopathy and valvular heart disease. The demographics of SCD are changing, and chronic congestive heart failure accounts for an increasing percentage of patients with sudden death. In these patients, an old myocardial infarct can serve as a focus for electrical instability, leading to fatal arrhythmias.[15] One third of patients with congestive heart failure die from acute coronary syndromes, which are not consistently recognized in patients dying suddenly.[16] Predisposing risk factors closely parallel those for coronary disease in general. These include male sex, age, cigarette smoking, hypertension, hyperlipidemia, and left ventricular hypertrophy. In several studies, smoking had a particularly strong relationship to the risk of sudden death.[15,17]

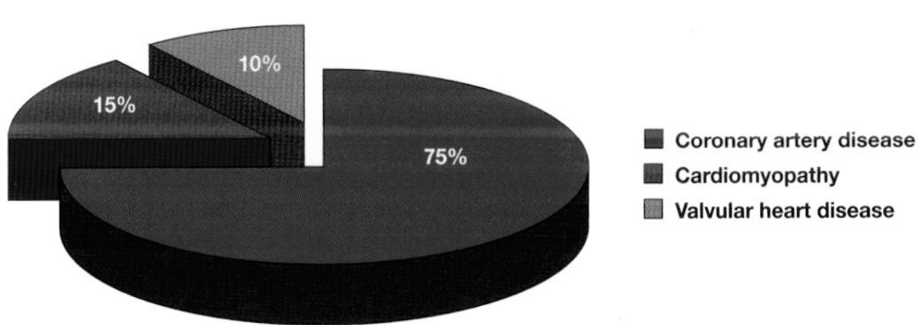

Figure 2. Major underlying etiologies of sudden cardiac death.

Sudden Deaths Caused by Noncardiac Causes

In the patient with sudden atraumatic death, the events around the event may provide some clues about the likely cause. Although cardiac disease is often present and may be the primary cause of arrest, other likely diagnoses must be considered and treated if necessary to revive the patient. Identifying special circumstances that require specific interventions may increase the victim's chance of survival when acted on in a timely and appropriate manner.

Strategies for Prevention and Treatment

A comprehensive strategy should be designed to modify risk factors, identify patients at high risk, and urgently treat patients with sudden arrest. Populations trained in CPR and a highly skilled and rapidly responding EMS system are essential for survival of the patient with cardiac arrest. Survival, however, is low, and many patients have advanced disease at the time of cardiac arrest. A strategy for primary and secondary prevention must be part of any public health policy if long-term goals are to be realized. Patients at high risk of sudden death should be identified and survivors of sudden death extensively evaluated and treated as part of a postarrest management plan.

The Adult Chain of Survival

When cardiac arrest occurs, an integrated set of coordinated actions must be done as rapidly as possible to achieve the greatest potential for survival. These actions are linked together in a Chain of Survival (Figure 3), and each link is critical. The links include

- Immediate **recognition** of cardiac arrest and **activation** of the emergency response system
- Early **CPR** with an emphasis on chest compressions
- Rapid **defibrillation**
- Effective **advanced life support**
- Integrated **post–cardiac arrest care**

Figure 3. The AHA adult Chain of Survival.

The First Link: Immediate Recognition of Cardiac Arrest and Activation of Emergency Response System

Immediate activation of the emergency response system encompasses the events initiated after the patient's collapse until the arrival of emergency personnel prepared to provide care. The following events, each of which must occur rapidly, make up the immediate recognition and activation link:

- Someone must immediately identify the patient's collapse or signs of emergency and activate the emergency response system.
- The emergency medical dispatcher or other individual receiving the request must rapidly recognize the potential cardiac arrest or emergency and immediately initiate an appropriate emergency response (BLS-level and ACLS-level personnel respond simultaneously).
- Properly equipped emergency responders must arrive rapidly at the patient's side.

Regardless of the setting, once a victim or patient becomes unresponsive with no breathing or no normal breathing (ie, only gasping), the first person on the scene should activate the appropriate emergency response system and start CPR.

Immediate recognition of early warning signs, such as chest discomfort and shortness of breath, enables patients or bystanders to activate the emergency response system before collapse. However, recognition of cardiac arrest is not always straightforward, especially for laypeople. A rescuer's confusion can result in a delay or failure to activate the emergency response system or to start CPR. In healthcare facilities such as hospitals, it is increasingly common to have a defined mechanism for patients, family members, and other laypeople to alert hospital staff about a potential emergency. In both out-of-hospital and in-hospital settings, the person receiving the call for assistance must immediately recognize the emergency and rapidly summon the appropriate assistance.

Dispatchers and the EMS System

Rapid emergency medical dispatch has emerged as a critical component of the immediate recognition link for out-of-hospital emergencies.[18] Use of a 3-digit, dedicated emergency number (eg, 911) has simplified and shortened access to emergency assistance. EMS dispatch systems must be able to immediately answer all emergency medical calls, quickly determine the nature of the emergency, identify the nearest appropriate EMS responder unit, rapidly dispatch the unit to the scene, and provide critical information to EMS responders. EMS systems that implement a rapidly responding first tier of personnel trained to provide early CPR and defibrillation and a second tier of ACLS-level responders have consistently reported the highest rates of survival to hospital discharge.[19] Trained dispatchers have a key role in shortening the time needed to complete the first step in the Chain of Survival.

The Second Link: Early CPR With an Emphasis on Chest Compressions

Effective chest compressions are essential for providing blood flow during CPR. For this reason all patients in cardiac arrest should receive chest compressions. Hospital systems should consider widespread BLS training of all employees so that anyone passing by the patient can initiate CPR. Healthcare providers should administer cycles of 30 compressions to 2 ventilations until an advanced airway is placed; and then continuous chest compressions with ventilations at a rate of 1 breath every 6 to 8 seconds (8 to 10 ventilations/min) should be performed. Healthcare providers should interrupt chest compressions as infrequently as possible and for no longer than 10 seconds.

Many review articles have compiled results of studies that consistently confirm the value of bystander-initiated CPR started immediately after the patient's collapse.[14-16] The probability of survival to hospital discharge can double when bystanders initiate early CPR.[16] For most adults with out-of-hospital cardiac arrest, bystander CPR with chest compression only (Hands-Only™ CPR) appears to achieve outcomes similar to those of conventional CPR (compressions with rescue breathing).[20-22] In addition, if the lay rescuer is trained and able to perform rescue breaths, he or she should add rescue breaths in a ratio of 30 compressions to 2 breaths. For children, as well as other victims with a high likelihood of asphyxia as the cause of arrest (eg, drowning and drug overdose), conventional CPR is superior to Hands-Only CPR.[23]

Among EMS-treated out-of-hospital cardiac arrests, 23% have an initial rhythm of VF or VT or are shockable by an automated external defibrillator. Among in-hospital cardiac arrests, 17.7% of adults had VF or pulseless VT as the first recorded rhythm.[4] For victims with VF, survival rates are highest when immediate bystander CPR is provided and defibrillation occurs within 3 to 5 minutes of collapse.[24-29] In monitored hospital patients, the time from VF to defibrillation should be under 3 minutes. Because the interval between a call to EMS and arrival of EMS personnel at the patient's side is typically longer than 5 minutes, achieving high survival rates depends on a public trained in CPR and on well-organized public-access defibrillation programs. In this situation, the most important link in the community is the layperson, who has the responsibility to activate the EMS system and initiate BLS. The best results of lay provider CPR programs have occurred in controlled environments with trained, motivated personnel and an automated external defibrillation program.[29,30]

> The first person on the scene of a cardiac arrest must perform the same interventions regardless of level of training: activate the emergency response system and begin chest compressions.

Dispatcher-Assisted CPR

In a prehospital setting, the dispatcher may need to provide CPR or defibrillation instructions to the individuals at the scene. EMS leaders developed the highly successful concept of *prearrival instructions* that the dispatcher gives to the caller during a 911 call in the late 1980s.[31] This concept of prearrival instructions from trained dispatchers has the potential to improve outcomes if widely implemented. The AHA recommends that 911 callers be formally and systematically questioned to determine whether the patient may have had a cardiac arrest, and when such is identified, that CPR prearrival instructions be immediately provided to assist bystanders if CPR is not already ongoing. These instructions should be provided in a confident and assertive manner and should include straightforward Hands-Only CPR instructions.[32]

The Third Link: Rapid Defibrillation

Rapid defibrillation is the treatment of choice for VF of short duration, such as for victims of witnessed out-of-hospital cardiac arrest or for hospitalized patients whose heart rhythm is monitored. Survival rates are highest with immediate CPR and defibrillation that occurs within 3 to 5 minutes of collapse.[24-29]

Any community that can achieve earlier defibrillation may improve its rate of survival from cardiac arrest.[33] Early CPR plus defibrillation within 3 to 5 minutes of collapse can produce survival rates as high as 41% to 74%.[34,35] The first 2 links (immediate recognition and early CPR) and the fourth link (early ACLS) cannot improve survival without early defibrillation in patients suffering from a VF cardiac arrest.

Several studies have documented the effects of time to defibrillation and the effects of bystander CPR on survival from sudden cardiac arrest (SCA). For every minute that passes between collapse and defibrillation without CPR, survival rates from witnessed VF SCA decrease 7% to 10% (Figure 4).[36] CPR provided by bystanders results in a more gradual decrease in survival rates that averages 3% to 4% per minute from collapse to defibrillation.[36,37] Additionally, early defibrillation alone can achieve remarkable survival rates, as demonstrated by placement of automated external defibrillators (AEDs) in commercial airplanes,[38-40] gambling casinos,[26] and terminals of major airports.[40,41] When an AED or defibrillator is not immediately available, however, a period of high-quality CPR may incrementally improve survival.

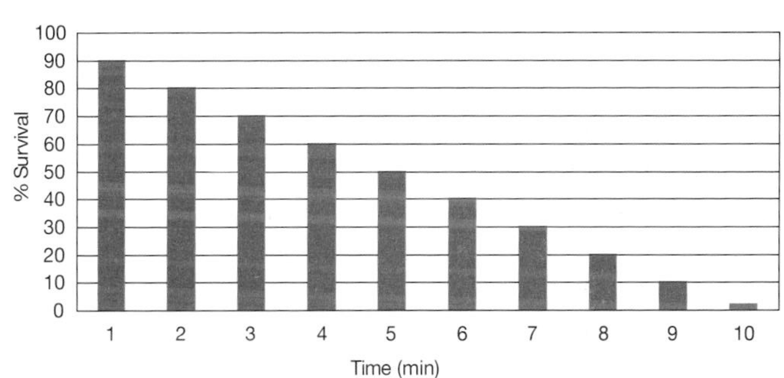

Figure 4. Relationship between survival from ventricular fibrillation sudden cardiac arrest and time from collapse to defibrillation.

The Principle of Early Defibrillation

The world's major resuscitation organizations, including the American Heart Association (AHA),[42-45] European Resuscitation Council,[46-48] and International Liaison Committee on Resuscitation,[49] have all endorsed the principle of early defibrillation. This has led to a recommendation that every emergency vehicle that responds to potential cardiac arrest patients or transports patients at risk for cardiac arrest should be equipped with a defibrillator and staffed with emergency personnel trained and permitted to use this device.

In several reports of unsuccessful early defibrillation initiatives, such as by police in Indiana[50] and firefighters in Tennessee,[51] responders did not rapidly deploy their AEDs. These reports teach a valuable lesson: if personnel hesitate or fail to use their AED, survival will not increase.[52]

AEDs alone are not enough to ensure survival. Responders need both BLS and early deployment of defibrillation. It is estimated that approximately 80% of out-of-hospital cardiac arrests occur in private or residential settings.[53] One study demonstrated that survival was not improved in homes of high-risk individuals equipped with AEDs compared with homes where only CPR training had been provided.[54]

Early defibrillation, however, has turned out to be a weak link and a significant problem for many hospitals. Some hospitals have been reluctant to acquire AEDs for in-hospital use.[55-57] This reluctance has led to collapse-to–first shock intervals in some larger hospitals as long as those seen in out-of-hospital settings.[56] In hospitals with onsite AEDs, healthcare providers should provide immediate CPR and should use the AED as soon as it becomes available.

The Fourth Link: Effective Advanced Life Support

ACLS affects multiple links in the Chain of Survival, including interventions to prevent and treat cardiac arrest and to improve outcomes of patients who achieve ROSC after cardiac arrest. Early effective ACLS is another critical link in the management of cardiac arrest; it should be seamlessly integrated with initial BLS efforts. EMS systems should have sufficient staff to provide at least one responder trained in ACLS. Because of the difficulties in treating cardiac arrest in the field, additional responders should be present when possible. In systems with survival rates of more than 20% for patients with VF, response teams usually have a minimum of 2 ACLS providers plus 2 BLS personnel at the scene.[58,59]

The in-hospital early ACLS link is provided by the code team, which is composed of personnel who arrive from various locations after being summoned by a hospital-wide loudspeaker announcement or by radio-controlled pager. In-hospital early ACLS is highly dependent on where the cardiac arrest occurs. This code team should not interrupt ongoing CPR but should complement and enhance the BLS response team, integrating seamlessly with the rest of the staff.

The Fifth Link: Integrated Post–Cardiac Arrest Care

Organized post–cardiac arrest care with an emphasis on multidisciplinary programs that focus on optimizing hemodynamic, neurologic, and metabolic function (including therapeutic hypothermia) may improve survival to hospital discharge among victims who achieve ROSC following cardiac arrest either in- or out-of-hospital.[60,61] Although it is not yet possible to determine the individual effect of many of these therapies, when bundled as an integrated system of care, their deployment may well improve outcomes.

Therapeutic hypothermia is one intervention that has been shown to improve outcome for comatose adult victims of witnessed out-of-hospital cardiac arrest when the presenting rhythm was VF.[62,63] Since 2005, 2 non-randomized studies with concurrent controls, as well as other studies using historic controls, have indicated the possible benefit of hypothermia following in- and out-of-hospital cardiac arrest from all other initial rhythms in adults.[60,64-68] Hypothermia has also been shown to be effective in improving intact neurologic survival in neonates with hypoxic-ischemic encephalopathy, and the results of a prospective multicenter pediatric study of therapeutic hypothermia after cardiac arrest are eagerly awaited.

The primary objectives of post–cardiac arrest care are to

1. Optimize cardiopulmonary function and vital organ perfusion
2. Transport the patient with out-of-hospital cardiac arrest to an appropriate hospital with a comprehensive post–cardiac arrest treatment system of care that includes acute coronary interventions, neurological care, goal-directed critical care, and hypothermia
3. Transport the in-hospital post–cardiac arrest patient to an appropriate critical care unit capable of providing comprehensive post–cardiac arrest care
4. Try to identify and treat the precipitating causes of the arrest and prevent recurrent arrest

The secondary objectives of post–cardiac arrest care are to

1. Control body temperature to optimize survival and neurological recovery
2. Identify and treat acute coronary syndromes (ACS)
3. Optimize mechanical ventilation to minimize secondary organ injury
4. Reduce the risk of multiorgan injury and support organ function
5. Objectively assess prognosis for recovery at an appropriate time
6. Assist survivors with rehabilitation services when required

Closing the Gaps

Quality Assessment, Review, and Translational Science

Every EMS and hospital system should perform continuous quality improvement (CQI) to assess its resuscitation interventions and outcomes through a defined process of data collection and review. There is now widespread consensus that the best way to improve either community or in-hospital survival from SCA is to start with the standard "quality improvement model" and then modify that model according to the Chain of Survival metaphor. Each link in the chain comprises structural, process, and outcome variables that can be examined, measured, and recorded. System managers can quickly identify gaps that exist between observed processes and outcomes and local expectations or published "gold standards."

Get With the Guidelines-Resuscitation

To prevent or intervene successfully in cardiac arrest, more data about in-hospital cardiac arrests are needed. In addition, in-hospital quality assurance systems require ongoing assessment of process and outcome for cardiac arrest. To aid and accomplish this effort, the AHA established a task force to develop a national registry of cardiopulmonary resuscitation called Get With the Guidelines®-Resuscitation. This program supports individual hospitals in conducting review, quality-assurance, and quality-improvement projects relating to resuscitation in the individual hospital. Today this registry is the largest repository of information on in-hospital cardiopulmonary arrest.[69] This registry has great practical value for establishing the resuscitation performance level for an individual hospital. That step can be followed by projects to improve the quality of resuscitation attempts and increase survival. In addition the database allows researchers to query HIPAA-compliant aggregated data to answer investigator-initiated research questions. This database has resulted in defining important outcomes and benchmarks for clinical care and research initiatives.

Identify Barriers That Delay the Implementation of AHA Guidelines in EMS Agencies

Out-of-hospital cardiac arrest (OHCA) affects over 359 000 people each year in the United States with a case fatality rate of 90.5%.[4] Prehospital providers, including lay responders and bystanders, are often the first to provide care for out-of-hospital patients. Previous research has determined that while 99% of EMS agencies participating in the Resuscitation Outcomes Consortium (ROC) implemented the 2005 AHA Guidelines, delay to implementation

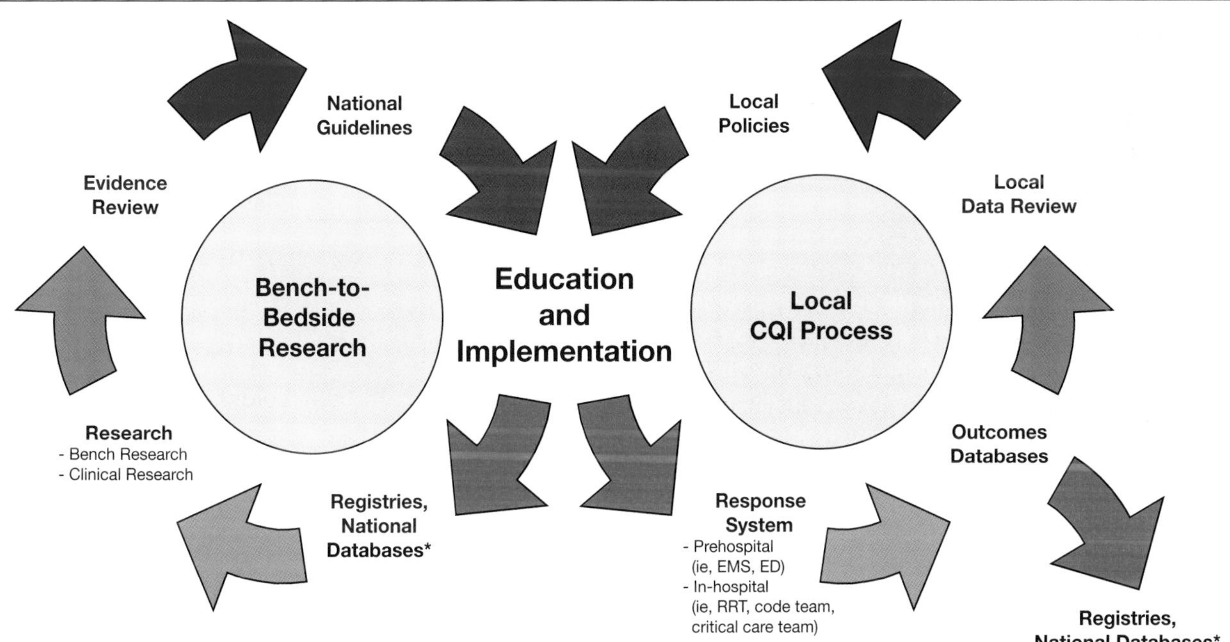

Figure 5. A continuous process evaluates and improves clinical care and generates new guidelines and therapy. Outcome data from cardiac arrest and periarrest periods are reviewed in a continuous quality improvement (CQI) process. Research and clinical initiatives are periodically reviewed in an evidence-based process. Experts then evaluate new therapy and make clinical and educational recommendations for patient care. The process is repeated, and continual progress and care improvements are generated.
*This is an overlap point in the cycle. That is, data come from outcomes databases (shown on the right) and go into registries and national databases (over on the left-hand cycle).
Abbreviations: ED, emergency department; EMS, emergency medical services; RRT, rapid response team.

was significant and highly variable (median 415 days, range: 49 to 750 days).[71] In 2010, 178 agencies were surveyed to identify the barriers to implementation of guidelines.[72] Ten barriers were identified and categorized under 3 themes:

- **Instruction delays** included 3 barriers: booking/training instructors (9%), receiving training materials (15%), and scheduling staff for training (18%).
- **Defibrillator delays** included 2 barriers: reprogramming defibrillators (24%) and receiving new defibrillators to replace nonupgradeable units (15%).
- **Decision making** included 5 barriers: coordinating with allied agencies (9%), government regulators, such as state and provincial health authorities (9%), medical direction and base hospitals (9%), ROC participation (9%), and internal crises (3%).

These identified barriers should be addressed proactively to facilitate rapid translation of science into clinical practice.

Translational Science—Bench to Bedside

Evidence-based guidelines are derived from a basic and clinical research structure designed to ask and investigate questions to improve clinical outcomes. Many of these questions are initially investigated in the laboratory and then in well-designed clinical trials. This ongoing investigative process is part of the continual process that improves recommendations and clinical outcomes (Figure 5). This process generates evidence that is reviewed by experts and then assigned a class of recommendation and level of evidence (Table 1). Periodically new evidence is reviewed and recommendations are updated.

Table 1. Applying Classification of Recommendations and Levels of Evidence

SIZE OF TREATMENT EFFECT (columns); ESTIMATE OF CERTAINTY (PRECISION) OF TREATMENT EFFECT (rows)

	CLASS I *Benefit >>> Risk* Procedure/Treatment **SHOULD** be performed/administered	**CLASS IIa** *Benefit >> Risk* *Additional studies with focused objectives needed* **IT IS REASONABLE** to perform procedure/administer treatment	**CLASS IIb** *Benefit ≥ Risk* *Additional studies with broad objectives needed; additional registry data would be helpful* Procedure/Treatment **MAY BE CONSIDERED**	**CLASS III** *No Benefit* or **CLASS III** *Harm* Procedure/Test / Treatment COR III: No benefit — Not Helpful / No Proven Benefit COR III: Harm — Excess Cost w/o Benefit or Harmful / Harmful to Patients
LEVEL A Multiple populations evaluated* Data derived from multiple randomized clinical trials or meta-analyses	■ Recommendation that procedure or treatment is useful/effective ■ Sufficient evidence from multiple randomized trials or meta-analyses	■ Recommendation in favor of treatment or procedure being useful/effective ■ Some conflicting evidence from multiple randomized trials or meta-analyses	■ Recommendation's usefulness/efficacy less well established ■ Greater conflicting evidence from multiple randomized trials or meta-analyses	■ Recommendation that procedure or treatment is not useful/effective and may be harmful ■ Sufficient evidence from multiple randomized trials or meta-analyses
LEVEL B Limited populations evaluated* Data derived from a single randomized trial or nonrandomized studies	■ Recommendation that procedure or treatment is useful/effective ■ Evidence from single randomized trial or nonrandomized studies	■ Recommendation in favor of treatment or procedure being useful/effective ■ Some conflicting evidence from single randomized trial or nonrandomized studies	■ Recommendation's usefulness/efficacy less well established ■ Greater conflicting evidence from single randomized trial or nonrandomized studies	■ Recommendation that procedure or treatment is not useful/effective and may be harmful ■ Evidence from single randomized trial or nonrandomized studies
LEVEL C Very limited populations evaluated* Only consensus opinion of experts, case studies, or standard of care	■ Recommendation that procedure or treatment is useful/effective ■ Only expert opinion, case studies, or standard of care	■ Recommendation in favor of treatment or procedure being useful/effective ■ Only diverging expert opinion, case studies, or standard of care	■ Recommendation's usefulness/efficacy less well established ■ Only diverging expert opinion, case studies, or standard of care	■ Recommendation that procedure or treatment is not useful/effective and may be harmful ■ Only expert opinion, case studies, or standard of care

A recommendation with Level of Evidence B or C does not imply that the recommendation is weak. Many important clinical questions addressed in the guidelines do not lend themselves to clinical trials. Although randomized trials are unavailable, there may be a very clear clinical consensus that a particular test or therapy is useful or effective.

*Data available from clinical trials or registries about the usefulness/efficacy in different subpopulations, such as sex, age, history of diabetes, history of prior myocardial infarction, history of heart failure, and prior aspirin use.

Science Behind the Guidelines—Why Do They Change?

Evidence-based medicine defines a practice that uses a drug, intervention, or strategy based on levels of evidence and consensus opinion. The *2010 AHA Guidelines for CPR and ECC* are based on the most current and comprehensive review of resuscitation literature ever published, the *2010 International Consensus on CPR and ECC Science With Treatment Recommendations.*[73] This publication serves as the foundation for guidelines published by many member councils of the International Liaison Committee on Resuscitation (ILCOR).[73] It is the product of the 2010 International Consensus Conference in which 356 resuscitation experts from 29 countries participated in a comprehensive process to evaluate the evidence pertaining to resuscitation and emergency cardiovascular care. In particular, they analyzed the sequence and priorities of the steps of CPR in light of current scientific advances to identify factors with the greatest potential impact on survival after cardiac arrest. These experts gathered and ranked the evidence, and then expert panels and committees made a class of recommendation based on this evidence. On the basis of the strength of the available evidence, these experts developed recommendations to support the interventions that showed the most promise. There was unanimous support for continued emphasis on providing high-quality CPR, with compressions of adequate rate and depth; allowing complete chest recoil; minimizing interruptions in chest compressions; and avoiding excessive ventilation. High-quality CPR is the cornerstone of a system of care that can optimize outcomes. Return to the prior quality of life and functional state of health is the ultimate goal of a resuscitation system of care.

The ILCOR evidence evaluation process is a continual one and repeats every 5 years. In this way new science can be incorporated into both the ILCOR consensus document and the AHA guidelines, and questions generated by evidence review will lead to new research and better recommendations with improved outcomes.

FAQ

What is cardiac arrest?

Cardiac arrest is defined as a sudden cessation of cardiac mechanical activity, confirmed by unresponsiveness; apnea or agonal, gasping respirations; and the absence of a detectable pulse.

How long should healthcare providers perform CPR before delivering the first shock?

Data is presently insufficient to determine the ideal duration of CPR before attempted defibrillation.

- In settings with lay rescuer AED programs (where the AED is onsite and available) and for in-hospital environments, or if the EMS rescuer witnesses the collapse, the rescuer should use the defibrillator as soon as it is available. There is insufficient evidence to recommend for or against delaying defibrillation to provide CPR for patients in VF/pulseless VT out-of-hospital cardiac arrest.
- In all cases where there is more than 1 rescuer, CPR should be performed while a defibrillator is being acquired or readied.

Can a rhythm and pulse check be performed after defibrillation?

- Pulse and rhythm checks are not recommended immediately after defibrillation. One study found that following defibrillation, 78% of patients developed PEA/asystole and 22% remained in VF.[74] Even in those instances where the myocardium regains an organized rhythm following defibrillation, the myocardium is not performing adequately and the patient is at risk for rearrest. Providing chest compressions improves cardiac output and allows time for the myocardial contractions to become more effective.
- In some circumstances, a physician team leader may modify the resuscitation sequence for particular purposes, with attention to minimal interruption in chest compressions. Healthcare providers should not interrupt chest compressions for longer than 10 seconds. Pulse checks are performed at the end of a 2-minute cycle of CPR and only if an organized rhythm is present.

Why do guidelines and recommendations continue to change?

An ongoing investigative process continually looks for interventions and strategies to improve outcome from cardiac arrest and emergency cardiovascular care. When some questions are answered, new ones may be generated. A process of evidence review and recommendations by international experts integrates science into treatment algorithms and strategies in a process of continuous quality improvement. As science changes, the guidelines are revised to reflect the changes.

References

1. Abella BS, Alvarado JP, Myklebust H, Edelson DP, Barry A, O'Hearn N, Vanden Hoek TL, Becker LB. Quality of cardiopulmonary resuscitation during in-hospital cardiac arrest. *JAMA.* 2005;293:305-310.
2. Stiell IG, Wells GA, Field B, Spaite DW, Nesbitt LP, De Maio VJ, Nichol G, Cousineau D, Blackburn J, Munkley D, Luinstra-Toohey L, Campeau T, Dagnone E, Lyver M. Advanced cardiac life support in out-of-hospital cardiac arrest. *N Engl J Med.* 2004;351:647-656.
3. Roger VL, Go AS, Lloyd-Jones DM, Benjamin EJ, Berry JD, Borden WB, Bravata DM, Dai S, Ford ES, Fox CS, Fullerton HJ, Gillespie C, Hailpern SM, Heit JA, Howard VJ, Kissela BM, Kittner SJ, Lackland DT, Lichtman JH, Lisabeth LD, Makuc DM, Marcus GM, Marelli A, Matchar DB, Moy CS, Mozaffarian D, Mussolino ME, Nichol G, Paynter NP, Soliman EZ, Sorlie PD, Sotoodehnia N, Turan TN, Virani SS, Wong ND, Woo D, Turner MB. Executive summary: heart disease and stroke statistics—2012 update. A report from the American Heart Association. *Circulation.* 2012;125:188-197.
4. Go AS, Mozaffarian D, Roger VL, Benjamin EJ, Berry JD, Borden WB, Bravata DM, Dai S, Ford ES, Fox CS, Franco S, Fullerton HJ, Gillespie C, Hailpern SM, Heit JA, Howard VJ, Huffman MD, Kissela BM, Kittner SJ, Lackland DT, Lichtman JH, Lisabeth LD, Magid D, Marcus GM, Marelli A, Matchar DB, McGuire D, Mohler E, Moy CS, Mussolino ME, Nichol G, Paynter NP, Schreiner PJ, Sorlie PD, Stein J, Turan TN, Virani SS, Wong ND, Woo D, Turner MB; on behalf of the American Heart Association Statistics Committee and Stroke Statistics Subcommittee. Heart disease and stroke statistics—2013 update: a report from the American Heart Association [published online ahead of print December 12, 2012]. *Circulation.* 2013. doi:10.1161/CIR.0b013e31828124ad.
5. Roger VL, Go AS, Lloyd-Jones DM, Benjamin EJ, Berry JD, Borden WB, Bravata DM, Dai S, Ford ES, Fox CS, Fullerton HJ, Gillespie C, Hailpern SM, Heit JA, Howard VJ, Kissela BM, Kittner SJ, Lackland DT, Lichtman JH, Lisabeth LD, Makuc DM, Marcus GM, Marelli A, Matchar DB, Moy CS, Mozaffarian D, Mussolino ME, Nichol G, Paynter NP, Soliman EZ, Sorlie PD, Sotoodehnia N, Turan TN, Virani SS, Wong ND, Woo D, Turner MB. Heart disease and stroke statistics—2012 update. A report from the American Heart Association. *Circulation.* 2012;125:e2-e220.
6. Edelson DP, Abella BS, Kramer-Johansen J, Wik L, Myklebust H, Barry AM, Merchant RM, Hoek TL, Steen PA, Becker LB. Effects of compression depth and pre-shock pauses predict defibrillation failure during cardiac arrest. *Resuscitation.* 2006;71:137-145.
7. Edelson DP, Litzinger B, Arora V, Walsh D, Kim S, Lauderdale DS, Vanden Hoek TL, Becker LB, Abella BS. Improving in-hospital cardiac arrest process and outcomes with performance debriefing. *Arch Intern Med.* 2008;168:1063-1069.
8. Wik L, Kramer-Johansen J, Myklebust H, Sorebo H, Svensson L, Fellows B, Steen PA. Quality of cardiopulmonary resuscitation during out-of-hospital cardiac arrest. *JAMA.* 2005;293:299-304.
9. Berg RA, Hemphill R, Abella BS, Aufderheide TP, Cave DM, Hazinski MF, Lerner EB, Rea TD, Sayre MR, Swor RA. Part 5: Adult basic life support: 2010 American Heart Association Guidelines for Cardiopulmonary Resuscitation and Emergency Cardiovascular Care. *Circulation.* 2010;122:S685-705.
10. Fox CS, Evans JC, Larson MG, Kannel WB, Levy D. Temporal trends in coronary heart disease mortality and sudden cardiac death from 1950 to 1999: The Framingham Heart Study. *Circulation.* 2004;110:522-527.
11. Cummins RO, Chamberlain DA, Abramson NS, Allen M, Baskett P, Becker L, Bossaert L, Delooz H, Dick W, Eisenberg M, et al. Recommended guidelines for uniform reporting of data from out-of-hospital cardiac arrest: the Utstein style. Task force of the American Heart Association, the European Resuscitation Council, the Heart and Stroke Foundation of Canada, and the Australian Resuscitation Council. *Ann Emerg Med.* 1991;20:861-874.
12. Myerburg RJ, Interian A, Simmons J, Castellanos A. Sudden cardiac death. In: Zipes DP, ed. *Cardiac Electrophysiology: From Cell to Bedside.* Philadelphia, PA: WB Saunders; 2004:720-731.
13. Burke AP, Farb A, Malcom GT, Liang YH, Smialek J, Virmani R. Coronary risk factors and plaque morphology in men with coronary disease who died suddenly. *N Engl J Med.* 1997;336:1276-1282.
14. Thom T, Kannel W, Silberschatz H, D'Agostino RB. Cardiovascular diseases in the United States and prevention approaches. In: Fuster V, Alexander RW, Schlant RC, O'Rourke RA, Roberts R, Sonnenblick EH, eds. *Hurst's the Heart.* New York, NY: McGraw-Hill; 2001:3-7.
15. Rajat D, Albert CM. Sudden cardiac death. Epidemiology and genetics of sudden cardiac death. *Circulation.* 2012;125:620-637.
16. Uretsky BF, Thygesen K, Armstrong PW, Cleland JG, Horowitz JD, Massie BM, Packer M, Poole-Wilson PA, Ryden L. Acute coronary findings at autopsy in heart failure patients with sudden death: results from the assessment of treatment with lisinopril and survival (ATLAS) trial. *Circulation.* 2000;102:611-616.
17. Albert CM, Chae CU, Grodstein F, Rose LM, Rexrode KM, Ruskin JN, Stampfer MJ, Manson JE. Prospective study of sudden cardiac death among women in the United States. *Circulation.* 2003;107:2096-2101.
18. Clawson JJ. Emergency medical dispatching. In: Roush WR, Aranosian RD, Blair TMH, Handal KA, Kellow RC, Steward RD, eds. *Principles of EMS Systems.* Dallas, TX: American College of Emergency Physicians; 1989:119-133.
19. Valenzuela TD, Roe DJ, Cretin S, Spaite DW, Larsen MP. Estimating effectiveness of cardiac arrest interventions: a logistic regression survival model. *Circulation.* 1997;96:3308-3313.
20. Iwami T, Kawamura T, Hiraide A, Berg RA, Hayashi Y, Nishiuchi T, Kajino K, Yonemoto N, Yukioka H, Sugimoto H, Kakuchi H, Sase K, Yokoyama H, Nonogi H. Effectiveness of bystander-initiated cardiac-only resuscitation for patients with out-of-hospital cardiac arrest. *Circulation.* 2007;116:2900-2907.
21. Cardiopulmonary resuscitation by bystanders with chest compression only (SOS-KANTO): an observational study. *Lancet.* 2007;369:920-926.
22. Ong ME, Ng FS, Anushia P, Tham LP, Leong BS, Ong VY, Tiah L, Lim SH, Anantharaman V. Comparison of chest compression only and standard cardiopulmonary resuscitation for out-of-hospital cardiac arrest in Singapore. *Resuscitation.* 2008;78:119-126.
23. Kitamura T, Iwami T, Kawamura T, Nagao K, Tanaka H, Nadkarni VM, Berg RA, Hiraide A. Conventional and chest-compression-only cardiopulmonary resuscitation by bystanders for children who have out-of-hospital cardiac arrests: a prospective, nationwide, population-based cohort study. *Lancet.* 2010;375:1347-1354.

24. Chan PS, Nichol G, Krumholz HM, Spertus JA, Nallamothu BK. Hospital variation in time to defibrillation after in-hospital cardiac arrest. *Arch Intern Med.* 2009;169:1265-1273.
25. Sasson C, Rogers MA, Dahl J, Kellermann AL. Predictors of survival from out-of-hospital cardiac arrest: a systematic review and meta-analysis. *Circ Cardiovasc Qual Outcomes.* 2010;3:63-81.
26. Valenzuela TD, Roe DJ, Nichol G, Clark LL, Spaite DW, Hardman RG. Outcomes of rapid defibrillation by security officers after cardiac arrest in casinos. *N Engl J Med.* 2000;343:1206-1209.
27. Agarwal DA, Hess EP, Atkinson EJ, White RD. Ventricular fibrillation in Rochester, Minnesota: experience over 18 years. *Resuscitation.* 2009;80:1253-1258.
28. Rea TD, Cook AJ, Stiell IG, Powell J, Bigham B, Callaway CW, Chugh S, Aufderheide TP, Morrison L, Terndrup TE, Beaudoin T, Wittwer L, Davis D, Idris A, Nichol G. Predicting survival after out-of-hospital cardiac arrest: role of the Utstein data elements. *Ann Emerg Med.* 2010;55:249-257.
29. Caffrey SL, Willoughby PJ, Pepe PE, Becker LB. Public use of automated external defibrillators. *N Engl J Med.* 2002;347:1242-1247.
30. Hallstrom AP, Ornato JP, Weisfeldt M, Travers A, Christenson J, McBurnie MA, Zalenski R, Becker LB, Schron EB, Proschan M. Public-access defibrillation and survival after out-of-hospital cardiac arrest. *N Engl J Med.* 2004;351:637-646.
31. Carter WB, Eisenberg MS, Hallstrom AP, Schaeffer S. Development and implementation of emergency CPR instruction via telephone. *Ann Emerg Med.* 1984;13:695-700.
32. Lerner EB, Rea TD, Bobrow BJ, Acker JE III, Berg RA, Brooks SC, Cone DC, Gay M, Gent LM, Mears G, Nadkarni VM, O'Connor RE, Potts J, Sayre MR, Swor RA, Travers AH. Emergency medical service dispatch cardiopulmonary resuscitation prearrival instructions to improve survival from out-of-hospital cardiac arrest: a scientific statement from the American Heart Association. *Circulation.* 2012;125:648-655.
33. Cummins RO, Ornato JP, Thies WH, Pepe PE. Improving survival from sudden cardiac arrest: the "chain of survival" concept. A statement for health professionals from the Advanced Cardiac Life Support Subcommittee and the Emergency Cardiac Care Committee, American Heart Association. *Circulation.* 1991;83:1832-1847.
34. England H, Hoffman C, Hodgman T, Singh S, Homoud M, Weinstock J, Link M, Estes NA III. Effectiveness of automated external defibrillators in high schools in greater Boston. *Am J Cardiol.* 2005;95:1484-1486.
35. Rea TD, Stickney RE, Doherty A, Lank P. Performance of chest compressions by laypersons during the public access defibrillation trial. *Resuscitation.* 2010;81:293-296.
36. Larsen MP, Eisenberg MS, Cummins RO, Hallstrom AP. Predicting survival from out-of-hospital cardiac arrest: a graphic model. *Ann Emerg Med.* 1993;22:1652-1658.
37. Chan PS, Krumholz HM, Nichol G, Nallamothu BK. Delayed time to defibrillation after in-hospital cardiac arrest. *N Engl J Med.* 2008;358:9-17.
38. O'Rourke MF, Donaldson E, Geddes JS. An airline cardiac arrest program. *Circulation.* 1997;96:2849-2853.
39. Page RL, Hamdan MH, McKenas DK. Defibrillation aboard a commercial aircraft. *Circulation.* 1998;97:1429-1430.
40. Page RL, Joglar JA, Kowal RC, Zagrodzky JD, Nelson LL, Ramaswamy K, Barbera SJ, Hamdan MH, McKenas DK. Use of automated external defibrillators by a US airline. *N Engl J Med.* 2000;343:1210-1216.
41. Robertson RM. Sudden death from cardiac arrest—improving the odds. *N Engl J Med.* 2000;343:1259-1260.
42. Kerber RE. Statement on early defibrillation from the Emergency Cardiac Care Committee, American Heart Association. *Circulation.* 1991;84:2233.
43. Cobb LA, Eliastam M, Kerber RE, Melker R, Moss AJ, Newell L, Paraskos JA, Weaver WD, Weil M, Weisfeldt ML. Report of the American Heart Association Task Force on the Future of Cardiopulmonary Resuscitation. *Circulation.* 1992;85:2346-2355.
44. Nichol G, Hallstrom AP, Kerber R, Moss AJ, Ornato JP, Palmer D, Riegel B, Smith S Jr, Weisfeldt ML. American Heart Association Report on the Second Public Access Defibrillation Conference, April 17-19, 1997. *Circulation.* 1998;97:1309-1314.
45. Weisfeldt ML, Kerber RE, McGoldrick RP, Moss AJ, Nichol G, Ornato JP, Palmer DG, Riegel B, Smith SC Jr. American Heart Association Report on the Public Access Defibrillation Conference December 8-10, 1994. Automatic external defibrillation task force. *Circulation.* 1995;92:2740-2747.
46. Bossaert L, Callanan V, Cummins RO. Early defibrillation. An advisory statement by the Advanced Life Support Working Group of the International Liaison Committee on Resuscitation. *Resuscitation.* 1997;34:113-114.
47. Bossaert L, Handley A, Marsden A, Arntz R, Chamberlain D, Ekstrom L, Evans T, Monsieurs K, Robertson C, Steen P. European Resuscitation Council guidelines for the use of automated external defibrillators by EMS providers and first responders: a statement from the Early Defibrillation Task Force, with contributions from the Working Groups on Basic and Advanced Life Support, and approved by the Executive Committee. *Resuscitation*. 1998;37:91-94.
48. Shuster M, Billi JE, Bossaert L, de Caen AR, Deakin CD, Eigel B, Hazinski MF, Hickey RW, Jacobs I, Kleinman ME, Koster RW, Mancini ME, Montgomery WH, Morley PT, Morrison LJ, Munoz H, Nadkarni VM, Nolan JP, O'Connor RE, Perlman JM, Richmond S, Sayre MR, Soar J, Wyllie J, Zideman D. Part 4: conflict of interest management before, during, and after the 2010 International Consensus Conference on Cardiopulmonary Resuscitation and Emergency Cardiovascular Care Science With Treatment Recommendations. *Resuscitation*. 2010;81(suppl 1):e41-e47.
49. Kloeck W, Cummins RO, Chamberlain D, Bossaert L, Callanan V, Carli P, Christenson J, Connolly B, Ornato JP, Sanders A, Steen P. Early defibrillation: an advisory statement from the Advanced Life Support Working Group of the International Liaison Committee on Resuscitation. *Circulation.* 1997;95:2183-2184.
50. Groh WJ, Newman MM, Beal PE, Fineberg NS, Zipes DP. Limited response to cardiac arrest by police equipped with automated external defibrillators: lack of survival benefit in suburban and rural Indiana—the police as responder automated defibrillation evaluation (PARADE). *Acad Emerg Med.* 2001;8:324-330.
51. Kellermann AL, Hackman BB, Somes G, Kreth TK, Nail L, Dobyns P. Impact of first-responder defibrillation in an urban emergency medical services system. *JAMA.* 1993;270:1708-1713.
52. Sweeney TA, Runge JW, Gibbs MA, Raymond JM, Schafermeyer RW, Norton HJ, Boyle-Whitesel MJ. EMT defibrillation does not increase survival from sudden cardiac death in a two-tiered urban-suburban EMS system. *Ann Emerg Med.* 1998;31:234-240.

53. Becker L, Eisenberg M, Fahrenbruch C, Cobb L. Public locations of cardiac arrest. Implications for public access defibrillation. *Circulation.* 1998;97:2106-2109.

54. Bardy GH, Lee KL, Mark DB, Poole JE, Toff WD, Tonkin AM, Smith W, Dorian P, Packer DL, White RD, Longstreth WT Jr, Anderson J, Johnson G, Bischoff E, Yallop JJ, McNulty S, Ray LD, Clapp-Channing NE, Rosenberg Y, Schron EB. Home use of automated external defibrillators for sudden cardiac arrest. *N Engl J Med.* 2008;358:1793-1804.

55. Kaye W, Mancini ME, Giuliano KK, Richards N, Nagid DM, Marler CA, Sawyer-Silva S. Strengthening the in-hospital chain of survival with rapid defibrillation by first responders using automated external defibrillators: training and retention issues. *Ann Emerg Med.* 1995;25:163-168.

56. Kaye W, Mancini ME. Improving outcome from cardiac arrest in the hospital with a reorganized and strengthened chain of survival: an American view. *Resuscitation.* 1996;31:181-186.

57. Benson D, Klain M, Braslow A, Cummins R, Grenvik A, Herlich A, Kampschulte S, Kaye W, Scarberry E. Future directions for resuscitation research. I. Advanced airway control measures. *Resuscitation.* 1996;32:51-62.

58. Jacobs I, Callanan V, Nichol G, Valenzuela T, Mason P, Jaffe AS, Landau W, Vetter N. The chain of survival. *Ann Emerg Med.* 2001;37:S5-S16.

59. Pepe PE, Bonnin MJ, Mattox KL. Regulating the scope of EMS. *Prehosp Disaster Med.* 1990;5:59-63.

60. Sunde K, Pytte M, Jacobsen D, Mangschau A, Jensen LP, Smedsrud C, Draegni T, Steen PA. Implementation of a standardised treatment protocol for post resuscitation care after out-of-hospital cardiac arrest. *Resuscitation.* 2007;73:29-39.

61. Rittenberger JC, Menegazzi JJ, Callaway CW. Association of delay to first intervention with return of spontaneous circulation in a swine model of cardiac arrest. *Resuscitation.* 2007;73:154-160.

62. Mild therapeutic hypothermia to improve the neurologic outcome after cardiac arrest. *N Engl J Med.* 2002;346:549-556.

63. Bernard SA, Gray TW, Buist MD, Jones BM, Silvester W, Gutteridge G, Smith K. Treatment of comatose survivors of out-of-hospital cardiac arrest with induced hypothermia. *N Engl J Med.* 2002;346:557-563.

64. Don CW, Longstreth WT Jr, Maynard C, Olsufka M, Nichol G, Ray T, Kupchik N, Deem S, Copass MK, Cobb LA, Kim F. Active surface cooling protocol to induce mild therapeutic hypothermia after out-of-hospital cardiac arrest: a retrospective before-and-after comparison in a single hospital. *Crit Care Med.* 2009;37:3062-3069.

65. Storm C, Steffen I, Schefold JC, Krueger A, Oppert M, Jorres A, Hasper D. Mild therapeutic hypothermia shortens intensive care unit stay of survivors after out-of-hospital cardiac arrest compared to historical controls. *Crit Care.* 2008;12:R78.

66. Busch M, Soreide E, Lossius HM, Lexow K, Dickstein K. Rapid implementation of therapeutic hypothermia in comatose out-of-hospital cardiac arrest survivors. *Acta Anaesthesiol Scand.* 2006;50:1277-1283.

67. Oddo M, Schaller MD, Feihl F, Ribordy V, Liaudet L. From evidence to clinical practice: effective implementation of therapeutic hypothermia to improve patient outcome after cardiac arrest. *Crit Care Med.* 2006;34:1865-1873.

68. Bernard SA, Jones BM, Horne MK. Clinical trial of induced hypothermia in comatose survivors of out-of-hospital cardiac arrest. *Ann Emerg Med.* 1997;30:146-153.

69. Peberdy MA, Kaye W, Ornato JP, Larkin GL, Nadkarni V, Mancini ME, Berg RA, Nichol G, Lane-Trultt T. Cardiopulmonary resuscitation of adults in the hospital: a report of 14720 cardiac arrests from the National Registry of Cardiopulmonary Resuscitation. *Resuscitation.* 2003;58:297-308.

70. Nichol G, Thomas E, Callaway CW, Hedges J, Powell JL, Aufderheide TP, Rea T, Lowe R, Brown T, Dreyer J, Davis D, Idris A, Stiell I. Regional variation in out-of-hospital cardiac arrest incidence and outcome. *JAMA.* 2008;300:1423-1431.

71. Bigham BL, Koprowicz K, Aufderheide TP, Davis DP, Donn S, Powell J, Suffoletto B, Nafziger S, Stouffer J, Idris A, Morrison LJ. Delayed prehospital implementation of the 2005 American Heart Association Guidelines for Cardiopulmonary Resuscitation and Emergency Cardiac Care. *Prehosp Emerg Care.* 2010;14:355-360.

72. Bigham BL, Aufderheide TP, Davis DP, Powell J, Donn S, Suffoletto B, Nafziger S, Stouffer J, Morrison LJ. Knowledge translation in emergency medical services: a qualitative survey of barriers to guideline implementation. *Resuscitation.* 2010;81:836-840.

73. Hazinski MF, Nolan JP, Billi JE, Bottiger BW, Bossaert L, de Caen AR, Deakin CD, Drajer S, Eigel B, Hickey RW, Jacobs I, Kleinman ME, Kloeck W, Koster RW, Lim SH, Mancini ME, Montgomery WH, Morley PT, Morrison LJ, Nadkarni VM, O'Connor RE, Okada K, Perlman JM, Sayre MR, Shuster M, Soar J, Sunde K, Travers AH, Wyllie J, Zideman D. Part 1: Executive Summary: 2010 International Consensus on Cardiopulmonary Resuscitation and Emergency Cardiovascular Care Science With Treatment Recommendations. *Circulation.* 2010;122:S250-S275.

74. Hess EP, White RD. Ventricular fibrillation is not provoked by chest compression during post-shock organized rhythms in out-of-hospital cardiac arrest. *Resuscitation.* 2005;66:7-11.

Chapter 2

The Expanded Systematic Approach

This Chapter

- The Systematic Approach
- The Expanded Systematic Approach (ACLS EP Survey)
- Critical Thinking

Overview

Healthcare providers use a systematic approach to assess and treat arrest and nonarrest patients for optimal care. The goal of the resuscitation team's interventions for a patient in respiratory or cardiac arrest is to support and restore effective oxygenation, ventilation, and circulation with return of intact neurologic function. An intermediate goal of resuscitation is the return of spontaneous circulation (ROSC). The actions used are guided by the following systematic approaches:

- **BLS Survey**
- **ACLS Survey**

The systematic approach first requires ACLS providers to determine the patient's level of consciousness (Figure 6). As you approach the patient:

- If the patient appears unconscious
  - Use the BLS Survey for the initial assessment.
  - After completing all of the appropriate steps of the BLS Survey, use the ACLS Survey for more advanced assessment and treatment.
- If the patient appears conscious
  - Use the ACLS Survey for your initial assessment.

Before conducting the BLS or ACLS Survey, make sure the scene is safe.

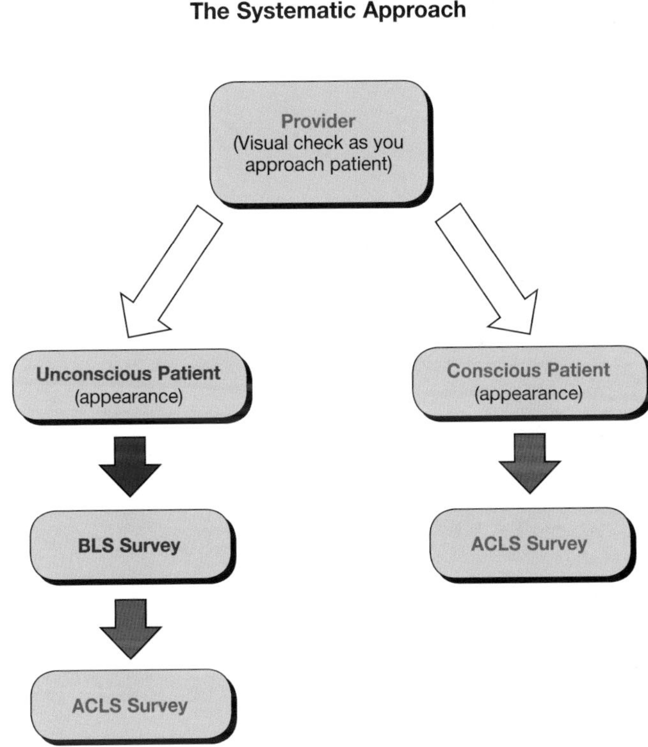

Figure 6. The Systematic Approach.

The Expanded Systematic Approach for Experienced Providers

The Expanded Systematic Approach consists of the BLS Survey and the ACLS EP Survey, which cover *assessments* and *actions* that apply to almost any emergency setting. The ACLS EP Survey expands on the ACLS Survey primarily in the "differential diagnosis" step. Experienced clinicians need to tailor the expanded systematic approach to the clinical situation. For example, cervical spine immobilization may need to be added to the BLS and ACLS Surveys for patients suffering from cardiac arrest associated with trauma, drowning, electric shock, or lightning strike. Modifications are also necessary when dealing with hypothermic cardiac arrest or cardiac arrest associated with pregnancy.

The BLS Survey is a systematic approach to basic life support that any trained healthcare provider can perform. This approach stresses *early CPR* and *early defibrillation*. It does not include advanced interventions, such as advanced airway techniques or drug administration. By using the BLS Survey, healthcare providers may achieve their goal of supporting or restoring effective oxygenation, ventilation, and circulation until ROSC or initiation of ACLS interventions.

Performing the actions in the BLS Survey substantially improves the patient's chance of survival and a good neurologic outcome. Although the BLS Survey requires no advanced equipment, healthcare providers can use any readily available universal precaution supplies or adjuncts, such as a pocket mask or bag-mask ventilation device. Whenever possible, place the patient on a firm surface in a supine position to maximize the effectiveness of chest compressions. Table 2 is an overview of the BLS Survey, and Figures 7 through 10 illustrate the steps needed during the BLS Survey.

BLS should not be interrupted because of the arrival of additional assistance such as the code team, paramedics, or other healthcare personnel. The ACLS team must reinforce this practice by integrating seamlessly into the ongoing resuscitation that is already under way.

The Expanded ACLS Survey (The ACLS EP Survey)

This survey addresses advanced airways, pharmacologic treatment of arrhythmias, intravenous (IV) and intraosseous (IO) routes, monitoring devices (such as waveform capnography), and a comprehensive set of vital signs that includes temperature and glucose. The experienced ACLS team leader also begins to think about the cause of the emergency, differential diagnoses, and alternative approaches to treatment (Table 3).

- **Airway:** Determine if initial airway techniques and ventilations are adequate (assessment); if inadequate, use airway adjuncts or place an advanced airway (action).
- **Breathing:** Check effectiveness of airway and breathing support, including oxygenation and ventilation. Place an advanced airway if bag-mask ventilation is inadequate (action). If an advanced airway is being used, use physical examination and continuous waveform capnography to check placement (assessment); provide positive-pressure ventilations but avoid excessive ventilation (action).

Critical Concept	If only 1 or 2 people are present for a patient in cardiopulmonary arrest, CPR must be provided regardless of the providers' training level or expertise. The first 2 healthcare providers on the scene should primarily focus on the proven lifesaving interventions of chest compressions and defibrillation until additional assistance arrives.

Critical Concept High-Quality CPR	• Compress the chest hard and fast. • Allow complete chest recoil after each compression. • Minimize interruptions in compressions (10 seconds or less). • Switch providers about every 2 minutes to avoid fatigue. • Avoid excessive ventilation.

Critical Concept Agonal Gasps	**Agonal gasps are not adequate breathing. They are a sign of cardiac arrest in an unresponsive patient.** A patient who gasps usually looks as if he is drawing air in very quickly. The patient may open his mouth or move his jaw, head, or neck. Gasps may appear forceful or weak, and some time may pass between gasps because they usually happen at a slow rate. The gasp may sound like a snort, snore, or groan. Gasping is not regular or normal breathing.

Table 2. The BLS Survey

	Assess	Assessment Technique and Action	
1	**Check responsiveness**	• Tap and shout, ***"Are you all right?"*** • Check for absent or abnormal breathing (no breathing or only gasping) by looking at or **scanning the chest for movement** (about 5 to 10 seconds)	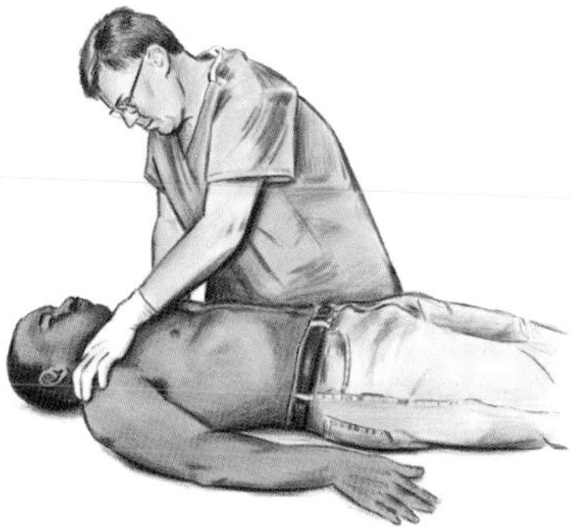 **Figure 7.** Check responsiveness.
2	**Activate the emergency response system/get AED**	• Activate the emergency response system and get an AED if one is available or send someone to activate the emergency response system and get an AED or defibrillator	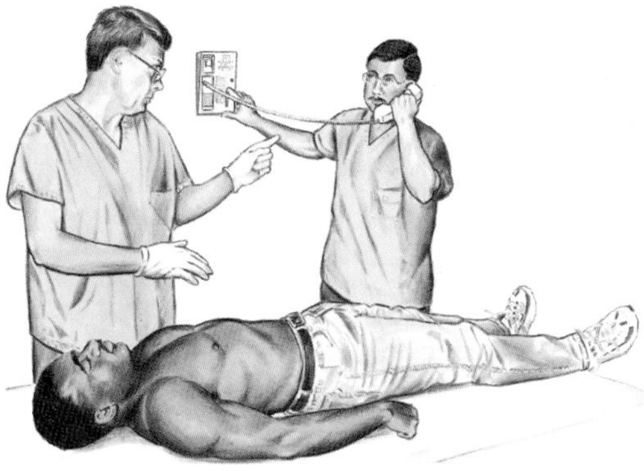 **Figure 8.** Activate the emergency response system.
3	**Circulation**	• **Check the carotid pulse** for 5 to 10 seconds • If no pulse within 10 seconds, start CPR (30:2) beginning with chest compressions – Compress the center of the chest (lower half of the sternum) hard and fast with at least 100 compressions per minute at a depth of at least 2 inches – Allow complete chest recoil after each compression – Minimize interruptions in compressions (10 seconds or less) – Switch providers about every 2 minutes to avoid fatigue – Avoid excessive ventilation • If there is a pulse, start rescue breathing at 1 breath every 5 to 6 seconds (10 to 12 breaths per minute). Check pulse about every 2 minutes.	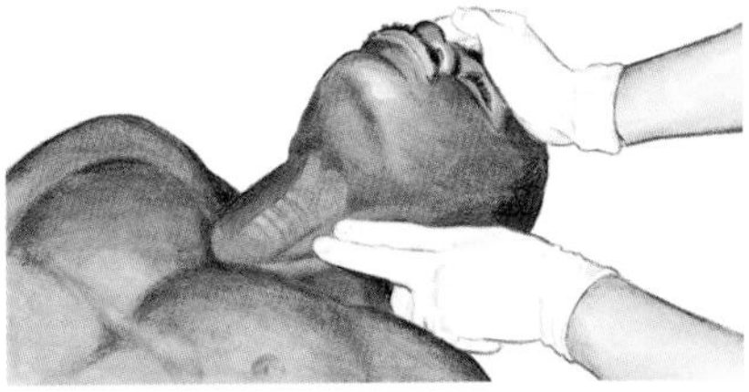 **Figure 9.** Check the carotid pulse.
4	**Defibrillation**	• If no pulse, check for a shockable rhythm with an AED/defibrillator as soon as it arrives • Provide shocks as indicated • Follow each shock immediately with CPR, beginning with compressions	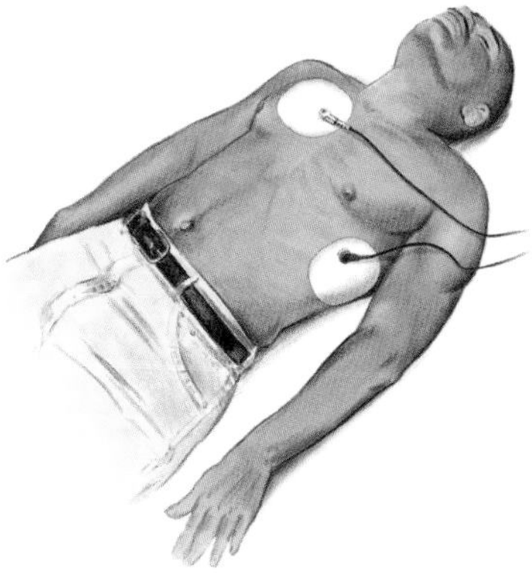 **Figure 10.** Defibrillation.

Table 3. ACLS EP Survey

Assess	Action as Appropriate
Airway – *Is the airway patent?* – *Is an advanced airway indicated?* – *Is proper placement of airway device confirmed?* – *Is tube secured and placement reconfirmed frequently?*	• **Maintain airway patency in unconscious patients** by use of the head tilt–chin lift, oropharyngeal airway (OPA), or nasopharyngeal airway (NPA). • **Use advanced airway management if needed** (eg, laryngeal mask airway, laryngeal tube, esophageal-tracheal tube, endotracheal tube [ET tube]). *Healthcare providers must weigh the benefit of advanced airway placement against the adverse effects of interrupting chest compressions. If bag-mask ventilation is adequate, healthcare providers may defer insertion of an advanced airway until the patient fails to respond to initial CPR and defibrillation or until spontaneous circulation returns. Advanced airway devices such as a laryngeal mask airway, laryngeal tube, or esophageal-tracheal tube can be placed while chest compressions continue.* If using advanced airway devices: • **Confirm proper integration of CPR and ventilation.** • **Confirm proper placement of advanced airway devices** by – Physical examination – Quantitative waveform capnography ▪ Is a Class I recommendation for use with an ET tube ▪ Is reasonable to use with supraglottic airways • **Secure the device to prevent dislodgment.** • **Monitor airway placement with continuous quantitative waveform capnography.**
Breathing – *Are ventilation and oxygenation adequate?* – *Are quantitative waveform capnography and oxyhemoglobin saturation monitored?*	• **Give supplementary oxygen when indicated** – For cardiac arrest patients, administer 100% oxygen. – For others, titrate oxygen administration to achieve oxygen saturation values of 94% or higher by pulse oximetry. • **Monitor the adequacy of ventilation and oxygenation by** – Clinical criteria (chest rise and cyanosis) – Quantitative waveform capnography – Oxygen saturation • **Avoid excessive ventilation.**
Circulation – *Are chest compressions effective?* – *What is the cardiac rhythm?* – *Is defibrillation or cardioversion indicated?* – *Has intravenous/intraosseous (IV/IO) access been established?* – *Is ROSC present?* – *Is the patient unstable?* – *Are medications needed for rhythm or blood pressure?* – *Does the patient need volume (fluid) for resuscitation?*	• **Monitor CPR quality:** – Quantitative waveform capnography (If P_{ETCO_2} is less than 10 mm Hg, attempt to improve CPR quality.) – Intra-arterial pressure (If relaxation phase [diastolic] pressure is less than 20 mm Hg, attempt to improve CPR quality.) • **Attach monitor/defibrillator for arrhythmias or cardiac arrest rhythms** (eg, VF, pulseless VT, asystole, and PEA). • **Provide defibrillation/cardioversion.** • **Obtain IV/IO access.** • **Give appropriate drugs** to manage rhythm and blood pressure. • **Give IV/IO fluids if needed.** • **Check vitals.** • **Check labs.** • **Obtain temperature and glucose readings.**
Differential diagnosis – *Why did this patient develop symptoms or arrest?* – *Is there a reversible cause that can be treated?* – ***What is the response to interventions and how does it alter the evaluation of the most likely diagnosis?***	• **Focused history** (SAMPLE) – **S**igns and Symptoms – **A**llergy – **M**edications – **P**ast Medical History – **L**ast Meal – **E**vents • **Search for, find, and treat reversible causes** (ie, definitive care): The H's and T's **H**ypovolemia — **T**ension pneumothorax **H**ypoxia — **T**amponade (cardiac) **H**ydrogen ion (acidosis) — **T**oxins **H**yper-/hypokalemia — **T**hrombosis (pulmonary) **H**ypothermia — **T**hrombosis (coronary) • **Perfusion problems** (volume, resistance, contractility, rate) – Intravascular volume problem – Peripheral vascular resistance problem – Cardiac contractility problem – Heart rate problem

P_{ETCO_2} is the partial pressure of CO_2 in exhaled air at the end of the exhalation phase.

Critical Concept Minimize Interruptions	**ACLS providers must make every effort to minimize any interruptions in chest compressions.** Try to limit interruptions in chest compressions (eg, defibrillation and advanced airway) to no longer than 10 seconds, except in extreme circumstances, such as removing the patient from a dangerous environment. When you stop chest compressions, blood flow to the brain and heart stops. **Avoid:** • Prolonged rhythm analysis • Frequent or inappropriate pulse checks • Taking too long to give breaths to the patient • Unnecessarily moving the patient

- **Circulation:** Vital signs are probably one of the most neglected areas in training for cardiopulmonary emergencies. The vital signs provide critical information needed to manage these patients and evaluate their response to therapy. Check heart rate and attach monitor leads to determine the rhythm (assessment); monitor CPR, establish IV/IO access to administer fluids and medications (action); administer vasopressors and rhythm-appropriate medications (action); obtain comprehensive vital signs and measure blood glucose level (action).
- **Differential diagnoses:** This essential part of the assessment of a cardiopulmonary emergency requires the experienced provider to engage in ***critical thinking***. Most other steps involve simple yes/no decision making. The experienced provider should think carefully and try to identify the cause of the periarrest or arrest.

As various causes are considered, think of the treatment for each cause using the following memory aids:

Focused history (SAMPLE) (Table 4).

- **S**igns and Symptoms
- **A**llergy
- **M**edications
- **P**ast Medical History
- **L**ast Meal
- **E**vents

The **H's and T's** are a memory aid for the most common and potentially reversible causes of periarrest and cardiopulmonary arrest (Table 5). The table also shows how the steps of *assessment* and *action* are linked with each differential diagnosis.

H's	T's
Hypovolemia	**T**ension pneumothorax
Hypoxia	**T**amponade (cardiac)
Hydrogen ion (acidosis)	**T**oxins
Hyper-/hypokalemia	**T**hrombosis (pulmonary)
Hypothermia	**T**hrombosis (coronary)

Perfusion assessment: If the patient has poor perfusion, what is the cause?

- Intravascular volume
- Peripheral vascular resistance
- Cardiac contractility
- Heart rate

By using critical thinking, the team leader reviews the patient's background, condition, and response to interventions in an ongoing manner to determine the most likely cause so that therapies can be tailored to the particular needs of the patient. If the team leader can step back and take in the big picture rather than performing specific treatment maneuvers, alternatives can be considered and contingencies can be planned.

Perfusion

Perfusion assessment is an important component of evaluation in every cardiovascular emergency. Determining the cause of shock or inadequate end-organ perfusion will guide the treatment priorities for the patient. The clinician should try to classify the patient's condition (if possible) into 1 or more categories of altered cardiovascular physiology: intravascular volume, peripheral vascular resistance, cardiac contractility, and heart rate:

- Intravascular volume problem: fluid loss, bleeding, gastrointestinal losses
- Peripheral vascular resistance problem: vasomotor tone, vasodilation, vasoconstriction, redistribution of blood flow, and cardiac output
- Cardiac contractility problem: either primary or secondary cardiac dysfunction
- Rate problem (the electrical system): either too fast or too slow

What Is Critical Thinking?

Critical Thinking and the Team Leader

"Critical thinking is best understood as the ability of thinkers to take charge of their own thinking. This requires that they develop sound criteria for analyzing and assessing their own thinking and routinely use those criteria and standards to improve its quality."[1]

One aspect of developing clinical expertise is learning to think critically about a medical problem or emergency healthcare event. Good team leaders know the protocols and checklists that help avoid missing steps and keep the team on track, but they also know when to think beyond established guidelines and how to reset priorities based on a particular situation or patient condition. Critical thinking draws on a combination of experience combined with reflection and education. Each individual component is important, but it is the deliberate combination of all 3 that leads to the development of expertise. As such, becoming an "expert" is not a title one achieves, but is rather a continual process of learning-reflecting-acting that allows one to continually improve above a baseline of competence.

To make the best decisions in a clinically urgent situation, experienced providers use their knowledge base combined with intuition and pattern recognition based on their prior experience. To avoid making a clinical error or omission, the experienced clinician must continually reassess, using checklists, input from team members, and response to interventions. This is a process Schön called reflection-in-action, an intentional, conscious, immediate, and ongoing skill of "thinking on your feet."[2]

The practice of reflection-on-action supports this skill and develops expertise as providers review and consider their experiences and the actions taken in light of the outcome achieved, enhanced with new knowledge, past similar experiences, and input from colleagues.[2,3]

The team leader should request input from the other team members to be sure that nothing is missed. If there are enough people, it is beneficial to designate one team member to continuously review the appropriate checklist to make sure all appropriate actions are covered. In many cases, the event recorder is an appropriate designee for this role; in other situations, a colleague is a good choice. This practice has the benefit of reducing the cognitive load of the team leader so that she can critically think about unfolding events without worrying that an important step might be inadvertently missed; this has the additional benefit of providing time to find creative or new solutions to solve problems that have not been previously encountered.

Although experience is an essential component of building expertise, experience alone is not enough.[4] The team leader should organize a debriefing after every event to foster reflection-on-action and to improve the team's function in future events. This may be possible immediately after an event; however, the timing must be determined based on team dynamics and patient care needs. Delayed debriefing is still beneficial.[5] The team leader is also responsible for making sure that lessons learned, particularly recommendations for system improvement, are communicated and followed up in the local, continual, quality-assurance process.

Table 4. Focused History: SAMPLE

Signs and **S**ymptoms	Signs and symptoms at onset of illness: • Chest discomfort or abdominal pain • Breathing difficulty (eg, cough, rapid breathing, increased respiratory effort, breathlessness, abnormal breathing pattern) • Decreased level of consciousness • Agitation, anxiety • Motor or sensory impairment • Fever • Diarrhea, vomiting • Bleeding • Fatigue • Time course of symptoms
Allergies	• Medications, foods, latex, among others
Medications	• Medications taken • Last dose and time of recent medications • Length of time on medication(s) • Any changes to the patient's medication(s) • Name and dose of any over-the-counter medications, herbals, vitamins, or nutritional supplements taken
Past Medical History	• Pertinent medical problems (eg, hypertension, asthma, chronic lung disease, congenital heart disease, arrhythmia, congenital airway abnormality, seizures, head injury, brain tumor, diabetes, neuromuscular disease) • Past surgeries • Risk factors (eg, smoking, drug use, overweight, obesity)
Last Meal	• Time and nature of last oral intake of liquid or food • Important to note in cases of food poisoning, bowel obstruction, allergies, etc.
Events	• Events leading to current illness or injury (eg, sudden or gradual onset, type of injury) • Hazards at scene • Treatment during interval from onset of disease or injury until evaluation • Estimated time of arrival or time to intervention

Table 5. The H's and T's*

The H's: Causes (Examples)	Assessments	Actions/Treatments
Hypovolemia • Occult bleeding • Anaphylaxis • Supine position in late-term pregnancy • Sepsis	• History • Physical exam: flat neck veins • Hematocrit • ECG: narrow complex, rapid rate	• Administer volume • Administer blood if needed • Turn the pregnant patient to her left side (see Chapter 18)
Hypoxia • Narcotic overdose • Drowning • Carbon monoxide poisoning • Methemoglobinemia	• History: airway problems • Physical exam: cyanosis, abnormal breath sounds • Pulse oximetry • Tube placement • Arterial blood gas • ECG: slow rate	• Oxygen • Ventilation • Advanced airway • Good CPR technique
Hydrogen ion (acidosis) • Respiratory or metabolic acidosis • DKA • Drug overdose, ingestion, exposure • Renal failure	• History: diabetes • Physical exam • Clinical setting • Arterial blood gas • Lab tests • ECG: smaller-amplitude QRS complexes	• Acid-base abnormalities: see Chapter 15 • Optimization of perfusion • Establishment of effective oxygen-ation and ventilation • Overdose: bicarbonate • Toxicologic causes, symptomatic and antidotal therapies: see Chapter 14
Hyper-/hypokalemia • Renal failure • Crush injury • Massive transfusion • Iatrogenic causes • Vomiting • Diarrhea	• History: diabetes, medications (diuretics) • Risk factors, eg, dialysis • Physical exam • ECG: both cause wide-complex QRS; flat-tened T waves, prominent U waves, prolonged QT; tachycardia may be seen in hypokalemia; peaked and tall T waves, small P waves, and sine wave may be seen in hyperkalemia	• Treatment of specific electrolyte imbalance: see Chapter 15 • Hypokalemia: potassium replacement • Hyperkalemia: may use calcium, bicarbonate, insulin, glucose
Hypothermia • Profound hypothermia	• History of exposure to cold • Physical exam: core body temperature • ECG: J or Osborne waves	• Hypothermia: see Chapter 21 • Active/passive, external/internal rewarming
The T's: Causes (Examples)	**Assessments**	**Actions/Treatments**
Tension pneumothorax • Asthma • Trauma • COPD • Ventilators plus positive pressures	• History • Risk factors • Physical exam: lung sounds diminished or unequal, tracheal deviation, neck-vein distention • No pulse felt with CPR • Difficult to ventilate patient • ECG: narrow complex, slow rate (hypoxia)	• Needle decompression • Chest tube thoracostomy
Tamponade (cardiac) • Trauma • Renal failure • Chest compressions • Carcinoma • Central-line perforations	• History: prearrest symptoms • Physical exam: neck-vein distention • Risk factors • No pulse felt with CPR • Bedside ultrasonography, echocardiography • ECG: narrow complex, rapid rate	• Administration of volume • Pericardiocentesis • Thoracotomy

(continued)

(continued)

The T's: Causes (Examples)	Assessments	Actions/Treatments
Toxins (drug overdose, ingestion, and exposure) • Acetaminophen • Amphetamines • Anticholinergic drugs • Antihistamines • Barbiturates • Calcium channel antagonists • Cocaine • Cyclic antidepressants • Digoxin • Isoniazid • Opioid narcotics • Salicylates • SSRI, serotonin syndrome, NMS • Toxic alcohols • Theophylline/caffeine • Withdrawal states	• History • Risk factors • Physical exam: bradycardia, pupils, neurologic exam • Toxidrome • Clues such as empty bottles at the scene • ECG: various effects, predominantly prolongation of QT interval	• Specific antidotes and more comprehensive list of therapies: see Chapter 14 • Possible volume therapy (titrate carefully) and vasopressors for hypotension • TCA overdose: bicarbonate • Calcium channel blocker or β-blocker overdose: glucagon, calcium • Cocaine overdose: benzodiazepines; do not give nonselective β-blockers • Prolonged CPR may be justified • Advanced airway management • Cardiopulmonary bypass
Thrombosis (coronary) • STEMI • Other acute coronary syndromes	• History: prearrest symptoms, chest pain • Physical exam • Serum cardiac markers • ECG: ST-segment changes, Q waves, T-wave inversions	• ACS: see Chapter 11 • Aspirin, oxygen, nitroglycerin, and morphine if no response to nitrates • Vasopressors • Emergent reperfusion (PCI or fibrinolytics) • IABP, CABG
Thrombosis (pulmonary) • Pulmonary embolism	• History • Risk factors: prior positive test for deep vein thrombosis or pulmonary embolism • Physical exam: neck-vein distention • Diagnostic imaging • ECG: narrow complex, rapid rate	• Administration of volume • Dopamine • Heparin • Fibrinolytics • Consider rtPA • Surgical embolectomy

Abbreviations: ACS, acute coronary syndromes; CABG, coronary artery bypass graft; COPD, chronic obstructive pulmonary disease; CPR, cardiopulmonary resuscitation; DKA, diabetic ketoacidosis; ECG, electrocardiogram; IABP, intra-aortic balloon pump; NMS, neuroleptic malignant syndrome; PCI, percutaneous coronary intervention; rtPA, recombinant tissue plasminogen activator; SSRI, selective serotonin reuptake inhibitor; STEMI, ST-segment elevation myocardial infarction; TCA, tricyclic antidepressant.

*The "H's and T's" provide an expanded list of possible causes of periarrest or cardiac arrest. The emphasis is on *reversible, treatable conditions*. The list contains examples and is not meant to be exhaustive or exclusive. The diagnostic test listed may not be useful during resuscitation, but results from recent studies or tests done after resuscitation may provide clinical clues or be diagnostic. Remember, diagnostic tests should never delay clinically indicated and necessary treatments and interventions. For example, fibrinolytics are administered on the basis of the patient's history, ECG, and clinical-risk stratification. There should be no delay waiting for cardiac biomarker results. Tension pneumothorax is treated on the basis of clinical examination, not the chest x-ray.

Critical Concepts **Diagnostic Tests**	Diagnostic tests should never delay clinically indicated and necessary treatments and interventions.

Multiple or Overlapping Problems

After identifying the patient's problem, the healthcare provider can select the appropriate therapy. The following priority of actions is recommended for perfusion problems:

- First, correct primary *rate* problems if present.
- Second, correct any *volume* problems with fluid or transfusions or diuresis. Always correct volume problems before treating resistance problems.
- Third, treat *contractility* problems with vasopressors, inotropic agents, or both.

Each patient requires individualized treatment. Three rules will help you avoid major errors:

- If the primary cause of hypotension is an arrhythmia, treat the rhythm first.
  - Identifying the rhythm problem can be challenging. One clue may be the duration of the arrhythmia.
  - Over 80% of atrial fibrillation with hypotension is associated with hypovolemia.[6] Hypovolemia is very rarely a primary rate problem.
  - Perform a fluid challenge with or without vasopressors while trying to identify the underlying problem.
- Do not use vasopressors alone to treat hypotension caused by hypovolemia (eg, shock due to gastrointestinal bleeding). Rapid volume administration should be the primary intervention. If the hypotension is so profound that eminent death might occur (eg, BP of 60/30 with thready pulse), starting vasopressors simultaneously with fluids is prudent.
- Contractility problems can include acute myocardial infarction, congestive heart failure, or cardiomyopathy with acute pulmonary edema. Treat contractility problems with inotropic agents rather than fluids. If the volume status is unclear during initial assessment, it may be prudent to administer a fluid bolus of 250 to 500 mL and serially evaluate the patient's clinical response.

Vasodilators may be needed to treat inadequate cardiac output with poor myocardial function. Ensure that blood pressure and intravascular volume are adequate before administering vasodilators, and be ready to administer additional volume if needed during vasodilator therapy.

Using the BLS and ACLS EP Surveys: Key Principles

- The survey sequence uses numbers and the alphabet as a memory aid to address problems in their order of importance.
- Figure 11 integrates the BLS and ACLS EP Surveys into 1 algorithm, the Systematic Approach for Experienced Providers Algorithm.
- Whenever you identify a problem, resolve it *immediately*. For example, if you are unable to make the chest rise with ventilation ("B" of the ACLS EP Survey), you must solve that problem before you start an IV and administer medications.
- The survey assessments and actions can be followed only as far as personnel and equipment resources allow. A single provider, for example, is limited to basic CPR and automated defibrillation until other help arrives.
- When additional personnel arrive, the survey sequence tells them exactly where to enter the resuscitative effort. To illustrate, personnel arriving to assist a lone provider doing CPR assume responsibility for defibrillation, advanced airway management, IV access, and medications—and in that order.
- If a sufficient number of skilled personnel are available, they can proceed with the survey steps simultaneously. But the surveys supply a useful review to make sure someone has responsibility for every task.

FAQ

What is the ACLS systematic approach?

The systematic approach first requires ACLS providers to determine the patient's level of consciousness. Approach to treatment will follow accordingly.

- If the patient appears unconscious
  - Use the BLS Survey for the initial assessment followed by the ACLS Survey for more advanced assessment and treatment.
- If the patient appears conscious
  - Use the ACLS Survey for your initial assessment.

What does the ACLS experienced provider have to do differently when applying the ACLS EP Survey?

The ACLS experienced provider should pause to think critically and use the following memory aid to try to identify the cause of the periarrest or arrest:

- "SAMPLE" to obtain a focused history
- "H's and T's" to identify the most common and potentially reversible causes of periarrest and cardiopulmonary arrest
- "Volume, resistance, contractility, and rate" for assessment of perfusion

What priority of action is recommended when there are multiple, overlapping perfusion problems?

- First, correct primary *rate* problems if present.
- Second, correct any *volume* problems with fluid or transfusions or diuresis.
- Third, treat *contractility* problems with vasopressors, inotropic agents, or both.

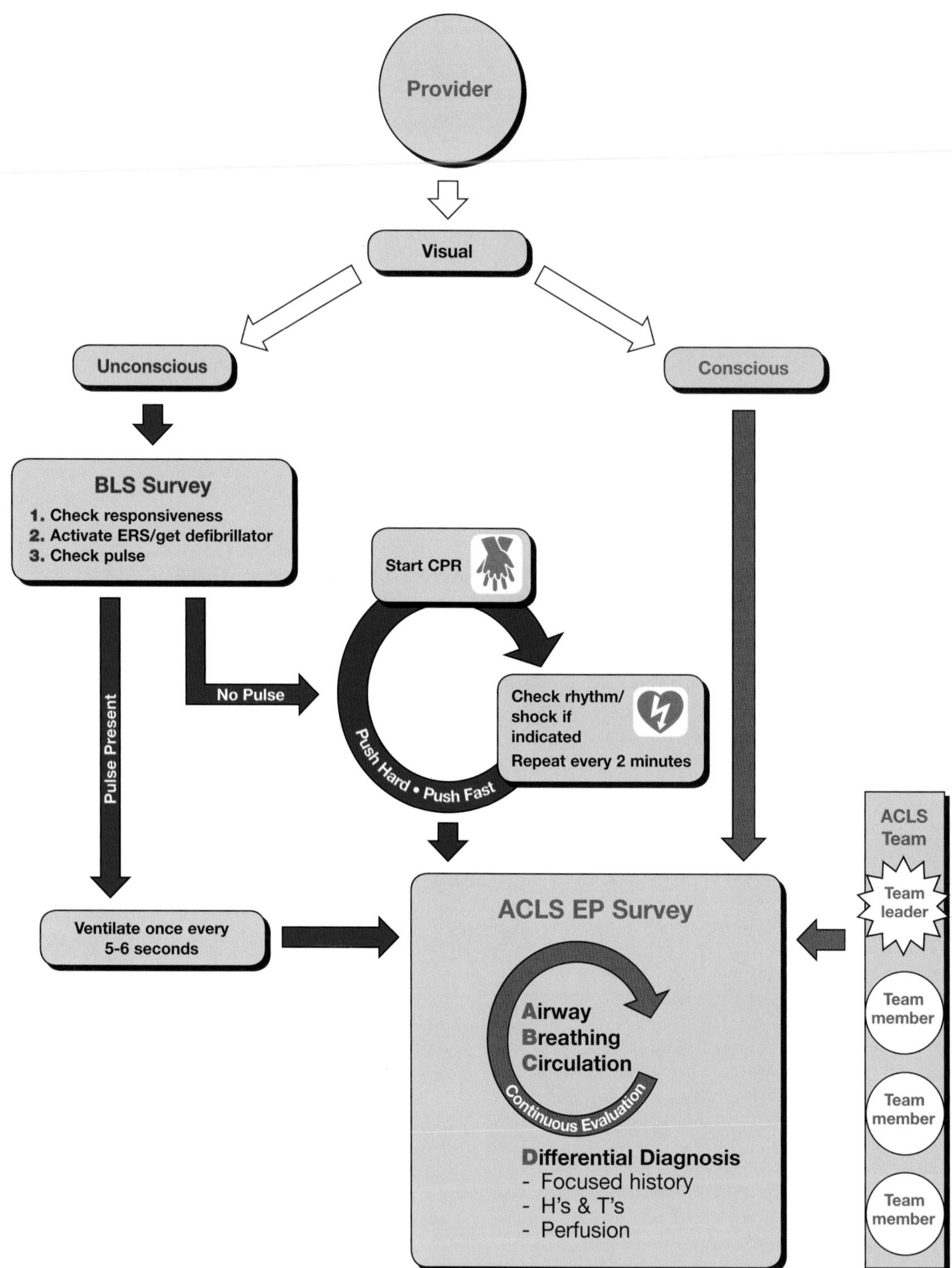

Figure 11. The Systematic Approach for Experienced Providers Algorithm.

References

1. Elder L, Paul R. Critical thinking: why we must transform our teaching. *J Dev Educ*. 1994;18:34-35.
2. Schön D. *Educating the Reflective Practitioner: Toward a New Design for Teaching and Learning in the Professions*. San Francisco, CA: Jossey-Bass; 1987.
3. Schön D. *The Reflective Practitioner: How Professionals Think in Action*. London, England: Temple Smith; 1983.
4. Ericsson KA. An expert-performance perspective of research on medical expertise: the study of clinical performance. *Med Educ*. 2007;41:1124-1130.
5. Edelson DP, Litzinger B, Arora V, Walsh D, Kim S, Lauderdale DS, Vanden Hoek TL, Becker LB, Abella BS. Improving in-hospital cardiac arrest process and outcomes with performance debriefing. *Arch Intern Med*. 2008;168:1063-1069.
6. Donnino MW, Miller JC, Bivens M, Cocchi MN, Salciccioli JD, Farris S, Gautam S, Cutlip D, Howell M. A pilot study examining the severity and outcome of the post-cardiac arrest syndrome: a comparative analysis of two geographically distinct hospitals. *Circulation*. 2012;126:1478-1483.

Chapter 3

Effective Resuscitation Team Dynamics

This Chapter

- **Roles of the Team Leader and Team Members**
- **Elements of Effective Resuscitation Team Dynamics**

Introduction

Successful resuscitation attempts often require healthcare providers to perform a variety of interventions simultaneously. Although a CPR-trained bystander working alone can resuscitate a patient within the first moments after collapse, most attempts require the concerted efforts of multiple healthcare providers. Effective teamwork divides the tasks while multiplying the chances of a successful outcome.

Successful teams not only have medical expertise and mastery of resuscitation skills, but they also demonstrate effective communication and team dynamics.

Roles of the Team Leader and Team Members

Role of the Team Leader

The role of the team leader is multifaceted. The team leader

- Organizes the group
- Monitors individual performance of team members
- Backs up team members
- Models excellent team behavior
- Trains and coaches
- Facilitates understanding
- Focuses on comprehensive patient care
- Employs critical thinking

Every resuscitation team needs a leader to organize the efforts of the group. The team leader is responsible for making sure everything is done at the right time in the right way by monitoring and integrating individual performance of team members. The role of the team leader is similar to that of an orchestra conductor who directs individual musicians. Like a conductor, the team leader does not play the instruments but instead knows how each member of the orchestra fits into the overall music.

The role of the team leader also includes modeling excellent team behavior and leadership skills for the team and other people involved or interested in the resuscitation. The team leader should serve as a teacher or guide to help train future team leaders and improve team effectiveness. After a resuscitation is performed, the team leader can facilitate analysis, criticism, and practice in preparation for the next resuscitation attempt.

The team leader also helps team members understand why they must perform certain tasks in a specific way. The team leader should be able to explain why it is essential to

- Push hard and fast
- Ensure complete chest recoil
- Minimize interruptions in chest compressions
- Avoid excessive ventilations

Whereas team members should focus on their individual tasks, the team leader must focus on comprehensive patient care. The experienced team leader knows the protocols and checklists that keep the team on track and knows when to think beyond established guidelines. Using critical thinking, the team leader should draw on a combination of experience, education, and reflection, using the input of the team to reset priorities based on a particular situation or patient condition. Experienced providers conduct a debriefing with the team after every event to foster reflection-on-action and to improve the team's function in future events. Lessons learned and recommendations for system improvement should be passed on to the local quality-assurance process.

Role of the Team Member

Team members must be proficient in performing the skills authorized by their scope of practice. It is essential to the success of the resuscitation attempt that team members are

- Clear about role assignments
- Prepared to fulfill their role responsibilities
- Well practiced in resuscitation skills
- Knowledgeable about the algorithms
- Committed to success

Elements of Effective Resuscitation Team Dynamics

Closed-Loop Communications

When communicating with resuscitation team members, the team leader should use closed-loop communication by taking these steps:

1. The team leader gives a message, order, or assignment to a team member.
2. By receiving a clear response and eye contact, the team leader confirms that the team member heard and understood the message.
3. The team leader listens for confirmation of task performance from the team member before assigning another task.

What to Do

Team leader	• Assign another task after receiving oral confirmation that a task has been completed, such as "Now that the IV is in, give 1 mg of epinephrine."
Team members	• Close the loop: inform the team leader when a task begins or ends, such as "The IV is in."

What Not to Do

Team leader	• Give more tasks to a team member without asking or receiving confirmation of a completed assignment
Team members	• Give drugs without verbally confirming the order with the team leader • Forget to inform the team leader after giving the drug or performing the procedure

Clear Messages

Clear messages consist of concise communication spoken with distinctive speech in a controlled tone of voice. All healthcare providers should deliver messages and orders in a calm and direct manner without yelling or shouting. Unclear communication can lead to unnecessary delays in treatment or to medication errors.

For example, "Did the patient get IV propofol so I can proceed with the cardioversion?" "No, I thought you said to give him *propranolol*."

Yelling or shouting can impair effective team interaction. Only one person should talk at any time.

What to Do

Team leader	• Encourage team members to speak clearly
Team members	• Repeat the medication order • Question an order if the slightest doubt exists

What Not to Do

Team leader	• Mumble or speak in incomplete sentences • Give unclear messages and drug/medication orders • Yell, scream, or shout
Team members	• Feel patronized by distinct and concise messages

Clear Roles and Responsibilities

Every member of the team should know his or her role and responsibilities. Just as pieces of different shapes make up a jigsaw puzzle, each team member's role is unique and critical to the effective performance of the team. Figure 12 identifies 6 team roles for resuscitation. When fewer than 6 people are present, all tasks must be assigned to the healthcare providers present.

When roles are unclear, team performance suffers. Signs of unclear roles include

- Performing the same task more than once
- Missing essential tasks
- Freelancing of team members

To avoid inefficiencies, the team leader must clearly delegate tasks. Team members should communicate when and if they can handle additional responsibilities. The team leader should encourage team members to participate in leadership and not simply follow directions blindly.

What to Do

Team leader	• Clearly define all team member roles in the clinical setting
Team members	• Seek out and perform clearly defined tasks appropriate to your level of competence • Ask for a new task or role if you are unable to perform your assigned task because it is beyond your level of experience or competence

What Not to Do

Team leader	• Neglect to assign tasks to all available team members • Assign tasks to team members who are unsure of their responsibilities • Distribute assignments unevenly, leaving some with too much to do and others with too little
Team members	• Avoid taking assignments • Take assignments beyond your level of competence or expertise

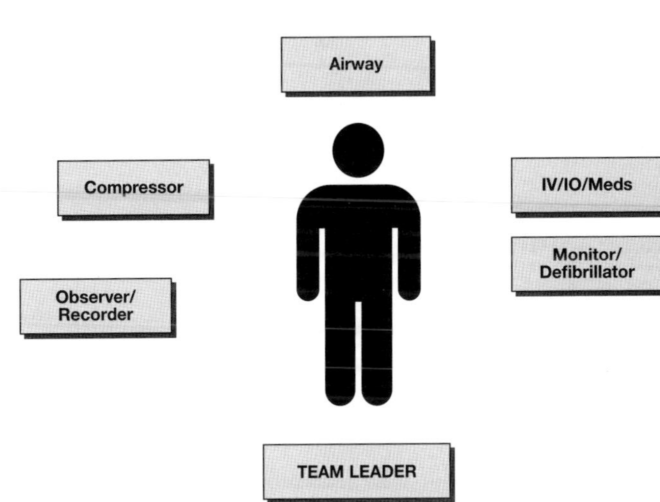

Figure 12. Suggested locations of team leader and team members during case simulations.

Knowing One's Limitations

Not only should everyone on the team know his or her own limitations and capabilities, but also the team leader should be aware of them. This allows the team leader to evaluate team resources and call for backup of team members when assistance is needed. Team members should anticipate situations in which they might require assistance and inform the team leader.

During the stress of an attempted resuscitation, do not practice or explore a new skill. If you need extra help, request it early. It is not a sign of weakness or incompetence to ask for help; it is better to have more help than needed rather than not enough help, which might negatively affect patient outcome.

What to Do

Team leader and team members	• Call for assistance early rather than waiting until the patient deteriorates to the point that help is critical • Seek advice from more experienced personnel when the patient's condition worsens despite primary treatment

What Not to Do

Team leader and team members	• Reject offers from others to carry out an assigned task you are unable to complete, especially if task completion is essential to treatment

Team members	• Use or start an unfamiliar treatment or therapy without seeking advice from more experienced personnel • Take on too many assignments at a time when assistance is readily available

Knowledge Sharing

Sharing information is a critical component of effective team performance. Team leaders may become trapped in a specific treatment or diagnostic approach; this common human error is called a fixation error. Examples of 3 common types of fixation errors are

- "Everything is okay."
- "This and only this is the correct path."
- "Anything but this."

When resuscitative efforts are ineffective, go back to the basics and talk as a team. "Well, we've gotten the following on the ACLS EP Survey… Have we missed something?"

Team members should inform the team leader of any changes in the patient's condition to ensure that decisions are made with all available information.

What to Do

Team leader	• Encourage an environment of information sharing and ask for suggestions if uncertain of the next best interventions • Ask for good ideas for differential diagnoses • Ask if anything has been overlooked (eg, IV access should have been obtained or drugs should have been administered)
Team members	• Share information with other team members

What Not to Do

Team leader	• Ignore others' suggestions for treatment • Overlook or fail to examine clinical signs that are relevant to the treatment
Team members	• Ignore important information to improve your role

Constructive Intervention

During a resuscitation attempt, the team leader or a team member may need to intervene if an action that is about to occur may be inappropriate at the time. Although constructive intervention is necessary, it should be tactful. Team leaders should avoid confrontation with team members. Instead conduct a debriefing afterward if constructive criticism is needed.

What to Do

Team leader	• Ask that a different intervention be started if it has a higher priority
Team members	• Suggest an alternative drug or dose in a confident manner • Question a colleague who is about to make a mistake

What Not to Do

Team leader	• Fail to reassign a team member who is trying to function beyond his or her level of skill
Team members	• Ignore a team member who is about to administer a drug incorrectly

Reevaluation and Summarizing

An essential role of the team leader is monitoring and reevaluating

- The patient's status
- Interventions that have been performed
- Assessment findings

A good practice is for the team leader to summarize this information out loud in a periodic update to the team. Review the status of the resuscitation attempt and announce the plan for the next few steps. Remember that the patient's condition can change. Remain flexible to changing treatment plans and revisiting the initial differential diagnosis. Ask for information and summaries from the code recorder as well.

What to Do

Team leader	• Draw continuous attention to decisions about differential diagnoses • Review or maintain an ongoing record of drugs and treatments administered and the patient's response
Team leader and team members	• Clearly draw attention to significant changes in the patient's clinical condition • Increase monitoring (eg, frequency of respirations and blood pressure) when the patient's condition deteriorates

What Not to Do

Team leader	• Fail to change a treatment strategy when new information supports such a change • Fail to inform arriving personnel of the current status and plans for further action

Mutual Respect

The best teams are composed of members who share a mutual respect for each other and work together in a collegial, supportive manner. To have a high-performing team, everyone must abandon ego and respect each other during the resuscitation attempt, regardless of any additional training or experience that the team leader or specific team members may have.

What to Do

Team leader and team members	• Speak in a friendly, controlled tone of voice • Avoid shouting or displaying aggression if you are not understood initially
Team leader	• Acknowledge correctly completed assignments by saying "Thanks—good job!"

What Not to Do

Team leader and team members	• Shout or yell at team members—when one person raises his voice, others will respond similarly • Behave aggressively, confusing directive behavior with aggression • Be uninterested in others

Chapter 3

Chapter 4

Systems of Care

This Chapter

- Systems of Care for CPR
- Systems of Care for Post–Cardiac Arrest Care
- Systems of Care for Acute Coronary Syndromes (ACS)
- Systems of Care for Stroke

Introduction

A system is a group of regularly interacting and interdependent components. The system provides the links for the chain and determines the strength of each link and the chain as a whole. By definition, the system determines the ultimate outcome and strength of the chain and provides collective support and organization. For patients with possible ACS, the system rapidly triages patients, determines a possible or provisional diagnosis, and initiates a strategy based on initial clinical characteristics.

Cardiopulmonary Resuscitation

Quality Improvement in Resuscitation Systems, Processes, and Outcomes

Cardiopulmonary resuscitation is a series of lifesaving actions that improve the chance of survival following cardiac arrest. Although the optimal approach to CPR may vary, depending on the rescuer, the patient, and the available resources, the fundamental challenge remains how to achieve early and effective CPR.

A Systems Approach

Successful resuscitation following cardiac arrest requires an integrated set of coordinated actions represented by the links in the adult Chain of Survival (Figure 13). The links include the following:

- Immediate recognition of cardiac arrest and activation of the emergency response system
- Early CPR with an emphasis on chest compressions
- Rapid defibrillation
- Effective advanced life support
- Integrated post–cardiac arrest care

Effective resuscitation requires an integrated response known as a system of care. Fundamental to a successful resuscitation system of care is the collective appreciation of the challenges and opportunities presented by the Chain of Survival: individuals and groups must work together, sharing ideas and information, to evaluate and improve their resuscitation system. Leadership and accountability are important components of this team approach.

To improve care, leaders must assess the performance of each system component. Only when performance is evaluated can participants in a system effectively intervene to improve care. This process of quality improvement consists of an iterative and continuous cycle of

- Systematic evaluation of resuscitation care and outcome
- Benchmarking with stakeholder feedback
- Strategic efforts to address identified deficiencies

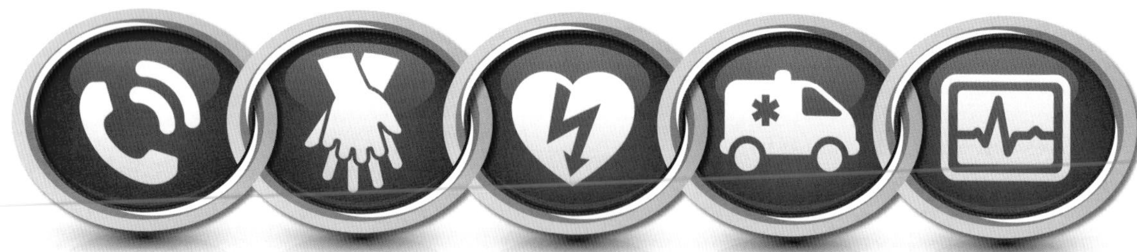

Figure 13. The AHA adult Chain of Survival.

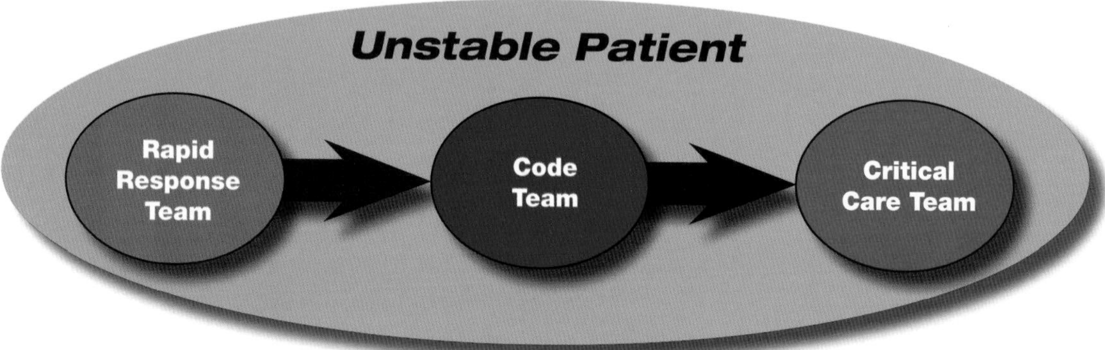

Figure 14. Management of life-threatening emergencies requires integration of multidisciplinary teams that can involve rapid response teams, cardiac arrest teams, and intensive care specialties to achieve survival of the patient. Team leaders have an essential role in coordination of care with team members and other specialists.

Many hospitals have implemented the use of medical emergency teams (METs) or rapid response teams (RRTs). The purpose of these teams is to improve patient outcomes by identifying and treating early clinical deterioration (Figure 14). In-hospital cardiac arrest is commonly preceded by physiologic changes. In one study, nearly 80% of hospitalized patients with cardiorespiratory arrest had abnormal vital signs documented for up to 8 hours before the actual arrest. Many of these changes can be recognized by monitoring routine vital signs. Intervention before clinical deterioration or cardiac arrest may be possible. Consider this question: "Would you have done anything differently if you knew 15 minutes before the arrest that . . .?"

Measurement

Quality improvement relies on valid assessment of resuscitation performance and outcome.

- The Utstein guidelines provide guidance for core performance measures, including
  - Rate of bystander CPR
  - Time to defibrillation
- Importance of information sharing among all links in the system of care include
  - Dispatch records
  - Emergency medical services (EMS) patient care report
  - Hospital records
- Survival to hospital discharge

Benchmarking and Feedback

Data should be systematically reviewed and compared internally with prior performance and externally with similar systems. Existing registries can facilitate this benchmarking effort. Examples include

- Resuscitation Outcomes Consortium (ROC) Cardiac Arrest Epidemiologic Registry (Epistry) and Cardiac Arrest Registry to Enhance Survival (CARES) for out-of-hospital cardiac arrest
- Get With the Guidelines®-Resuscitation program for in-hospital cardiac arrest
- Mission: Lifeline® for ST-segment elevation myocardial infarction (STEMI) and cardiac resuscitation systems of care

Change

Simply measuring and benchmarking care can positively influence outcome. However, ongoing review and interpretation are necessary to identify areas for improvement, such as

- Increased bystander CPR response rates
- Improved CPR performance
- Shortened time to defibrillation
- Citizen awareness
- Citizen and healthcare professional education and training

Summary

Over the past 50 years, basic life support fundamentals of early recognition and activation, early CPR, and early defibrillation have saved hundreds of thousands of lives around the world. However, we still have a long road to travel if we are to fulfill the potential offered by the Chain of Survival. Survival disparities present a generation ago appear to persist. Fortunately we currently possess the knowledge and tools—represented by the Chain of Survival—to address many of these care gaps, and future discoveries will offer opportunities to improve rates of survival.

Post–Cardiac Arrest Care

The healthcare system should implement a comprehensive, structured, multidisciplinary system of care in a consistent manner for the treatment of post–cardiac arrest patients. Programs should address therapeutic hypothermia, hemodynamic and ventilation optimization, immediate coronary reperfusion with percutaneous coronary intervention (PCI), glycemic control, neurologic care and prognostication, and other structured interventions.

Individual hospitals with a high frequency of treating cardiac arrest patients show an increased likelihood of survival when these interventions are provided.

Therapeutic Hypothermia

The *2010 AHA Guidelines for CPR and ECC* recommend cooling comatose (ie, lack of meaningful response to verbal commands) adult patients with return of spontaneous circulation (ROSC) after out-of-hospital VF cardiac arrest to 32°C to 34°C (89.6°F to 93.2°F) for 12 to 24 hours. Healthcare providers should also consider induced hypothermia for comatose adult patients with ROSC after in-hospital cardiac arrest of any initial rhythm or after out-of-hospital cardiac arrest with an initial rhythm of pulseless electrical activity or asystole.

Hemodynamic and Ventilation Optimization

Although providers often use 100% oxygen while performing the initial resuscitation, providers should titrate inspired oxygen during the post–cardiac arrest phase to the lowest level required to achieve an arterial oxygen saturation of 94% or higher. This helps to avoid any potential complications associated with oxygen toxicity.

Avoid excessive ventilation of the patient because of potential adverse hemodynamic effects when intrathoracic pressures are increased and because of potential decreases in cerebral blood flow when $Pa{CO_2}$ decreases.

Healthcare providers may start ventilation rates at 10 to 12 breaths per minute and titrate to achieve a $PET{CO_2}$ of 35 to 40 mm Hg or a $Pa{CO_2}$ of 40 to 45 mm Hg.

Healthcare providers should titrate fluid administration and vasoactive or inotropic agents as needed to optimize blood pressure, cardiac output, and systemic perfusion. The optimal post–cardiac arrest blood pressure remains unknown; however, a mean arterial pressure of 65 mm Hg or higher is a reasonable goal.

Immediate Coronary Reperfusion With PCI

Following ROSC, rescuers should transport the patient to a facility capable of reliably providing coronary reperfusion (eg, PCI) and other goal-directed postarrest care therapies. The decision to perform PCI can be made irrespective of the presence of coma or the decision to induce hypothermia because concurrent PCI and hypothermia are reported to be feasible, safe, and effective.

Glycemic Control

Consider strategies to target moderate glycemic control (144 to 180 mg/dL [8 to 10 mmol/L]) in adult patients with ROSC after cardiac arrest.

Healthcare providers should not attempt to alter glucose concentration within a lower range (80 to 110 mg/dL [4.4 to 6.1 mmol/L]) due to the increased risk of hypoglycemia.

Neurologic Care and Prognostication

The goal of post–cardiac arrest management is to return patients to their prearrest functional level. Reliable early prognostication of neurologic outcome is an essential component of post–cardiac arrest care. Most important, when considering decisions to limit or withdraw life-sustaining care, tools used to prognosticate poor outcome must be accurate and reliable, with a false-positive rate approaching 0%. Durations of observation greater than 72 hours after

ROSC should be considered before predicting poor outcome in patients treated with hypothermia.

ACS

The primary goals of therapy for patients with ACS are to

- Reduce the amount of myocardial necrosis that occurs in patients with acute myocardial infarction (AMI), thus preserving left ventricular (LV) function, preventing heart failure, and limiting other cardiovascular complications
- Prevent major adverse cardiac events (MACE): death, nonfatal MI, and the need for urgent revascularization
- Treat acute, life-threatening complications of ACS, such as VF, pulseless VT, unstable tachycardias, symptomatic bradycardias, pulmonary edema, cardiogenic shock, and mechanical complications of AMI

Starts "On the Phone" With Activation of EMS

Prompt diagnosis and treatment offer the greatest potential benefit for myocardial salvage. Thus, it is imperative that healthcare providers recognize patients with potential ACS in order to initiate evaluation, appropriate triage, and management as expeditiously as possible.

EMS Components

- Prehospital ECGs
- Notification of the receiving facility of a patient with possible ST-segment elevation myocardial infarction ("STEMI alert")
- Activation of the cardiac catheterization team to shorten reperfusion time
- Continuous review and quality improvement

Hospital-Based Components

- **Emergency department (ED) protocols**
  - Activation of the cardiac catheterization laboratory
  - Admission to the coronary intensive care unit (ICU)
  - Quality assurance, real-time feedback, and healthcare provider education
- **Emergency physician**
  - Empowerment to select the most appropriate reperfusion strategy
  - Empowerment to activate the cardiac catheterization team as indicated
- **Hospital leadership**
  - Involvement in the process and commitment to support rapid access to STEMI reperfusion therapy

Adult Stroke

The healthcare system has achieved significant improvements in stroke care through integration of public education, emergency dispatch, prehospital detection and triage, development of hospital stroke systems, and management of stroke units. Not only have the rates of appropriate fibrinolytic therapy increased over the past 5 years, but overall stroke care has also improved, in part through the creation of stroke centers.

Regionalization of Stroke Care

These advances in stroke care will have the greatest effect on stroke outcome if care is delivered within a regional stroke system designed to improve both efficiency and effectiveness. The ultimate goal of stroke care is to minimize ongoing injury, emergently recanalize acute vascular occlusions, and begin secondary measures to maximize functional recovery. These efforts will provide stroke patients with the greatest opportunity for a return to previous quality of life and decrease the overall societal burden of stroke.

With the National Institute of Neurological Disorders and Stroke (NINDS) recombinant tissue plasminogen activator (rtPA) trial,[1] the crucial need for local partnerships between academic medical centers and community hospitals became clear. The time-sensitive nature of stroke requires such an approach, even in densely populated metropolitan centers.

Community and Professional Education

Community and professional education is essential and has successfully increased the proportion of stroke patients treated with fibrinolytic therapy.

- Patient education efforts are most effective when the message is clear and succinct.
- Educational efforts need to couple the knowledge of the signs and symptoms of stroke with action—activate the emergency response system.

EMS

The integration of EMS into regional stroke models is crucial for improvement of patient outcomes.[2] It is recommended that all paramedics and emergency medical technicians-basic (EMT-basic) be trained in recognition of stroke using a validated, abbreviated out-of-hospital screening tool such as the Cincinnati Prehospital Stroke Scale or the Los Angeles Prehospital Stroke Screen.

Stroke Centers

In 2000, the Brain Attack Coalition provided a description of "primary stroke centers," which would ensure that best practices for stroke care (acute and beyond) would be offered in an organized fashion.[3] The logic of having a multitiered system such as that provided for trauma was evident. In 2005, the Brain Attack Coalition followed the statement on primary stroke centers with recommendations for comprehensive stroke centers.[4] Following the establishment of primary stroke centers and comprehensive stroke centers, the new concept of a stroke-prepared hospital has recently emerged. This stroke-prepared hospital can access stroke expertise via telemedicine. The comparison with a trauma system with Level 1, 2, and 3 centers is rational and quite intuitive to emergency care providers familiar with such configurations.

Education, Implementation, and Teams

The Chain of Survival is a metaphor used to organize and describe the integrated set of time-sensitive coordinated actions necessary to maximize survival from cardiac arrest. The use of evidence-based education and implementation strategies can optimize the links in the chain.

The Need for Teams

Mortality from in-hospital cardiac arrest remains high. The average survival rate is approximately 24% despite significant advances in treatments. Survival rates are particularly poor for arrest associated with rhythms other than VF/VT. Non-VF/VT rhythms are present in more than 82% of arrests in the hospital.[5]

Many in-hospital arrests are preceded by easily recognizable physiologic changes, many of which are evident with routine monitoring of vital signs. In recent studies, nearly 80% of hospitalized patients with cardiorespiratory arrest had abnormal vital signs documented for up to 8 hours before the actual arrest. This finding suggests that there is a period of increasing instability before the arrest.

Of the small percentage of in-hospital cardiac arrest patients who experience ROSC and are admitted to the ICU, 80% ultimately die before discharge. In comparison, only 44% of nonarrest patients admitted to intensive care urgently from the floor (ie, before an arrest occurs) die before discharge.

Cardiac Arrest Teams (In-Hospital)

Cardiac arrest teams are unlikely to prevent arrests because their focus has traditionally been to respond only after the arrest has occurred. Unfortunately the mortality rate is over 75% once the arrest occurs.[5] Rather than focus solely on resuscitation, hospitals have now developed a more comprehensive approach to cardiac arrest prevention and care, including RRTs, high-quality CPR, and better teamwork across healthcare disciplines. The best way to improve a patient's chance of survival from a cardiorespiratory arrest is to prevent the arrest from happening.

The majority of cardiorespiratory arrests in the hospital should be classified as a "failure to rescue" rather than as isolated, unexpected, random occurrences. Doing so requires a significant cultural shift within institutions. Actions and interventions need to be proactive with the goal of improving rates of morbidity and mortality rather than reacting to a catastrophic event.

Rapid assessment and intervention for many abnormal physiologic variables can decrease the number of arrests occurring in the hospital.

Rapid Response System

Over the past decade, hospitals in several countries have designed systems to identify and treat early clinical deterioration in patients. The purpose of these rapid response systems is to improve patient outcomes by bringing critical care expertise to ward patients. The rapid response system has several components:

- Event-detection and response-triggering arm
- A planned response arm, such as the MET or RRT
- Quality monitoring
- Administrative support

Many rapid response systems allow activation by a nurse, physician, or family member who is concerned that the patient is deteriorating. Some rapid response systems use specific physiologic criteria to determine when to call the team. The following list gives examples of such criteria for adult patients:

- Threatened airway
- Respiratory rate less than 6 or more than 30 breaths per minute
- Heart rate slower than 40/min or faster than 140/min
- Systolic blood pressure (SBP) lower than 90 mm Hg
- Symptomatic hypertension
- Unexpected decrease in level of consciousness
- Unexplained agitation
- Seizure
- Significant fall in urine output
- Subjective concern about the patient

Medical Emergency Teams and Rapid Response Teams

There are several names for rapid response systems, including medical emergency team, rapid response team, and rapid assessment team.

The rapid response system is critically dependent on early identification and activation to immediately summon the team to the patient's bedside. These teams typically consist of healthcare providers with both the critical care or emergency care experience and skills needed to support immediate intervention for life-threatening situations. These teams are responsible for performing a rapid patient assessment and initiating appropriate treatment to reverse physiologic deterioration and prevent a poor outcome.

Regional Systems of (Emergency) Cardiovascular Care

Hospitals with larger patient volumes have a better survival-to–hospital discharge rate than low-volume centers for patients treated for either in- or out-of-hospital cardiac arrest.[6]

Published Studies

The majority of published "before and after" studies of METs or rapid response systems have reported a 17% to 65% drop in the rate of cardiac arrests after the intervention. Other documented benefits of these systems include

- A decrease in unplanned emergency transfers to the ICU
- Decreased ICU and total hospital length of stay
- Reductions in postoperative morbidity and mortality rates
- Improved rates of survival from cardiac arrest

The recently published MERIT trial is the only randomized controlled trial comparing hospitals with a MET and those without one. The study did not show a difference in the composite primary outcome (cardiac arrest, unexpected death, unplanned ICU admission) between the 12 hospitals in which a MET system was introduced and 11 hospitals that had no MET system in place. Further research is needed about the critical details of implementation and the potential effectiveness of METs in preventing cardiac arrest or improving other important patient outcomes.

Implementation of a Rapid Response System

Implementing any type of rapid response system will require a significant cultural change in most hospitals. Those who design and manage the system must pay particular attention to issues that may prevent the system from being used effectively. Examples of such issues are insufficient resources, poor education, fear of calling the team, fear of losing control over patient care, and resistance from team members.

Implementation of a rapid response system requires ongoing education, impeccable data collection and review, and feedback. Development and maintenance of these programs require a long-term cultural and financial commitment from the hospital administration, which must understand that the potential benefits from the system (decreased resource use and improved survival rates) may have independent positive financial ramifications. Hospital administrators and healthcare professionals need to reorient their approach to emergency medical events and develop a culture of patient safety with a primary goal of decreasing morbidity and mortality.

References

1. Tissue plasminogen activator for acute ischemic stroke. The National Institute of Neurological Disorders and Stroke rt-PA Stroke Study Group. *N Engl J Med*. 1995;333:1581-1587.
2. Acker JE, Pancioli AM, Crocco TJ, Eckstein MK, Jauch EC, Larrabee H, Meltzer NM, Mergendahl WC, Munn JW, Prentiss SM, Sand C, Saver JL, Eigel B, Gilpin BR, Schoeberl M, Solis P, Bailey JR, Horton KB, Stranne SK. Implementation strategies for emergency medical services within stroke systems of care: a policy statement from the American Heart Association/American Stroke Association Expert Panel on Emergency Medical Services Systems and the Stroke Council. *Stroke*. 2007;38:3097-3115.
3. Alberts MJ, Hademenos G, Latchaw RE, Jagoda A, Marler JR, Mayberg MR, Starke RD, Todd HW, Viste KM, Girgus M, Shephard T, Emr M, Shwayder P, Walker MD. Recommendations for the establishment of primary stroke centers. Brain Attack Coalition. *JAMA*. 2000;283:3102-3109.
4. Alberts MJ, Latchaw RE, Selman WR, Shephard T, Hadley MN, Brass LM, Koroshetz W, Marler JR, Booss J, Zorowitz RD, Croft JB, Magnis E, Mulligan D, Jagoda A, O'Connor R, Cawley CM, Connors JJ, Rose-DeRenzy JA, Emr M, Warren M, Walker MD. Recommendations for comprehensive stroke centers: a consensus statement from the Brain Attack Coalition. *Stroke*. 2005;36:1597-1616.
5. Go AS, Mozaffarian D, Roger VL, Benjamin EJ, Berry JD, Borden WB, Bravata DM, Dai S, Ford ES, Fox CS, Franco S, Fullerton HJ, Gillespie C, Hailpern SM, Heit JA, Howard VJ, Huffman MD, Kissela BM, Kittner SJ, Lackland DT, Lichtman JH, Lisabeth LD, Magid D, Marcus GM, Marelli A, Matchar DB, McGuire D, Mohler E, Moy CS, Mussolino ME, Nichol G, Paynter NP, Schreiner PJ, Sorlie PD, Stein J, Turan TN, Virani SS, Wong ND, Woo D, Turner MB; on behalf of the American Heart Association Statistics Committee and Stroke Statistics Subcommittee. Heart disease and stroke statistics—2013 update: a report from the American Heart Association [published online ahead of print December 12, 2012]. *Circulation*. 2013. doi:10.1161/CIR.0b013e31828124ad.
6. Carr BG, Kahn JM, Merchant RM, Kramer AA, Neumar RW. Inter-hospital variability in post-cardiac arrest mortality. *Resuscitation*. 2009;80:30-34.

Chapter 5

CPR Techniques and Devices

This Chapter

- CPR Techniques
- CPR Devices: Current and New
- Devices That Support Ventilation
- Devices That Support Circulation

Overview

In the past 25 years researchers have developed a variety of alternatives to conventional (manual) cardiopulmonary resuscitation (CPR) in an effort to enhance perfusion during attempted resuscitation from cardiac arrest and to improve survival. Compared with conventional CPR, these techniques and devices typically require more personnel, training, and equipment, or they apply to a specific setting. Because use of these devices has the potential to delay or interrupt CPR, rescuers should be trained to minimize any interruption of chest compressions or defibrillation and should be retrained as needed. This chapter will discuss the various techniques and devices used in CPR.

To date no adjunct has consistently been shown to be superior to standard, conventional CPR for out-of-hospital basic life support (BLS), and no device other than a defibrillator has consistently improved long-term survival from out-of-hospital cardiac arrest.

CPR Techniques

High-Frequency Chest Compression

High-frequency chest compression, which is typically conducted at a frequency of more than 120/min, is a technique used to improve resuscitation from cardiac arrest.[1] Studies showed that a compression frequency of 120/min improved hemodynamics compared with conventional chest compressions[2,3]; however, no change in clinical outcome was reported. Therefore, the *2010 AHA Guidelines for CPR and ECC* recommend compressions at a rate of at least 100/min.

Open-Chest CPR

In open-chest CPR, compression of the heart is conducted through a thoracotomy, which is typically created through the fifth left intercostal space. Compression is performed with the thumb and fingers, or with the palm and extended fingers, against the sternum. The forward blood flow and coronary perfusion pressure generated by this technique exceed those generated by closed chest compressions. This technique improves coronary perfusion pressure and/or return of spontaneous circulation (ROSC) in both in-hospital[4] and out-of-hospital environments.[5] Cardiac arrest patients who were treated with open-chest CPR after blunt[6] or penetrating trauma[7,8] survived with mild or no neurological deficit. Open-chest CPR can be useful in the following circumstances:

- If cardiac arrest develops during surgery when the chest or abdomen is already open
- In the early postoperative period after cardiothoracic surgery
- In selected circumstances with penetrating trauma, if the transport time to a trauma facility is short[9]

Interposed Abdominal Compression-CPR

Interposed abdominal compression (IAC)-CPR is a 3-rescuer technique that includes conventional chest compressions combined with alternating abdominal compressions in addition to ventilation. In this technique, the abdomen is compressed midway between the xiphoid and the umbilicus during the relaxation phase of chest compression. Hand position, depth, rhythm, and rate of abdominal compressions are similar to those for chest compressions. The force required for abdominal compression is similar to that used to palpate the abdominal aorta. Generally, an endotracheal tube is placed before or shortly after initiation of IAC-CPR. The IAC-CPR technique increases diastolic aortic pressure and venous return, resulting in improved coronary perfusion pressure and blood flow to other vital organs. Results of clinical studies are conflicting.[10-12] Therefore, IAC-CPR may be considered during in-hospital resuscitation when a sufficient number of personnel trained in its use are available.

"Cough" CPR

"Cough" CPR is the use of forceful voluntary coughs every 1 to 3 seconds in conscious patients shortly after the onset of a witnessed nonperfusing cardiac rhythm in a controlled environment, such as the cardiac catheterization laboratory. Coughing increases the intrathoracic pressure, and it can increase systemic blood pressures to higher levels than those generated by conventional chest compressions.[13] Coughing can allow patients to maintain consciousness for a brief (up to 92 seconds) arrhythmic interval.[14] "Cough" CPR may be considered in settings such as the cardiac catheterization laboratory for a conscious, supine, and monitored patient if the patient can be instructed and coached to cough forcefully. However, not all victims are able to produce hemodynamically effective coughs.[15] Therefore, when used, "cough" CPR should not delay definitive treatment.

Prone CPR

When the patient cannot be placed in the supine position, rescuers may provide CPR with the patient in the prone position, particularly in hospitalized patients with an advanced airway in place.[16,17]

Precordial Thump

Precordial thump is a procedure performed by highly trained providers who strike a single, very carefully aimed blow with the fist to a specific place on the patient's sternum. Precordial thump converted ventricular tachyarrhythmias in several studies; however, other studies found precordial thump to be ineffective in more than 98% of cases of malignant ventricular arrhythmias.[18,19] Moreover, precordial thump was associated with complications in adults and children, such as sternal fracture, osteomyelitis, stroke, and the triggering of malignant arrhythmias.[20-22] Therefore, precordial thump should not be used for unwitnessed out-of-hospital cardiac arrest but may be considered for patients with witnessed, monitored, unstable ventricular tachycardia (VT) including pulseless VT, if a defibrillator is not immediately ready for use. Precordial thump should not delay CPR and shock delivery.[23]

Percussion Pacing

Percussion (eg, fist) pacing refers to the use of regular, rhythmic, and forceful percussion of the chest with the rescuer's fist in an attempt to pace the myocardium. There is insufficient evidence to recommend percussion pacing during typical attempted resuscitation from cardiac arrest.

CPR Devices

Automatic Transport Ventilators

Automatic transport ventilators (ATVs) are pneumatically powered and time- or pressure-cycled devices that are used during prolonged resuscitation efforts to provide ventilation and oxygenation similar to those delivered with a manual resuscitation bag while allowing the emergency medical services (EMS) team to perform other tasks. Some of the disadvantages of ATVs include the need for oxygen and a power source. Therefore, providers should always have a bag-mask device available as a manual ventilation backup. Detailed information regarding support of airway and ventilation in adults is discussed in Chapter 6.

Manually Triggered, Oxygen-Powered, Flow-Limited Resuscitators

Compared with bag-mask ventilation, anesthetized patients without an advanced airway (ie, endotracheal tube) have less gastric inflation when ventilated with manually triggered, oxygen-powered flow-limited resuscitators.[24] Rescuers should avoid using the automatic mode of the device during CPR because it may generate high positive end-expiratory pressure (PEEP) that may impede venous return during chest compressions and compromise forward blood flow.[25]

Devices to Support Circulation

Active Compression-Decompression CPR

Active compression-decompression CPR (ACD-CPR) is performed with a device that includes a suction cup to actively lift the anterior chest during decompression. The application of external negative suction during the decompression phase of CPR creates negative intrathoracic pressure, potentially enhancing the venous return to the heart. When used, the device is positioned at midsternum on the chest. Studies on the use of ACD-CPR have shown mixed results, with some studies reporting improved ROSC and short-term survival, including improvement in neurologically intact survival compared with conventional CPR.[26] In contrast, one Cochrane meta-analysis of 10 studies involving both in-hospital and out-of-hospital arrest showed no difference in ROSC or survival and did not report any increase in ACD-CPR–related complications.[27] This procedure may be considered for use when providers are adequately trained and monitored.

Phased Thoracic-Abdominal Compression-Decompression CPR With a Handheld Device

Phased thoracic-abdominal compression-decompression CPR (PTACD-CPR) combines the concepts of IAC-CPR and ACD-CPR. A handheld device alternates chest compression and abdominal decompression with chest decompression and abdominal compression. There are no data suggesting improvement in survival to hospital discharge with the use of PTACD-CPR during out-of-hospital cardiac arrest.

Impedance Threshold Device

The impedance threshold device (ITD) is a pressure-sensitive valve that is attached to an endotracheal tube, supraglottic airway, or face mask. The ITD limits air entry into the lungs during the decompression phase of CPR, creating negative intrathoracic pressure and improving venous return to the heart and cardiac output during CPR. ITD does so without impeding positive-pressure ventilation or passive exhalation. The ITD and ACD-CPR devices are thought to act synergistically to enhance venous return. Addition of ITD during ACD-CPR had no effect on survival in one randomized study,[28] whereas in another randomized study the addition of an ITD improved short-term survival (24-hour survival and survival to ICU admission).[29] The ITD is used also during conventional CPR with an endotracheal tube or with a face mask if a tight seal is maintained. One meta-analysis reported improved ROSC and short-term survival with the use of an ITD in the management of adult out-of-hospital cardiac arrest patients.[30] No significant improvement in either survival to hospital discharge or neurologically intact survival to discharge was reported.[30] The use of the ITD may be considered by trained personnel as a CPR adjunct in adult cardiac arrest.

Mechanical Piston Devices

A mechanical piston device consists of a compressed gas or electric-powered plunger mounted on a backboard, and the piston device depresses the sternum. Some devices incorporate a suction cup in the piston device. The use of a mechanical piston device for CPR has been shown to improve end-tidal CO_2 and mean arterial pressure during resuscitation from adult cardiac arrest. However, compared with manual CPR, no improvement in short- and long-term survival in adult patients was demonstrated.[31,32] Mechanical piston devices interrupt CPR during initiation and removal of the device.

The Lund University Cardiac Arrest System (LUCAS) is a gas- (oxygen or air) or electric-powered piston device that produces a consistent chest compression rate and depth. It incorporates a suction cup attached to the sternum that returns the sternum to the starting position. Use of LUCAS showed no benefit over conventional CPR for out-of-hospital witnessed cardiac arrest.[33] Mechanical piston devices may be considered for use by properly trained personnel in specific settings for the treatment of adult cardiac arrest in circumstances that make manual resuscitation difficult (eg, during diagnostic and interventional procedures). When used, rescuers should attempt to limit substantial interruptions in CPR during deployment. The device should be programmed to deliver high-quality CPR, ensuring an adequate compression depth of at least 2 inches (5 cm) (this may require conversion from a percent of chest depth), a rate of at least 100 compressions per minute, and compression duration of approximately 50% of the cycle length.

Load-Distributing Band CPR or Vest CPR

The load-distributing band (LDB) is a circumferential chest compression device composed of a pneumatically or electrically actuated constricting band and backboard. The LDB demonstrated improvement in hemodynamics, ROSC, and survival to hospital discharge in patients with cardiac arrest; however, the use of LDB-CPR was associated with lower odds of 30-day survival (odds ratio 0.4).[34] When compared with manual CPR, LDB-CPR for out-of-hospital cardiac arrest showed no improvement in 4-hour survival and a worse neurologic outcome.[35] These results raised concerns about possible harm with use of this device. The LDB may be considered for use by properly trained personnel in specific settings but not for the routine use in the treatment of cardiac arrest.

Extracorporeal Techniques and Invasive Perfusion Devices

Extracorporeal membrane oxygenation (ECMO) and cardiopulmonary bypass are different forms of extracorporeal CPR (ECPR; an alternative term may be extracorporeal life support or ECLS) when used for resuscitation for cardiac arrest. Both are sophisticated techniques for circulating blood outside the body with or without extracorporeal oxygenation, with the goal of supporting the body's circulation in the absence of an adequately functioning cardiac pump. The initiation of ECPR and the management of a patient on ECPR require highly trained personnel and specialized equipment. The use of ECPR for in-hospital[36,37] and out-of-hospital[38-40] cardiac arrest has been associated with improved survival when compared with conventional CPR in patients younger than 75 years of age with potentially correctable conditions. ECPR is safe and feasible when used in highly specialized centers.[40,41] ECPR may be considered when the time without blood flow is brief and the condition leading to the cardiac arrest is reversible (eg, accidental hypothermia or drug intoxication) or amenable to heart transplantation (eg, myocarditis) or revascularization (eg, acute myocardial infarction).

Cardiac Mechanical Assist Devices for Cardiogenic Shock

Intra-aortic Balloon Pump Counterpulsation

The most frequently used mechanical assist device for cardiogenic shock is the intra-aortic balloon pump (IABP). This device improves coronary and peripheral perfusion and augments left ventricular performance through balloon counterpulsation, which is timed to coincide with specific points in the cardiac cycle. A flexible catheter with 2 lumens is placed into the descending thoracic aorta via a femoral artery. One lumen allows for either distal aspiration and flushing or pressure monitoring. A second lumen permits the periodic delivery and removal of helium gas to a closed balloon near the end of the catheter. Phased inflation and deflation is synchronized to the patient's ECG. The balloon inflates during diastole just as the aortic valve closes, which increases blood pressure and flow upstream to the coronary arteries and brain and downstream to the vital organs and peripheral circulation. The balloon then quickly deflates during systole to decrease afterload and reduce the work of the left ventricle. The net result is a 10% to 20% increase in cardiac output, decreased heart rate, and improved perfusion usually.[42]

IABPs are commonly used for patients in cardiogenic shock before, during, and after cardiac procedures. In some cases they have been used as a bridge to transplant or to provide temporary assistance for an injured heart to recover. Absolute contraindications for use of an IABP include aortic insufficiency and irreversible cardiac disease. Aortic aneurysm and severe peripheral vascular disease are relative contraindications because these conditions increase the risk of the procedure and tachyarrhythmias interfere with the timing of the balloon counterpulsation. Although the outcome data on the use of IABPs are somewhat mixed, the 2013 ACCF/AHA Guideline for the Management of ST-Elevation Myocardial Infarction states that the use of IABP counterpulsation can be useful for patients with cardiogenic shock after STEMI who do not quickly stabilize with pharmacologic therapy.[43]

Ventricular Assist Devices

A percutaneous ventricular assist device (VAD) is a mechanical pump that assists the heart in pumping blood and is often used for short-term support following heart surgery or a myocardial infarction to allow the heart to recover. ECMO can be added with some devices to assist with oxygenation as well. Implantable VADs have been used for patients awaiting a heart transplant. These devices can now be considered for "destination therapy" (ie, permanent treatment) for patients who need long-term therapy and are not candidates for heart transplant. Implanted VADs typically use outflow cannulae from the left ventricle to the aorta with an implanted pump.

References

1. Ornato JP, Gonzalez ER, Garnett AR, Levine RL, McClung BK. Effect of cardiopulmonary resuscitation compression rate on end-tidal carbon dioxide concentration and arterial pressure in man. *Crit Care Med.* 1988;16:241-245.
2. Swenson RD, Weaver WD, Niskanen RA, Martin J, Dahlberg S. Hemodynamics in humans during conventional and experimental methods of cardiopulmonary resuscitation. *Circulation.* 1988;78:630-639.
3. Kern KB, Sanders AB, Raife J, Milander MM, Otto CW, Ewy GA. A study of chest compression rates during cardiopulmonary resuscitation in humans. The importance of rate-directed chest compressions. *Arch Intern Med.* 1992;152:145-149.
4. Anthi A, Tzelepis GE, Alivizatos P, Michalis A, Palatianos GM, Geroulanos S. Unexpected cardiac arrest after cardiac surgery: incidence, predisposing causes, and outcome of open chest cardiopulmonary resuscitation. *Chest.* 1998;113:15-19.
5. Hachimi-Idrissi S, Leeman J, Hubloue Y, Huyghens L, Corne L. Open chest cardiopulmonary resuscitation in out-of-hospital cardiac arrest. *Resuscitation.* 1997;35:151-156.
6. Fialka C, Sebok C, Kemetzhofer P, Kwasny O, Sterz F, Vecsei V. Open-chest cardiopulmonary resuscitation after cardiac arrest in cases of blunt chest or abdominal trauma: a consecutive series of 38 cases. *J Trauma.* 2004;57:809-814.
7. Sheppard FR, Cothren CC, Moore EE, Orfanakis A, Ciesla DJ, Johnson JL, Burch JM. Emergency department resuscitative thoracotomy for nontorso injuries. *Surgery.* 2006;139:574-576.
8. Seamon MJ, Fisher CA, Gaughan JP, Kulp H, Dempsey DT, Goldberg AJ. Emergency department thoracotomy: survival of the least expected. *World J Surg.* 2008;32:604-612.
9. Powell RW, Gill EA, Jurkovich GJ, Ramenofsky ML. Resuscitative thoracotomy in children and adolescents. *Am Surg.* 1988;54:188-191.
10. Sack JB, Kesselbrenner MB, Jarrad A. Interposed abdominal compression-cardiopulmonary resuscitation and resuscitation outcome during asystole and electromechanical dissociation. *Circulation.* 1992;86:1692-1700.
11. Mateer JR, Stueven HA, Thompson BM, Aprahamian C, Darin JC. Pre-hospital IAC-CPR versus standard CPR: paramedic resuscitation of cardiac arrests. *Am J Emerg Med.* 1985;3:143-146.
12. Waldman PJ, Walters BL, Grunau CF. Pancreatic injury associated with interposed abdominal compressions in pediatric cardiopulmonary resuscitation. *Am J Emerg Med.* 1984;2:510-512.
13. Keeble W, Tymchak WJ. Triggering of the Bezold Jarisch Reflex by reperfusion during primary PCI with maintenance of consciousness by cough CPR: a case report and review of pathophysiology. *J Invasive Cardiol.* 2008;20:E239-E242.
14. Niemann JT, Rosborough J, Hausknecht M, Brown D, Criley JM. Cough-CPR: documentation of systemic perfusion in man and in an experimental model: a "window" to the mechanism of blood flow in external CPR. *Crit Care Med.* 1980;8:141-146.

15. Criley JM, Blaufuss AH, Kissel GL. Cough-induced cardiac compression: self-administered from of cardiopulmonary resuscitation. *JAMA.* 1976;236:1246-1250.

16. Mazer SP, Weisfeldt M, Bai D, Cardinale C, Arora R, Ma C, Sciacca RR, Chong D, Rabbani LE. Reverse CPR: a pilot study of CPR in the prone position. *Resuscitation.* 2003;57:279-285.

17. Brown J, Rogers J, Soar J. Cardiac arrest during surgery and ventilation in the prone position: a case report and systematic review. *Resuscitation.* 2001;50:233-238.

18. Amir O, Schliamser JE, Nemer S, Arie M. Ineffectiveness of precordial thump for cardioversion of malignant ventricular tachyarrhythmias. *Pacing Clin Electrophysiol.* 2007;30:153-156.

19. Haman L, Parizek P, Vojacek J. Precordial thump efficacy in termination of induced ventricular arrhythmias. *Resuscitation.* 2009;80:14-16.

20. Ahmar W, Morley P, Marasco S, Chan W, Aggarwal A. Sternal fracture and osteomyelitis: an unusual complication of a precordial thump. *Resuscitation.* 2007;75:540-542.

21. Miller J, Tresch D, Horwitz L, Thompson BM, Aprahamian C, Darin JC. The precordial thump. *Ann Emerg Med.* 1984;13:791-794.

22. Muller GI, Ulmer HE, Bauer JA. Complications of chest thump for termination of supraventricular tachycardia in children. *Eur J Pediatr.* 1992;151:12-14.

23. Shuster M, Lim SH, Deakin CD, Kleinman ME, Koster RW, Morrison LJ, Nolan JP, Sayre MR. Part 7: CPR techniques and devices: 2010 International Consensus on Cardiopulmonary Resuscitation and Emergency Cardiovascular Care Science With Treatment Recommendations. *Circulation.* 2010;122:S338-S344.

24. Noordergraaf GJ, van Dun PJ, Kramer BP, Schors MP, Hornman HP, de Jong W, Noordergraaf A. Can first responders achieve and maintain normocapnia when sequentially ventilating with a bag-valve device and two oxygen-driven resuscitators? A controlled clinical trial in 104 patients. *Eur J Anaesthesiol.* 2004;21:367-372.

25. Hevesi ZG, Thrush DN, Downs JB, Smith RA. Cardiopulmonary resuscitation: effect of CPAP on gas exchange during chest compressions. *Anesthesiology.* 1999;90:1078-1083.

26. Plaisance P, Lurie KG, Vicaut E, Adnet F, Petit JL, Epain D, Ecollan P, Gruat R, Cavagna P, Biens J, Payen D. A comparison of standard cardiopulmonary resuscitation and active compression-decompression resuscitation for out-of-hospital cardiac arrest. French Active Compression-Decompression Cardiopulmonary Resuscitation Study Group. *N Engl J Med.* 1999;341:569-575.

27. Lafuente-Lafuente C, Melero-Bascones M. Active chest compression-decompression for cardiopulmonary resuscitation. *Cochrane Database Syst Rev.* 2004:CD002751.

28. Plaisance P, Lurie KG, Payen D. Inspiratory impedance during active compression-decompression cardiopulmonary resuscitation: a randomized evaluation in patients in cardiac arrest. *Circulation.* 2000;101:989-994.

29. Plaisance P, Lurie KG, Vicaut E, Martin D, Gueugniaud PY, Petit JL, Payen D. Evaluation of an impedance threshold device in patients receiving active compression-decompression cardiopulmonary resuscitation for out of hospital cardiac arrest. *Resuscitation.* 2004;61:265-271.

30. Cabrini L, Beccaria P, Landoni G, Biondi-Zoccai GG, Sheiban I, Cristofolini M, Fochi O, Maj G, Zangrillo A. Impact of impedance threshold devices on cardiopulmonary resuscitation: a systematic review and meta-analysis of randomized controlled studies. *Crit Care Med.* 2008;36:1625-1632.

31. Dickinson ET, Verdile VP, Schneider RM, Salluzzo RF. Effectiveness of mechanical versus manual chest compressions in out-of-hospital cardiac arrest resuscitation: a pilot study. *Am J Emerg Med.* 1998;16:289-292.

32. Wang HC, Chiang WC, Chen SY, Ke YL, Chi CL, Yang CW, Lin PC, Ko PC, Wang YC, Tsai TC, Huang CH, Hsiung KH, Ma MH, Chen SC, Chen WJ, Lin FY. Video-recording and time-motion analyses of manual versus mechanical cardiopulmonary resuscitation during ambulance transport. *Resuscitation.* 2007;74:453-460.

33. Axelsson C, Nestin J, Svensson L, Axelsson AB, Herlitz J. Clinical consequences of the introduction of mechanical chest compression in the EMS system for treatment of out-of-hospital cardiac arrest-a pilot study. *Resuscitation.* 2006;71:47-55.

34. Steinmetz J, Barnung S, Nielsen SL, Risom M, Rasmussen LS. Improved survival after an out-of-hospital cardiac arrest using new guidelines. *Acta Anaesthesiol Scand.* 2008;52:908-913.

35. Hallstrom A, Rea TD, Sayre MR, Christenson J, Anton AR, Mosesso VN Jr, Van Ottingham L, Olsufka M, Pennington S, White LJ, Yahn S, Husar J, Morris MF, Cobb LA. Manual chest compression vs use of an automated chest compression device during resuscitation following out-of-hospital cardiac arrest: a randomized trial. *JAMA.* 2006;295:2620-2628.

36. Chen YS, Lin JW, Yu HY, Ko WJ, Jerng JS, Chang WT, Chen WJ, Huang SC, Chi NH, Wang CH, Chen LC, Tsai PR, Wang SS, Hwang JJ, Lin FY. Cardiopulmonary resuscitation with assisted extracorporeal life-support versus conventional cardiopulmonary resuscitation in adults with in-hospital cardiac arrest: an observational study and propensity analysis. *Lancet.* 2008;372:554-561.

37. Athanasuleas CL, Buckberg GD, Allen BS, Beyersdorf F, Kirsh MM. Sudden cardiac death: directing the scope of resuscitation towards the heart and brain. *Resuscitation.* 2006;70:44-51.

38. Tanno K, Itoh Y, Takeyama Y, Nara S, Mori K, Asai Y. Utstein style study of cardiopulmonary bypass after cardiac arrest. *Am J Emerg Med.* 2008;26:649-654.

39. Krarup NH, Terkelsen CJ, Johnsen SP, Clemmensen P, Olivecrona GK, Hansen TM, Trautner S, Lassen JF. Quality of cardiopulmonary resuscitation in out-of-hospital cardiac arrest is hampered by interruptions in chest compressions—a nationwide prospective feasibility study. *Resuscitation.* 2011;82:263-269.

40. Nagao K, Kikushima K, Watanabe K, Tachibana E, Tominaga Y, Tada K, Ishii M, Chiba N, Kasai A, Soga T, Matsuzaki M, Nishikawa K, Tateda Y, Ikeda H, Yagi T. Early induction of hypothermia during cardiac arrest improves neurological outcomes in patients with out-of-hospital cardiac arrest who undergo emergency cardiopulmonary bypass and percutaneous coronary intervention. *Circ J.* 2010;74:77-85.

41. Chen YS, Yu HY, Huang SC, Lin JW, Chi NH, Wang CH, Wang SS, Lin FY, Ko WJ. Extracorporeal membrane oxygenation support can extend the duration of cardiopulmonary resuscitation. *Crit Care Med.* 2008;36:2529-2535.

42. Kar B, Basra SS, Shah NR, Loyalka P. Percutaneous circulatory support in cardiogenic shock: interventional bridge to recovery. *Circulation.* 2012;125:1809-1817.

43. O'Gara PT, Kushner FG, Ascheim DD, Casey DE Jr, Chung MK, de Lemos JA, Ettinger SM, Fang JC, Fesmire FM, Franklin BA, Granger CB, Krumholz HM, Linderbaum JA, Morrow DA, Newby LK, Ornato JP, Ou N, Radford MJ, Tamis-Holland JE, Tommaso CL, Tracy CM, Woo YJ, Zhao DX. 2013 ACCF/AHA guideline for the management of ST-elevation myocardial infarction: a report of the American College of Cardiology Foundation/American Heart Association Task Force on Practice Guidelines [published online ahead of print December 17, 2012]. *Circulation.* 2013. doi:10.1161/CIR.0b013e3182742cf6.

Chapter 6

Airway Management

This Chapter

- Oxygenation and Ventilation
- Basic Airway Adjuncts: Oropharyngeal and Nasopharyngeal Airways
- Pulse Oximetry and Waveform Capnography
- Advanced Airways
- Airway Management in Patients With Severe Trauma

Overview

A major emphasis of the *2010 AHA Guidelines for Cardiopulmonary Resuscitation and Emergency Cardiovascular Care* is high-quality chest compressions with minimal interruption. There has been a decreased emphasis on early advanced airway insertion and increased emphasis on consideration of the risk-benefit ratio for the interruption of chest compressions to place an advanced airway. Such risks are affected by the condition of the patient and the provider's expertise in airway control. Because insertion of an advanced airway may require interruption of chest compressions for many seconds, the need for uninterrupted compressions is weighed against the need for insertion of an advanced airway. Providers may defer insertion of an advanced airway until the patient fails to respond to initial cardiopulmonary resuscitation (CPR) and defibrillation attempts or demonstrates return of spontaneous circulation (ROSC).

Oxygenation and Ventilation

Oxygen administration is often necessary for patients with acute cardiac disease, respiratory distress, or stroke. Supplementary oxygen administration, ideally, should be titrated to the lowest concentration required to maintain Spo_2 at 94% or higher. Various devices can deliver supplementary oxygen from 21% to 100% (Table 6). This section describes 4 devices used to provide supplementary oxygen:

- Nasal cannula
- Simple oxygen face mask
- Venturi mask
- Face mask with O_2 reservoir

Whenever you care for a patient receiving supplementary oxygen, quickly verify the proper function of the oxygen delivery system in use. *Oxygen supply* refers to an oxygen cylinder or wall unit that connects to an administration device to deliver oxygen to the patient. When the patient is receiving oxygen from one of these systems, be sure to check the following equipment:

- Oxygen administration device
- Valve handles to open the cylinder
- Pressure gauge
- Flow meter
- Tubing connecting the oxygen supply to the patient's oxygen administration device

Trained ACLS providers should be sure they are familiar with all emergency equipment before an emergency arises.

Healthcare providers should administer *oxygen* if the patient is dyspneic, hypoxemic, has obvious signs of heart failure, has an arterial oxygen saturation less than 94%, or if the oxygen saturation is unknown. Providers should titrate

Table 6. Delivery of Supplementary Oxygen: Flow Rates and Percentage of Oxygen Delivered

Device	Flow Rates (L/min)	Delivered O_2 (%)*
Nasal cannula	1 2 3 4 5 6	21 to 24 25 to 28 29 to 32 33 to 36 37 to 40 41 to 44
Simple oxygen face mask	6 to 10	35 to 60
Venturi mask	4 to 8 10 to 12	24 to 40 40 to 50
Face mask with oxygen reservoir (nonrebreathing mask)	6 7 8 9 10 to 15	60 70 80 90 95 to 100

*Percentages are approximate.

therapy to achieve an oxyhemoglobin saturation of 94% or higher based on noninvasive monitoring of oxyhemoglobin saturation.

During CPR the purpose of ventilation is to maintain adequate oxygenation, but the optimal tidal volume, respiratory rate, and inspired oxygen concentration to achieve this are unknown. During the first minutes of sudden cardiac arrest due to ventricular fibrillation (VF), the oxygen level in the blood remains high. To improve oxygenation, healthcare providers may give 100% inspired oxygen (FIO_2 = 1.0) during basic life support, and give advanced cardiovascular life support as soon as it becomes available. High inspired-oxygen tension will tend to maximize arterial oxygen saturation and, in turn, arterial oxygen content. This will help support oxygen delivery (cardiac output × arterial oxygen content) when cardiac output is limited. There is insufficient evidence to indicate that short-term oxygen therapy produces oxygen toxicity.

Clues to Suspect Airway Obstruction

Significant partial upper airway obstruction typically causes noisy airflow during inspiration (stridor or "crowing") and cyanosis (late sign). Another sign of airway obstruction is use of accessory muscles, indicated by retractions of the suprasternal, supraclavicular, and intercostal spaces. If the patient is not making spontaneous breathing efforts, airway obstruction becomes more difficult to recognize. Occasionally, isolated bradycardia, secondary to occult hypoxemia, provides an early sign of airway obstruction. Figure 15 demonstrates the anatomy of the airway. The most common cause of upper airway obstruction in the unconscious/unresponsive patient is loss of tone in the throat muscles. In this case, the tongue falls back and occludes the airway at the level of the pharynx (Figure 16A). Basic airway-opening techniques will effectively relieve airway obstruction caused either by the tongue or from relaxation of muscles in the upper airway. The basic airway-opening technique is head tilt with anterior displacement of the mandible, ie, head tilt–chin lift (Figure 16B). In the trauma patient with suspected neck injury, use jaw thrust without head extension (Figure 16C). Because maintaining an open airway and providing ventilation are a priority, use a head tilt–chin lift maneuver if the jaw thrust does not open the airway. ACLS providers should be aware that BLS training courses no longer teach the jaw thrust technique to lay rescuers. Proper airway positioning may be all that is required for patients who can breathe spontaneously. In patients who are unconscious with no cough or gag reflex, insert an oropharyngeal (OPA) or nasopharyngeal airway (NPA) to maintain airway patency.

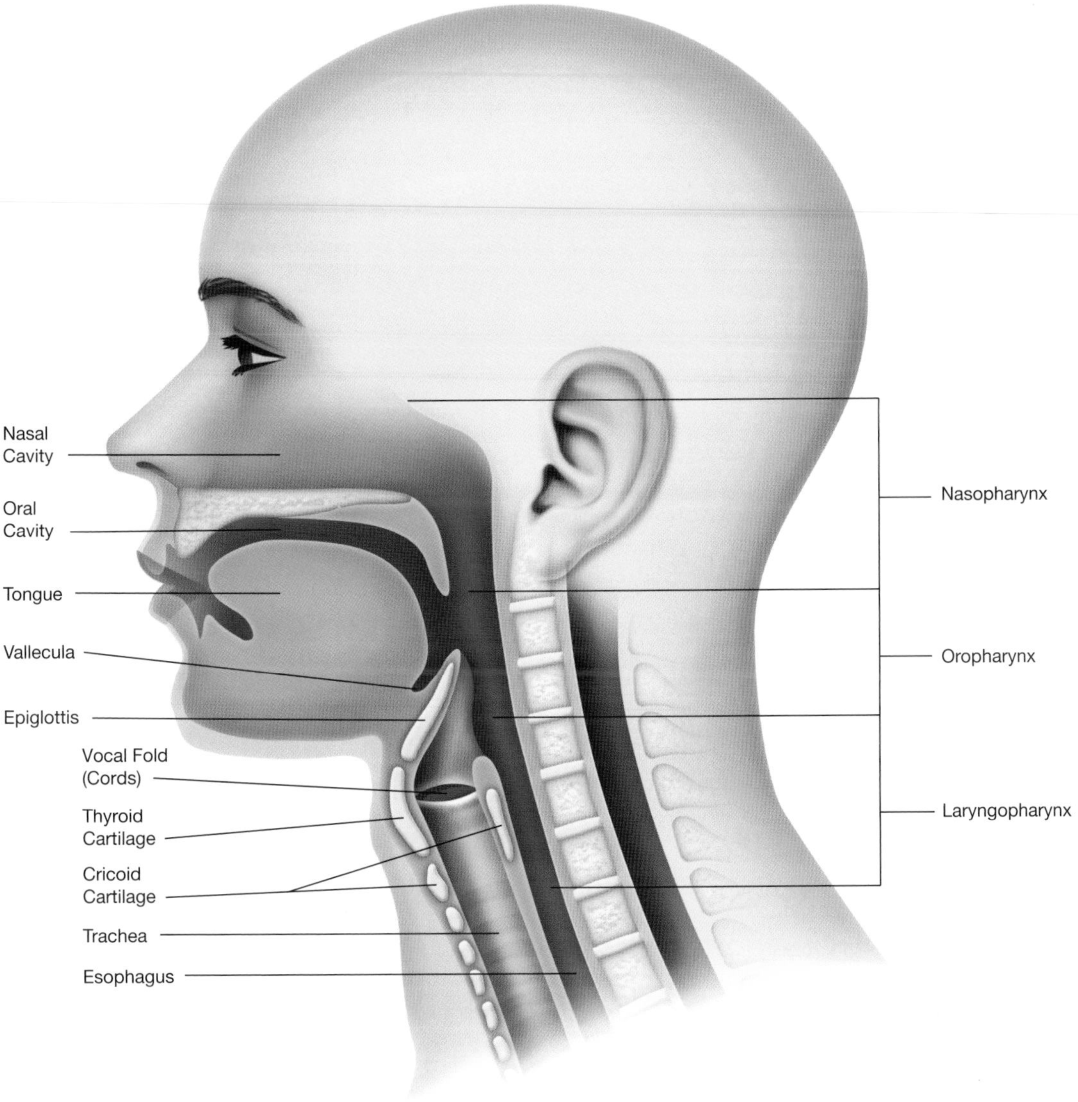

Nasal Cavity
Oral Cavity
Tongue
Vallecula
Epiglottis
Vocal Fold (Cords)
Thyroid Cartilage
Cricoid Cartilage
Trachea
Esophagus
Nasopharynx
Oropharynx
Laryngopharynx

Figure 15. Anatomy of the airway.

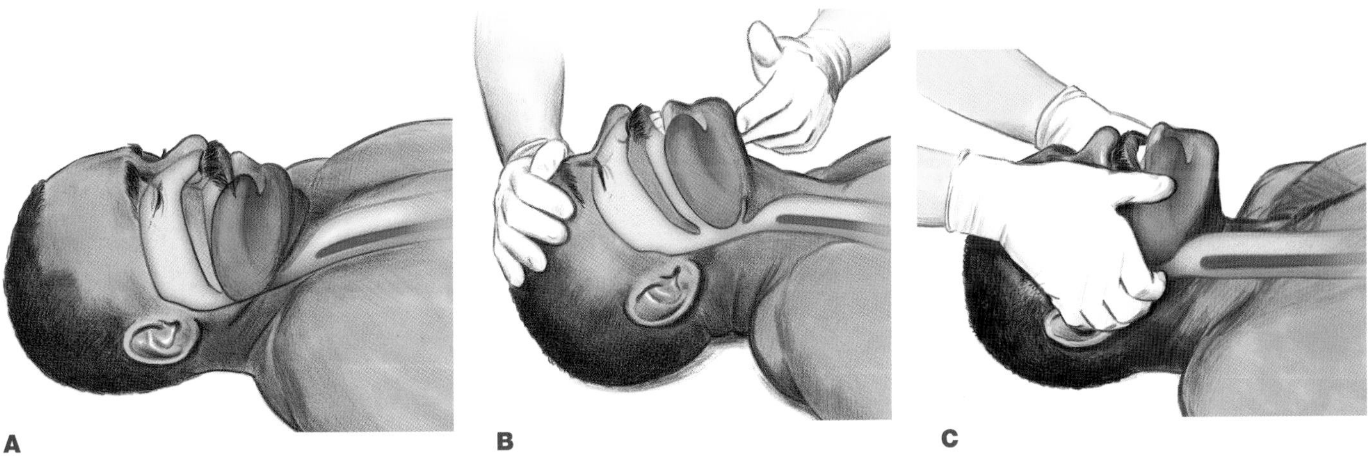

Figure 16. Obstruction of the airway by the tongue and epiglottis. When a patient is unresponsive, the tongue can obstruct the airway. The head tilt–chin lift relieves obstruction in the unresponsive patient. **A,** The tongue is obstructing the airway. **B,** The head tilt–chin lift maneuver lifts the tongue, relieving the obstruction. **C,** If healthcare providers suspect cervical spine trauma, use the jaw thrust without head extension.

Basic Airway Adjuncts: Oropharyngeal and Nasopharyngeal Airways

Oropharyngeal Airway

The OPA is used in patients who are at risk for developing airway obstruction from the tongue or from relaxed upper airway muscles. This J-shaped device (Figure 17) fits over the tongue to hold it and the soft hypopharyngeal structures away from the posterior wall of the pharynx.

The OPA is used in *unconscious* patients if procedures to open the airway (eg, head tilt–chin lift or jaw thrust) fail to provide and maintain a clear, unobstructed airway. *An OPA should not be used in a conscious or semiconscious patient* because it may stimulate gagging and vomiting. The key assessment is to check whether the patient has an intact cough and gag reflex. If so, do not use an OPA.

The OPA may be used to keep the airway open during bag-mask ventilation when providers might unknowingly push down on the chin, blocking the airway. The OPA is also used during suctioning of the mouth and throat and in intubated patients to prevent them from biting and occluding the endotracheal (ET) tube. After insertion of an OPA, monitor the patient. Keep the head and jaw positioned properly to maintain a patent airway. Suction the airway as needed.

Technique

1. Use a rigid pharyngeal suction tip (Yankauer) to clear the mouth and pharynx of secretions, blood, or vomitus.
2. Turn the airway so that it enters the mouth either inverted or on its side.
3. As the airway transverses the oral cavity and approaches the posterior wall of the pharynx, rotate the airway into proper position (Figure 17).
4. Alternatively, use a tongue depressor to move the tongue downward before inserting the airway. Be careful not to obstruct the airway by pushing the tongue back into the throat.

Complications

Successful use of the oropharyngeal airway without complications requires adequate initial training, frequent practice, and timely retraining.

- If the OPA is too long, it may press the epiglottis against the laryngeal entry, where it can cause complete airway obstruction.
- If the OPA is inserted incorrectly or is too small, it may push the tongue posteriorly into the hypopharynx, thereby aggravating upper airway obstruction.

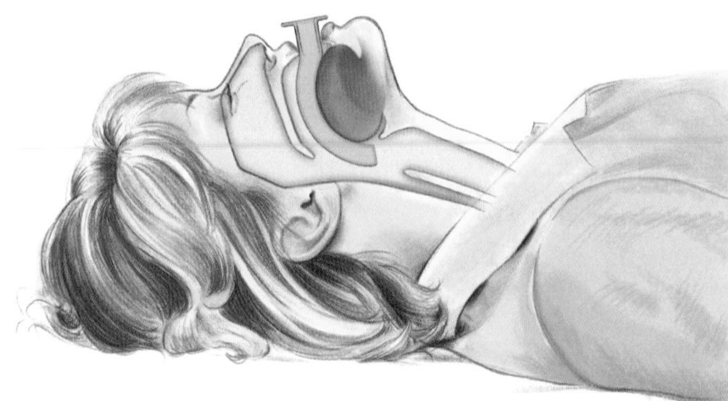

Figure 17. Oropharyngeal airway device inserted.

- The patient's lips and tongue can be lacerated if they are caught between the teeth and the oral airway.
- Attempts to insert the airway in a patient with intact cough and gag reflexes may stimulate vomiting and laryngospasm.

Nasopharyngeal Airway

The NPA is used as an alternative to an OPA in patients who need a basic airway management adjunct. The NPA is a soft rubber or plastic uncuffed tube (Figure 18) that provides a conduit for airflow between the nares and the pharynx.

Unlike oral airways, NPAs may be used in conscious or semiconscious patients (patients with an intact cough and gag reflex). The NPA is indicated when insertion of an OPA is technically difficult or dangerous. Examples include patients with a gag reflex, trismus, massive trauma around the mouth, or wiring of the jaws. The NPA may also be used in patients who are neurologically impaired with poor pharyngeal tone or coordination leading to upper airway obstruction.

Insertion Technique

1. Lubricate the appropriate size airway with a water-soluble lubricant or anesthetic jelly.
2. Gently insert the airway close to the midline, along the floor of the nostril, into the posterior pharynx behind the tongue.
3. If you encounter resistance, slightly rotate the tube to facilitate insertion at the angle of the nasal passage and nasopharynx.
4. Maintain head tilt; maintain anterior mandible displacement by chin lift or, if necessary, jaw thrust (without head extension if cervical spine injury is possible).

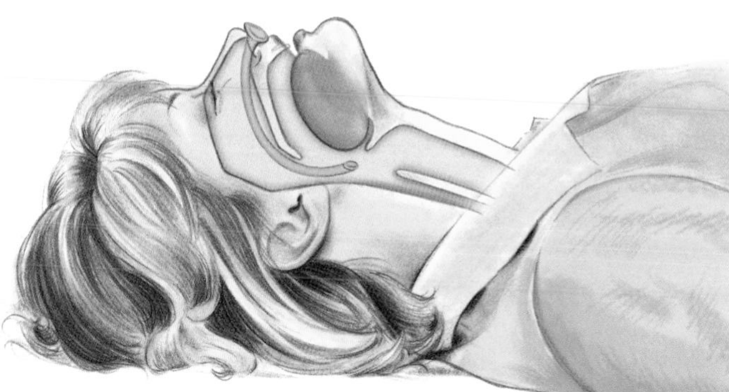

Figure 18. Nasopharyngeal airway device inserted.

Reevaluate frequently. Maintain head tilt by providing anterior displacement of the mandible using chin lift or jaw thrust. Mucus, blood, vomit, or the soft tissues of the pharynx can obstruct the NPA, which has a small internal diameter. Frequent evaluation and suctioning of the airway may be necessary to ensure patency.

Complications

Successful use of the nasopharyngeal airway without complications requires adequate initial training, frequent practice, and timely retraining.

- If the nasopharyngeal tube is *too long,* the tube may injure the epiglottis or vocal cords or may cause bradycardia through vagal stimulation. If assisted ventilation is required, the tube will facilitate air entry into the esophagus, causing gastric inflation and possible hypoventilation.
- If the patient has an intact cough and gag reflex, tube insertion may provoke laryngospasm and vomiting.
- Insertion of the tube may injure the nasal mucosa, causing bleeding. Aspiration of a clot into the trachea is possible.
- Insertion of a nasopharyngeal tube stimulates excessive secretions that may require suctioning.
- If adequate spontaneous respirations do not resume after 15 to 30 seconds, the tube may be malpositioned or obstructed. If this occurs, remove the tube and reattempt proper placement.
- If the patient has occult basilar skull fractures or previous maxillofacial surgery, insertion of a nasopharyngeal tube is contraindicated because a tear in the dura may enable the tube to enter the brain.

Suctioning

Suctioning is an essential component of maintaining a patient's airway. Providers should suction the airway immediately if there are copious secretions, blood, or vomit. Suction devices consist of both portable and wall-mounted units.

- Portable suction devices are easy to transport but may not provide adequate suction power. A suction force of −80 to −120 mm Hg is generally necessary.
- Wall-mounted suction units should be capable of providing an airflow of more than 40 L/min at the end of the delivery tube and a vacuum of more than −300 mm Hg when the tube is clamped at full suction.
- Adjust the amount of suction force for use in children and intubated patients.

Both soft flexible and rigid suctioning catheters are available:

- *Soft flexible catheters* may be used in the mouth or nose. Soft flexible catheters are available in sterile wrappers and can also be used for deep suctioning of an ET tube.
- *Rigid catheters* (eg, Yankauer) are used to suction the oropharynx. These are better for suctioning thick secretions and particulate matter.

Catheter Type	Use For
Soft	• Aspirating thin secretions from the oropharynx and nasopharynx • Performing intratracheal suctioning • Suctioning through an in-place airway (ie, NPA) to access the back of the pharynx in a patient with clenched teeth
Rigid	• More effective suctioning of the oropharynx, particularly if there is thick particulate matter

Critical Concept

Precautions While Suctioning

- Monitor the patient's heart rate, pulse, oxygen saturation, and clinical appearance during suctioning.
- If bradycardia develops, oxygen saturation drops, or clinical appearance deteriorates, interrupt suctioning at once. Administer high-flow oxygen until the heart rate returns to normal and the clinical condition improves. Assist ventilation as needed.

Bag-Mask Ventilation

Bag-Mask Device

The bag-mask device typically consists of a self-inflating bag and a nonrebreathing valve; it may be used with a face mask or an advanced airway (Figure 19). Masks are made of transparent material to allow detection of regurgitation. They should be capable of creating a tight seal on the face, covering both mouth and nose. Bag-masks are available in adult and pediatric sizes. These devices are used to deliver high concentrations of oxygen by positive pressure to a patient who is not breathing. Some devices have a port to add positive end-expiratory pressure (PEEP).

Bag-mask ventilation is a challenging skill that requires considerable practice for competency. Bag-mask ventilation is not the recommended method of ventilation for a lone rescuer during CPR. It is easier for 2 trained and experienced rescuers to provide. One rescuer opens the airway and seals the mask to the face while the other squeezes the bag, with both rescuers watching for visible chest rise. Healthcare providers can provide bag-mask ventilation with room air or oxygen if they use a self-inflating bag. This device provides positive-pressure ventilation when used without an advanced airway and, therefore, may produce gastric inflation and its consequent complications.

- Insert an OPA as soon as possible if the patient has no cough or gag reflex to help maintain the airway.
- Use an adult (1- to 2-L) bag to deliver approximately 600 mL tidal volume for adult patients. This amount is usually sufficient to produce visible chest rise and maintain oxygenation and normal carbon dioxide levels in apneic patients.
- To create a leakproof mask seal, perform and maintain a head tilt, and then use the thumb and index finger to make a "C," pressing the edges of the mask to the face. Next use the remaining fingers to lift the angle of the jaw and open the airway (Figure 19A).
- To create an effective mask seal, the hand holding the mask must perform multiple tasks simultaneously: maintaining the head-tilt position, pressing the mask against the face, and lifting the jaw.
- Two well-trained, experienced healthcare providers are preferred during bag-mask ventilation (Figure 19B).

The seal and volume problems do not occur when the bag-mask device is attached to the end of an advanced airway device (eg, laryngeal mask airway, laryngeal tube, esophageal-tracheal tube, or ET tube).

Precaution

Bag-mask ventilation can produce gastric inflation with complications, including regurgitation, aspiration, and pneumonia. Gastric inflation can elevate the diaphragm, restrict lung movement, and decrease respiratory system compliance.

A

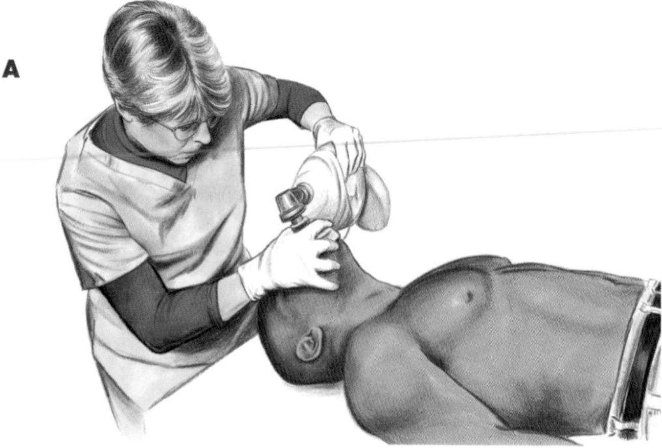

B

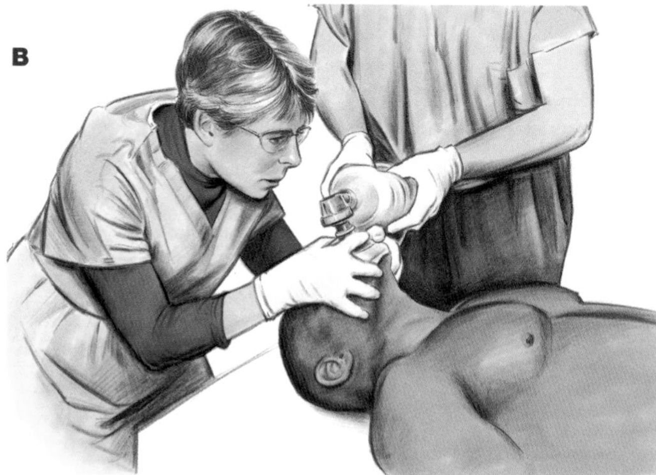

Figure 19. **A,** E-C clamp technique of holding mask while lifting the jaw. Position yourself at the patient's head. Circle the thumb and first finger around the top of the mask (forming a "C") while using the third, fourth, and fifth fingers (forming an "E") to lift the jaw. **B,** Two-rescuer use of the bag-mask. The rescuer at the patient's head tilts the patient's head and seals the mask against the patient's face with the thumb and first finger of each hand creating a "C" to provide a complete seal around the edges of the mask. The rescuer uses the remaining 3 fingers (the "E") to lift the jaw (this holds the airway open). The second rescuer slowly squeezes the bag (over 1 second) until the chest rises. Both rescuers should observe chest rise.

Assessing Ventilation and Oxygenation

Providers must be able to accurately assess *oxygenation* and *ventilation* to detect and treat respiratory distress and failure. The 2 major functions of respiration are to achieve

- Oxygenation (oxygenate arterial blood):
  - Evaluate oxygenation with pulse oximetry.
- Ventilation (remove carbon dioxide from venous blood):
  - Evaluate ventilation with capnography (can use capnometry if capnography is not available).

Oximetry—Basic Principles

To understand the clinical utility of oximetry—as well as its limitations and pitfalls—one must understand the physics involved in measurement and the clinical principles of adequate tissue oxygenation. Here too, "treat the patient and not the number" is most important.

Basic Physics of Pulse Oximetry

The concentration of a substance in a fluid can be determined by its ability to transmit light. Oxygenated hemoglobin absorbs and reflects red and infrared light differently than nonoxygenated hemoglobin. Oxygenated hemoglobin in a pulsatile tissue bed primarily absorbs *infrared* light; reduced (nonoxygenated) hemoglobin in a pulsatile tissue bed primarily absorbs *red* light. In pulse oximetry red and infrared light are passed through a pulsatile tissue bed, and a photodetector captures any nonabsorbed light on the other side of the tissue bed. A microprocessor calculates the relative absorption of red and infrared light that occurred as it passed through the tissue bed and can determine the percentage of oxygenated and nonoxygenated hemoglobin present in that tissue bed. In this way pulse oximeters calculate the *percent of hemoglobin that is saturated with oxygen (percent saturation, Spo_2).* In the absence of abnormal hemoglobins, such as carboxyhemoglobin or methemoglobin, if the arterial oxygen saturation is greater than 70%, there should be no more than 3% variance between pulse oximetry and the arterial oxyhemoglobin saturation measured by co-oximeter used in arterial blood gas determinations. Studies have shown pulse oximetry to be an accurate and useful guide for patient care in the in-hospital setting as well as in the prehospital EMS setting,[1-4] including transport by rotary-wing aircraft.[5] The presence of a plethysmograph waveform on pulse oximetry is potentially valuable in detecting ROSC, and pulse oximetry is useful to ensure appropriate oxygenation after ROSC.

Hemoglobin and Tissue Oxygen Delivery

Analysis of arterial blood is an invasive procedure, and arterial blood gases are infrequently ordered, available, or clinically useful during cardiac arrest. *Pulse oximetry* was developed to provide a noninvasive, painless approximation of the percent of hemoglobin saturated with oxygen (percent Sao_2). During cardiac arrest, pulse oximetry will not function (and should not be measured) because pulsatile blood flow is inadequate for measurement in peripheral tissue beds. But pulse oximetry is commonly used for monitoring patients who are not in arrest because it provides a simple, continuous method of tracking oxyhemoglobin saturation. There are 3 major determinants of adequate tissue oxygenation:

- Adequate amount of oxygen to saturate the hemoglobin molecules
- Enough hemoglobin to carry adequate oxygen
- Cardiac output sufficient to deliver the saturated hemoglobin to peripheral tissues

Arterial oxygen content is determined by the hemoglobin concentration and its saturation with oxygen. Normal pulse oximetry saturation, however, does not ensure adequate systemic *oxygen delivery* because it does not calculate the total oxygen content (O_2 bound to hemoglobin + dissolved O_2) *and* adequacy of blood flow (cardiac output).

Normal oxygen content is 18 to 20 mL/dL of blood.

Measurement of the arterial oxygen content of blood is only part of the determination of effective oxygenation. The oxygen present needs to be delivered to the tissues for use. Peripheral cells need to be able to uptake and use oxygen for cellular metabolism. Oxygen delivery is defined by how much oxygen is present and how much of it is delivered to the body. It is defined by the second equation below.

Pulse Oximetry Precautions and Limitations

Pulse oximetry readings, even those that appear to be accurate, do not always correlate with cardiac output and oxygen delivery. When clinically evaluating a patient's cardiac output and oxygen delivery, always assess systemic perfusion and be aware of the hemoglobin concentration. If cardiac output or hemoglobin concentration is low, oxygen delivery can be inadequate even if oxyhemoglobin saturation is normal.

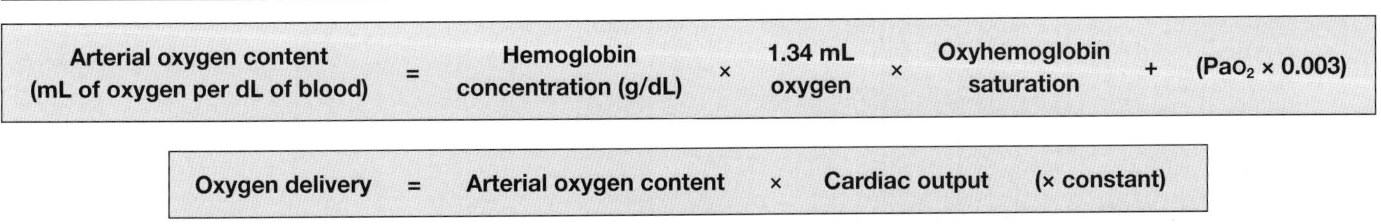

Arterial oxygen content (mL of oxygen per dL of blood) = Hemoglobin concentration (g/dL) × 1.34 mL oxygen × Oxyhemoglobin saturation + (PaO2 × 0.003)
Oxygen delivery = Arterial oxygen content × Cardiac output (× constant)

Abnormal Hemoglobins (eg, Carbon Monoxide Poisoning)

The light absorption of carboxyhemoglobin (carbon monoxide) and of methemoglobin (cyanide) differs from that of normal hemoglobin, so carboxyhemoglobin and methemoglobin are *not* recognized by pulse oximeters. If these altered forms of hemoglobin are present, the Spo_2 calculated by the pulse oximeters will be falsely high because most pulse oximeters calculate the percent of *normal* hemoglobin that is saturated with oxygen rather than the percent of *total* hemoglobin that is saturated with oxygen. When you suspect the presence of carbon monoxide poisoning or methemoglobin toxicity, you should measure the oxyhemoglobin saturation with a co-oximeter (this requires arterial blood sampling). Most of the newer generation field monitor/defibrillators are equipped with co-oximeters.

Abnormal Conditions Affecting Pulse Oximetry

In several clinical situations abnormal or inaccurate oximetry readings may occur. Major sources of error are finger thickness, hemoglobin level, skin color, and peripheral temperature.[6,7]

- Motion artifact and low perfusion are the most common sources of Spo_2 inaccuracies. Motion artifacts can occur with patient transport, movement, twitching, and agitation.
- When the systolic blood pressure is low, oximetry becomes inaccurate because of decreased pulsatile flow, response time, or calibration characteristics of the instrument.
- Oximetry may read falsely high when the Sao_2 is less than 70% or may become inaccurate when the hemoglobin level is very low (2 to 3 g/dL).
- Peripheral hypoperfusion from hypothermia, low cardiac output, or vasoconstrictive drugs may cause or increase inaccuracies.
- Very dark skin, fingernail polish, and fungal infections of the nails (onychomycosis) may cause spuriously low readings when digital monitors are used.

Safety Considerations

Some safety precautions regarding use of the pulse oximetry equipment are

- Do not use oximetry probes with broken or cracked casings. Burns have been reported when the lights from the probes came into direct contact with the skin.
- Do not connect the probes from one manufacturer to base units made by another manufacturer.

Waveform Capnography

End-tidal CO_2 is the concentration of carbon dioxide in exhaled air at the end of expiration. It is typically expressed as a partial pressure in millimeters of mercury (P_{ETCO_2}). Waveform capnography directly measures end-tidal CO_2. Because CO_2 is a trace gas in atmospheric air, waveform capnography also indirectly measures the production of CO_2 by the body and delivery of CO_2 to the lungs by the circulatory system. Cardiac output is the major determinant of CO_2 delivery to the lungs. If ventilation is relatively constant, P_{ETCO_2} correlates well with cardiac output during CPR. Providers should observe a persistent capnographic waveform with ventilation to confirm and monitor ET tube placement in the field (Figure 20), in the transport vehicle, on arrival at the hospital, and after any patient transfer to reduce the risk of unrecognized tube misplacement or displacement. Continuous waveform capnography is recommended in addition to clinical assessment as the most reliable method of confirming and monitoring correct placement of an ET tube (Class I, LOE A).

Although capnography to confirm and monitor correct placement of supraglottic airways (eg, laryngeal mask airway, laryngeal tube, esophageal-tracheal tube) has not been studied, effective ventilation through a supraglottic airway device should result in a capnography waveform during CPR and after ROSC.

Some *capnography devices* are infrared devices in which a light-emitting diode is used to measure the intensity of light transmitted across a short distance, usually the diameter of an ET tube. The measured light absorption varies inversely with the concentration of CO_2 passing through the ET tube. When attached to the end of an ET tube, these infrared devices are called *mainstream capnometers*. These devices readily reveal low exhaled CO_2 indicative of esophageal intubation, and they can provide estimates of the adequacy of ventilation and the effectiveness of circulation during CPR.

Capnography devices provide a continuous readout of the concentration of exhaled CO_2. They are used to monitor the quality of ventilation in nonarrest patients. Because of their high degree of sensitivity to expired CO_2, however, capnographs can often detect a sufficient quantity of CO_2 to indicate the presence of a tracheal tube in the trachea even when cardiac arrest is present. Continuous capnography monitoring devices can identify and signal a fall in exhaled CO_2 consistent with tracheal tube dislodgment. This may be very helpful in emergencies.

Critical Concept **Waveform Capnography**	In addition to monitoring ET tube position, quantitative waveform capnography allows healthcare personnel to monitor CPR quality, optimize chest compressions, and detect ROSC during chest compressions or when a rhythm check reveals an organized rhythm.

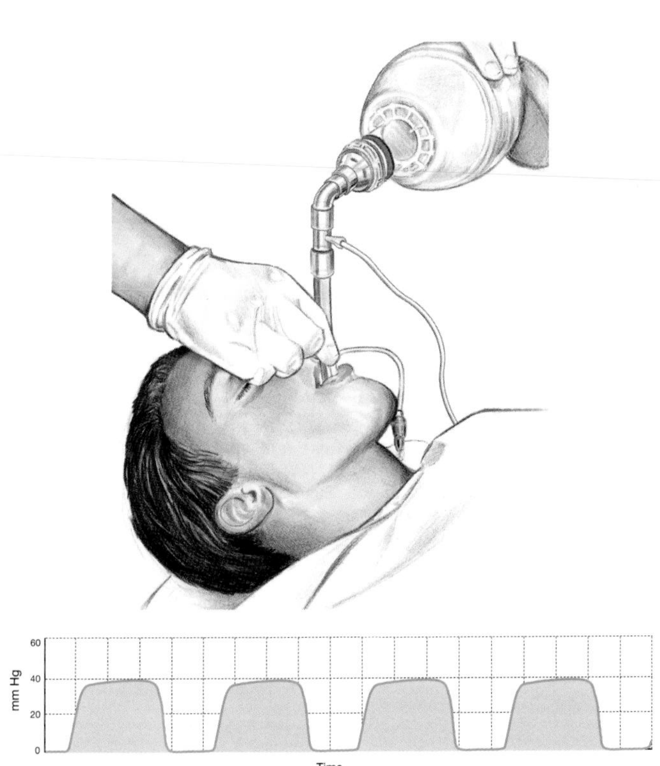

Figure 20. Waveform capnography with an ET tube showing a normal (adequate) ventilation pattern: PETCO$_2$ 35 to 40 mm Hg.

Waveform capnography devices which display both a waveform and a number will give you the most comprehensive information. The waveform is a graphic demonstration of the carbon dioxide exhaled with every breath. Humans with healthy lungs have a characteristic waveform (Figure 21A) that corresponds to inspiration and expiration. The highest value in this curve is the end-tidal CO_2.

In the patient with adequate circulation, the key uses for waveform capnography include the placement and monitoring of an advanced airway and the management of ventilation. In this patient, the healthcare provider should target a PETCO$_2$ of 35 to 40 mm Hg.

In the cardiac arrest patient, waveform capnography primarily monitors the effectiveness of chest compressions during CPR (Figure 21B) and signals ROSC. The higher the end-tidal CO_2 levels are, the higher the cardiac output is during resuscitation. A reading of less than 10 mm Hg indicates that the cardiac output is insufficient to achieve ROSC and that CPR quality should be improved. An abrupt sustained increase in PETCO$_2$ (typically 40 mm Hg or more) may indicate ROSC.

A decrease to zero (Figure 21C) indicates that there is no gas exchange occurring or no carbon dioxide delivery, such as when an ET tube is incorrectly placed or dislodged.

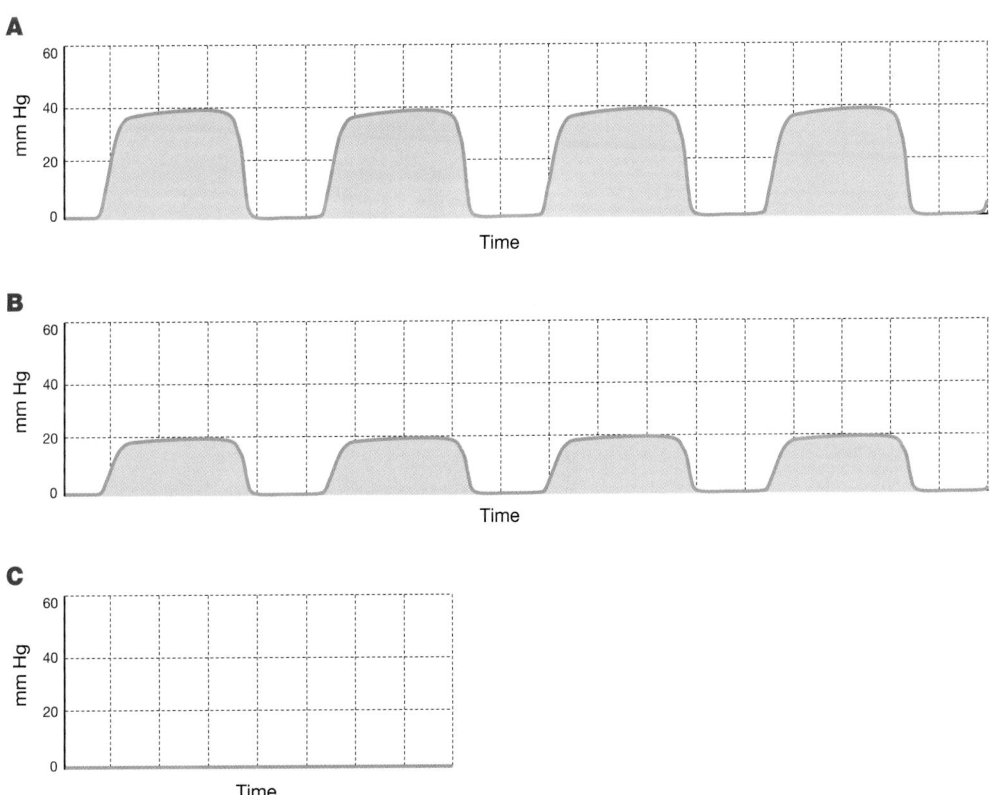

Figure 21. Waveform capnography. **A,** Normal range (approximately 35 to 40 mm Hg). **B,** Expected waveform with adequate chest compressions in cardiac arrest (approximately 20 mm Hg). **C,** ET tube incorrectly placed or dislodged (0 mm Hg).

Advanced Airways

Selection of an appropriate advanced airway device depends on the training, scope of practice, and equipment of the providers on the resuscitation team. Advanced airways include

- Laryngeal mask airway
- Laryngeal tube
- Esophageal-tracheal tube
- ET tube

When the patient has an advanced airway in place, 2 providers no longer deliver *cycles* of CPR (ie, compressions interrupted by pauses for ventilation). Instead, the compressing provider gives continuous chest compressions at a rate of at least 100/min without pauses for ventilation. The provider delivering ventilation provides 8 to 10 breaths per minute or 1 ventilation every 6 to 8 seconds. Providers should change compressor and ventilator roles approximately every 2 minutes to prevent compressor fatigue and deterioration in quality and rate of CPR. When multiple providers are present, they should rotate the compressor role about every 2 minutes.

Ventilation Rates

Airway Devices	Ventilations During Cardiac Arrest	Ventilations During Respiratory Arrest
Bag-mask	2 ventilations after every 30 compressions	**1 ventilation every 5 to 6 seconds** (10 to 12 breaths per minute)
Any advanced airway	**1 ventilation every 6 to 8 seconds** (8 to 10 breaths per minute)	

ET Tube

An ET tube is a single-use, cuffed tube that facilitates delivery of a high concentration of oxygen and selected tidal volume to maintain adequate ventilation; placement requires visualization of the patients' vocal cords.

The advantages of ET tube insertion are

- Maintains patent airway
- May protect the airway from aspiration of stomach contents or other substances in the mouth, throat, or the upper airway
- Permits effective suctioning of the trachea
- Facilitates delivery of PEEP
- Provides alternative route for administration of some resuscitation medications when intravenous (IV) or intraosseous (IO) access cannot be obtained

Although endotracheal administration of some resuscitation drugs is possible, IV or IO drug administration is preferred because it will provide more predictable drug delivery and pharmacologic effect. However, if IV or IO access cannot be established, epinephrine, vasopressin, and lidocaine may be administered by the endotracheal route during cardiac arrest (Class IIb, LOE B). Moreover, providers should use the memory aid *NAVEL* to recall the emergency medications that can be administered by ET tube: naloxone, atropine, vasopressin, epinephrine, and lidocaine. There were no data regarding endotracheal administration of amiodarone at the time of writing the *2010 AHA Guidelines for CPR and ECC.*

- The optimal endotracheal dose of most drugs is unknown, but typically the dose given by the endotracheal route is 2 to 2½ times the recommended IV dose.
- Mix the dose of drug with 5 to 10 mL of normal saline or sterile water.[8] Studies with epinephrine[9] and lidocaine[10] showed that dilution with water instead of 0.9% saline may achieve better drug absorption.
- Once medication has been administered through the ET tube, perform 1 to 2 ventilations to facilitate deposition of the drug into the airways.

The following are indications for endotracheal intubation:

- Cardiac arrest when bag-mask ventilation is not possible or is ineffective.
- Responsive patient in respiratory compromise who is unable to oxygenate adequately despite noninvasive ventilator measures.
- Patient is unable to protect airway (eg, coma, areflexia, or cardiac arrest).

Endotracheal intubation was once considered the optimal method of managing the airway during cardiac arrest. However, intubation attempts by unskilled providers can produce complications, the incidence of which is unacceptably high (see "Cautions and Minimizing Interruptions to CPR" below). Therefore esophageal-tracheal tubes, laryngeal mask airway, and laryngeal tube are now considered acceptable alternatives to the ET tube for advanced airway management.

Misplacement of an ET tube can result in severe, even fatal, complications. For this reason, only skilled, experienced personnel should perform endotracheal intubation. In most states, medical practice acts specify the level of personnel allowed to perform this procedure. For clinical reasons intubation should be restricted to healthcare providers who meet the following criteria:

- Personnel are well trained.
- Personnel perform intubation frequently.
- Personnel receive frequent refresher training in this skill.
- ET tube placement is included in the scope of practice defined by governmental regulations.

and

- Personnel participate in a process of continuous quality improvement to detect frequency of complications and minimize those complications.

Step	Action
1	*Patient preparation:* Provide oxygenation and ventilation, and position the patient. Assess the likelihood of difficult ET tube placement based on the patient's anatomy.
2	*Equipment preparation:* Assemble and check all necessary equipment (ET tube and laryngoscope).
3	*Insertion technique:* • Choose appropriate size ET tube. In general, an 8-mm internal diameter tube is used for adult males, and a 7-mm internal diameter tube is used for adult females. • Choose appropriate type (straight or curved) and size of laryngoscope blade (Figure 22). • Test ET tube cuff integrity. • Lubricate and secure stylet inside ET tube. • Place head in neutral position. • Open the mouth of the patient by using the "thumb and index finger" technique. • Insert laryngoscope blade and visualize glottic opening (Figure 22). • Clear airway if needed. • Insert ET tube (Figure 23) and watch it pass through the vocal cords. • Inflate ET tube cuff to achieve proper seal. • Remove laryngoscope blade from the mouth. • Hold tube with one hand and remove stylet with other hand. • Insert bite-block. • Attach bag to tube. • Squeeze the bag to give breaths (1 second each) while watching for chest rise. • Assess proper placement by both clinical assessment and device confirmation: – Auscultate for breath sounds. – Confirm correct positioning of ET tube by quantitative waveform capnography or, if not available, an exhaled CO_2 or esophageal detector device (EDD). • Secure ET tube in place. • Provide ventilation, and continue to monitor the patient's condition and the position of the ET tube using continuous waveform capnography.

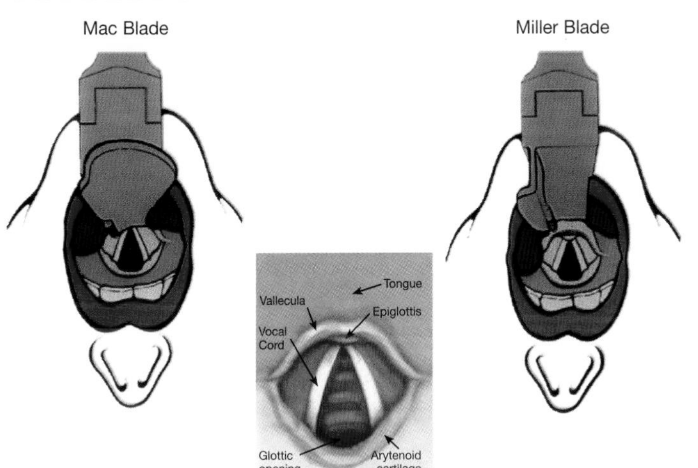

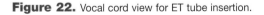

Figure 22. Vocal cord view for ET tube insertion.

Figure 23. ET tube inserted.

Placement of an ET tube is an important part of a resuscitation attempt. But it is a much lower priority than providing high-quality continuous chest compressions with few interruptions and delivering defibrillation.

Many ACLS providers do not perform intubation because of the professional restrictions noted above. Nonetheless, all members of the resuscitation team must understand the *concept* of endotracheal intubation. Team members may assist with endotracheal intubation and must know how to integrate compressions and ventilations when an ET tube is placed. This knowledge is often more important than knowing how to perform the procedure itself.

Cautions and Minimizing Interruptions to CPR

The incidence of complications is unacceptably high when intubation is performed by inexperienced providers or monitoring of tube placement is inadequate. Detailed assessment of out-of-hospital intubation attempts has concluded that ET tubes are much more difficult to place properly in that setting and highly susceptible to dislodgment.

Healthcare providers can minimize interruptions in chest compressions for endotracheal intubation with advanced preparation. Insert the laryngoscope blade with the tube ready at hand as soon as compressions are paused. Interrupt compressions only to visualize the vocal cords and insert the tube; this is ideally less than 10 seconds. Chest compressions should resume immediately after passing the tube between the vocal cords. If the initial intubation attempt is unsuccessful, healthcare providers may make a second attempt, but should consider using a supraglottic airway.

Tube Trauma and Adverse Effects

Endotracheal intubation can cause significant trauma to the patient, including

- Lacerated lips or tongue from forceful pressure between the laryngoscope blade and the tongue or cheek
- Chipped teeth
- Lacerated pharynx or trachea from the end of the stylet or ET tube
- Injury to the vocal cords
- Pharyngeal-esophageal perforation

Other complications associated with endotracheal intubation include

- Vomiting and aspiration of gastric contents into the lower airway
- Release of high levels of epinephrine and norepinephrine, which can cause elevated blood pressures, tachycardia, or arrhythmias

If the ET tube is inserted into the esophagus, the patient will receive no ventilation or oxygenation unless he or she is still breathing spontaneously. If you or your team fails to recognize esophageal intubation, the patient could suffer permanent brain damage or die.

Insertion of ET Tube Into One Bronchus

Insertion of the ET tube into the right or left main bronchus is a frequent complication. Unrecognized and uncorrected intubation of a bronchus can result in hypoxemia due to underinflation of the uninvolved lung or overinflation of the ventilated lung.

To determine if the ET tube has been inserted into a bronchus, listen to the chest for bilateral breath sounds. Also look for equal expansion of both sides during ventilation.

If you suspect that the tube has been inserted into either the left or right main bronchus, take these actions:

1. Deflate the tube cuff.
2. Withdraw the tube back 1 to 2 cm.
3. Confirm correct tube placement by both clinical assessment and device confirmation.
4. Reinflate the cuff and secure ET tube in place.
5. Recheck the patient's clinical signs, including chest expansion, breath sounds, and evidence of oxygenation.

Even when the ET tube is seen to pass through the vocal cords and tube position is verified by chest expansion and auscultation during positive-pressure ventilation, you should obtain additional confirmation of placement using waveform capnography or esophageal detector device (EDD).

Once the patient is more stable, an x-ray may be obtained to optimize ET tube position and assess lung pathology. An x-ray takes too long to be used as a means of confirming tracheal placement of an ET tube. Recognizing misplacement of an ET tube is a clinical responsibility.

After inserting and confirming correct placement of an ET tube, you should record the depth of the tube as marked at the front teeth or gums and secure it. Because there is significant potential for ET tube movement with head flexion and extension and when the patient is moved from one location to another, secure the ET tube with tape or a commercial device. Devices and tape should be applied in a manner that avoids compression of the front and sides of the neck to protect against impairment of venous return from the brain.

Laryngeal Mask Airway

The laryngeal mask airway is composed of a tube with a cuffed mask-like projection at the end of the tube. The laryngeal mask airway is an advanced airway device that is considered an acceptable alternative to the ET tube. When compared with the ET tube, the laryngeal mask airway provided equivalent ventilation[11]; successful ventilation during CPR was reported in 73% to 98% of patients.[12,13] A small proportion of patients cannot be ventilated with the laryngeal mask airway. Therefore it is important for providers to have an alternative strategy for airway management.

The advantages of laryngeal mask airway:

- Regurgitation is less likely with the laryngeal mask airway than with the bag-mask device.

The steps for insertion of the laryngeal mask airway (Figure 24) are as follows:

Step	Action
1	*Patient preparation:* Provide oxygenation and ventilation, and position the patient.
2	*Equipment preparation:* Check the integrity of the mask and tube according to the manufacturer's instructions. Lubricate only the posterior surface of the cuff to avoid blocking the airway aperture.
3	*Insertion technique:* • Introduce the laryngeal mask airway into the pharynx and advance it blindly until you feel resistance. Resistance indicates that the distal end of the tube has reached the hypopharynx. • Inflate the cuff of the mask. Cuff inflation pushes the mask up against the tracheal opening, allowing air to flow through the tube and into the trachea. • Ventilation through the tube is ultimately delivered to the opening in the center of the mask and into the trachea. • To avoid trauma, do not use force at any time during insertion of the laryngeal mask airway. • Avoid overinflating the cuff. Excessive intracuff pressure can result in misplacement of the device. It also can cause pharyngolaryngeal injury (eg, sore throat, dysphagia, or nerve injury).
4	Insert a bite-block (if the laryngeal mask airway does not have intrinsic bite-block), provide ventilation, and continue to monitor the patient's condition and the position of the laryngeal mask airway. A bite-block reduces the possibility of airway obstruction and tube damage. Keep the bite-block in place until you remove the laryngeal mask airway. **Figure 24.** Insertion of the laryngeal mask airway.

- Aspiration is uncommon with laryngeal mask airways.
- Because insertion of the laryngeal mask airway does not require laryngoscopy and visualization of the vocal cords, training in its placement and use is simpler than for endotracheal intubation.
- Laryngeal mask airway insertion is easier than ET tube insertion when access to the patient is limited, there is a possibility of unstable neck injury, or appropriate positioning of the patient for endotracheal intubation is impossible.

Cautions/Additional Information

Do not apply cricoid pressure because it may hinder the insertion of the laryngeal mask airway. Eight studies in anesthetized adults showed that when cricoid pressure was used before insertion of a laryngeal mask airway, the proportion of tubes correctly positioned decreased, and the incidence of failed insertion and impaired ventilation once the laryngeal mask airway had been placed increased.[14]

- In general, size 5 fits adult males and size 4 fits adult females.
- You may note a smooth swelling at the level of the cricoid cartilage in the neck. This is normal, and it confirms the proper positioning of the device.
- If you hear an air leak during ventilation with a bag for the next 3 or 4 breaths, reevaluate the position of the laryngeal mask airway for possible misplacement.
- To avoid displacement, limit the patient's head movement and avoid suctioning secretions in the pharynx once the laryngeal mask airway is in place.

Disadvantages

A small proportion of patients cannot be ventilated with the laryngeal mask airway; therefore it is important for providers to have an alternative strategy for airway management.

Laryngeal Tube

The laryngeal tube is a supraglottic airway device that is considered an acceptable alternative to an ET tube. The laryngeal tube is available in single and dual lumen versions. Only experienced providers should perform laryngeal tube insertion.

The steps for insertion of the laryngeal tube are as follows:

Step	Action
1	*Patient preparation:* Provide oxygenation and ventilation, and position the patient.
2	*Equipment preparation:* Check the integrity of the laryngeal tube according to the manufacturer's instructions.
3	*Insertion technique:* • Inspect the mouth and larynx of the patient before insertion of the laryngeal tube. • Open the mouth of the patient by approximately 2 to 3 cm using the "thumb and index finger" technique. • Use a laryngoscope to facilitate insertion. • Insert the laryngeal tube (Figure 25) in the midline of the mouth along the palate until a slight resistance is felt. • In some cases a slight head extension can facilitate mouth opening and tube placement. • Ensure that the ventilation holes of the laryngeal tube lie in front of the laryngeal inlet. • The insertion depth can be verified according to the teeth marks at the upper end of the tube. • The laryngeal tube is available in different sizes. **Figure 25.** Insertion of the laryngeal tube.

At the time of writing the *2010 AHA Guidelines for CPR and ECC*, there were limited data published on the use of the laryngeal tube in cardiac arrest. In one case series assessing 40 out-of-hospital cardiac arrest patients, insertion of the laryngeal tube by trained paramedics was successful and ventilation was effective in 85% of patients.[15] Another out-of-hospital assessment of 157 attempts at laryngeal tube placement revealed a 97% success rate in a mixed population of cardiac arrest and noncardiac arrest patients.[16]

The advantages of the laryngeal tube are ease of training and ease of insertion due to the compact size of the tube. In addition, the tube isolates the airway, reduces the risk of aspiration, and provides reliable ventilation. Trained healthcare professionals may consider the laryngeal tube as an alternative to bag-mask ventilation or endotracheal intubation for airway management in cardiac arrest.

Esophageal-Tracheal Tube

The esophageal-tracheal tube is an advanced airway that is an acceptable alternative to the ET tube. The esophageal-tracheal tube is an invasive airway device with 2 inflatable balloon cuffs. The tube is more likely to enter the esophagus than the trachea, thereby allowing ventilation to occur through side openings in the device adjacent to the vocal cords and trachea. If the tube enters the trachea, ventilation can still occur by an opening in the end of the tube.

Studies show that healthcare providers with all levels of experience can insert the esophageal-tracheal tube and deliver ventilation comparable to that achieved with endotracheal intubation.[17] Compared with bag-mask ventilation, the esophageal-tracheal tube is advantageous because it isolates the airway, reduces the risk of aspiration, and provides more reliable ventilation. The advantages of the esophageal-tracheal tube are chiefly related to ease of training when compared with the training needed for endotracheal intubation.[18,19] Only providers trained and experienced with the use of the esophageal-tracheal tube should insert the device because fatal complications are possible if the position of the distal lumen of the esophageal-tracheal tube in the esophagus or trachea is identified incorrectly. Other possible complications related to the use of the esophageal-tracheal tube are esophageal trauma, including lacerations, bruising, and subcutaneous emphysema.[20-22] The esophageal-tracheal tube is supplied in 2 sizes: the smaller size (37F) is used in patients 4 to 5½ feet tall, and the larger size (41F) is used in patients more than 5 feet tall.

Contraindications

- Responsive patients with cough or gag reflex
- Age: 16 years or younger
- Height: 4 feet or shorter
- Known or suspected esophageal disease
- Ingestion of a caustic substance

The steps for insertion of the esophageal-tracheal tube are as follows:

Step	Action
1	*Patient preparation:* Provide oxygenation and ventilation, and position the patient. Rule out the contraindications to insertion of the esophageal-tracheal tube.
2	*Equipment preparation:* Check the integrity of both cuffs according to the manufacturer's instructions and lubricate the tube.
3	*Insertion technique:* • Hold the device with cuffs deflated so that the curvature of the tube matches the curvature of the pharynx. • Lift the jaw and insert the tube gently until the black lines on the tube (Figure 26) are positioned between the patient's upper teeth. Do not force insertion and do not attempt for more than 30 seconds. • Inflate the proximal/pharyngeal (blue) cuff with 100 mL of air. (Inflate with 85 mL for the smaller esophageal-tracheal tube.) Then inflate the distal (white or clear) cuff with 15 mL of air. (Inflate with 12 mL for the smaller esophageal-tracheal tube.) **Figure 26.** Insertion of the esophageal-tracheal tube.
4	Confirm tube location and select the lumen for ventilation. To select the appropriate lumen to use for ventilation, you must determine where the tip of the tube is located. The tip of the tube can rest in either the esophagus or the trachea. • *Esophageal placement:* To confirm esophageal placement, attach the bag-mask device to the blue (proximal/pharyngeal) lumen. Squeezing the bag provides ventilation by forcing air through the openings in the tube between the 2 inflated cuffs. This action produces bilateral breath sounds. Epigastric sounds do not occur because the distal cuff, once inflated, obstructs the esophagus, thereby preventing airflow into the stomach. Because the tip of the tube rests in the esophagus, do not use the distal (white or clear) tube for ventilation. • *Tracheal placement:* If squeezing the bag attached to the blue (proximal/pharyngeal lumen) does not produce breath sounds, immediately disconnect the bag and reattach it to the distal (white or clear) lumen. Squeezing the bag should now produce breath sounds because this lumen goes to the trachea. With endotracheal placement of the tube, the distal cuff performs the same function as a cuff on an ET tube. Detection of exhaled CO_2 (through the ventilating lumen) should be used for confirmation, particularly if the patient has a perfusing rhythm. • *Unknown placement:* If you are unable to hear breath sounds, deflate both cuffs and withdraw the tube slightly. Reinflate both cuffs (see steps above) and attempt to ventilate the patient. If breath sounds and epigastric sounds are still absent, remove the tube.

Caution

Do not apply cricoid pressure during insertion because it may hinder the insertion of the esophageal-tracheal tube.

Disadvantages

- Insertion of an esophageal-tracheal tube may cause esophageal trauma, including lacerations, bruising, and subcutaneous emphysema.
- The esophageal-tracheal tube is available in only 2 sizes and cannot be used in any patient less than 4 feet tall.

Cricoid Pressure

Cricoid pressure in nonarrest patients may offer some measure of protection to the airway from aspiration and gastric insufflation during bag-mask ventilation.[23-26] However, it also may impede ventilation and interfere with placement of a supraglottic airway or intubation.[14,27-32] If cricoid pressure is used in special circumstances during cardiac arrest, the pressure should be adjusted, relaxed, or released if it impedes ventilation or advanced airway placement. Because the role of cricoid pressure during out-of-hospital cardiac arrest and in-hospital cardiac arrest has not been studied, routine use of cricoid pressure in cardiac arrest is not recommended.

Clinical Assessment to Confirm Tube Placement

Providers should perform a thorough assessment of ET tube position immediately after placement. This assessment should not require interruption of chest compressions.

Assessment by physical examination consists of visualizing chest expansion bilaterally and listening over the epigastrium (breath sounds should not be heard) and the lung fields bilaterally (breath sounds should be equal and adequate). If there is doubt about correct tube placement, use the laryngoscope to visualize the tube passing through the vocal cords. If still in doubt, remove the tube and provide bag-mask ventilation until the tube can be replaced.

Use of Devices to Confirm Tube Placement

The body eliminates CO_2 through *ventilation*. When blood passes through the lungs, CO_2 moves from the blood, across the alveolar capillary membrane into the alveoli, and then into the airways and is exhaled. Alveolar P_{CO_2} should be approximately equal to pulmonary venous, left atrial, and arterial P_{CO_2}. If there is a good match of ventilation and perfusion in the lungs and if there is no airway obstruction, exhaled CO_2 should correlate well with arterial P_{CO_2}, and exhaled CO_2 can be used to estimate arterial CO_2 tension and to follow trends over time.

ACLS providers should always use *both* clinical assessment and devices to confirm ET tube location immediately after placement and each time the patient is moved. No study, however, has identified a single device as both sensitive and specific for ET tube placement in the trachea or esophagus. The *2010 AHA Guidelines for CPR and ECC* recommend the use of continuous waveform capnography in addition to clinical assessment as the most reliable method of confirming and monitoring correct placement of an ET tube. Providers should observe a persistent capnographic waveform with ventilation to confirm and monitor ET tube placement in the field, in the transport vehicle, on arrival at the hospital, and after any patient transfer to reduce the risk of unrecognized tube misplacement or displacement.

Exhaled CO_2 Detectors

Detection of exhaled CO_2 is one of several independent methods of confirming ET tube position. Given the simplicity of the colorimetric and nonwaveform exhaled CO_2 detector, these methods can be used in addition to clinical assessment as the initial method for detecting correct tube placement in a patient in cardiac arrest when waveform capnography is not available (Class IIa, LOE B) (See "Use of Devices to Confirm Tube Placement"). However, studies indicate that these devices are no more accurate than auscultation and direct visualization for confirming the tracheal position of an ET tube in victims of cardiac arrest. Use of CO_2 detecting devices to determine the correct placement of other advanced airways (eg, laryngeal tube, laryngeal mask airway, esophageal-tracheal tube) has not been adequately studied.

Esophageal Detector Devices

One type of esophageal detector device (EDD) consists of a bulb that is compressed and attached to the ET tube. If the tube is in the esophagus (positive result for an EDD), the suction created by the EDD will collapse the lumen of the esophagus or pull the esophageal tissue against the tip of the tube and the bulb will not reexpand. Another type of EDD consists of a syringe that is attached to the ET tube; the provider tries to pull the barrel of the syringe. If the tube is in the esophagus, it will not be possible to pull the barrel (aspirate air) with the syringe. An EDD can be used to confirm ET tube placement if waveform capnography is not available, although studies indicate that these devices are no more accurate than watching for chest rise and other clinical observations in victims of cardiac arrest.[33-36]

Misleading Results of Colorimetric End-Tidal CO_2 Detectors

- CO_2 can be detected when the tube is either in the trachea (positive results) or in the esophagus or hypopharynx (false positive).
  - The reasons for the false positive results include distended stomach, recent ingestion of carbonated beverages, or nonpulmonary source of CO_2.
  - Unrecognized esophageal intubation can lead to iatrogenic death.
- No CO_2 detection might occur while the tube is in the trachea (false negative results) or if the tube is not in the trachea (ie, tube is in the esophagus; negative results).
  - The reasons for false negative results include low or no blood flow state (eg, cardiac arrest); and any cardiac arrest with no, prolonged, or poor CPR.

Critical Concept **Advanced Airway Confirmation**	The AHA recommends continuous waveform capnography in addition to clinical assessment as the most reliable method of confirming and monitoring correct placement of an ET tube: • Clinical assessment immediately after placement • Waveform capnography immediately after placement It is reasonable to use waveform capnography in addition to clinical assessment for supraglottic airways.

- False negative results might lead to unnecessary removal of properly inserted ET tube and reintubation attempts, which might increase chances of other adverse events.
- For these reasons, if CO_2 is not detected, it is recommended that a second method be used to confirm ET tube placement, such as direct visualization or the esophageal detector device.

Misleading Results of EDD

Results may suggest that the tube is in the esophagus when the tube is either in the esophagus (positive results) or in the trachea instead of the esophagus (false positive results). The reasons for false positive results include secretion in the trachea (eg, mucus, gastric contents, acute pulmonary edema); insertion in right main bronchus; pliable trachea (eg, morbid obesity, late-term pregnancy); or status asthmaticus.

Secure the Airway

After inserting the advanced airway and confirming correct placement, the provider should record the depth of the tube (as marked at the front teeth) and secure it. Because there is significant potential for ET tube movement with head flexion and extension,[37-39] ongoing monitoring of ET tube placement is essential during transport, particularly when the patient is moved from one location to another.[40,41] Providers should verify correct placement of all advanced airways immediately after insertion and whenever the patient is moved.

Secure the ET tube with tape or a commercial device. Placing the patient on a backboard, securing the ET tube, and other strategies provide an equivalent method for preventing accidental tube displacement when compared with traditional methods of securing the tube (tape).[42,43] These strategies may be considered during patient transport. Devices and tape should be applied in a manner that avoids compression of the front[44] and sides of the neck, which may impair venous return from the brain. After tube confirmation and fixation, obtain a chest x-ray (when feasible) to confirm that the end of the ET tube is properly positioned above the carina. A chest x-ray is never used as a primary method for confirmation of ET tube position.

Avoid Excessive Ventilations

During CPR, blood flow to the lungs is substantially reduced, so an adequate ventilation-perfusion ratio can be maintained with lower tidal volumes and respiratory rates than normal. Providers should not hyperventilate the patient (too many breaths per minute or too large a volume per breath). Excessive ventilation is unnecessary and is harmful because it increases intrathoracic pressure, decreases venous return to the heart, and diminishes cardiac output and survival.

In case of a patient in respiratory arrest with a pulse, give 1 breath every 5 to 6 seconds (10 to 12 breaths/min) with bag-mask ventilation or with any advanced airway device. Recheck the pulse about every 2 minutes. Take at least 5 seconds but no more than 10 seconds for a pulse check. Take special precautions when providing ventilation for patients with suspected cervical spine trauma as described below.

Airway Management in Patients With Severe Trauma

Trauma poses special problems in airway control. In the patient with vertebral injury, excessive movement of the spine may produce or exacerbate a spinal cord injury. A possible spine injury is suspected based on other apparent injuries (multiple trauma, head or neck injury, or facial trauma) and the type and mechanism of injury (eg, motor vehicle crash, fall from a height). If suspected, appropriate immobilization precautions are taken until qualified personnel can evaluate the patient properly.

Techniques

Only providers experienced in these procedures should attempt them.

1. The initial step in a patient with a suspected neck injury is chin lift or jaw thrust *without* head extension.

Critical Concept **Avoid Excessive Ventilation**	When using any form of assisted ventilation, you must avoid delivering excessive ventilation (too many breaths per minute or too large a volume per breath). Excessive ventilation can be harmful because it increases intrathoracic pressure, decreases venous return to the heart, and diminishes cardiac output. It may also cause gastric inflation and predispose the patient to vomiting and aspiration of gastric contents.

Critical Concept **Securing an Advanced Airway**	When securing an advanced airway, avoid using ties that pass circumferentially around the patient's neck, thereby obstructing venous return from the brain.

2. If the airway remains obstructed, add head tilt slowly and carefully until the airway is open.

3. Then stabilize the head in a neutral position. A trained provider should stabilize the patient's head during any airway manipulation to prevent excessive flexion, extension, or lateral movement of the head during airway control.

4. Nasotracheal intubation is relatively contraindicated in a patient with facial fractures or fractures at the base of the skull. Direct orotracheal intubation becomes the technique of choice in such circumstances. A second provider is needed to provide manual immobilization of the head and neck during intubation attempts.

If the patient is breathing spontaneously and requires intubation but oral intubation is not possible, the experienced provider may attempt *"blind" nasotracheal intubation*. This technique, however, is rarely indicated and should be attempted only by personnel with experience in the technique. A second provider must provide head and neck immobilization during the intubation attempt to prevent reactive neck movement.

- Be prepared to provide immediate suctioning of the upper airway if necessary.
- When endotracheal intubation cannot be performed, experienced experts should achieve airway control using alternative airway devices or perform cricothyrotomy.

FAQ

When is an advanced airway inserted or required?

There is inadequate evidence to define the optimal timing of advanced airway placement in relation to other interventions during resuscitation from cardiac arrest. The provider should weigh the need for continuous compressions against the need for an advanced airway. If advanced airway placement will interrupt chest compressions, providers may consider deferring insertion of the airway until the patient fails to respond to initial CPR and defibrillation attempts or demonstrates ROSC. Some advanced airways can be performed without interruption of chest compressions. The risks and benefits are affected by

- The condition of the patient
- The provider's expertise in airway control
- The ability to ventilate the patient with a bag-mask device

References

1. Carlson KA, Jahr JS. An update on pulse oximetry. Part II: limitations and future applications. *Anesthesiol Rev*. 1994;21:41-46.
2. Aughey K, Hess D, Eitel D, Bleecher K, Cooley M, Ogden C, Sabulsky N. An evaluation of pulse oximetry in prehospital care. *Ann Emerg Med*. 1991;20:887-891.
3. Bota GW, Rowe BH. Continuous monitoring of oxygen saturation in prehospital patients with severe illness: the problem of unrecognized hypoxemia. *J Emerg Med*. 1995;13:305-311.
4. Brown LH, Manring EA, Kornegay HB, Prasad NH. Can prehospital personnel detect hypoxemia without the aid of pulse oximeters? *Am J Emerg Med*. 1996;14:43-44.
5. Valko PC, Campbell JP, McCarty DL, Martin D, Turnbull J. Prehospital use of pulse oximetry in rotary-wing aircraft. *Prehosp Disaster Med*. 1991;6:421-428.
6. Gehring H, Duembgen L, Peterlein M, Hagelberg S, Dibbelt L. Hemoximetry as the "gold standard"? Error assessment based on differences among identical blood gas analyzer devices of five manufacturers. *Anesth Analg*. 2007;105:S24-S30.
7. Feiner JR, Severinghaus JW, Bickler PE. Dark skin decreases the accuracy of pulse oximeters at low oxygen saturation: the effects of oximeter probe type and gender. *Anesth Analg*. 2007;105:S18-S23.
8. Jasani MS, Nadkarni VM, Finkelstein MS, Mandell GA, Salzman SK, Norman ME. Effects of different techniques of endotracheal epinephrine administration in pediatric porcine hypoxic-hypercarbic cardiopulmonary arrest. *Crit Care Med*. 1994;22:1174-1180.
9. Naganobu K, Hasebe Y, Uchiyama Y, Hagio M, Ogawa H. A comparison of distilled water and normal saline as diluents for endobronchial administration of epinephrine in the dog. *Anesth Analg*. 2000;91:317-321.
10. Hahnel JH, Lindner KH, Schurmann C, Prengel A, Ahnefeld FW. Plasma lidocaine levels and PaO_2 with endobronchial administration: dilution with normal saline or distilled water? *Ann Emerg Med*. 1990;19:1314-1317.
11. Samarkandi AH, Seraj MA, el Dawlatly A, Mastan M, Bakhamees HB. The role of laryngeal mask airway in cardiopulmonary resuscitation. *Resuscitation*. 1994;28:103-106.
12. Rumball CJ, MacDonald D. The PTL, Combitube, laryngeal mask, and oral airway: a randomized prehospital comparative study of ventilatory device effectiveness and cost-effectiveness in 470 cases of cardiorespiratory arrest. *Prehosp Emerg Care*. 1997;1:1-10.
13. Kokkinis K. The use of the laryngeal mask airway in CPR. *Resuscitation*. 1994;27:9-12.
14. Asai T, Goy RW, Liu EH. Cricoid pressure prevents placement of the laryngeal tube and laryngeal tube-suction II. *Br J Anaesth*. 2007;99:282-285.
15. Heuer JF, Barwing J, Eich C, Quintel M, Crozier TA, Roessler M. Initial ventilation through laryngeal tube instead of face mask in out-of-hospital cardiopulmonary arrest is effective and safe. *Eur J Emerg Med*. 2010;17:10-15.
16. Schalk R, Byhahn C, Fausel F, Egner A, Oberndorfer D, Walcher F, Latasch L. Out-of-hospital airway management by paramedics and emergency physicians using laryngeal tubes. *Resuscitation*. 2010;81:323-326.

17. Tanigawa K, Shigematsu A. Choice of airway devices for 12,020 cases of nontraumatic cardiac arrest in Japan. *Prehosp Emerg Care*. 1998;2:96-100.

18. Lefrancois DP, Dufour DG. Use of the esophageal tracheal combitube by basic emergency medical technicians. *Resuscitation*. 2002;52:77-83.

19. Dorges V, Wenzel V, Knacke P, Gerlach K. Comparison of different airway management strategies to ventilate apneic, nonpreoxygenated patients. *Crit Care Med*. 2003;31:800-804.

20. Atherton GL, Johnson JC. Ability of paramedics to use the Combitube in prehospital cardiac arrest. *Ann Emerg Med*. 1993;22:1263-1268.

21. Rabitsch W, Krafft P, Lackner FX, Frenzer R, Hofbauer R, Sherif C, Frass M. Evaluation of the oesophageal-tracheal double-lumen tube (Combitube) during general anaesthesia. *Wien Klin Wochenschr*. 2004;116:90-93.

22. Vezina D, Lessard MR, Bussieres J, Topping C, Trepanier CA. Complications associated with the use of the Esophageal-Tracheal Combitube. *Can J Anaesth*. 1998;45:76-80.

23. Petito SP, Russell WJ. The prevention of gastric inflation—a neglected benefit of cricoid pressure. *Anaesth Intensive Care*. 1988;16:139-143.

24. Lawes EG, Campbell I, Mercer D. Inflation pressure, gastric insufflation and rapid sequence induction. *Br J Anaesth*. 1987;59:315-318.

25. Salem MR, Wong AY, Mani M, Sellick BA. Efficacy of cricoid pressure in preventing gastric inflation during bag-mask ventilation in pediatric patients. *Anesthesiology*. 1974;40:96-98.

26. Moynihan RJ, Brock-Utne JG, Archer JH, Feld LH, Kreitzman TR. The effect of cricoid pressure on preventing gastric insufflation in infants and children. *Anesthesiology*. 1993;78:652-656.

27. Turgeon AF, Nicole PC, Trepanier CA, Marcoux S, Lessard MR. Cricoid pressure does not increase the rate of failed intubation by direct laryngoscopy in adults. *Anesthesiology*. 2005;102:315-319.

28. Allman KG. The effect of cricoid pressure application on airway patency. *J Clin Anesth*. 1995;7:197-199.

29. Brimacombe J, White A, Berry A. Effect of cricoid pressure on ease of insertion of the laryngeal mask airway. *Br J Anaesth*. 1993;71:800-802.

30. McNelis U, Syndercombe A, Harper I, Duggan J. The effect of cricoid pressure on intubation facilitated by the gum elastic bougie. *Anaesthesia*. 2007;62:456-459.

31. Hartsilver EL, Vanner RG. Airway obstruction with cricoid pressure. *Anaesthesia*. 2000;55:208-211.

32. Hocking G, Roberts FL, Thew ME. Airway obstruction with cricoid pressure and lateral tilt. *Anaesthesia*. 2001;56:825-828.

33. Takeda T, Tanigawa K, Tanaka H, Hayashi Y, Goto E, Tanaka K. The assessment of three methods to verify tracheal tube placement in the emergency setting. *Resuscitation*. 2003;56:153-157.

34. Tanigawa K, Takeda T, Goto E, Tanaka K. The efficacy of esophageal detector devices in verifying tracheal tube placement: a randomized cross-over study of out-of-hospital cardiac arrest patients. *Anesth Analg*. 2001;92:375-378.

35. Tanigawa K, Takeda T, Goto E, Tanaka K. Accuracy and reliability of the self-inflating bulb to verify tracheal intubation in out-of-hospital cardiac arrest patients. *Anesthesiology*. 2000;93:1432-1436.

36. Pelucio M, Halligan L, Dhindsa H. Out-of-hospital experience with the syringe esophageal detector device. *Acad Emerg Med*. 1997;4:563-568.

37. Yap SJ, Morris RW, Pybus DA. Alterations in endotracheal tube position during general anaesthesia. *Anaesth Intensive Care*. 1994;22:586-588.

38. Sugiyama K, Yokoyama K. Displacement of the endotracheal tube caused by change of head position in pediatric anesthesia: evaluation by fiberoptic bronchoscopy. *Anesth Analg*. 1996;82:251-253.

39. King HK. A new device: Tube Securer. An endotracheal tube holder with integrated bite-block. *Acta Anaesthesiol Sin*. 1997;35:257-259.

40. Falk JL, Sayre MR. Confirmation of airway placement. *Prehosp Emerg Care*. 1999;3:273-278.

41. Wang HE, Kupas DF, Paris PM, Bates RR, Yealy DM. Preliminary experience with a prospective, multi-centered evaluation of out-of-hospital endotracheal intubation. *Resuscitation*. 2003;58:49-58.

42. Kupas DF, Kauffman KF, Wang HE. Effect of airway-securing method on prehospital endotracheal tube dislodgment. *Prehosp Emerg Care*. 2010;14:26-30.

43. Levy H, Griego L. A comparative study of oral endotracheal tube securing methods. *Chest*. 1993;104:1537-1540.

44. Tasota FJ, Hoffman LA, Zullo TG, Jamison G. Evaluation of two methods used to stabilize oral endotracheal tubes. *Heart Lung*. 1987;16:140-146.

Chapter 7

Electrical Therapies

This Chapter

- Principle of Defibrillation
- Automated External Defibrillators
- Manual Defibrillation

Overview

Defibrillation involves the delivery of electrical current through the chest and heart to depolarize myocardial cells and eliminate ventricular fibrillation (VF). The technique of delivering electrical current to the heart to terminate arrhythmias dates to Kouwenhoven, Zoll, and Lown over one-half century ago.[1] Initially the use of defibrillators was restricted to the operating suite. Now automated external defibrillators (AEDs) are found in virtually all emergency medical services (EMS) systems and many large public buildings, and they can be used with minimal or no prior training. Defibrillation is a critical component of the Chain of Survival, and its integration with cardiopulmonary resuscitation (CPR), especially chest compressions, is crucial. AEDs may be used by lay rescuers and healthcare providers as part of basic life support. Manual defibrillation, cardioversion, and pacing are advanced life support therapies. The use of a defibrillator alone does not guarantee success or survival.

Principle of Defibrillation

Definition

In cardiac arrest, VF is the presenting rhythm most often associated with survival. Time to defibrillation is a critical determinant of the outcome of resuscitation attempts. A defibrillator is a device that administers a controlled electrical shock to patients to terminate a cardiac arrhythmia, usually VF. The technique of administering the electrical shock is usually referred to as *defibrillation* if the shock is used to successfully terminate VF. Defibrillators can be synchronized to an organized rhythm for shock delivery to perform *cardioversion* (eg, for atrial fibrillation, atrial flutter, or stable ventricular tachycardia [VT] with pulses); thus some healthcare providers use the term *cardioverters.* Devices that are implanted in high-risk patients so they can pace, detect a cardiac arrhythmia, and automatically perform defibrillation or cardioversion are called *implantable cardioverter/defibrillators*—or *ICDs* for short.

Defibrillatory shocks deliver massive amounts of electrical energy over a few milliseconds. Passing between positive and negative defibrillatory pads placed on the chest or paddles pressed against the chest, this electrical energy flows through the interposed, fibrillating heart (Figure 27). The split-second flow of current does not "jump-start" the heart. Instead the current flow totally depolarizes, or *stuns,* the entire myocardium, producing complete electrical silence, or *asystole*. This brief period of electrical silence allows spontaneously repolarizing *pacemaking* cells within the heart to recover. The regular cycles of repolarization/depolarization of these pacemaker cells allow coordinated contractile activity to resume if the cells are not stunned or damaged.

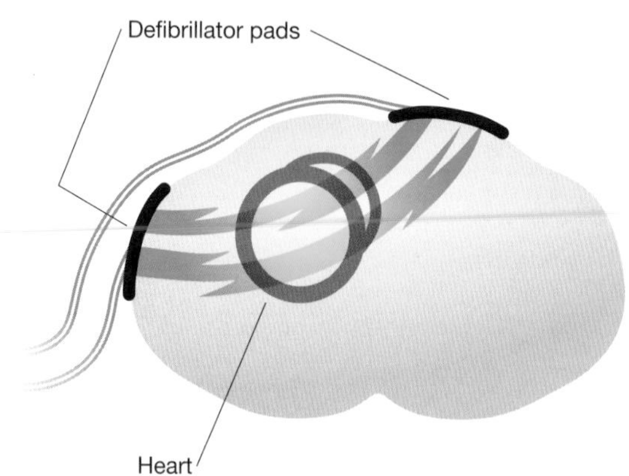

Figure 27. Pathway of electrical energy through the chest and heart with placement of pads (or paddles) for defibrillation. Modified from Ewy GA, Bressler R, eds. *Cardiovascular Drugs and the Management of Heart Disease.* New York, NY: Raven Press; 1982.

Recipe for Success and Survival

The Scientific Evidence for Early Defibrillation

The most critical interventions during the first minutes of VF or pulseless VT are immediate CPR, with minimal interruption in chest compressions, and defibrillation as soon as it can be accomplished. A significant body of research supports the concept that defibrillation must be performed as early as possible for adult patients with sudden cardiac arrest (SCA):

- VF is a frequent initial rhythm in out-of-hospital witnessed SCA.
- Pulseless VT rapidly deteriorates to VF.
- When VF is present, the heart quivers and does not pump blood.
- The only effective treatment for VF is electrical defibrillation (delivery of a shock to stop the VF).
- The probability of successful defibrillation decreases quickly over time.
- VF deteriorates to asystole if not treated.

The earlier defibrillation occurs, the higher the survival rate. When VF is present, CPR can provide a small amount of blood flow to the heart and brain but cannot directly restore an organized rhythm. Restoration of a perfusing rhythm requires immediate CPR and defibrillation within a few minutes of the initial arrest.

For every minute that passes between collapse and defibrillation, the chance of survival from a witnessed VF SCA declines by 7% to 10% per minute if no bystander CPR is provided.[2] When bystanders perform CPR, the decline is more gradual and averages 3% to 4% per minute.[2-5] CPR performed early can double[2,6] or triple[7] survival from witnessed SCA at most defibrillation intervals. Lay rescuer AED programs increase the likelihood of CPR and attempted defibrillation.

Evidence: Survival Before and After Early Defibrillation Programs

In the 1980s communities with no out-of-hospital ACLS services and defibrillation programs began to perform "before-and-after" studies. EMS systems invariably reported improved survival rates for cardiac arrest patients when the community added *any* type of program that resulted in earlier defibrillation (Table 7). Impressive results were reported from early studies in King County, Washington, where the odds ratio for improved survival (comparing the odds of survival after versus before the addition of an early defibrillation program) was 3.7,[8] and rural Iowa, where the odds ratio was 6.3.[9] That is, a person was about 4 to 6 times more likely to survive a VF arrest after institution of an early defibrillation program.

Evidence continued to accumulate during the 1980s; investigators reported positive odds ratios for improved survival of 4.3 in rural communities of southeastern Minnesota,[10] 5.0 in northeastern Minnesota,[11] and 3.3 in Wisconsin.[12]

When the survival rates were examined by the type of system deployed across larger geographic areas, that same pattern emerged. The system organized to get the defibrillator there the fastest—independent of the arrival of personnel to perform endotracheal intubation and provide intravenous (IV) medications—achieved better survival rates (Table 8). If early defibrillation was combined with early advanced airway placement and IV medications, survival rates were even higher.

By the end of the 1980s, evidence had confirmed the importance of each link in the Chain of Survival. Figure 28 illustrates this concept in a different way. The figure gives

Critical Concept **Integrated CPR and Defibrillation**	To give the patient with VF SCA the best chance of survival, 3 actions must occur within the first moments of cardiac arrest: • Activation of the EMS system • High-quality CPR, starting with chest compressions • Operation of an AED/defibrillator

Table 7. Effectiveness of Early Defibrillation Programs by Community

Location	% Survival Before Early Defibrillation		% Survival After Early Defibrillation		Odds Ratio for Improved Survival
King County, Washington	7	(4/56)	26	(10/38)	3.7
Iowa	3	(1/31)	19	(12/64)	6.3
Southeast Minnesota	4	(1/27)	17	(6/36)	4.3
Northeast Minnesota	2	(3/118)	10	(8/81)	5.0
Wisconsin	4	(32/893)	11	(33/304)	3.3

*Values represent survival rate (in percent); numbers in parentheses represent actual fraction of patients who had ventricular fibrillation.

Reproduced from Cummins,[13] with permission from Elsevier.

general estimates of survival among patients who receive different interventions ("links in the chain") at different intervals. Figure 28A shows what happens when the patient receives no CPR and delayed defibrillation is provided 10 minutes after collapse. A dismal survival rate of 0% to 2% is all that can be expected. Figure 28B shows an improvement in survival to 2% to 8% because a witness started CPR 2 minutes after collapse, but early defibrillation was still missing. Figure 28C shows a jump in survival to 20% because the witness who called 911 started CPR and because this particular community had an early defibrillation program that delivered the first shock at 6 to 7 minutes. Figure 28D demonstrates what can occur with a very early public defibrillation program. The witness calls 911, starts CPR, and delivers the first shock using an AED, at 4 to 5 minutes. Estimates are based on a large number of published studies, which were collectively reviewed by Eisenberg et al.[14,15]

Some EMS systems organized in this manner have reported survival rates as high as 30%, and studies of lay provider AED programs in airports and casinos and first-responder programs with police officers have demonstrated 41% to 74% survival from out-of-hospital witnessed VF SCA when immediate bystander CPR is provided and defibrillation occurs within 3 to 5 minutes of collapse.[16,17] These high survival rates, however, are not attained in programs that fail to reduce time to defibrillation.[13-15]

Time: The Major Determinant of Survival

The major determinant of survival in each study in Tables 7 and 8 was time, or more precisely, the interval between collapse and delivery of the first shock. It is now well established that the earlier defibrillation occurs, the better the prognosis. Emergency personnel have only a few minutes after the collapse of a patient to reestablish a perfusing rhythm. Restoration of a sustained adequate perfusing rhythm requires defibrillation, which must be administered within a few minutes of the initial arrest, and advanced cardiac care provided in a timely manner.

Immediate CPR for Witnessed Arrest

Survival rates from cardiac arrest can be remarkably high if the event is witnessed. For example, when people in supervised cardiac rehabilitation programs suffer a witnessed cardiac arrest, defibrillation is usually performed within the first minutes after VF has occurred. In studies of cardiac arrest in this setting, approximately 90% of patients were resuscitated.[18,19] No other studies with a defined out-of-hospital population have observed survival rates this high.

If bystanders provide immediate CPR, many adults in VF can survive with intact neurologic function, especially if defibrillation is performed within 5 to 10 minutes after SCA. CPR prolongs VF, delays the onset of asystole, and extends the window of time during which defibrillation can occur. Basic CPR alone, however, will not terminate VF and restore a perfusing rhythm.

Critical Concept **Time From Collapse to Shock**	The major determinant of survival in early studies was the interval between collapse and delivery of the first shock. It is now well established that the earlier defibrillation occurs, the better the prognosis.

Table 8. Survival to Hospital Discharge From Cardiac Arrest by System Type: Data From 29 Locations*

System Type	Survival: All Rhythms	Weighted Average	Survival: Ventricular Fibrillation	Weighted Average
EMT only	2-9	5	3-20	12
EMT-D	4-19	10	6-26	16
Paramedic	7-18	10	13-30	17
EMT/paramedic	4-26	17	23-33	26
EMT-D/paramedic	13-18	17	27-29	29

Abbreviations: EMT, emergency medical technician; EMT-D, emergency medical technician-defibrillation.

*Values are the range of survival rates (%) for all rhythms and ventricular fibrillation and the weighted average of each range.

Data from Eisenberg et al.[14]

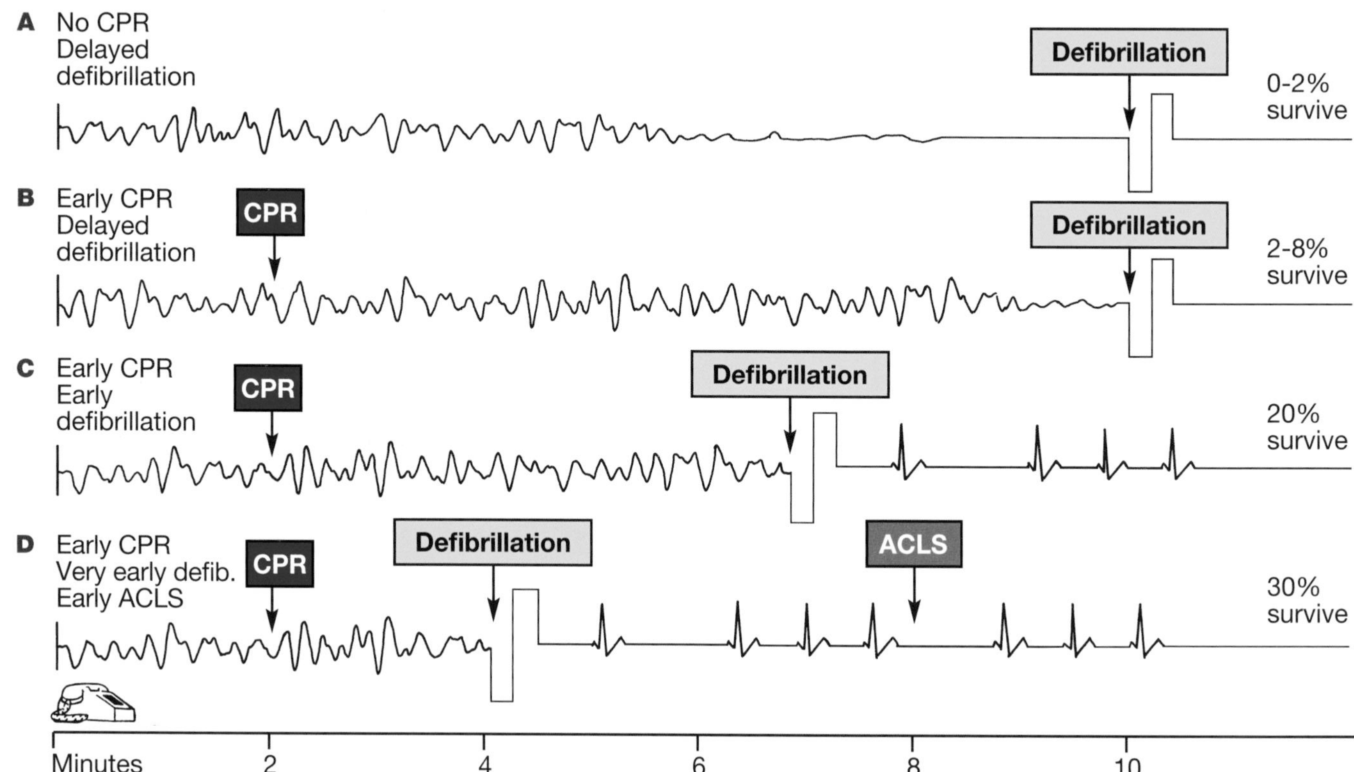

Figure 28. Estimated rates of survival to hospital discharge for patients with witnessed ventricular fibrillation arrest based on presence or absence of Chain of Survival links.

The 3-Phase Model of Cardiac Arrest

When VF causes cardiac arrest, 3 general phases of arrest occur: an electrical phase, a hemodynamic phase, and a metabolic phase (Figure 29).[20] Early defibrillation is critical in the electrical phase. In the hemodynamic phase, perfusion pressure to the heart and brain are very important. A brief period of CPR may "prime the pump" and provide a small but significant amount of oxygen and energy substrate. In the metabolic phase, the cardiac energy stores—adenosine triphosphate (ATP)—are depleted, and cellular damage and stunning are present.

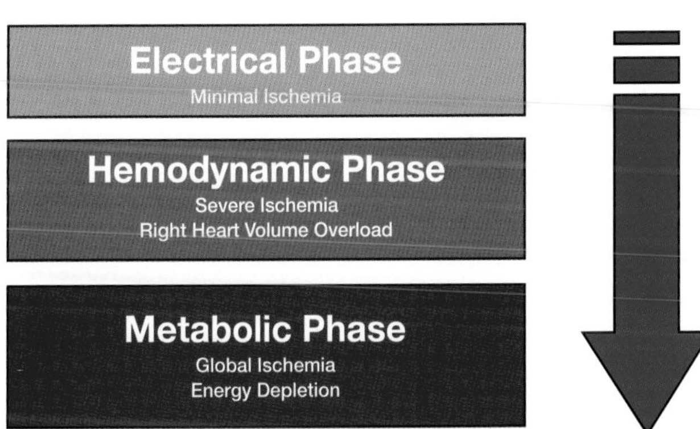

Figure 29. When cardiac arrest occurs due to ventricular fibrillation (VF), 3 phases can be proposed: an initial electrical phase, when early defibrillation is critical; a hemodynamic phase, when perfusion pressure to the heart and brain is very important; and a metabolic phase, when adenosine triphosphate is depleted and cellular damage and stunning are present. Adapted from Weisfeldt and Becker.[20]

Successful defibrillation depends on the electrical and metabolic state of the myocardium, the amount of myocardial damage that occurs during hypoxic arrest, the prior functional state of the heart, and the cause of VF. From a metabolic perspective, VF depletes more ATP per minute than does normal sinus rhythm. Prolonged VF will exhaust the energy stores of ATP in the myocardium, particularly in the cardiac pacemaker cells. The longer VF persists, the greater the myocardial deterioration as energy stores become exhausted. In a heart stunned into electrical silence by a defibrillatory shock, no spontaneous contractions will resume if the fibrillating myocardium has consumed all its energy stores. In the metabolic phase, when ATP is depleted and cellular functions are disrupted, shocks are more likely to convert VF to asystole than to a spontaneous rhythm because no "fuel" remains to support spontaneous depolarization in the pacemaker tissues or the contracting myocardium. With depleted reserves of energy, any postshock *asystole* or *agonal rhythms* will be permanent, not temporary. For this reason, VF of short duration is much more likely to respond to a shock delivered soon after VF starts.

An important objective for resuscitation and for any effort to improve outcome is shortening the interval between the onset of VF and the first shock. Therefore, rapid defibrillation is the treatment of choice for VF of short duration, such as for victims of witnessed out-of-hospital cardiac arrest or for hospitalized patients whose heart rhythm is being monitored. The *2010 AHA Guidelines for CPR and ECC* state that survival rates from VF are highest when immediate CPR is provided and defibrillation occurs within 3 to 5 minutes of collapse. In monitored patients, the time from VF to defibrillation should be under 3 minutes.

VF—Shock First or CPR First?

A healthcare provider should start CPR and use the AED as soon as possible when that provider

- Treats cardiac arrest in hospitals and other facilities where AEDs are onsite
- Witnesses an out-of-hospital arrest, and an AED is immediately available onsite

This recommendation will provide early CPR and early defibrillation during the electrical phase and possibly prolong the period when immediate defibrillation has the best chance of success. However, there is insufficient evidence to recommend for or against delaying defibrillation to provide CPR for patients in VF/pulseless VT out-of-hospital cardiac arrest. In all cases where there is more than one rescuer, CPR should be performed while a defibrillator is being acquired or readied.

For an out-of-hospital cardiac arrest that is not witnessed by EMS personnel, the *2010 AHA Guidelines for CPR and ECC* recommend that EMS personnel may give 5 cycles (about 2 minutes) of CPR before checking the ECG rhythm and attempting defibrillation. One cycle of CPR consists of 30 compressions and 2 breaths. When compressions are delivered at a rate of at least 100/min, 5 cycles of CPR should take roughly 2 minutes. This recommendation takes into account the delay inherent in the EMS call time and response. Almost all patients treated out of hospital by EMS providers will be in the hemodynamic or metabolic phase of cardiac arrest. EMS system medical directors may consider implementing a protocol that would allow EMS responders to provide 5 cycles of CPR before defibrillation of patients found by EMS personnel to be in VF.

Two studies showed that, when EMS call-to-arrival intervals were 4 to 5 minutes or longer, patients who had received 1½ to 3 minutes of CPR before defibrillation had higher rates of initial resuscitation, survival to hospital discharge, and 1-year

Critical Concept **Shock First or CPR First?**	• When any provider witnesses an out-of-hospital or in-hospital cardiac arrest and an AED is immediately available onsite, the provider should start CPR and use the AED as soon as possible. • When an out-of-hospital cardiac arrest is not witnessed by EMS personnel, EMS personnel may give about 5 cycles (about 2 minutes) of CPR before checking the ECG rhythm and attempting defibrillation.

survival when compared with those who had received immediate defibrillation for VF SCA.[21,22] More evaluation is needed, however, because 1 randomized study found no benefit to CPR before defibrillation for non–paramedic-witnessed SCA.[23]

Cobb et al noted that as more first responders were equipped with AEDs, survival rates from SCA unexpectedly fell.[21] This decline was attributed to a reduced emphasis on CPR, and there is growing evidence to support this view.

AEDs

AEDs are sophisticated, reliable computerized devices that use voice and visual prompts to guide lay providers and healthcare providers to defibrillate VF SCA safely. Modified prototype AEDs that record information about the frequency and depth of chest compressions during CPR are being tested. If such devices become commercially available, AEDs may one day prompt providers to improve CPR performance and provide high-quality chest compressions with minimal interruption. An analysis of the VF waveform may also guide whether to perform CPR first or provide an immediate shock.

AEDs have microprocessors that analyze multiple features of the surface ECG signal that is displayed as a rhythm on a monitor. This signal is complex and includes frequency, amplitude, and some integration of frequency and amplitude, such as slope or wave morphology. Filters check for artifacts such as QRS-like signals, radio transmission, or 50-cycle or 60-cycle interference, as well as loose electrodes and poor electrode contact (Figure 30).

AEDs have been tested extensively, both in experiments using libraries of recorded cardiac rhythms and clinically in many field trials in both adults and children. They are extremely accurate in rhythm analysis. AEDs are not designed to deliver synchronized shocks and will not perform cardioversion (eg, for VT with pulses or supraventricular tachycardia [SVT]). AEDs will recommend a shock (nonsynchronized) for monomorphic and polymorphic VT if the rate and R-wave morphology exceed preset values.

Manual Defibrillation

Successful defibrillation requires the delivery of enough energy to generate sufficient current flow through the heart to terminate VF, but the operator must avoid delivering excess current, which may cause significant myocardial damage. Myocardial damage or stunning may cause postarrest myocardial dysfunction. A few terms in basic electricity help with understanding defibrillation and these concepts (Table 9 and Figure 31). A defibrillatory shock passes a large flow of charged particles (electrons) through the heart over a brief period. This flow of electricity is called *current*, which is measured in *amperes*. The *pressure* pushing this flow of electrons is the electrical *potential*, measured in *volts*. There is always a *resistance* to this flow of electrons, called *impedance*, measured in *ohms*. In short, electrons flow (*current, amperes*) with a *pressure (volts)* for a period of *time* (usually *milliseconds*) through a substance that has *resistance (impedance, ohms)*. A typical shock will terminate VF within 400 to 500 milliseconds of shock delivery.

Table 9. Electrical Nomenclature and Equations to Help Understand Defibrillation

Ohm's Law: the potential must overcome impedance or no electrons will flow (current):
Current (amperes) = Potential (volts) ÷ Impedance (ohms)
Power is a measure of the current flowing with a certain force:
Power (watts) = Potential (volts) × Current (amperes)
Energy is a measure of power delivered over a period of time:
Energy (joules) = Power (watts) × Duration (seconds)
OR
Energy (joules) = Potential (volts) × Current (amperes) × Duration (seconds)

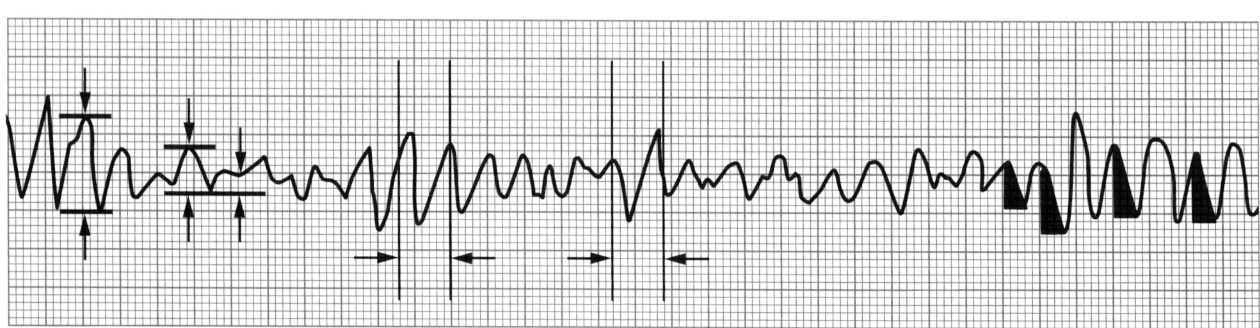

Figure 30. Features of the surface electrocardiogram analyzed by automated external defibrillators. Vertical arrows indicate amplitude, horizontal arrows indicate frequency, and black wedges indicate morphology.

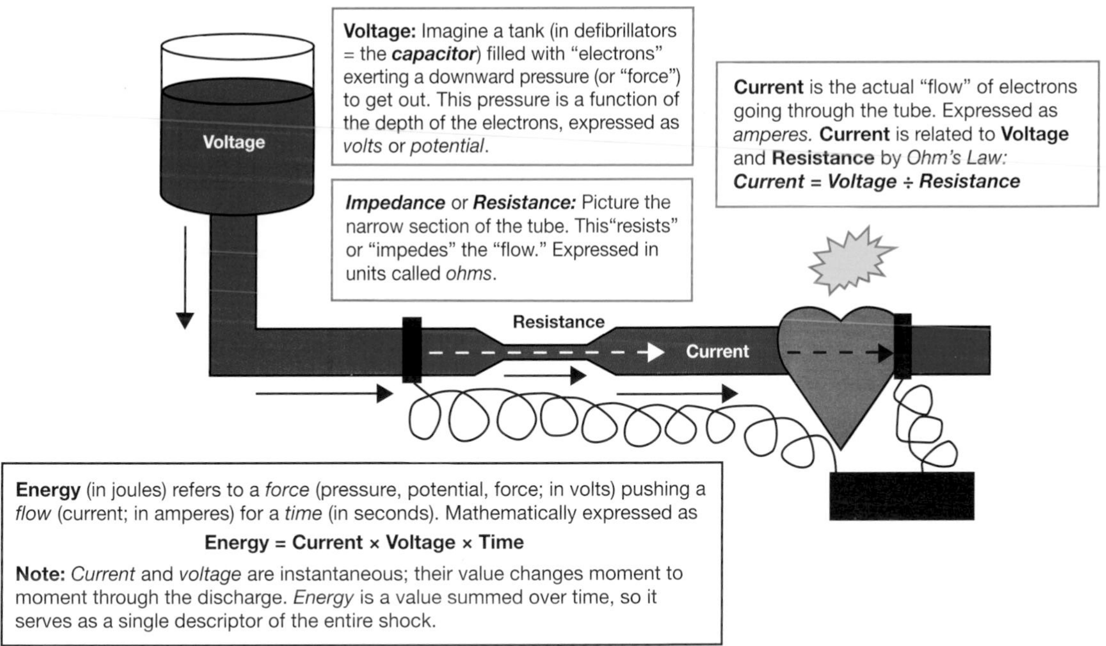

Voltage: Imagine a tank (in defibrillators = the capacitor) filled with "electrons" exerting a downward pressure (or "force") to get out. This pressure is a function of the depth of the electrons, expressed as volts or potential.
Current is the actual "flow" of electrons going through the tube. Expressed as amperes. Current is related to Voltage and Resistance by Ohm's Law: Current = Voltage ÷ Resistance
Voltage
Impedance or Resistance: Picture the narrow section of the tube. This"resists" or "impedes" the "flow." Expressed in units called ohms.
Resistance
Current
Energy (in joules) refers to a force (pressure, potential, force; in volts) pushing a flow (current; in amperes) for a time (in seconds). Mathematically expressed as
Energy = Current × Voltage × Time
Note: Current and voltage are instantaneous; their value changes moment to moment through the discharge. Energy is a value summed over time, so it serves as a single descriptor of the entire shock.

Figure 31. This diagram depicts some basic principles of electricity. This physics model has been called the "hydraulic model" of electricity because it depicts the flow of electrons during electrical current as the flow of water through a series of pipes. This model is a metaphorical memory aid only. It would be incorrect to think that the heart between 2 paddles in the figure has water flowing through it.

What Really Defibrillates the Heart?

Although the defibrillator operator selects the shock energy (in joules), it is the current flow (in amperes) through the heart that actually defibrillates. Defibrillation is achieved by generating an amplitude of current flow and sustaining that flow for a time interval. Current amplitude, shock duration, and how the current amplitude changes over that interval interact in complex ways to determine how a given shock will defibrillate.

Scientific researchers in this area speak more precisely in terms of *current density* as the key to defibrillation. Current density is the ratio of the magnitude of current flowing through a conductor to the cross-sectional area perpendicular to the current flow; it is expressed as current flow per unit of area (amperes/cm^2). Current density is a concept that will help in understanding the differences in defibrillation efficacy among different types of waveforms, such as monophasic and biphasic, discussed later in this chapter. Current density, in part dependent on the selected shock dose, differs from the amount of current passing through the heart. This *fractional transmyocardial current* is completely independent of the selected shock dose; it is determined more by pad- or paddle-position and thoracic anatomy.

Some of the nomenclature used in association with defibrillation can be confusing. VF is defined as chaotic, disorganized, and rapid depolarizations and repolarizations in multiple locations throughout the ventricles. The term *defibrillation* (shock success) is typically defined as termination of VF for at least 5 seconds following the shock, and it should not be equated with resuscitation success. The dominant hypothesis of the mechanism of defibrillation holds that a shock totally depolarizes every myocardial cellular membrane. When the shock achieves this total electrical neutrality across most or all of the heart, VF is abolished and *defibrillation* has been achieved.

In the strictest sense, *success* for a shock that attempts defibrillation is simply termination of VF; it has nothing to do with return of spontaneous electrical complexes, cardiac contractions, and circulation. Although return of spontaneous circulation (ROSC) is a critical point in the resuscitation process, it is influenced by multiple factors besides the ability of a shock to terminate fibrillation.

Transthoracic Impedance

Ohm's Law defines a relationship between current, voltage, and impedance (Current = Voltage ÷ Impedance). A study of this relationship reveals that the operator can have more of a direct effect on transthoracic impedance than on any other aspect of defibrillation. Many factors determine transthoracic impedance. The factors that affect current transmission through the chest include energy selected, electrode size, quality of electrode-to-skin contact, number and time interval of previous shocks, electrode-skin coupling material, phase of ventilation, distance between electrodes (size of the chest), and electrode-to-chest contact pressure. Studies have established a wide range of normal for human transthoracic impedance (15 to 150 ohms); the average for an adult is about 70 to 80 ohms. If transthoracic impedance is too high, a low-energy shock will not generate enough current passing through the chest and heart to achieve defibrillation.

Defibrillation Waveforms and Energy Requirements for Defibrillation of VF

Defibrillation success, as defined and discussed above, depends on selecting an appropriate energy setting to generate a sufficient current density throughout the heart to stop the fibrillation while causing minimal electrical injury. Electrical injury is important because it can cause postarrest myocardial dysfunction. Because the fractional transmyocardial current will affect the current density generated throughout the heart, positioning of the defibrillation pads or paddles is critically important. (This topic is discussed in more detail later in this chapter.) A shock will not terminate the arrhythmia if the selected energy and the resulting transmyocardial current flow are too low, yet functional and histologic damage may result if the energy and current are too high.

Selection of the appropriate current will both reduce the need for multiple shocks and limit the myocardial damage per shock. Although the relationship between body size and energy requirements for defibrillation has been hotly debated for decades, there is no fixed relationship. The critical relationships have to do with the fractional transmyocardial current (defined by the thoracic pathway between the 2 defibrillator electrodes and the position of the heart in that pathway) and the impedance to current flow from pad to pad. These relationships in combination determine the current density throughout the heart and thus the ultimate effect of the shock. In adults the body mass surrounding the thoracic current pathway plays only a minimal role.

Defibrillation Waveforms Overview

Modern defibrillators, including AEDs, deliver energy or current in *waveforms*. There are 2 broad categories of waveforms, monophasic and biphasic (Figure 32). Energy settings and their associated delivered current levels vary with the type of device and type of waveform. Monophasic waveforms (Figure 32A) deliver current in primarily one direction (polarity). Biphasic waveforms deliver current that flows in a positive direction for a specified duration. The current then reverses and flows in a negative direction for the remaining milliseconds of the electrical discharge (Figure 32B and 32C). The first phase of the biphasic waveform "prepares" the cell membrane for uniform depolarization when the second phase occurs.

Defibrillators can also vary the speed of both waveform rise and return to zero voltage point. A monophasic waveform that rises sharply and returns gradually is a *damped sinusoidal waveform* (Figure 32A). A waveform that rises sharply and then is cut off abruptly is a *truncated exponential waveform* (Figure 32C). Few monophasic waveform defibrillators are being manufactured, but many are still in use, and most use *monophasic damped sinusoidal waveforms*.

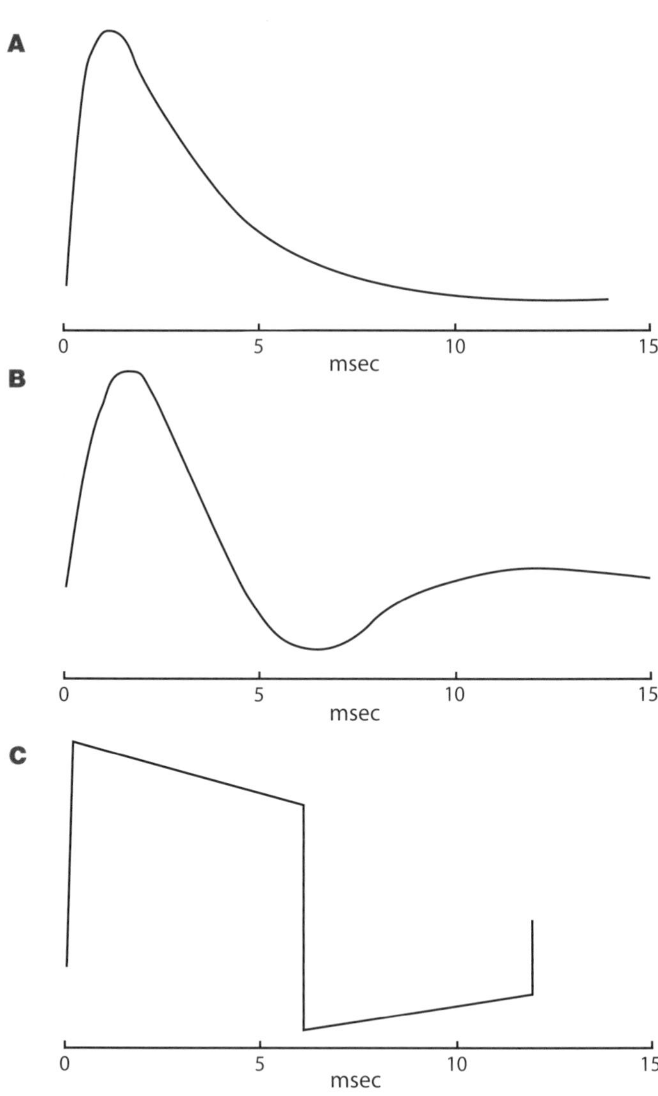

Figure 32. Voltage transition of 3 different defibrillation waveforms. **A,** Critically damped, sinusoidal monophasic; **B,** quasi-sinusoidal biphasic; and **C,** truncated exponential biphasic. Reproduced from Walcott et al.[24]

Biphasic waveforms were proven superior to monophasic waveforms when used in implantable defibrillators. The mechanisms underlying the superiority and greater efficacy of biphasic waveforms are still a subject of scientific investigation and debate. The most salient characteristic of biphasic waveforms is their ability to defibrillate with a significantly lower myocardial current density than monophasic waveforms. This characteristic provides a distinct advantage in transthoracic defibrillation, where the factors affecting the biphasic truncated exponential current density are either imprecise, such as pad position, or unknown, such as the exact intrathoracic anatomy or current pathways. No specific waveform (either monophasic or biphasic), however, is consistently associated with a higher rate of ROSC or rates of survival to hospital discharge after cardiac arrest.

Monophasic Waveform Defibrillators

Monophasic waveforms deliver current of one polarity (ie, direction of current flow). Monophasic waveforms can be further categorized by the rate at which the current pulse decreases to zero. The monophasic damped sinusoidal (MDS) waveform returns to zero gradually; whereas the monophasic truncated exponential (MTE) waveform abruptly returns to zero. Rescuers using monophasic defibrillators should give an initial shock of 360 J; if VF persists after the first shock, second and subsequent shocks of 360 J should be given. This single dose for monophasic shocks is designed to simplify instructions to rescuers but is not a mandate to recall monophasic AEDs for reprogramming. After shock delivery, rescuers should not delay resumption of chest compression. After 5 cycles of CPR, the AED should then analyze the cardiac rhythm and deliver another shock if indicated.

Shortening the interval between the last compression and the shock by even a few seconds can improve shock success (defibrillation and ROSC). Therefore, healthcare providers should practice efficient coordination between CPR and defibrillation to minimize the hands-off interval between stopping compression and administering shock. For example, when 2 rescuers are present, the rescuer operating the AED should be prepared to deliver a shock as soon as the compressor removes his or her hands from the victim's chest and all rescuers are "clear" of contact with the victim. Additionally, rescue breathing prior to the shock will increase the time from compression to shock, and thus it is reasonable to proceed immediately to shock without rescue breathing.

Few monophasic waveform defibrillators are being manufactured, but many are still in use. Most of these use MDS waveforms. Research indicates, however, that when doses equivalent to, or lower than, monophasic doses are used, biphasic waveform shocks are safe and effective for termination of VF.

Biphasic Waveform Defibrillators

Researchers have collected data from both out-of-hospital and in-hospital studies (electrophysiologic studies and ICD testing and evaluation). Overall this research indicates that lower-energy biphasic waveform shocks have equivalent or higher success for termination of VF than either MDS or MTE waveform shocks delivering escalating energy (200 J, 300 J, and 360 J) with successive shocks. No direct comparison of the different biphasic waveforms has been made.

The optimal energy for first-shock biphasic waveform defibrillation that yields the highest termination rate for VF has not been determined. Several randomized and observational studies have shown that defibrillation with biphasic waveforms of relatively low energy (200 J or less) is safe and has equivalent or higher efficacy for termination of VF than monophasic waveform shocks of equivalent or higher energy. Until more is known, providers should consult the recommendations of the manufacturer of their biphasic defibrillator.

Compensation for patient-to-patient differences in impedance may be achieved by changes in duration and voltage of shocks or by releasing the residual membrane charge (called *burping*). Whether there is an optimal ratio of first-phase to second-phase duration and leading-edge amplitude is unclear. It is unknown whether a waveform more effective for *immediate outcomes* (defibrillation) and *short-term outcomes* (ROSC, survival to hospital admission) results in better *long-term outcomes* (survival to hospital discharge, survival for 1 year). Given the high efficacy of all biphasic waveforms, other determinants of survival (eg, interval from collapse to CPR or defibrillation) are likely to supersede the impact of specific waveforms or energies.

Because different biphasic waveforms have not been compared in humans with regard to efficacy, providers should use the manufacturer's recommended energy dose (120 to 200 J). If the manufacturer's recommended dose is not known, the provider should consider defibrillation at the maximum dose. In the absence of biphasic defibrillators, the use of monophasic defibrillators is acceptable.

Commercially available biphasic AEDs provide either fixed or escalating energy levels. Multiple prospective and retrospective human clinical studies[25-33] have failed to identify an optimal biphasic energy level for first or subsequent shocks. However, human studies[33,34] did not demonstrate evidence of harm from any biphasic waveform defibrillation energy up to 360 J. Harm was defined as elevated biomarker levels, ECG findings, and reduced ejection fraction. Conversely, several animal studies[35-37] have shown the potential for myocardial damage with much higher energy shocks. Therefore, no definitive recommendation for the selected energy for subsequent biphasic defibrillation has been made. However, based on available evidence, the AHA recommends that second and subsequent energy levels should be at least equivalent, and higher energy levels, if available, may be considered.

Current-based defibrillation has been assessed and in one study was superior to energy-based defibrillation with monophasic waveforms.[38] The range of current necessary to achieve defibrillation and cardioversion by using MDS waveform shocks appears to be 30 to 40 A MDS. Comparable information on current dose for biphasic waveform shocks is under investigation. Transition to current-based defibrillation is timely and should be encouraged.

Pads, Paddles, and Positions

Placement of pads or paddles for defibrillation and cardioversion is an important, but often neglected, topic. Pads should be placed in a position that will maximize current flow through the myocardium. This fractional transmyocardial current affects the current density generated in the heart. It has been estimated that even with properly placed paddles, only 4% to 25% of the delivered current actually passes through the heart. The recommended placement is termed either *sternal-apical* or *anterior-apex* (Figure 33). The sternal (or anterior) electrode is placed to the right of the upper part of the sternum below the clavicle.

An acceptable alternative approach is to place one paddle anteriorly over the left apex (precordium) and the other posteriorly behind the heart, in the left infrascapular location. Either pathway will maximize current flow through the cardiac chambers and is reasonable for defibrillation, but for ease of placement and education, anterolateral is a reasonable default electrode placement. Alternative pad positions may be considered based on individual patient characteristics.

Defibrillation Considerations for Patients With a Pacemaker or ICD

When performing cardioversion or defibrillation in patients with permanent pacemakers or ICDs, do not place the electrodes over or in close proximity to the device generator, because defibrillation can cause pacemaker malfunction. A pacemaker or ICD (indicated by a lump or scar) also may block some current to the myocardium during defibrillation, causing delivery of suboptimal energy to the heart.

Previous recommendations for electrode pads recommended placement of the pad at least 1 inch (2.5 cm) away from the device. Finally, because some of the defibrillation current flows down the pacemaker leads, permanent pacemakers and ICDs should be reevaluated after the patient receives a shock.

A recent study evaluated the safety of external electrical cardioversion of atrial fibrillation in patients having a variety of permanent pacemakers and ICDs that had been implanted in either the right or left infraclavicular regions. Cardioversion electrodes were uniformly placed strictly in the anterior-posterior position (to the right of the sternum with the upper edge of the electrode at the fourth anterior

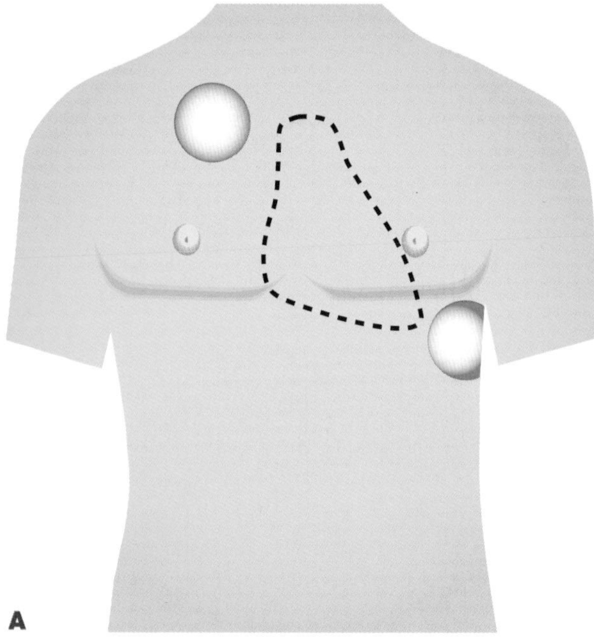

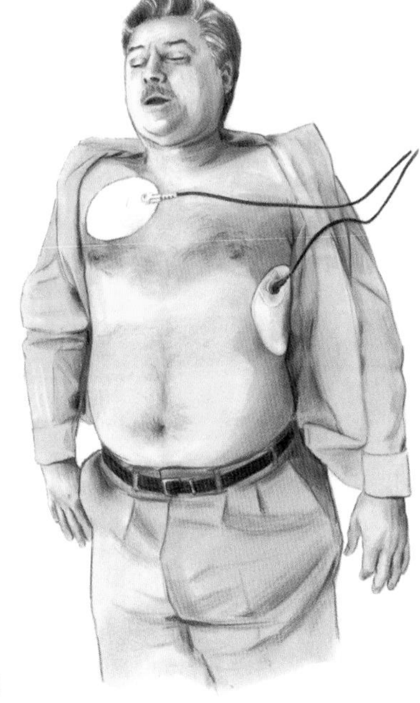

Figure 33. **A** and **B,** Recommended sternal-apex positions for placement of adhesive defibrillation pads or defibrillation paddles. Place the anterior electrode to the right of the upper sternum below the clavicle. Place the apex electrode to the left of the nipple with the center of the electrode in the midaxillary line.

intercostal space; and to the left of the patient's spine at the midscapular level posteriorly). In addition, the anterior electrode was kept a minimum of 8 cm (approximately 3 inches) away from the implanted device. These precautions assured both a safe distance of shock electrodes away from the pacemaker or ICD and a shock direction that was perpendicular to the orientation of the implanted lead systems. Both biphasic and monophasic waveform escalating synchronized shocks were deployed, ranging from 100 to 200 J and 200 to 360 J, respectively, including multiple shocks, if required, each separated by a 5-minute interval. No device or lead dysfunction resulting from cardioversion was observed in any patient.[39]

Placement of external shock electrodes in patients with an ICD is identical to those having a permanent pacemaker, described above. Some patients with older ICD systems may have epicardial defibrillation electrodes and an ICD generator implanted in the abdomen rather than a pectoral location. In this instance, external defibrillator electrodes may be placed in their traditional (right anterior to left anterolateral [at the heart apex]) positions, so long as each is a safe distance from the ICD generator, without the need for other special precautions. A theoretical concern in this instance is whether the epicardial defibrillator electrodes may insulate the heart from external shock and require higher energy settings in order to defibrillate successfully. In such instances, external cardioversion or defibrillation should default to using high energy settings.

If the patient has an ICD that is delivering shocks (ie, the patient's muscles contract as they do during external defibrillation), allow 30 to 60 seconds for the ICD to complete the treatment cycle before attaching a defibrillator. In general an ICD will likely have delivered its full complement of therapies within a few minutes of the patient's collapse. Thus, when encountering an unconscious, pulseless patient with an ICD, the most likely scenario is that the device has exhausted all of its therapies and failed to terminate the arrhythmia. All standard treatment measures should be initiated by providers, as though an implanted device were not present, including external defibrillation. However, ICDs require the same precautions as those required for patients with pacemakers when external shocks are administered. In particular, providers should note where the ICD generator and leads are located and place external defibrillation electrodes accordingly. Although ICD generators, unlike pacemakers, are better protected from high-energy shock by specialized high-voltage circuitry, they are nonetheless susceptible to the same spectrum of damage. It is therefore advised by manufacturers, as with pacemakers, that defibrillator electrodes should be placed at least 8 cm away from the ICD when possible, and shocks should be administered perpendicular to the orientation of the ICD leads and the heart.

Occasionally the analysis and shock cycles of ICDs and AEDs will conflict. ICDs and AEDs both deploy automated arrhythmia detection algorithms. This can lead to "back-to-back" shocks should the ICD and AED simultaneously detect a shockable arrhythmia. In such instances, providers should recognize the sudden muscular contraction that identifies receipt of an ICD shock and, if possible, be prepared to inhibit AED shock delivery. In addition, ICDs deploy both bradycardia pacing and antitachycardia pacing, which can in theory mislead the AED detection algorithm as to the nature of the patient's rhythm. Switching to a manual external defibrillator mode can circumvent such issues once providers with rhythm recognition skills are on scene.

In-Hospital Use of AEDs

Higher rates of survival to hospital discharge were reported when AEDs were used to treat adult VF or pulseless VT in the hospital. Defibrillation may be delayed when patients develop SCA in unmonitored hospital beds and in outpatient and diagnostic facilities. In such areas, several minutes may elapse before centralized response teams arrive with the defibrillator, attach it, and deliver shocks. Early defibrillation capability should be available in ambulatory care facilities, as well as throughout hospital inpatient areas. A study of 11 695 hospitalized patients with cardiac arrests at 204 US hospitals following the introduction of AEDs on general hospital wards found that AED use was not associated with improved survival to discharge in hospitalized patients with cardiac arrest. AED use was associated with a lower rate of survival in cardiac arrests due to nonshockable rhythms (80% of the in-hospital SCA) and was not linked to improved survival or shorter times to defibrillation in cardiac arrests due to shockable rhythms.[40] The authors indicated that earlier studies had conflicting results probably because they were limited by the small samples studied. Hospitals should monitor collapse-to–first shock intervals and resuscitation outcomes. The goal should be to provide the first shock for any SCA within 3 minutes of collapse.

Mistakes in Pad Position

One of the most common errors in pad placement is placing the pads too close together. In Figure 34A the apex paddle is in the proper position in the midaxillary line, which allows all the current to flow through the myocardium to achieve defibrillation. Figure 34B displays a cross-section of the heart and thorax showing how most of the current bypasses the heart when the paddles are placed too close together. Notice also that the sternal paddle is indeed over the sternum, which blocks much of the current flow.

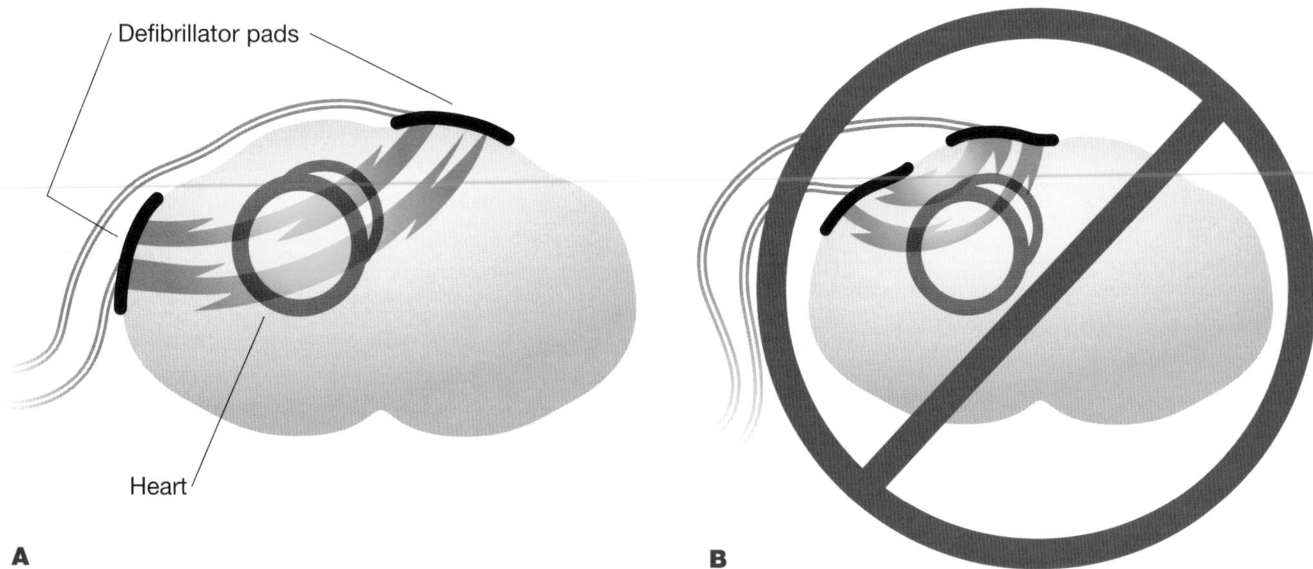

Figure 34. **A,** Current pathway through the chest and heart with placement of pads (or paddles) for defibrillation. **B,** Current pathway when the paddles are placed too closely together. Modified from Ewy GA, Bressler R, eds. *Cardiovascular Drugs and the Management of Heart Disease*. New York, NY: Raven Press; 1982.

Electrode Size

For adult defibrillation, both handheld paddle electrodes and self-adhesive pad electrodes 8 to 12 cm in diameter perform well, although defibrillation success may be higher with electrodes 12 cm in diameter rather than with those 8 cm in diameter. Small electrodes (4.3 cm) may be harmful and may cause myocardial necrosis. When using handheld paddles and gel or pads, rescuers must ensure that the paddle is in full contact with the skin. Even smaller pads have been found to be effective in VF of brief duration. Use of the smallest (pediatric) pads, however, can result in unacceptably high transthoracic impedance in larger children.

Synchronized Cardioversion

Synchronized cardioversion is shock delivery that is timed (synchronized) with the QRS complex. This synchronization avoids shock delivery during the relative refractory portion of the cardiac cycle, when a shock could produce VF. Synchronized cardioversion is recommended to treat SVT due to reentry, atrial fibrillation, atrial flutter, and atrial tachycardia. Electrical therapy for VT is discussed in Chapter 8: Part 1.

Pacing

Pacing is not effective for asystolic cardiac arrest and may delay or interrupt the delivery of chest compressions. Healthcare providers should be prepared to initiate pacing in patients who do not respond to atropine (or second-line drugs if these do not delay definitive management). If the patient does not respond to drugs or transcutaneous pacing, it is reasonable to initiate transvenous pacing. Pacing is discussed in Chapter 8: Part 2, Chapter 9, and Chapter 10.

Safety During Operation of a Defibrillator

Providers should make sure that the pads are separate and not touching. Touching pads or smearing of the paste or gel may allow current to follow a superficial pathway (arc) along the chest wall, "missing" the heart. Self-adhesive monitor/defibrillator electrode pads are as effective as gel pads or paste, and they can be placed before cardiac arrest to allow for monitoring and then rapid administration of an initial shock when necessary.[41] As a result, self-adhesive pads should be used routinely instead of standard paddles. Remember that the principles discussed above for correct placement also apply to pads. An improperly placed pad can decrease chances of successful defibrillation.

Do not place electrodes directly on top of a transdermal medication patch (eg, patches containing nitroglycerin, nicotine, analgesics, hormone replacements, or antihypertensives), because the patch may block delivery of energy from the electrode pad to the heart and may cause small burns to the skin. Remove medication patches and wipe the area before attaching the electrode pad.

If an unresponsive patient is lying in water or the chest is covered with water, remove the patient from the water and briskly wipe the chest dry before attaching electrode pads and attempting defibrillation. Defibrillation can be accomplished when a patient is lying on snow or ice.

Attempt to remove excess chest hair by briskly removing an electrode pad (which will remove some hair) or by rapidly shaving the chest in that area, provided chest compressions are not interrupted and defibrillation is not delayed.

Safety Concerns With an ICD in Place

Unlike external defibrillation, which typically deploys 150 to 360 J, the maximum shock output from an ICD is only a fraction of this level and ranges from 30 to 40 J, depending on the manufacturer. However, approximately 20% of an ICD's shock voltage may reach the patient's surface. Such voltage is not sufficient to cause harm to providers or others who are in contact with the patient at the time of ICD shock but may nonetheless be felt by them. The voltage is sufficiently small that the provider is more likely to feel the effect of abrupt muscle contraction when the patient is shocked than the electrical impulse itself. However, the degree of discomfort felt depends on where and how the provider may be in contact with the patient at the time of shock. Transmission of shock from the patient to the provider requires a 2-point contact to complete the electrical circuit, and a conductor (such as defibrillator paddle gel) that facilitates transmission of current between the patient and provider. Contact at only 1 location is unlikely to transmit shock to the provider unless, in addition, the provider and patient are grounded to one another (for example, both on a wet surface). For the typical "heel of hand" on the chest, with the second hand overlying the first during CPR, a relatively small single area is in contact with the patient, and shock risk is minimal. In addition, providers who use protective gloves during resuscitation are insulated from the patient and are unlikely to experience shock unless the integrity of the glove has been compromised. As a rule, apart from the location where defibrillator electrodes are placed, the presence of an ICD should not alter the handling of the patient in cardiac arrest.

Fire Hazard and Prevention

Several case reports have described fires ignited by sparks from poorly applied defibrillator paddles in the presence of an oxygen-enriched atmosphere. Severe fires have been reported when ventilator tubing is disconnected from the endotracheal tube and then left adjacent to the patient's head, blowing oxygen across the chest during attempted defibrillation.

The use of self-adhesive defibrillation pads is probably the best way to minimize the risk of sparks igniting during defibrillation. If manual paddles are used, gel pads are preferable to electrode pastes and gels because the pastes and gels can spread between the 2 paddles, creating the potential for a spark. Do not use medical gels or pastes with poor electrical conductivity, such as ultrasound gel.

Providers should take precautions to minimize sparking during attempted defibrillation; try to ensure that defibrillation is not attempted in an oxygen-enriched atmosphere. When ventilation is interrupted for shock delivery, providers should try to ensure that oxygen does not flow across the patient's chest during defibrillation attempts.

Defibrillator fires in oxygen-enriched environments, although rare, are an unacceptable danger to patients and healthcare providers. A defibrillator fire requires 3 fire-critical ingredients: an agent for flame propagation, an oxygen-enriched atmosphere close to the arc, and a source of ignition (an electrical arc). If any one is lacking, a fire cannot occur. Prevention of defibrillator fires is relatively simple: prevent a defibrillation error *or* prevent an oxygen-supply error. See "Recommendations for Prevention" in Table 10.[42,43]

Proposals to routinely turn off or disconnect the oxygen supply immediately before defibrillation[43] have generated controversy,[44] primarily because supplying oxygen is considered a higher priority than instituting time-consuming steps simply to prevent fires.[45] Much of this controversy loses clinical relevancy when providers focus on proper defibrillation techniques to prevent an electrical arc from ever occurring. As noted in Table 10, oxygen flow should be turned off and airway adjuncts disconnected for patients at higher risk for electrical arc formation. All ACLS providers and instructors can help generate greater awareness of this danger. Most important, though, is the lesson that simply by performing resuscitation procedures properly and effectively, defibrillator-associated fires will remain rare.

Maintaining Devices in a State of Readiness

Failure to properly maintain the defibrillator or power supply is responsible for the majority of reported malfunctions. Many currently available defibrillators do an automated check and display readiness. Checklists are useful when designed to identify and prevent such deficiencies; therefore, maintaining devices in a state of readiness is recommended.

Critical Concept **Defibrillation and High-Quality CPR**	Whenever defibrillation is attempted, rescuers must coordinate high-quality CPR with defibrillation to minimize interruptions in chest compressions and to ensure immediate resumption of chest compressions after shock delivery.

Table 10. Three Fire-Critical Ingredients: Common Errors That Supply Ingredients and Recommendations for Prevention

Required Ingredients	Ingredient Sources and Common Errors That Yield Ingredients	Recommendations for Prevention
1. Agent for flame propagation	• Fine surface body hair • Surface nap fibers on most fabrics • Fibers, dust, particulate matter suspended in the ambient air	• Move gown, pajamas from resuscitation area • Move bedding, drapes, curtains from immediate vicinity
2. Oxygen-enriched atmosphere close to electrical arc *("vicinity of potential ignition point")*	• Device for oxygen administration: – Left connected to open oxygen source – Placed close to defibrillation area *or* – Disconnected from oxygen source – Open oxygen source directed close to defibrillation area • "Pockets" of high oxygen concentration allowed to collect close to defibrillation area	• Always properly connect an airway adjunct to open oxygen supply lines • If oxygen is not properly connected to an airway adjunct or if the airway adjunct is not in use, then TURN OFF OXYGEN • If an airway device with oxygen flow must be set aside urgently, place it as far away from the chest as practical • Never let oxygen flow directly onto the chest surface during defibrillation • Consider turning off oxygen supply or disconnecting ventilation bag immediately before shock delivery • Always turn off and disconnect oxygen source in clinical scenarios with high risk of electrical arc (eg, irregular chest surface)
3. Electrical arc *("source of ignition")*	• Paddles not pushed evenly down against skin with force • Paddles "tipped" (paddle surface not parallel to skin surface) • No (or insufficient) conductive gel • Too much gel (smears across skin surface, contacting other paddle, ECG wires, or electrodes) • Hairy chest (pockets of air and gaps within hair between skin and paddles) • Irregular chest surface (eg, highly curved thorax, pectus excavatum, or depressed intercostal spaces between ribs secondary to cachexia) • Paddles or pads placed on or close to wires or monitoring electrodes • Adhesive pads for "hands-free" remote defibrillation dried out, folded, or not pressed down firmly • Adhesive metal "target pads" (on which paddles are placed): paddle overlaps edge of pad; pads dried out, folded, or not pressed down firmly • Prolonged resuscitations: gel rubs off; pads dry out	• Push paddles down firmly with at least 25 pounds of pressure • Make sure paddles are parallel to skin surface with no "tipping" or angles • Carefully apply sufficient conductive gel, specifically formulated for defibrillation, to cover paddle surface • Avoid excessive gel that spreads beyond the edges of the paddles • If excessive chest hair interferes with paddle-skin contact, clip or shave chest hair or consider extra gel (can sometimes fill in the spaces between skin, hair, and paddles) • For patients with an irregular chest surface, check carefully for gaps between paddle surface and skin • If gaps are not corrected by firmer paddle pressure, try kneading conductive gel into several 4" × 4" saline-moistened gauze pads; try defibrillation if "conductive gauze" bridges gaps • Avoid placing paddles or pads over or adjacent to ECG wires or electrodes • Make sure pads for "hands-free" defibrillation or metal "target" pads are not dried out, have no folds, and are at least the size of the defibrillator paddles (avoid overlap)

FAQ

Can you defibrillate in snow or ice or if the patient is wet?

If an unresponsive victim is lying in water or if the victim's chest is covered with water or the victim is extremely diaphoretic, it may be reasonable to remove the victim from water and briskly wipe the chest before attaching electrode pads and attempting defibrillation. Defibrillation can be accomplished when a patient is lying on snow or ice.

References

1. Kouwenhoven WB, Milnor WR, Knickerbocker GG, Chesnut WR. Closed chest defibrillation of the heart. *Surgery*. 1957;42:550-561.
2. Larsen MP, Eisenberg MS, Cummins RO, Hallstrom AP. Predicting survival from out-of-hospital cardiac arrest: a graphic model. *Ann Emerg Med*. 1993;22:1652-1658.
3. Valenzuela TD, Roe DJ, Cretin S, Spaite DW, Larsen MP. Estimating effectiveness of cardiac arrest interventions: a logistic regression survival model. *Circulation*. 1997;96:3308-3313.
4. Chan PS, Krumholz HM, Nichol G, Nallamothu BK. Delayed time to defibrillation after in-hospital cardiac arrest. *N Engl J Med*. 2008;358:9-17.
5. Stiell IG, Wells GA, Field B, Spaite DW, Nesbitt LP, De Maio VJ, Nichol G, Cousineau D, Blackburn J, Munkley D, Luinstra-Toohey L, Campeau T, Dagnone E, Lyver M. Advanced cardiac life support in out-of-hospital cardiac arrest. *N Engl J Med*. 2004;351:647-656.
6. Swor RA, Jackson RE, Cynar M, Sadler E, Basse E, Boji B, Rivera-Rivera EJ, Maher A, Grubb W, Jacobson R, et al. Bystander CPR, ventricular fibrillation, and survival in witnessed, unmonitored out-of-hospital cardiac arrest. *Ann Emerg Med*. 1995;25:780-784.
7. Holmberg M, Holmberg S, Herlitz J. Incidence, duration and survival of ventricular fibrillation in out-of-hospital cardiac arrest patients in Sweden. *Resuscitation*. 2000;44:7-17.
8. Eisenberg MS, Cummins RO. Defibrillation performed by the emergency medical technician. *Circulation*. 1986;74:IV9-IV12.
9. Stults KR, Brown DD, Schug VL, Bean JA. Prehospital defibrillation performed by emergency medical technicians in rural communities. *N Engl J Med*. 1984;310:219-223.
10. Vukov LF, White RD, Bachman JW, O'Brien PC. New perspectives on rural EMT defibrillation. *Ann Emerg Med*. 1988;17:318-321.
11. Bachman JW, McDonald GS, O'Brien PC. A study of out-of-hospital cardiac arrests in northeastern Minnesota. *JAMA*. 1986;256:477-483.
12. Olson DW, LaRochelle J, Fark D, Aprahamian C, Aufderheide TP, Mateer JR, Hargarten KM, Stueven HA. EMT-defibrillation: the Wisconsin experience. *Ann Emerg Med*. 1989;18:806-811.
13. Cummins RO. From concept to standard-of-care? Review of the clinical experience with automated external defibrillators. *Ann Emerg Med*. 1989;18:1269-1275.
14. Eisenberg MS, Horwood BT, Cummins RO, Reynolds-Haertle R, Hearne TR. Cardiac arrest and resuscitation: a tale of 29 cities. *Ann Emerg Med*. 1990;19:179-186.
15. Eisenberg MS, Cummins RO, Damon S, Larsen MP, Hearne TR. Survival rates from out-of-hospital cardiac arrest: recommendations for uniform definitions and data to report. *Ann Emerg Med*. 1990;19:1249-1259.
16. England H, Hoffman C, Hodgman T, Singh S, Homoud M, Weinstock J, Link M, Estes NA III. Effectiveness of automated external defibrillators in high schools in greater Boston. *Am J Cardiol*. 2005;95:1484-1486.
17. Rea TD, Olsufka M, Bemis B, White L, Yin L, Becker L, Copass M, Eisenberg M, Cobb L. A population-based investigation of public access defibrillation: role of emergency medical services care. *Resuscitation*. 2010;81:163-167.
18. Van Camp SP, Peterson RA. Cardiovascular complications of outpatient cardiac rehabilitation programs. *JAMA*. 1986;256:1160-1163.
19. Fletcher GF, Cantwell JD. Ventricular fibrillation in a medically supervised cardiac exercise program. Clinical, angiographic, and surgical correlations. *JAMA*. 1977;238:2627-2629.
20. Weisfeldt ML, Becker LB. Resuscitation after cardiac arrest: a 3-phase time-sensitive model. *JAMA*. 2002;288:3035-3038.
21. Cobb LA, Fahrenbruch CE, Walsh TR, Copass MK, Olsufka M, Breskin M, Hallstrom AP. Influence of cardiopulmonary resuscitation prior to defibrillation in patients with out-of-hospital ventricular fibrillation. *JAMA*. 1999;281:1182-1188.
22. Wik L, Hansen TB, Fylling F, Steen T, Vaagenes P, Auestad BH, Steen PA. Delaying defibrillation to give basic cardiopulmonary resuscitation to patients with out-of-hospital ventricular fibrillation: a randomized trial. *JAMA*. 2003;289:1389-1395.
23. Jacobs IG, Finn JC, Oxer HF, Jelinek GA. CPR before defibrillation in out-of-hospital cardiac arrest: a randomized trial. *Emerg Med Australas*. 2005;17:39-45.
24. Walcott GP, Melnick SB, Chapman FW, Jones JL, Smith WM, Ideker RE. Relative efficacy of monophasic and biphasic waveforms for transthoracic defibrillation after short and long durations of ventricular defibrillation. *Circulation*. 1998;98:2210-2215.
25. van Alem AP, Chapman FW, Lank P, Hart AA, Koster RW. A prospective, randomised and blinded comparison of first shock success of monophasic and biphasic waveforms in out-of-hospital cardiac arrest. *Resuscitation*. 2003;58:17-24.
26. Carpenter J, Rea TD, Murray JA, Kudenchuk PJ, Eisenberg MS. Defibrillation waveform and post-shock rhythm in out-of-hospital ventricular fibrillation cardiac arrest. *Resuscitation*. 2003;59:189-196.
27. Morrison LJ, Dorian P, Long J, Vermeulen M, Schwartz B, Sawadsky B, Frank J, Cameron B, Burgess R, Shield J, Bagley P, Mausz V, Brewer JE, Lerman BB. Out-of-hospital cardiac arrest rectilinear biphasic to monophasic damped sine defibrillation waveforms with advanced life support intervention trial (ORBIT). *Resuscitation*. 2005;66:149-157.
28. Schneider T, Martens PR, Paschen H, Kuisma M, Wolcke B, Gliner BE, Russell JK, Weaver WD, Bossaert L, Chamberlain D. Multicenter, randomized, controlled trial of 150-J biphasic shocks compared with 200- to 360-J monophasic shocks in the resuscitation of out-of-hospital cardiac arrest victims. Optimized Response to Cardiac Arrest (ORCA) Investigators. *Circulation*. 2000;102:1780-1787.
29. Stothert JC, Hatcher TS, Gupton CL, Love JE, Brewer JE. Rectilinear biphasic waveform defibrillation of out-of-hospital cardiac arrest. *Prehosp Emerg Care*. 2004;8:388-392.
30. Walsh SJ, McClelland AJ, Owens CG, Allen J, Anderson JM, Turner C, Adgey AA. Efficacy of distinct energy delivery protocols comparing two biphasic defibrillators for cardiac arrest. *Am J Cardiol*. 2004;94:378-380.

31. Gliner BE, Jorgenson DB, Poole JE, White RD, Kanz KG, Lyster TD, Leyde KW, Powers DJ, Morgan CB, Kronmal RA, Bardy GH. Treatment of out-of-hospital cardiac arrest with a low-energy impedance-compensating biphasic waveform automatic external defibrillator. The LIFE Investigators. *Biomed Instrum Technol*. 1998;32:631-644.
32. White RD, Russell JK. Refibrillation, resuscitation and survival in out-of-hospital sudden cardiac arrest victims treated with biphasic automated external defibrillators. *Resuscitation*. 2002;55:17-23.
33. Stiell IG, Walker RG, Nesbitt LP, Chapman FW, Cousineau D, Christenson J, Bradford P, Sookram S, Berringer R, Lank P, Wells GA. BIPHASIC Trial: a randomized comparison of fixed lower versus escalating higher energy levels for defibrillation in out-of-hospital cardiac arrest. *Circulation*. 2007;115:1511-1517.
34. Higgins SL, Herre JM, Epstein AE, Greer GS, Friedman PL, Gleva ML, Porterfield JG, Chapman FW, Finkel ES, Schmitt PW, Nova RC, Greene HL. A comparison of biphasic and monophasic shocks for external defibrillation. Physio-Control Biphasic Investigators. *Prehosp Emerg Care*. 2000;4:305-313.
35. Berg RA, Samson RA, Berg MD, Chapman FW, Hilwig RW, Banville I, Walker RG, Nova RC, Anavy N, Kern KB. Better outcome after pediatric defibrillation dosage than adult dosage in a swine model of pediatric ventricular fibrillation. *J Am Coll Cardiol*. 2005;45:786-789.
36. Killingsworth CR, Melnick SB, Chapman FW, Walker RG, Smith WM, Ideker RE, Walcott GP. Defibrillation threshold and cardiac responses using an external biphasic defibrillator with pediatric and adult adhesive patches in pediatric-sized piglets. *Resuscitation*. 2002;55:177-185.
37. Tang W, Weil MH, Sun S, Jorgenson D, Morgan C, Klouche K, Snyder D. The effects of biphasic waveform design on post-resuscitation myocardial function. *J Am Coll Cardiol*. 2004;43:1228-1235.
38. Kerber RE, Kieso RA, Kienzle MG, Olshansky B, Waldo AL, Carlson MD, Wilber DJ, Aschoff AM, Birger S, Charbonnier F. Current-based transthoracic defibrillation. *Am J Cardiol*. 1996;78:1113-1118.
39. Manegold JC, Israel CW, Ehrlich JR, Duray G, Pajitnev D, Wegener FT, Hohnloser SH. External cardioversion of atrial fibrillation in patients with implanted pacemaker or cardioverter-defibrillator systems: a randomized comparison of monophasic and biphasic shock energy application. *Eur Heart J*. 2007;28:1731-1738.
40. Chan PS, Krumholz HM, Spertus JA, Jones PG, Cram P, Berg RA, Peberdy MA, Nadkarni V, Mancini ME, Nallamothu BK. Automated external defibrillators and survival after in-hospital cardiac arrest. *JAMA*. 2010;304:2129-2136.
41. Perkins GD, Roberts C, Gao F. Delays in defibrillation: influence of different monitoring techniques. *Br J Anaesth*. 2002;89:405-408.
42. ECRI. Defibrillation in oxygen-enriched environments. *Health Devices*. 1987;16:113-114.
43. ECRI. Fires from defibrillation during oxygen administration. *Health Devices*. 1994;23:307-309.
44. Lefever J, Smith A. Risk of fire when using defibrillation in an oxygen enriched atmosphere. *Medical Devices Agency Safety Notices*. 1995;3:1-3.
45. McAnulty GR, Robertshaw H. Risk of fire outweighed by need for oxygen and defibrillation. *J Accid Emerg Med*. 1999;16:77.

Chapter 8

Cardiac Arrest, Part 1: VF/Pulseless VT

This Part

- **Application of the Cardiac Arrest Algorithm: VF/VT Pathway**
- **Vasopressors and Antiarrhythmics**
- **Access for Parenteral Medications During Cardiac Arrest**
- **Advanced Airway**
- **Monitoring During CPR**

Overview of Cardiac Arrest

The Cardiac Arrest Algorithm (Figure 35) outlines the assessment and management steps for the pulseless patient who does not initially respond to basic life support (BLS) interventions. This algorithm emphasizes the importance of minimally interrupted high-quality cardiopulmonary resuscitation (CPR). The algorithm consists of 2 pathways for a cardiac arrest:

- A shockable rhythm (**VF/pulseless VT**) displayed on the left side of the algorithm (discussed in Part 1 of this chapter)
- A nonshockable rhythm (**asystole/PEA**) displayed on the right side of the algorithm (discussed in Part 2 of this chapter)

Ventricular fibrillation (VF) represents disorganized electric activity, whereas pulseless ventricular tachycardia (VT) represents organized electric activity of the ventricular myocardium. Neither of these rhythms generates significant forward blood flow. Survival from these arrest rhythms requires immediate BLS, early defibrillation, prioritized advanced cardiovascular life support (ACLS), and post–cardiac arrest care. The *2010 AHA Guidelines for CPR and ECC* added a new circular algorithm to the original box algorithm (Figure 36).

Application of the Cardiac Arrest Algorithm: VF/VT Pathway

The foundation of ACLS care is continued high-quality CPR, starting with compressions for VF/pulseless VT and attempted defibrillation within minutes of collapse. For victims of witnessed VF arrest, prompt bystander CPR and early defibrillation can significantly increase the chance of survival to hospital discharge. In comparison, typical ACLS therapies, such as insertion of advanced airways and pharmacologic support of circulation, have not been shown to increase the rate of survival to hospital discharge. This chapter details the initial general care of a patient in VF/pulseless VT cardiac arrest and provides an overview of the ACLS Cardiac Arrest Algorithms (Figures 35 and 36).

After completing the BLS Survey, including activation of the emergency response system, performing high-quality CPR, attaching the manual defibrillator, and delivering the first shock (Numbers 1 through 4), the ACLS resuscitation team now intervenes and conducts the ACLS Survey. In this case, team members should continue to perform high-quality CPR while additional measures are taken to address the potential underlying cause. The team leader coordinates the efforts of the resuscitation team members as they perform the steps listed in the VF/VT pathway on the left side of the Cardiac Arrest Algorithm. The team leader assigns roles and responsibilities and organizes interventions to minimize interruptions (Figure 37) in chest compressions. This accomplishes the most critical interventions for VF or pulseless VT: CPR with minimal interruptions in chest compressions and defibrillation during the first minutes of arrest.

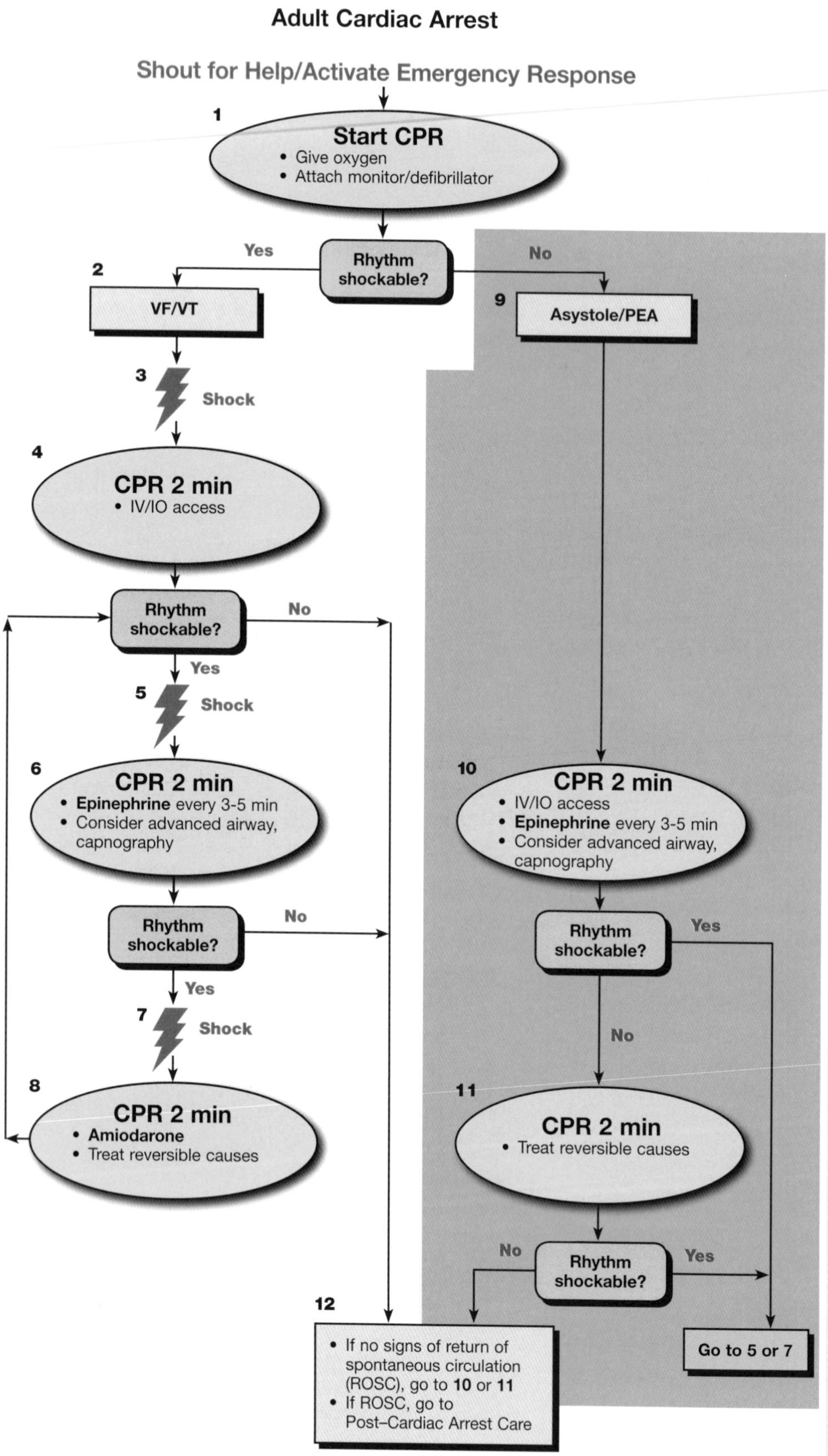

Adult Cardiac Arrest

Shout for Help/Activate Emergency Response

1 **Start CPR**
- Give oxygen
- Attach monitor/defibrillator

Rhythm shockable?

Yes → 2 VF/VT

No → 9 Asystole/PEA

3 Shock

4 **CPR 2 min**
- IV/IO access

Rhythm shockable? (No → 12)

Yes

5 Shock

6 **CPR 2 min**
- **Epinephrine** every 3-5 min
- Consider advanced airway, capnography

Rhythm shockable? (No → 12)

Yes

7 Shock

8 **CPR 2 min**
- **Amiodarone**
- Treat reversible causes

10 **CPR 2 min**
- IV/IO access
- **Epinephrine** every 3-5 min
- Consider advanced airway, capnography

Rhythm shockable? (Yes → Go to 5 or 7)

No

11 **CPR 2 min**
- Treat reversible causes

Rhythm shockable?

No → 12; Yes → Go to 5 or 7

12
- If no signs of return of spontaneous circulation (ROSC), go to **10** or **11**
- If ROSC, go to Post–Cardiac Arrest Care

Go to 5 or 7

CPR Quality
- Push hard (≥2 inches [5 cm]) and fast (≥100/min) and allow complete chest recoil
- Minimize interruptions in compressions
- Avoid excessive ventilation
- Rotate compressor every 2 minutes
- If no advanced airway, 30:2 compression-ventilation ratio
- Quantitative waveform capnography
  - If P_{ETCO_2} <10 mm Hg, attempt to improve CPR quality
- Intra-arterial pressure
  - If relaxation phase (diastolic) pressure <20 mm Hg, attempt to improve CPR quality

Return of Spontaneous Circulation (ROSC)
- Pulse and blood pressure
- Abrupt sustained increase in P_{ETCO_2} (typically ≥40 mm Hg)
- Spontaneous arterial pressure waves with intra-arterial monitoring

Shock Energy
- **Biphasic:** Manufacturer recommendation (eg, initial dose of 120-200 J); if unknown, use maximum available. Second and subsequent doses should be equivalent, and higher doses may be considered.
- **Monophasic:** 360 J

Drug Therapy
- **Epinephrine IV/IO Dose:** 1 mg every 3-5 minutes
- **Vasopressin IV/IO Dose:** 40 units can replace first or second dose of epinephrine
- **Amiodarone IV/IO Dose:** First dose: 300 mg bolus. Second dose: 150 mg.

Advanced Airway
- Supraglottic advanced airway or endotracheal intubation
- Waveform capnography to confirm and monitor ET tube placement
- 8-10 breaths per minute with continuous chest compressions

Reversible Causes
- **H**ypovolemia
- **H**ypoxia
- **H**ydrogen ion (acidosis)
- **H**ypo-/hyperkalemia
- **H**ypothermia
- **T**ension pneumothorax
- **T**amponade, cardiac
- **T**oxins
- **T**hrombosis, pulmonary
- **T**hrombosis, coronary

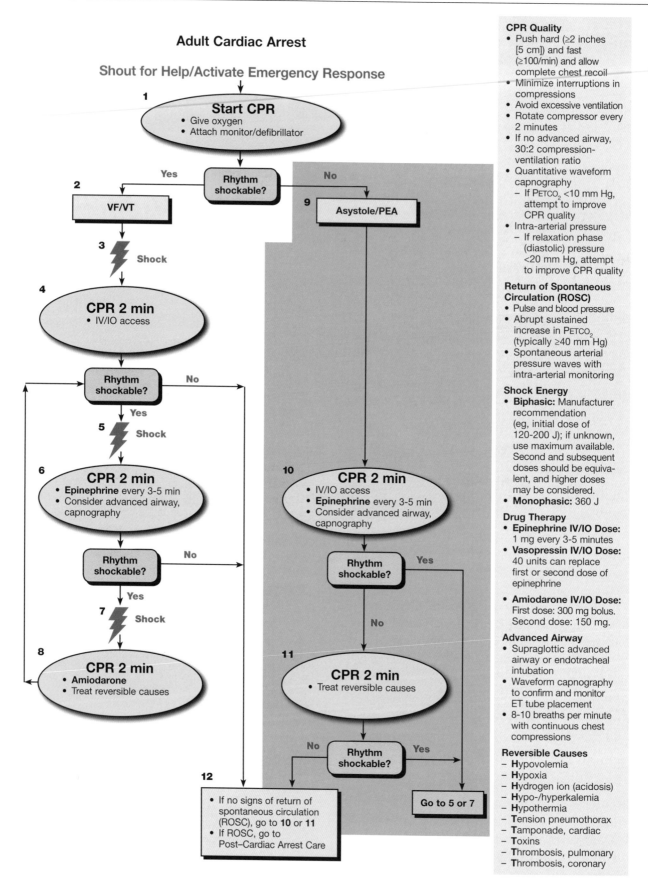

Figure 35. The Cardiac Arrest Algorithm.

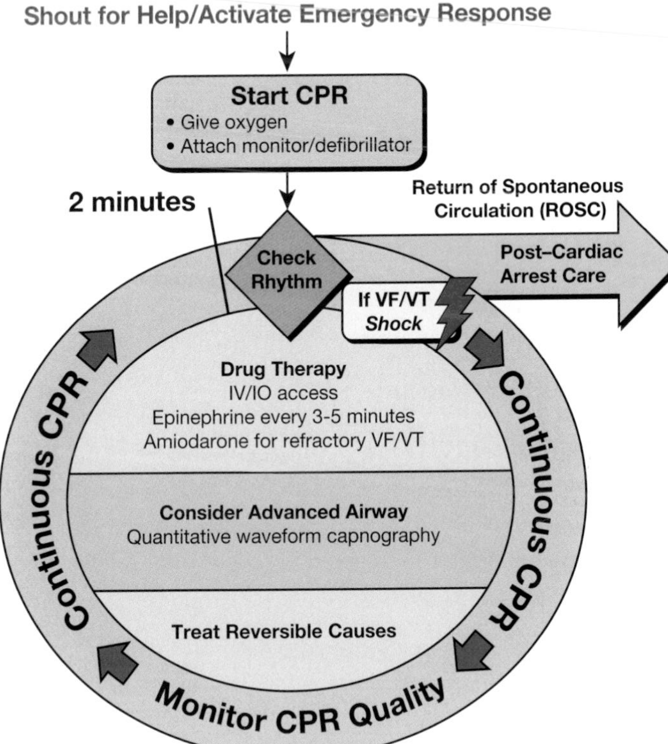

CPR Quality
- Push hard (≥2 inches [5 cm]) and fast (≥100/min) and allow complete chest recoil
- Minimize interruptions in compressions
- Avoid excessive ventilation
- Rotate compressor every 2 minutes
- If no advanced airway, 30:2 compression-ventilation ratio
- Quantitative waveform capnography
  - If P_{ETCO_2} <10 mm Hg, attempt to improve CPR quality
- Intra-arterial pressure
  - If relaxation phase (diastolic) pressure <20 mm Hg, attempt to improve CPR quality

Return of Spontaneous Circulation (ROSC)
- Pulse and blood pressure
- Abrupt sustained increase in P_{ETCO_2} (typically ≥40 mm Hg)
- Spontaneous arterial pressure waves with intra-arterial monitoring

Shock Energy
- **Biphasic:** Manufacturer recommendation (eg, initial dose of 120-200 J); if unknown, use maximum available. Second and subsequent doses should be equivalent, and higher doses may be considered.
- **Monophasic:** 360 J

Drug Therapy
- **Epinephrine IV/IO Dose:** 1 mg every 3-5 minutes
- **Vasopressin IV/IO Dose:** 40 units can replace first or second dose of epinephrine
- **Amiodarone IV/IO Dose:** First dose: 300 mg bolus. Second dose: 150 mg.

Advanced Airway
- Supraglottic advanced airway or endotracheal intubation
- Waveform capnography to confirm and monitor ET tube placement
- 8-10 breaths per minute with continuous chest compressions

Reversible Causes

– **H**ypovolemia	– **T**ension pneumothorax
– **H**ypoxia	– **T**amponade, cardiac
– **H**ydrogen ion (acidosis)	– **T**oxins
– **H**ypo-/hyperkalemia	– **T**hrombosis, pulmonary
– **H**ypothermia	– **T**hrombosis, coronary

Figure 36. The Cardiac Arrest Circular Algorithm. Do not delay shock. Continue CPR while preparing and administering drugs and charging the defibrillator. Interrupt chest compressions only for the minimum amount of time required for ventilation (until advanced airway placed), rhythm check, and actual shock delivery.

The team leader must concurrently consider the potential underlying causes for the arrest based on the patient's presentation and response to interventions.

Coronary perfusion pressure (CPP) is aortic relaxation “diastolic” pressure minus right atrial relaxation “diastolic” pressure. During CPR, CPP correlates with both myocardial blood flow and return of spontaneous circulation (ROSC). In 1 human study ROSC did not occur unless a CPP 15 mm Hg or higher was achieved during CPR.[1]

Number 3 directs you to deliver 1 shock.

If you are using a *monophasic* defibrillator, give a single 360-J shock. Use the same energy dose for subsequent shocks.

Biphasic defibrillators use a variety of waveforms, each of which is effective for terminating VF over a specific dose range. When using biphasic defibrillators, providers should use the manufacturer's recommended energy dose (eg, initial dose of 120 to 200 J). Many biphasic defibrillator manufacturers display the effective energy dose range on the face of the device. If you do not know the effective dose range, deliver the maximum energy dose available on the machine for the first and all subsequent shocks.

If the initial shock terminates VF but the arrhythmia recurs later in the resuscitation attempt, deliver subsequent shocks at the previously successful energy level.

Immediately after the first shock, resume CPR, beginning with chest compressions.

- Do not perform a rhythm or pulse check at this point.
- Establish intravenous/intraosseous (IV/IO) access during compressions.

To ensure safety during defibrillation, always announce the shock warning. State the warning firmly and in a forceful voice before delivering each shock (this entire sequence should take less than 5 seconds). Conduct a rhythm check after 2 minutes (about 5 cycles) of CPR. Be careful to minimize interruptions in chest compressions.

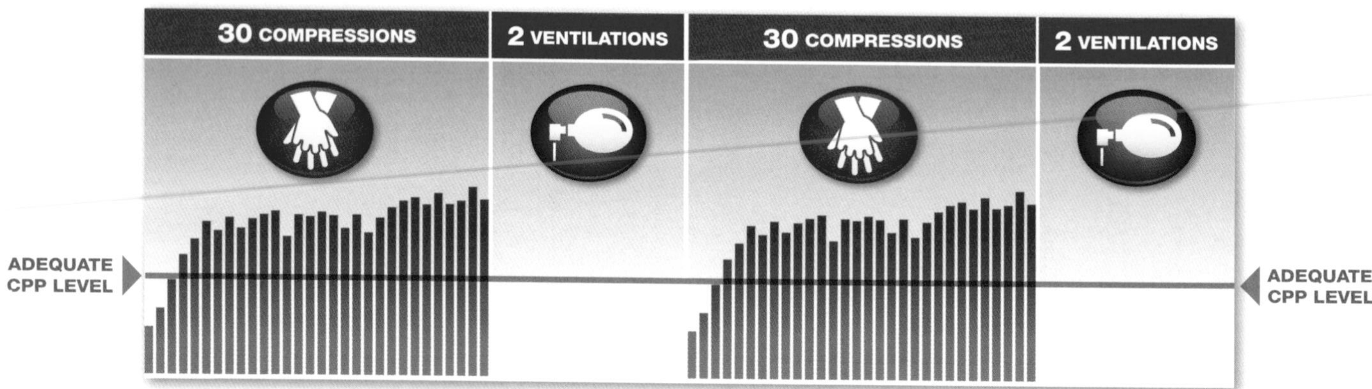

Figure 37. The relationship of quality CPR to coronary perfusion pressure (CPP) demonstrates the need for minimizing interruptions in compressions.

- If a nonshockable rhythm is present and the rhythm is organized (regular and narrow complexes), a team member should try to palpate a pulse. If there is any doubt about the presence of a pulse, immediately resume CPR.
  Remember: *Perform a pulse check—preferably during rhythm analysis—only if an organized rhythm is present.*
- If the rhythm is organized and there is a palpable pulse, proceed to post–cardiac arrest care.
- If the rhythm check reveals a nonshockable rhythm and there is no pulse, then proceed along the asystole/PEA pathway on the right side of the Cardiac Arrest Algorithm (Numbers 9 through 11).
- If the rhythm check reveals a shockable rhythm, give 1 shock and resume CPR immediately for 2 minutes after the shock (Number 6).

For persistent VF/pulseless VT, give 1 shock and resume CPR immediately for 2 minutes (about 5 cycles) after the shock. When IV/IO access is available, give a vasopressor dose during CPR (either before or after the shock) as follows:

- **Epinephrine** 1 mg IV/IO—repeat every 3 to 5 minutes

OR

- **Vasopressin** 40 units IV/IO—may substitute for the first or second dose of epinephrine

Note: If additional team members are available, they should anticipate the need for drugs and prepare them in advance.

Epinephrine hydrochloride is used during resuscitation primarily for its α-adrenergic effects, ie, vasoconstriction. Vasoconstriction increases cerebral and coronary blood flow during CPR by increasing mean arterial pressure and aortic diastolic pressure. In previous studies, escalating and high-dose epinephrine administration did not improve survival to discharge or neurologic outcome after resuscitation from cardiac arrest.[2-7]

Vasopressin is a nonadrenergic peripheral vasoconstrictor. A meta-analysis of 5 randomized trials found no difference between vasopressin and epinephrine for ROSC, 24-hour survival, or survival to hospital discharge.[8]

Conduct a rhythm check after 2 minutes (about 5 cycles) of CPR. Be careful to minimize interruptions in chest compressions.

- If a nonshockable rhythm is present and the rhythm is organized (regular and narrow complexes), a team member should try to palpate a pulse. If there is any doubt about the presence of a pulse, immediately resume CPR.
- If the rhythm is organized and there is a palpable pulse, proceed to post–cardiac arrest care.
- If the rhythm check reveals a nonshockable rhythm and there is no pulse, then proceed along the asystole/PEA pathway on the right side of the Cardiac Arrest Algorithm (Numbers 9 through 11).
- If the rhythm check reveals a shockable rhythm, resume chest compressions if indicated while the defibrillator is charging (Number 8). The team leader is responsible for team safety while compressions are being performed and the defibrillator is charging.

Give 1 shock and resume CPR beginning with chest compressions for 2 minutes (about 5 cycles) immediately after the shock.

Critical Concept Immediately After the Shock	• **Immediately** after the shock, resume CPR, beginning with chest compressions. Give 2 minutes (about 5 cycles) of CPR before reassessing the rhythm. • **The pause in chest compressions to check the rhythm should not exceed 10 seconds.**

Healthcare providers may consider giving antiarrhythmic drugs, either before or after the shock; however, there is no evidence that any antiarrhythmic drug given during cardiac arrest increases survival to hospital discharge. If administered, amiodarone is the first-line antiarrhythmic agent given in cardiac arrest because it has been clinically demonstrated that it improves the rate of ROSC and hospital admission in adults with refractory VF/pulseless VT.[9,10]

- **Amiodarone** 300 mg IV/IO bolus and then consider an additional 150 mg IV/IO once

If amiodarone is not available, providers may administer lidocaine.

- **Lidocaine** 1 to 1.5 mg/kg IV/IO first dose and then 0.5 to 0.75 mg/kg IV/IO at 5- to 10-minute intervals, to a maximum dose of 3 mg/kg

Providers should consider magnesium sulfate for torsades de pointes associated with a long QT interval.

- **Magnesium sulfate** for torsades de pointes, loading dose 1 to 2 g IV/IO diluted in 10 mL of D_5W given as IV/IO bolus, typically over 5 to 20 minutes

Routine administration of magnesium sulfate in cardiac arrest is not recommended unless torsades de pointes is present.

Search for and treat any treatable underlying cause of cardiac arrest. See column on the right of the algorithm.

ROSC

If the patient has ROSC, post–cardiac arrest care should be started (Chapter 13). Of particular importance are treatment of hypoxemia and hypotension, early diagnosis and treatment of ST-segment elevation myocardial infarction (STEMI), and therapeutic hypothermia in comatose patients.

VF and the Importance of Early Recognition

VF is the single most important rhythm for the ECC provider to recognize. In VF multiple areas within the ventricles display marked variation in depolarization and repolarization. There is no organized ventricular depolarization. Some have described VF as "myocardial chaos." The ventricles do not contract as a unit, and they produce no effective cardiac output. The initial, specific treatment for VF and pulseless VT is always CPR and immediate electrical defibrillation.

Coarse Versus Fine VF: Significance of VF Frequency

When myocardial ischemia or infarction causes sudden cardiac arrest, it is most often through the mechanism of VF. The terms *coarse* and *fine* have been used to describe the amplitude of the waveforms in VF (Figures 38 and 39). *Coarse* VF generally indicates VF that has been present only a short time, usually less than 3 to 5 minutes. High-amplitude, *coarse* VF requires significant levels of high-energy adenosine triphosphate (ATP) to persist. If the heart receives defibrillatory shocks before these energy stores are exhausted, spontaneous, organized contractions are more likely to resume after the myocardial "stunning" from a direct-current shock. The presence of *fine* VF that resembles asystole indicates "old" or "exhausted" VF. Often considerable delay—and no CPR—have followed patient collapse; high-energy phosphate stores and myocardial oxygen are depleted, and postshock resumption of spontaneous circulation becomes very unlikely.

The value of VF waveform analysis to guide management of defibrillation in adults with in-hospital and out-of-hospital cardiac arrest is uncertain. Providers could be prompted to continue with CPR for longer periods or to start other interventions before attempting defibrillation if informed by an AED or defibrillator that a shock is more likely to produce asystole. A complex analysis of central frequency, peak power frequency, spectral flatness, and energy has already achieved high levels of discrimination between rhythms that, when shocked, are followed by ROSC and rhythms that, when shocked, are followed by asystole.

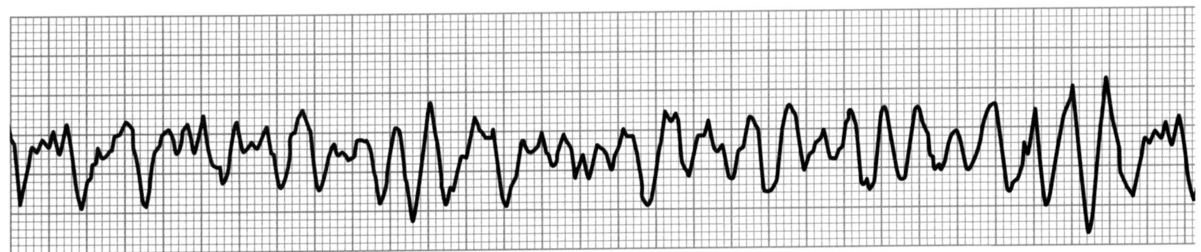

Figure 38. Coarse VF. Note high-amplitude waveforms, which vary in size, shape, and rhythm, representing chaotic ventricular electrical activity. The ECG criteria for VF are as follows: (1) QRS complexes: no normal-looking QRS complexes are recognizable; a regular "negative-positive-negative" pattern (Q-R-S) cannot be seen. (2) Rate: uncountable; electrical deflections are very rapid and too disorganized to count. (3) Rhythm: no regular rhythmic pattern can be discerned; the electrical waveforms vary in size and shape; the pattern is completely disorganized.

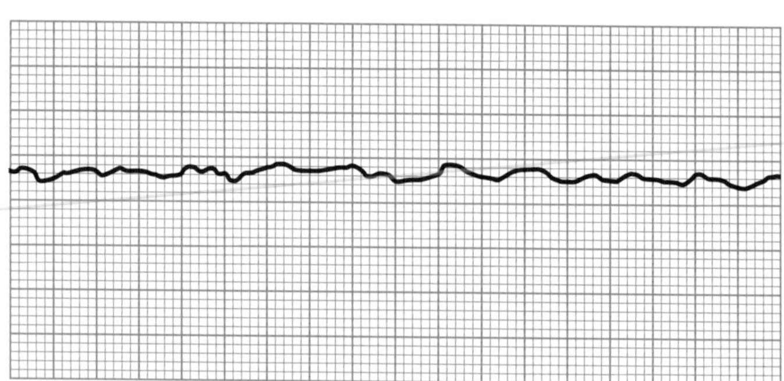

Figure 39. Fine VF. In comparison with Figure 38, the amplitude of electrical activity is much reduced. Note the complete absence of QRS complexes. In terms of electrophysiology, prognosis, and the likely clinical response to attempted defibrillation, adrenergic agents, or antiarrhythmics, this rhythm pattern may be difficult to distinguish from that of asystole.

Persistent, Refractory, Recurrent, and Shock-Resistant VF

Except for shocks from implantable defibrillators, it is unusual for a single shock to immediately return VF to a perfusing rhythm. In fact, this situation is uncommon, and almost all postshock rhythms are nonperfusing. After a shock, VF may be persistent, refractory to subsequent shocks, or recurrent after successful termination of VF.

- *Persistent* or *shock-resistant VF:* VF that persists after a defibrillatory shock
- *Refractory VF:* VF that persists after shocks, adrenergic agents, airway control, and antiarrhythmics
- *Recurrent or intermittent VF:* VF that recurs after 5 seconds following elimination (definition of successful defibrillation) or returns after an intervening restoration of a spontaneous perfusing rhythm

These distinctions are intended to remind clinicians to consider broader differential diagnoses and alternative or additional therapeutic strategies.

Defibrillation Strategies

- If a biphasic defibrillator is available, providers should use the manufacturer's recommended energy dose (120 to 200 J) for terminating VF.
  - If the provider is unaware of the effective dose range, the provider may use the maximum dose.
  - Second and subsequent energy levels should be at least equivalent to first shock, and higher energy levels may be considered if available.
  - If a monophasic defibrillator is used, providers should deliver an initial shock of 360 J and use that dose for all subsequent shocks.

If VF is terminated by a shock but then recurs later in the arrest, deliver subsequent shocks at the previously successful energy level.

Differential Diagnosis

Diagnosis and treatment of the underlying cause (H's and T's) is fundamental to management of all cardiac arrest rhythms. This is of paramount importance when dealing with asystolic and pulseless electrical activity (PEA) cardiac arrest. See Part 2 of this chapter for a detailed discussion of this topic.

H's	T's
Hypovolemia	**T**ension pneumothorax
Hypoxia	**T**amponade (cardiac)
Hydrogen ion (acidosis)	**T**oxins
Hyper-/hypokalemia	**T**hrombosis (pulmonary)
Hypothermia	**T**hrombosis (coronary)

Correct Priorities: Access and Airway

During cardiac arrest, provision of high-quality CPR and rapid defibrillation are of primary importance, and drug administration is of secondary importance. After beginning CPR and attempting defibrillation for identified VF or pulseless VT, providers can establish IV or IO access. This should be performed without interrupting chest compressions. The primary purpose of IV/IO access during cardiac arrest is to provide drug therapy. Although time to drug treatment appears to have importance, there is insufficient evidence to specify exact time parameters or the precise sequence with which drugs should be administered during cardiac arrest.

ACLS providers must be aware of the risks and benefits of insertion of an advanced airway during a resuscitation attempt. Such risks are affected by the condition of the patient and the provider's expertise in airway control. Because insertion of an endotracheal tube may require interruption of chest compressions for many seconds, the ACLS team leader should weigh the need for compressions against the need for insertion of an endotracheal tube. In some cases, an alternative advanced airway may be placed without any interruption in chest compressions. If adequate ventilations can be achieved with a bag-mask device, the team leader may defer insertion of an advanced airway until the patient fails to respond to initial CPR and defibrillation attempts or demonstrates ROSC.

Vasopressors and Antiarrhythmics

Because defibrillation is the definitive therapy for VF, vasopressors and antiarrhythmic agents should be given only when defibrillation and CPR are ineffective, and VF or pulseless VT persists. The Cardiac Arrest Algorithm (Figure 35) directs providers to administer a vasopressor and consider antiarrhythmia therapy after shocks and CPR fail to restore a perfusing rhythm. For patients with shock-refractory arrhythmias, providers should consider pharmacologic therapies sooner rather than later because the likelihood of benefit, if any, declines rapidly with increasing duration of VF; however, the administration of an antiarrhythmic should not delay or interfere with other more critical therapies. Amiodarone is the only antiarrhythmic shown to improve survival to hospital admission.[11]

Remember, priority is given to high-quality CPR with minimal interruption rather than to detailed rhythm analysis, pulse evaluation, and debate about drug administration.

- To date no placebo-controlled trials have shown that administration of any vasopressor or antiarrhythmic agent at any stage during management of VF or pulseless VT increases the rate of *neurologically intact survival* to hospital discharge. There is evidence, however, that the use of vasopressors may improve initial ROSC.[12]
- In addition, there is no evidence that any antiarrhythmic drug given routinely during human cardiac arrest increases *survival to hospital discharge*. Amiodarone, however, has been shown to increase short-term survival to hospital admission when compared with placebo or lidocaine.[9,10]

Vasopressors

Epinephrine or vasopressin is administered when VF or pulseless VT persists despite CPR and shock. Epinephrine hydrochloride produces beneficial physiological effects in patients during cardiac arrest, primarily because of its α-adrenergic receptor–stimulating (ie, vasoconstrictor) properties.[13] The α-adrenergic effects of epinephrine can increase myocardial and cerebral perfusion pressure during CPR.[14] The value and safety of the β-adrenergic effects of epinephrine are controversial because those effects may increase myocardial work and reduce subendocardial perfusion.[15] Vasopressin is a nonadrenergic peripheral vasoconstrictor that also causes vasoconstriction but lacks β-adrenergic side effects.[16,17]

Adrenergic and nonadrenergic vasopressors increase aortic diastolic pressure, which increases CPP. During cardiopulmonary arrest, CPP produced by CPR becomes the major determinant of successful resuscitation.[18] Cerebral perfusion pressure becomes the major determinant of successful neurologic resuscitation.[19] There is evidence that the use of vasopressor agents is associated with an increased rate of ROSC.

Abnormal cardiac output (Cardiac output = Heart rate × Stroke volume) and distribution and compromised oxygen delivery to tissues may be present before a cardiac arrest. Almost certainly they will be present during and immediately after a cardiac arrest. When cardiac output falls before or during cardiac arrest, peripheral vascular resistance initially increases in an attempt to compensate for the fall in mean arterial pressure. However, a measurable blood pressure (Blood pressure = Cardiac output × Systemic vascular resistance) or palpable peripheral pulse during CPR does not necessarily mean that cardiac output and peripheral perfusion are adequate. Remember, blood pressure is only a surrogate measure of cardiac function. Also, a measurable cardiac output does not necessarily mean that tissue oxygen delivery and oxygen uptake and utilization at the cellular level are adequate. Oxygen delivery may also be compromised by a decrease in hemoglobin concentration, in arterial oxygen tension, or in cardiac output. Distribution of blood flow and use of oxygen may be compromised in patients with diseases such as sepsis.

Mechanism of Action

Receptor Physiology: Signal Transduction

A *receptor* is a molecule or molecular complex that interacts with a stimulus called an *agonist*. Agonists are mediators such as hormones or neurotransmitters that bind selectively to a receptor, inducing a series of cellular changes that produce a biological response.

Autonomic (sympathetic) agonists in the cardiovascular system include epinephrine, released from the adrenal gland, and norepinephrine, released from adrenergic nerve terminals. When these agonists activate receptors, a second (intracellular) messenger alters intracellular calcium

Critical Concept **Success of Resuscitation Attempts**	The success of any resuscitation attempt is built on a strong base of high-quality CPR and defibrillation when required by the patient's ECG rhythm.

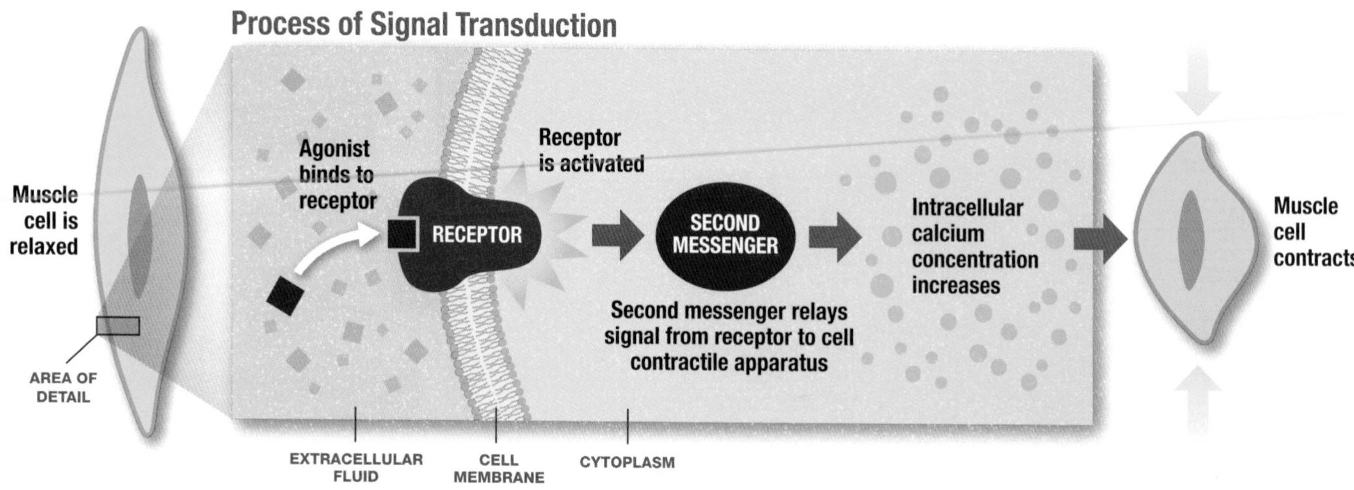

Figure 40. Process of signal transduction.

concentration. In muscle cells this increase of intracellular calcium interacts with the contractile apparatus of the cell, producing the biologic effect of a muscle contraction. The following diagram illustrates this sequence:

Process of Signal Transduction (Figure 40)

Agonist (eg, epinephrine)

- Leads to receptor binding and activation

↓

- Which causes an increase in intracellular calcium concentration

↓

- Which causes an interaction with cell contractile apparatus

↓

- Which produces a biologic effect (muscle contraction)

Adrenergic Receptors

Adrenergic receptors regulate cardiac, vascular, bronchiolar, and gastrointestinal smooth muscle tone.[20] The major classes of adrenergic receptors are

- α-Adrenergic (α_1 and α_2) receptors
- β-Adrenergic (β_1 and β_2) receptors
- Dopaminergic (DA) receptors

α-Adrenergic receptors predominantly regulate vascular smooth muscle tone and are important during resuscitation and the postarrest period. When α-adrenergic agonists stimulate vascular α-receptors, vasoconstriction occurs. This increases blood pressure during hypotension and cardiac arrest. The potency of the major α-adrenergic agonists (catecholamines) is as follows:

Norepinephrine	++++
Epinephrine	+++
Dopamine	++
Phenylephrine	+

α-Adrenergic receptors are also located in myocardial muscle cells, and stimulation of these receptors increases cardiac inotropic (force of contraction) function. This α-adrenergic inotropic effect, however, is not as significant as the β_1-adrenergic effect on myocardial function. The β_1-adrenergic effect increases myocardial oxygen requirements and is not beneficial during ischemia.

β_1 and β_2 are the most important types of β-adrenergic receptors:

- β_1-Adrenergic receptors are concentrated in the sinus node and ventricles of the heart. β_1-Adrenergic receptors are excitatory. When agonists stimulate these receptors, the heart responds with an increase in rate plus an increase in strength of contractility.
- β_2-Adrenergic receptors are found throughout the body acting primarily to cause smooth muscle relaxation. Some of the important effects of β_2 agonists include vasodilation and bronchodilation.

Dopaminergic receptors are located in smooth muscle cells in the cerebral, coronary, renal, and splanchnic vascular beds. Dopaminergic receptors are also present in proximal renal tubular cells and in the pituitary gland. Activation of dopaminergic receptors in the smooth muscle cells results in cerebral, coronary, renal, and splanchnic vasodilation. Activation of the dopaminergic cells in the proximal renal tubular cells results in inhibition of sodium ion reabsorption from tubular fluid, so renal sodium excretion increases. Activation of pituitary dopaminergic receptors modulates thyroid and prolactin hormone release. The most significant effect of dopaminergic receptor activation is increased blood flow to the cerebral, coronary, renal, and splanchnic circulations.[21]

Adrenergic Agonists and Vasoactive Drugs: Pharmacologic Effects

The clinical effects of a specific dose of adrenergic agonists may vary widely from patient to patient because the pharmacokinetics (relationship between drug dose and plasma concentration) and pharmacodynamics (relationship between plasma concentration and clinical effects) of these agents are influenced by a wide variety of factors. For example, the class of receptor, drug distribution factors, the large variety of drugs and hormones that influence the receptors, and the potential physical effects of receptor stimulation all play a role in how these agents work in an individual patient. Table 11 presents the overlapping effects of the adrenergic agonists. Note that most vasoactive drugs affect several types of adrenergic receptors (β_1, β_2, α, and DA). The receptors are affected by varying degrees of *receptor selectivity* (ie, the *binding affinity* of agonists for one type of receptor over another).

Other factors that contribute to the net effect of these drugs include

- Receptor density (a variety of clinical conditions influence the number of receptors present on the cell surface) and function (may be affected by activation of other receptors and other body processes)
- Parasympathetic nervous system
- Vasoactive platelet–mediated products such as thromboxane A_2 and prostacyclin
- Endothelial function (dysfunction may cause paradoxical responses to vasodilating stimuli)
- Loss of vasodilating substances such as endothelium relaxing factor

The interaction of a drug with receptors is complex. It varies from person to person and is further influenced by disease states, drug dose, drug distribution, receptors, pH, and whether the patient is in cardiac arrest.

Table 11. Adrenergic Receptor Subtypes: Anatomic Location, Response to Activation, and Effects of Selective Adrenergic Agonists

<table>
<tr><th>Receptors</th><th>α_1</th><th>β_1</th><th colspan="2">β_2</th><th>Dopaminergic</th></tr>
<tr><th>Receptor location</th><th>Arteries</th><th>Heart</th><th>Arteries</th><th>Bronchi</th><th>Kidney</th></tr>
<tr><td>Response to receptor activation</td><td>Constriction</td><td>Increased heart rate, contractions, and AV conduction</td><td>Dilation</td><td>Dilation</td><td>Dilation of renal vasculature</td></tr>
<tr><td></td><td colspan="4">← Epinephrine →</td><td></td></tr>
<tr><td></td><td colspan="2">← Norepinephrine →</td><td></td><td></td><td></td></tr>
<tr><td></td><td></td><td colspan="3">← Isoproterenol →</td><td></td></tr>
<tr><td></td><td></td><td>Dobutamine*</td><td></td><td></td><td></td></tr>
<tr><td></td><td>Dopamine (at high or "vasopressor" doses) ↔</td><td>Dopamine (at moderate or "cardiac" doses) ↔</td><td></td><td></td><td>Dopamine (at low, formerly "renal," doses) ↔</td></tr>
<tr><td></td><td>Phenylephrine</td><td></td><td></td><td></td><td></td></tr>
</table>

Abbreviation: AV, atrioventricular.

*Dobutamine has theoretical α-adrenergic agonist effects, but a major metabolite of dobutamine inhibits α-adrenergic receptors. In addition, any α-adrenergic effects are balanced by minimal activation of β_2-adrenergic receptors. These complex interactions of dobutamine result in net β_1-adrenergic effects.

Epinephrine: Double-Edged Sword

Both beneficial and toxic physiologic effects of epinephrine administration during CPR have been shown in animal and human studies.[22-24] Epinephrine produces significant renal vasoconstriction even at very low doses, causing decreased renal blood flow and urine output.[25] It increases heart rate by increasing the spontaneous depolarization rate of the sinoatrial node. The refractory periods of some cardiac conduction and myocardial cells can be decreased, and these effects may increase the likelihood of arrhythmias and contribute to a hyper-adrenergic state after resuscitation. Epinephrine does increase coronary artery blood flow, but its β-adrenergic effects increase myocardial work and reduce subendocardial perfusion. The net effect may be a greater increase in oxygen demand than oxygen delivery to the myocardium.

A prospective, nonrandomized, observational study evaluated the association between epinephrine use before hospital arrival and the short- and long-term mortality in patients with cardiac arrest. The study analyzed data from 417 188 out-of-hospital cardiac arrest patients in Japan. Patients were treated with or without epinephrine by emergency medical services (EMS) personnel on the scene and were transported to the hospital. Prehospital treatment with epinephrine was significantly ($P<0.001$) associated with increased chance of ROSC before hospital arrival. However, the prehospital administration of epinephrine was significantly ($P<0.001$) associated with decreased chance of both survival and good functional outcomes (cerebral and neurological performance) 1 month after the event.[26]

The ACLS provider should recognize that clinical response to adrenergic vasoactive drugs is variable, so these drugs must be titrated at the bedside with close observation of patient response. Table 11 is an attempt to simplify the clinical selection of vasoactive drugs. This table summarizes the major receptor sites of each drug and the net effect each agent has on arterial constriction or dilation, heart rate and contractility, bronchial constriction, potential for arrhythmias, and renal blood flow. Careful selection of agents, dose titration, and serial monitoring of patients are essential.

Epinephrine in Cardiac Arrest

Epinephrine is a natural catecholamine with both α- and β-adrenergic agonist activity. The beneficial effects of epinephrine during cardiac arrest come from its α-adrenergic effects. During resuscitation, epinephrine increases peripheral vasoconstriction and improves coronary artery perfusion pressure. As a result, stimulation of α-adrenergic receptors during CPR increases myocardial and cerebral blood flow.[14]

Overall epinephrine makes VF more responsive to direct-current shock. Although epinephrine has been used universally in resuscitation, there is a paucity of evidence to show that it improves outcomes in humans.

IV administration of epinephrine can increase

- Systemic vascular resistance
- Systolic and diastolic blood pressures
- Electrical activity in the myocardium
- Coronary and cerebral blood flow
- Strength of myocardial contraction
- Myocardial oxygen requirements
- Automaticity

Epinephrine is indicated in the following conditions:

- Cardiac arrest: VF and pulseless VT unresponsive to initial shocks
- Symptomatic bradycardia: After atropine has failed (see Chapter 9)
- Severe hypotension: Low blood pressure from shock, although its effects on myocardial oxygen demand may limit its usefulness in adults with coronary artery disease (see Chapter 11)
- Anaphylaxis, severe allergic reactions: Combine epinephrine with large fluid volume administration, corticosteroids, and antihistamines (see Chapter 17)

For the past 2 decades researchers and clinicians have attempted to determine the optimal dose of epinephrine for CPR. The "standard" dose of epinephrine (1 mg) is not based on body weight. Historically, resuscitation of dogs subjected to 10 minutes of circulatory arrest due to VF was successful when 1 mg of epinephrine was used with artificial ventilation of the lungs, external cardiac massage, and external electrical countershock.[27] A standard dose of 1 mg epinephrine was used in operating rooms for intracardiac injections.[22-24] Surgeons observed that 1 to 3 mg of *intracardiac* epinephrine was effective in restarting the arrested adult heart. When these and other experts first produced resuscitation guidelines in the 1970s, they assumed that 1 mg of *intravenous* epinephrine would work similarly to 1 mg of *intracardiac* epinephrine without any adjustment for patient weight.

It is reasonable to consider administering a dose of 1 mg epinephrine IV/IO every 3 to 5 minutes during adult cardiac arrest (Class IIb, LOE A). Initial or escalating high-dose epinephrine has occasionally improved initial ROSC and early survival rates. But in 8 randomized clinical studies involving more than 9000 cardiac arrest patients, high-dose

Critical Concept **Peripheral Injection of Epinephrine**	Follow each dose given by peripheral injection with 20 mL flush of IV fluid, and elevate the extremity above the level of the heart for 10 to 20 seconds.

epinephrine produced no improvement in survival to hospital discharge rates or neurologic outcomes when compared with standard doses, even in subgroups initially given high-dose epinephrine.[2,4] Higher doses were previously used and advocated by some clinicians, but evidence has accumulated that higher doses have no incremental benefit.

In theory higher doses may have the potential to cause harm. Careful laboratory studies corroborate both beneficial and harmful physiologic effects and outcomes. High-dose epinephrine may improve coronary perfusion and increase vascular resistance to promote initial ROSC during CPR. But these same effects may lead to increased myocardial dysfunction and occasionally a severely toxic hyperadrenergic state in the postresuscitation period. Higher doses may be indicated to treat specific problems, such as β-blocker or calcium channel blocker overdose, as discussed in Chapter 13 of this text. Higher doses can also be considered if guided by hemodynamic monitoring, such as arterial relaxation "diastolic" pressure or CPP. If IV/IO access is delayed or cannot be established, epinephrine may be given endotracheally at a dose of 2 to 2.5 mg.

Vasopressin in Cardiac Arrest

Vasopressin is a nonadrenergic peripheral vasoconstrictor that also causes coronary and renal vasoconstriction.[17,28] Two large randomized controlled human trials[29,30] failed to show an increase in rates of ROSC or survival when vasopressin (40 units, with the dose repeated in 1 study) was compared with epinephrine (1 mg, repeated) as the initial vasopressor for treatment of cardiac arrest. In the multicenter trial involving 1186 out-of-hospital cardiac arrests[30] with all rhythms, a *post hoc* analysis of patients with asystole showed significant improvement in survival to hospital discharge but not neurologically intact survival when 40 units (repeated once if necessary) of vasopressin was used as the initial vasopressor compared with epinephrine (1 mg, repeated if necessary). Because the effects of vasopressin have not been shown to differ from those of epinephrine in cardiac arrest, 1 dose of vasopressin 40 units IV/IO may replace either the first or second dose of epinephrine in the treatment of cardiac arrest (Class IIb, LOE A).

Arginine vasopressin is a naturally occurring hormone, also known as antidiuretic hormone. Endogenous vasopressin levels in patients undergoing CPR are significantly higher in patients who survive than in patients who have no ROSC. This finding stimulated interest in evaluation of vasopressin as a vasoconstrictor during cardiac arrest. It was hypothesized that vasopressin might be beneficial and avoid the harmful physiologic effects of epinephrine.

After a short duration of VF, vasopressin administration during CPR has been shown to increase

- CPP
- Vital organ blood flow
- Median frequency of VF
- Cerebral oxygen delivery

In higher doses than needed for its antidiuretic action, vasopressin is a nonadrenergic peripheral vasoconstrictor. Vasopressin causes vasoconstriction by directly stimulating smooth muscle V_1 receptors. A potential advantage is that vasopressin does not increase myocardial oxygen consumption during CPR because it has no β-adrenergic activity. The half-life of vasopressin in animal models with intact circulation is 10 to 20 minutes, which is longer than the half-life of epinephrine during CPR.

Principles of Pharmacologic Treatment of VF

For patients in VF arrest, providers administer the drugs during VF. Effective CPR must be performed to deliver drug therapy to the myocardium. Even with CPR, coronary blood flow is severely compromised (at no more than 15% to 25% of normal). In theory some drug-myocardium interaction occurs between attempted defibrillatory shocks in persistent VF. When a subsequent shock completely depolarizes the heart, there is a brief period of electrically *silent* asystole. During these few seconds of asystole before VF resumes, it is assumed that the antiarrhythmic drug in the tissues accomplishes 2 unlikely tasks:

- Selective suppression of myocardial action potentials related to fibrillation
- Selective facilitation of myocardial action potentials related to coordinated contractions

Antifibrillatory drugs have not been shown to improve survival to hospital discharge in any animal or human study. Historically lidocaine has been the drug most often used as an antifibrillatory agent, having entered VF/pulseless VT resuscitation protocols decades ago via empirical reasoning. Over years of use, lidocaine acquired a "grandfather" status. Lacking human evidence of any long-term or short-term efficacy from lidocaine administration in VF cardiac arrest or pulseless VT, experts at the International Guidelines 2000

Conference ranked lidocaine as Class Indeterminate. At the 2010 International Consensus Conference, experts reiterated that "there is inadequate evidence to support or refute the use of lidocaine" in cardiac arrest.

Studies to date of antiarrhythmic drugs for VF/pulseless VT arrest have been able to detect outcome differences for only short-term outcomes, such as ROSC or admission alive to the hospital.[9,10] Observed improvements in intermediate outcomes have not translated into observed improvements in longer-term outcomes. Because the circumstances of each patient's arrest vary and because the care a patient receives after ROSC is known to be critical to the patient's outcome, it is methodologically difficult to determine small but genuine benefits from out-of-hospital interventions.

Administration of antiarrhythmics for persistent VF should not take priority over established interventions such as uninterrupted high-quality CPR and attempts at defibrillation. Intravenous administration of drugs requires time and personnel. The team leader should direct these decisions to ensure minimal interruption in chest compressions and anticipate sequential drug dosing.

When the established benefits of defibrillation and high-quality chest compressions are balanced against the uncertain long-term benefits of antiarrhythmic agents, a clear choice emerges: *never delay the definitive benefits of defibrillation to attempt to provide the questionable long-term benefits of antiarrhythmics.* Equally clear is the corollary that, for patients with VF refractory to repeated defibrillation attempts, healthcare providers should proceed expeditiously with use of pharmacologic interventions because any beneficial effect decreases rapidly with time.

Antiarrhythmics to Consider for VF/VT: Amiodarone

When high-quality CPR, shocks, and a vasopressor have failed to terminate pulseless VF or VT, the use of antiarrhythmic agents can be considered. Amiodarone is the first-line antiarrhythmic agent given during cardiac arrest because it has been clinically demonstrated to improve the rate of ROSC and hospital admission in adults with refractory VF/pulseless VT.[9,10] During cardiac arrest, consider amiodarone 300 mg IV/IO push for the first dose. If VF/pulseless VT persists, consider giving a second dose of 150 mg IV/IO in 3 to 5 minutes. If amiodarone is unavailable, lidocaine may be considered (Class IIb, LOE B), but in clinical studies lidocaine has not been demonstrated to improve rates of ROSC and hospital admission compared with amiodarone.

More than a decade ago, data from a small European trial suggested that amiodarone may be more effective than lidocaine in improving short-term outcome from cardiac arrest.[9] In a large series of patients with nonarrest VT unresponsive to lidocaine, procainamide, or bretylium, the response rate for amiodarone was 40%.[10] In a head-to-head, randomized, controlled trial, amiodarone and bretylium were found to be equally effective in reducing recurrent, hemodynamically significant ventricular tachyarrhythmias in patients who did not respond to lidocaine and procainamide.[10] The incidence of significant hypotension, however, was much lower with amiodarone.

Amiodarone was reported to have higher incidence of bradycardia and hypotension when compared with placebo in an out-of-hospital cardiac arrest study.[9] This has been attributed to the presence of vasoactive solvents (polysorbate 80 and benzyl alcohol) used in the original formulation. A new water-soluble formulation of IV amiodarone is now available in the United States. Data from 4 clinical trials using amiodarone products without these solvents have shown similar incidence of hypotension to lidocaine.[31]

Premixed infusions of water-soluble amiodarone are available; however, at the time of this writing, no prefilled syringes for emergency bolus administration were available. Of note, amiodarone may adsorb to plastic tubing and bags, leading to the delivery of a reduced dose of the drug. Moreover, several critical compatibility issues may occur with amiodarone. For example, precipitation occurs when amiodarone is mixed with heparin or sodium bicarbonate.

Other Antiarrhythmics to Consider: Lidocaine

A retrospective review demonstrated an association between improved hospital admission rates and use of lidocaine (compared with standard treatment) in patients with out-of-hospital VF cardiac arrest.[32] But there is inadequate evidence to recommend the use of lidocaine in patients who have refractory VT/VF, which is defined as VT/VF that is not terminated by defibrillation or that continues to recur after defibrillation during out-of-hospital cardiac arrest or in-hospital cardiac arrest.

Lidocaine is an alternative antiarrhythmic of long-standing and widespread familiarity that has fewer immediate side effects than may be encountered with other antiarrhythmics. Lidocaine, however, has no proven short- or long-term efficacy in cardiac arrest. Lidocaine may be considered if amiodarone is not available (Class IIb, LOE B). The initial dose is 1 to 1.5 mg/kg IV. If VF/pulseless VT persists, additional doses of 0.5 to 0.75 mg/kg IV push may be administered at 5- to 10-minute intervals to a maximum dose of 3 mg/kg. If no IV/IO access is available, the dose for endotracheal administration is 2 to 4 mg/kg.

The use of lidocaine for ventricular arrhythmias was initially supported by evidence from animal studies and by extrapolation from the historical use of lidocaine to suppress premature ventricular contractions and to prevent VF after acute myocardial infarction. Administration of lidocaine improved rates of resuscitation and admission alive to the hospital in one retrospective prehospital study. But other trials of lidocaine and comparisons of lidocaine and bretylium (no longer available or recommended) found no statistically significant differences in outcomes. One small randomized comparison of amiodarone and lidocaine found a greater likelihood of successful resuscitation with amiodarone. A randomized comparison of lidocaine and epinephrine demonstrated a higher incidence of asystole with lidocaine use and no difference in ROSC. In an in-hospital Canadian study, investigators observed an association between the use of lidocaine and a lower rate of short-term resuscitation success. But this study, a retrospective, uncontrolled study, was flawed by the phenomenon that patients destined not to be resuscitated during a resuscitation attempt are treated for much longer periods; the longer patients are treated, the more medications they receive. As a result, researchers can observe an association between the use of pharmacologic agents and a negative outcome. This association must not be misinterpreted as a cause-and-effect relationship.

When administering lidocaine, healthcare providers should be aware of the following contraindications and precautions:

- Lidocaine is not recommended for prophylactic use in acute myocardial infarction.
- Reduce dose in hepatic failure or congestive heart failure.
- Stop infusion if neurologic abnormalities develop.

Magnesium

Magnesium is recommended for use in patients with persistent VF/VT arrest who are known or *suspected* to be in a hypomagnesemic state. Clinicians probably administer magnesium less frequently than indicated because of failure to suspect hypomagnesemia in patient groups known to be at high risk for the condition (ie, the elderly, those who abuse alcohol, and those with chronic malnutrition). Risk factors for hypomagnesemia may be noted in the medical record, which can be reviewed during the course of resuscitation, or elicited from family members (ie, patient history). Hypomagnesemia may also be evident on the ECG (prior prolongation of the QT_c interval).

IV/IO magnesium can terminate torsades de pointes (irregular/polymorphic VT). Magnesium is unlikely to be effective in terminating irregular/polymorphic VT in patients with a normal QT interval. Routine administration of magnesium sulfate in cardiac arrest is not recommended unless torsades de pointes is present; however, administration might be indicated in the absence of torsades in cases such as VF refractory to all other therapies.

When VF/pulseless VT cardiac arrest is associated with torsades de pointes, providers may administer an IV/IO bolus of magnesium sulfate at a dose of 1 to 2 g in 10 mL diluents (eg, D_5W, normal saline) (Class IIb, LOE C).

Evidence on the value of magnesium in cardiac arrest has been gathered, but the study investigators concluded that magnesium has no particular positive effects.[33] Thus, routine administration of magnesium sulfate in cardiac arrest is not recommended (Class III, LOE A) unless torsades de pointes is present or hypomagnesemia is suspected. Magnesium administration in resuscitation may be associated with a higher incidence of hypotension despite a potential for improved neurologic outcome in survivors.

Antiarrhythmic Cocktails and Combinations

There is no evidence supporting combination therapy, such as amiodarone alternating with lidocaine. Combination therapy has no proven benefit and could be harmful because of the proarrhythmic effects that can occur when agents are administered in combination. Most important, interruption of CPR to assess rhythm and administer antiarrhythmic agents is discouraged.

Atropine

Atropine sulfate reverses cholinergic-mediated decreases in heart rate and atrioventricular nodal conduction. No prospective controlled clinical trials have examined the use of atropine in asystole or bradycardic PEA cardiac arrest. There is no evidence that atropine has detrimental effects during bradycardic or asystolic cardiac arrest. Available evidence suggests that routine use of atropine during PEA or asystole is unlikely to have a therapeutic benefit (Class IIb, LOE B). *For this reason atropine has been removed from the cardiac arrest algorithm.*

Sodium Bicarbonate

Tissue acidosis and the resulting acidemia during cardiac arrest and resuscitation are dynamic processes resulting from no blood flow during arrest and low blood flow during CPR. These processes are affected by the duration of cardiac arrest, level of blood flow, and arterial oxygen content during CPR. Restoration of oxygen content with appropriate ventilation with oxygen, support of some tissue perfusion and some cardiac output with high-quality chest compressions, and then rapid ROSC are the mainstays of restoring acid-base balance during cardiac arrest. Two studies demonstrated increased ROSC, hospital admission, and survival to hospital discharge associated with use of bicarbonate.[34,35] However, the majority of studies showed no benefit or found a relationship with poor outcome. There are few data to support therapy with buffers during cardiac arrest. Routine use of sodium bicarbonate is not recommended for patients in cardiac arrest. In some special resuscitation situations, such as preexisting metabolic acidosis, hyperkalemia, or tricyclic antidepressant overdose, bicarbonate can be beneficial. When bicarbonate is used for special situations, an initial dose of 1 mEq/kg is typical.

Calcium

Studies of calcium during cardiac arrest have found variable results on ROSC, and no trial has found a beneficial effect on survival either in or out of hospital. Routine administration of calcium for treatment of in-hospital and out-of-hospital cardiac arrest is not recommended (Class III, LOE B); however, it is appropriate when the underlying cause of the arrest is hyperkalemia.

Fibrinolysis

Fibrinolytic therapy was proposed for use during cardiac arrest to treat both coronary thrombosis (acute coronary syndrome [ACS]) with presumably complete occlusion of a proximal coronary artery and major life-threatening pulmonary embolism. Ongoing CPR is not an absolute contraindication to fibrinolysis. Initial studies were promising and suggested benefit from fibrinolytic therapy in the treatment of victims of cardiopulmonary arrest unresponsive to standard therapy.[36,37] However, later studies showed no benefit.[38] Fibrinolytic therapy should not be routinely used in cardiac arrest. When pulmonary embolism is presumed or known to be the cause of cardiac arrest, empirical fibrinolytic therapy can be considered. Fibrinolytic therapy is discussed in Chapter 11.

No published human study directly compares the outcome of routine IV fluid administration to no fluid administration during CPR. If cardiac arrest is associated with hypovolemia, intravascular volume should be promptly restored.

Prophylactic Use of Antiarrhythmic Medications After Cardiac Arrest

Because of methodological challenges and sample-size barriers, researchers have been unable to complete studies that address the value of prophylactic antiarrhythmic drugs after shock-terminated VF/VT. Both experts and clinicians have argued that, if VF/VT is successfully terminated after antiarrhythmic agents have been administered, then the same antiarrhythmic agents should be continued for the next 6 to 24 hours. The rationale contends that this therapy reduces the probability of recurrent arrhythmias. There is no evidence to support or refute continued or prophylactic administration of these medications.[39-44] If VF, VT, or frequent ventricular premature beats occur, consider causes such as ischemia, electrolyte imbalance, and hypoxia.

Identify and Treat or Eliminate the Arrhythmia Trigger?

One important question after resuscitation from cardiac arrest involves the etiology, or trigger, of the arrest rhythm. In adults, ACS is a leading cause and precipitates cardiac arrest by ischemia. Frequent causes of malignant arrhythmias in addition to ischemia include electrolyte abnormalities, hypoxemia, hypotension, and drug-induced arrhythmias (including proarrhythmic effects of drugs). In patients with STEMI, treatment involves consideration of reperfusion therapy. The risk-benefit ratio for fibrinolytics and the logistical considerations for percutaneous coronary intervention are complicated. Alternatively, in the absence of ischemia, a "substrate" of electrical instability can cause cardiac arrest, impacting both short-term and long-term management. For these reasons consultations with cardiology and electrophysiology specialists are important early after resuscitation.

Access for Parenteral Medications During Cardiac Arrest

During cardiac arrest, provision of high-quality CPR and rapid defibrillation are of primary importance, and drug administration is of secondary importance. After beginning CPR and attempting defibrillation for identified VF or pulseless VT, providers can establish IV or IO access. This should be performed without interrupting chest compressions.

Peripheral IV Drug Delivery

If a resuscitation drug is administered by a peripheral venous route, it should be administered by bolus injection and followed with a 20-mL bolus of IV fluid to facilitate the drug flow from the extremity into the central circulation. Briefly elevating the extremity (10 to 20 seconds) during and after drug administration theoretically may recruit the benefit of gravity to facilitate delivery to the central circulation, but this technique has not been systematically studied.

Intraosseous Drug Delivery

IO cannulation provides access to a noncollapsible venous plexus, enabling drug delivery similar to that achieved by peripheral venous access at comparable doses. IO access can be established efficiently; is safe and effective for fluid resuscitation, drug delivery, and blood sampling for laboratory evaluation; and is attainable in all age groups. Although virtually all ACLS drugs have been given intraosseously in the clinical setting without known ill effects, there are few studies on the efficacy and effectiveness of such administration in clinical cardiac arrest during ongoing CPR. Therefore it is reasonable for providers to establish IO access if IV access is not readily available. Commercially available kits can facilitate IO access in adults.

Central IV Drug Delivery

The appropriately trained provider may consider placement of a central line (internal jugular or subclavian) during cardiac arrest, unless there are contraindications. The primary advantage of a central line is that peak drug concentrations are higher and drug circulation times shorter compared with drugs administered through a peripheral IV catheter. In addition, a central line extending into the superior vena cava can be used to monitor central venous oxygen saturation ($Scvo_2$) and estimate CPP during CPR, both of which are predictive of ROSC. However, central-line placement can interrupt CPR. Central venous catheterization is a relative (but not absolute) contraindication for fibrinolytic therapy in patients with ACS. Placement of central venous access carries additional risks that are not present with peripheral venous access.

Endotracheal Drug Delivery

Studies in adults, children, and animals have shown that lidocaine, epinephrine, atropine, naloxone, and vasopressin are absorbed via the trachea.[45-56] Although there are no data regarding endotracheal administration of amiodarone, it is generally not recommended. Administration of resuscitation drugs into the trachea results in lower blood concentrations than when the same dose is given intravascularly. Furthermore, the lower epinephrine concentrations achieved when the drug is delivered endotracheally may produce transient β-adrenergic effects, resulting in vasodilatation. These effects can be detrimental, causing hypotension, lower CPP and flow, and reduced potential for ROSC. Thus, although endotracheal administration of some resuscitation drugs is possible, IV or IO drug administration is preferred because it will provide more predictable drug delivery and pharmacologic effect. If IV or IO access cannot be established, epinephrine, vasopressin, and lidocaine may be administered by the endotracheal route during cardiac arrest.

The optimal endotracheal dose of most drugs is unknown, but typically the dose given by the endotracheal route is 2 to 2.5 times the recommended IV dose. Providers should dilute the recommended dose in 5 to 10 mL of sterile water or normal saline and inject the drug directly into the endotracheal tube; dilution with sterile water instead of 0.9% saline may achieve better drug absorption.

Advanced Airway

There is inadequate evidence to define the optimal timing of advanced airway placement in relation to other interventions during resuscitation from cardiac arrest. There are no prospective studies that directly address the relationship between timing or type of advanced airway placement during CPR and outcomes. In an urban out-of-hospital setting, intubation in less than 12 minutes has been associated with a better rate of survival than intubation in 13 minutes or more.[57] In a registry study of 25 006 in-hospital cardiac arrests, earlier time to advanced airway (less than 5 minutes) was not associated with increased ROSC but was associated with improved 24-hour survival.[58] In out-of-hospital urban and rural settings, patients intubated during resuscitation had better survival rates than patients who were not intubated.[59] In an in-hospital setting, patients requiring intubation during CPR had worse survival rates.[60] A recent study found that delayed endotracheal intubation combined with passive oxygen delivery and minimally interrupted chest compressions was associated with improved neurologically intact survival after out-of-hospital cardiac arrest in patients with witnessed VF/VT.[61]

Some of the advantages of advanced airway placement include elimination of the need for pauses in chest compressions for ventilation and ability to use quantitative waveform capnography to monitor quality of CPR, optimize chest compressions, and detect ROSC during chest compressions or when a rhythm check reveals an organized rhythm. The primary disadvantages are interruptions in chest compressions during placement and the risk of unrecognized esophageal intubation.

It is reasonable to place a supraglottic airway while chest compressions are underway to avoid interruptions in chest compressions. When an advanced airway (eg, endotracheal tube or supraglottic airway) is placed, the provider performing compressions should deliver at least 100 compressions per minute continuously without pauses for ventilation. The provider delivering ventilations should give 1 breath every 6 to 8 seconds (8 to 10 breaths per minute) and should be careful to avoid overventilation.

Physiologic Monitoring During CPR

Mechanical Parameters

CPR quality can be improved by using a number of nonphysiologic techniques that help the provider adhere to recommended CPR parameters such as rate and depth of compression and rate of ventilation.

- The simplest are auditory or visual metronomes to guide providers in performing the recommended rate of chest compressions or ventilations.
- More sophisticated devices actually monitor chest compression rate, depth, relaxation, and pauses in real time and provide visual and auditory feedback.
- When recorded, this information can also be useful in providing feedback to the entire team of providers after the resuscitation has ended.

Physiologic Parameters

Human cardiac arrest is the most critically ill condition, yet it is typically monitored by rhythm assessment using selected ECG leads and pulse checks as the only physiologic parameters to guide therapy. Animal and human studies indicate that monitoring of end-tidal CO_2 ($PETCO_2$), CPP, and $ScvO_2$ provides valuable information on both the patient's condition and response to therapy. Although no clinical study has examined whether titrating resuscitative efforts to these or other physiologic parameters improves outcome, it is reasonable to consider using these parameters when feasible to optimize chest compressions and guide vasopressor therapy during cardiac arrest.

Pulse

Clinicians frequently try to palpate arterial pulses during chest compressions to assess the effectiveness of compressions. Carotid pulsations during CPR do not indicate the efficacy of myocardial or cerebral perfusion during CPR. Palpation of a pulse when chest compressions are paused is a reliable indicator of ROSC but is potentially less sensitive than other physiologic measures discussed below. Healthcare providers also may take too long to check for a pulse and have difficulty determining if a pulse is present or absent. Because delays in chest compressions should be minimized, the healthcare provider should take no more than 10 seconds to check for a pulse, and if there is any doubt as to whether a pulse is felt within that time period, chest compressions should be started/resumed.

End-Tidal CO_2

End-tidal CO_2 is the concentration of carbon dioxide in exhaled air at the end of expiration. Because CO_2 is a trace gas in atmospheric air, CO_2 detected by capnography in exhaled air is produced in the body and delivered to the lungs by circulating blood. The main determinant to $PETCO_2$ during CPR is blood delivery to the lungs. Therefore, it is reasonable to consider using quantitative waveform capnography in intubated patients to monitor CPR quality, optimize chest compressions, and detect ROSC during chest compressions or when rhythm check reveals an organized rhythm (Figure 41).

If $PETCO_2$ abruptly increases to a normal value (35 to 40 mm Hg) or higher, it is reasonable to consider that this is an indicator of ROSC.

- If $PETCO_2$ is below 10 mm Hg, consider improving the quality of CPR by optimizing chest compression parameters or giving a vasopressor or both (Figure 42B).
- Persistently low $PETCO_2$ values (below 10 mm Hg) during CPR in intubated patients suggest that ROSC is unlikely.

CPP or Arterial Relaxation Pressure

Relaxation pressure during CPR is the trough of the pressure waveform during the relaxation phase of chest compressions and is analogous to diastolic pressure when the heart is beating. Increased CPP or arterial relaxation ("diastolic") pressure correlates with both myocardial blood flow and ROSC during CPR. CPP *equals* aortic relaxation ("diastolic") pressure *minus* right atrial relaxation ("diastolic") pressure during CPR. In one human study ROSC did not occur unless a CPP 15 mm Hg or higher was achieved during CPR.[1] Monitoring of CPP during CPR is rarely available clinically because measurement and calculation require simultaneous recording of aortic and central venous pressure. A reasonable surrogate for CPP during CPR is arterial relaxation pressure, which can be measured by using a radial, brachial, or femoral artery catheter.[11] Arterial pressure monitoring can also be used to detect ROSC during chest compressions or when a rhythm check reveals an organized rhythm. A specific target arterial relaxation pressure that optimizes the chance of ROSC has not been established. If intra-arterial relaxation pressure is below 20 mm Hg, it is reasonable to try to improve chest compressions and provide vasopressor therapy (Figure 42B).

Central Venous Oxygen Saturation

If oxygen consumption, arterial oxygen saturation, and hemoglobin are constant, changes in $ScvO_2$ reflect changes in oxygen delivery due to changes in cardiac output. Therefore it is reasonable to consider using continuous $ScvO_2$ measurement to monitor quality of CPR, optimize chest compressions, and detect ROSC during chest compressions or when rhythm check reveals an organized rhythm. $ScvO_2$ can be measured continuously by using oximetric tipped central venous catheters placed in the superior vena cava or pulmonary artery.

- Normal ranges of $ScvO_2$ are 60% to 80%.
- During cardiac arrest and CPR, these values range from 25% to 35%, indicating the inadequacy of blood flow produced during CPR.
- If the $ScvO_2$ is less than 30%, it is reasonable to try to improve chest compressions and provide vasopressor therapy.

Pulse Oximetry

During cardiac arrest, pulse oximetry typically does not provide a reliable signal because pulsatile blood flow is inadequate in peripheral tissue beds. However, the presence of a plethysmograph waveform on pulse oximetry is potentially valuable in detecting ROSC and in ensuring appropriate oxygenation after ROSC.

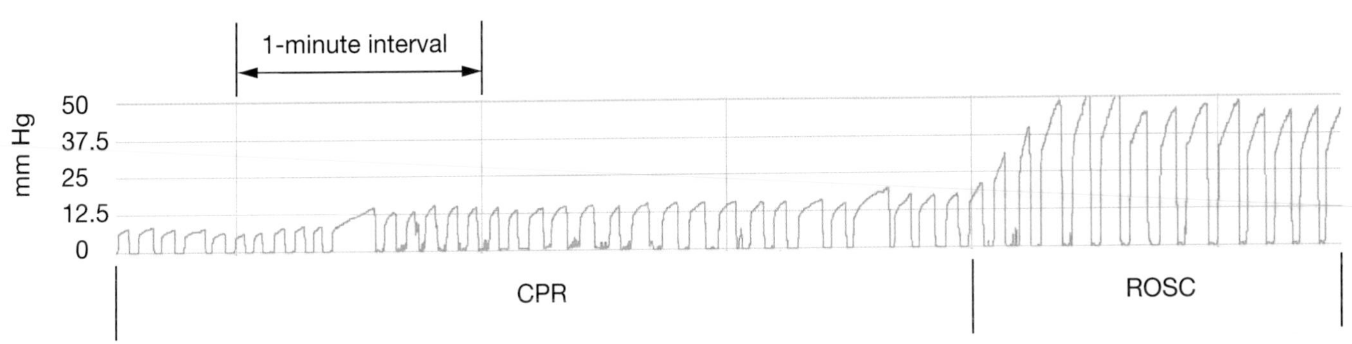

Figure 41. Waveform capnography during CPR with ROSC. This capnography tracing displays P_{ETCO_2} in millimeters of mercury on the vertical axis over time. This patient is intubated and receiving CPR. Note that the ventilation rate is approximately 8 to 10 breaths per minute. Chest compressions are given continuously at a rate slightly faster than 100/min but are not visible with this tracing. The initial P_{ETCO_2} is below 12.5 mm Hg during the first minute, indicating very low blood flow. P_{ETCO_2} increases to between 12.5 and 25 mm Hg during the second and third minutes, consistent with the increase in blood flow with ongoing resuscitation. ROSC occurs during the fourth minute. ROSC is recognized by the abrupt increase in P_{ETCO_2} (visible just after the fourth vertical line) to more than 50 mm Hg, which is consistent with a substantial improvement in blood flow.

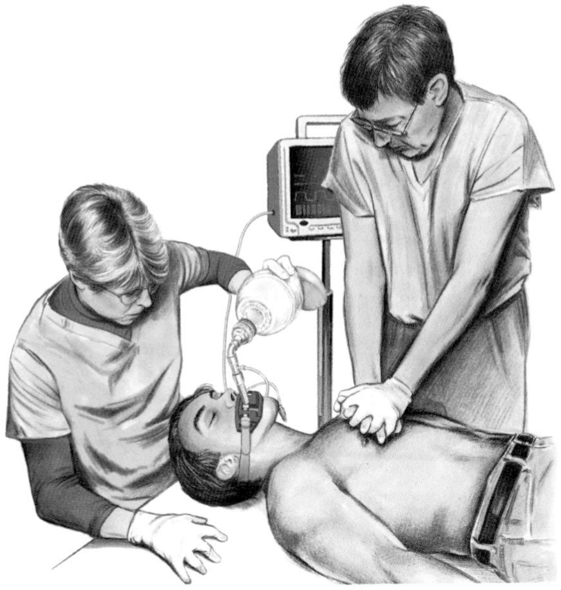

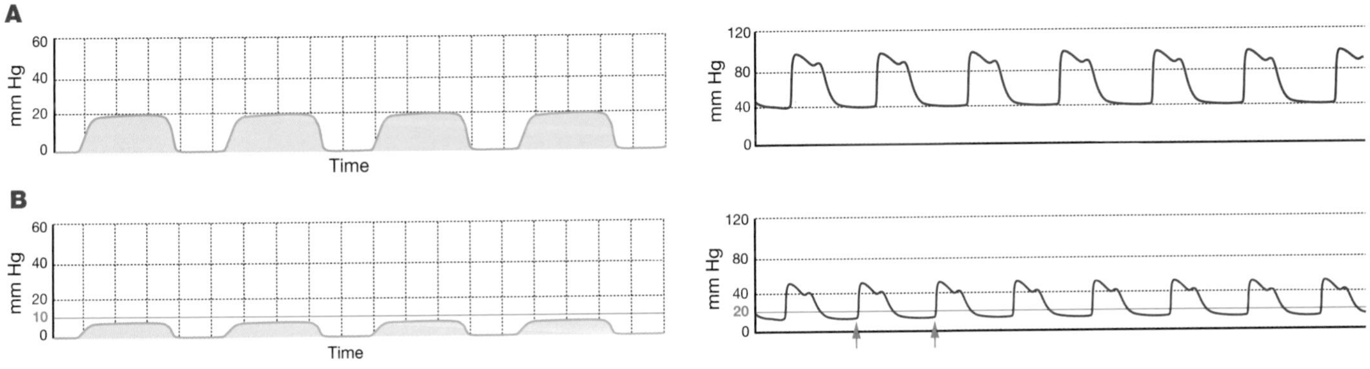

Figure 42. Physiologic monitoring during CPR. **A,** High-quality compressions are shown through waveform capnography and intra-arterial relaxation pressure. P_{ETCO_2} values below 10 mm Hg in intubated patients or intra-arterial relaxation pressures below 20 mm Hg indicate that cardiac output is inadequate to achieve ROSC. In either of those cases it is reasonable to consider trying to improve quality of CPR by optimizing chest compression parameters or giving a vasopressor or both. **B,** Ineffective CPR compressions shown through waveform capnography and intra-arterial relaxation pressure.

Arterial Blood Gases

Arterial blood gas monitoring during CPR is not a reliable indicator of the severity of tissue hypoxemia, hypercarbia (and, therefore, adequacy of ventilation during CPR), or tissue acidosis. Routine measurement of arterial blood gases during CPR has uncertain value.

Special Considerations

Topics such as duration of resuscitative efforts, when to terminate efforts, and providing emotional support to the family during a resuscitation attempt are covered at the end of Part 2 of this chapter.

FAQ

Will resumption of CPR provoke VF if an organized rhythm is present?

Concern that chest compressions might provoke recurrent VF in the presence of a postshock organized rhythm does not appear to be warranted. When VF/pulseless VT is present, 1 shock is delivered and CPR is immediately resumed, beginning with chest compressions. After 5 cycles (about 2 minutes) of CPR, the automated external defibrillator (AED) or ACLS provider should analyze the cardiac rhythm and deliver another shock if indicated.

Why was first-shock energy (monophasic) increased? Is immediate replacement of monophasic defibrillators recommended?

Experts weighed the potential negative effects of high first-shock energy versus the negative effects of prolonged VF:

- The consensus was that providers using monophasic AEDs should give an initial shock of 360 J.
- This single dose for monophasic shocks is designed to simplify instructions to providers; it is not a mandate to recall monophasic AEDs for reprogramming or to replace monophasic defibrillators.

Should I use a fixed dose or escalating dose for repeat biphasic shocks?

Second and subsequent energy levels should be at least equivalent to first-shock energy level, and higher energy levels may be considered if available. If VF is terminated by a shock but then recurs later in the arrest, deliver subsequent shocks at the previously successful energy level.

Are high or escalating doses of epinephrine still recommended?

High- or escalating-dose epinephrine is no longer recommended. Initial or escalating high-dose epinephrine has occasionally improved initial ROSC and early survival rates, but high-dose epinephrine has produced no improvement in survival to hospital discharge rates or neurologic outcomes when compared with standard doses, even in subgroups initially given high-dose epinephrine.[2-7]

Must you wait 10 to 15 minutes before giving epinephrine after vasopressin?

No. A vasopressor is given every 3 to 5 minutes during cardiac arrest.

- One dose of vasopressin 40 units may replace either the first or second dose of epinephrine.
- Epinephrine is administered 3 to 5 minutes after the dose of vasopressin if there is a continuing need for a vasopressor.

Can amiodarone be repeated during cardiac arrest?

Amiodarone may be administered for VF or pulseless VT unresponsive to CPR, shock, and vasopressors. *An initial dose of 300 mg IV/IO can be followed by 1 dose of 150 mg IV/IO. Due to uncertain efficacy and unknown drug-drug interactions, amiodarone and lidocaine are not used concomitantly.*

Can amiodarone and lidocaine be alternated?

Combination therapy has no proven benefit and could be harmful because of the proarrhythmic effects that can occur when agents are given in combination. Most important, interruption of CPR to assess rhythm and administer antiarrhythmic agents is discouraged.

If a rhythm and pulse check is not performed after shock administration, is drug administration harmful?

In balance, no drug has been demonstrated to improve survival to hospital discharge, but interruption of chest compressions will definitely decrease the chance of survival.

- Administer vasopressors or antiarrhythmics anytime during the 2-minute cycle as long as the administration does not interrupt compressions or interfere with the next rhythm check. It will take time for the drug to be circulated by compressions and for the drug to take effect.
- Amiodarone administration is associated with improved survival to hospital admission; however, the effects of the agent are not observed until the *next* cycle of rhythm assessment because the chest compressions are needed to move the agent into the central circulation. So shock success initially is independent of amiodarone effect. Amiodarone may facilitate shock conversion of VF during arrest, although improved survival to hospital admission may be due to prevention of rearrest independent of VF shock conversion.

Chapter 8

Cardiac Arrest, Part 2: PEA/Asystole

This Part

- Application of the Cardiac Arrest Algorithm: PEA/Asystole Pathway
- Enhanced Discussion of the H's and T's
- Correlation Between Response to Chest Compressions and Likely Cause of Arrest

Overview

Asystole, or more appropriately ventricular asystole, is often a terminal or end-stage rhythm with a poor prognosis and outcome. Pulseless electrical activity (PEA) is not a single rhythm but any organized rhythm having lack of pulse as a feature. Any measurable blood pressure is also absent, although this should never be measured in an unresponsive patient without a pulse. This heterogeneous group of pulseless rhythms includes idioventricular rhythms, ventricular escape rhythms, postdefibrillation idioventricular rhythms, and sinus rhythm. Pulseless rhythms that are excluded by definition include VF, VT, and asystole. Asystole and PEA are discussed together because they often occur during cardiac arrest and their treatments are similar. Survival from these arrest rhythms requires both immediate basic life support (BLS), early defibrillation if indicated, prioritized advanced cardiovascular life support (ACLS), and post–cardiac arrest care. Asystole and PEA rhythms and their management appear on the right side of the Cardiac Arrest Algorithm (Figure 43).

Application of the Cardiac Arrest Algorithm: PEA/Asystole Pathway

The right side of the algorithm (Numbers 9 through 11) outlines treatment for a nonshockable rhythm (asystole/PEA). In both pathways, therapies are organized around periods (2 minutes or 5 cycles) of uninterrupted, high-quality CPR. The ability to achieve a good resuscitation outcome with return of a perfusing rhythm and spontaneous respirations depends on the ability of the resuscitation team to provide effective CPR and to identify and correct a cause of PEA if present. Everyone on the resuscitation team must carry out the steps outlined in the algorithm and at the same time focus on the *identification and treatment of reversible causes of the arrest.* The team leader now directs the team in the steps outlined in the PEA pathway of the Cardiac Arrest Algorithm (Figure 43), beginning with Number 10.

Conduct a rhythm check and give 2 minutes (about 5 cycles) of CPR after administration of the drugs. Be careful to minimize interruptions in chest compressions.

- If *no electrical activity is present* (asystole), go back to Number 10.
- If organized electrical activity is present, try to palpate a pulse. Take at least 5 seconds but do not take more than 10 seconds to check for a pulse.
- If *no pulse is present*, or if there is any doubt about the presence of a pulse, immediately resume CPR for 2 minutes, starting with chest compressions. Go back to Number 10 and repeat the sequence.
- If a palpable pulse is present and the rhythm is organized, begin post–cardiac arrest care (Chapter 13 of this text).
- If the rhythm check reveals a shockable rhythm, resume CPR with chest compressions while the defibrillator is charging if possible.

Adult Cardiac Arrest

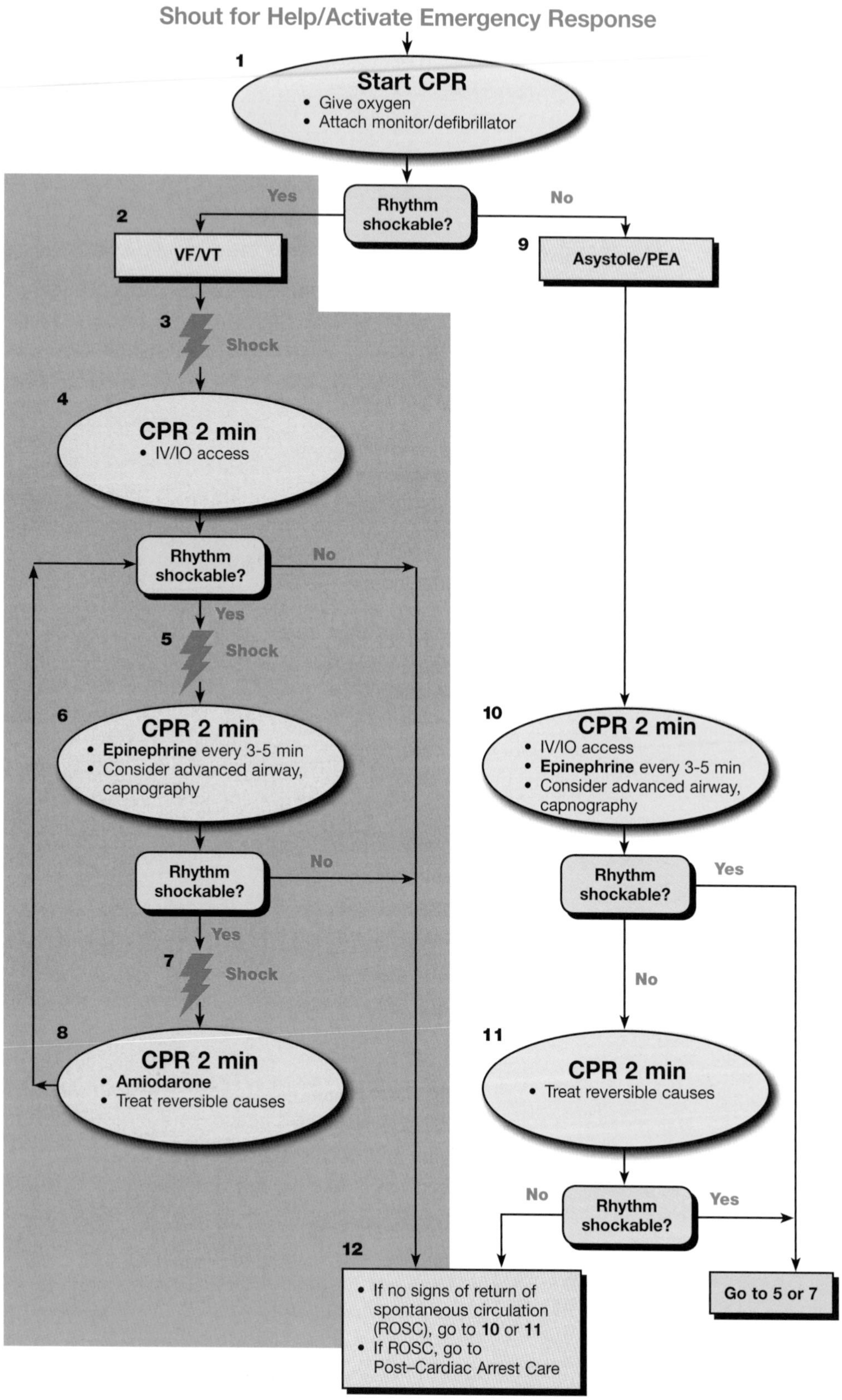

CPR Quality
- Push hard (≥2 inches [5 cm]) and fast (≥100/min) and allow complete chest recoil
- Minimize interruptions in compressions
- Avoid excessive ventilation
- Rotate compressor every 2 minutes
- If no advanced airway, 30:2 compression-ventilation ratio
- Quantitative waveform capnography
  - If P_{ETCO_2} <10 mm Hg, attempt to improve CPR quality
- Intra-arterial pressure
  - If relaxation phase (diastolic) pressure <20 mm Hg, attempt to improve CPR quality

Return of Spontaneous Circulation (ROSC)
- Pulse and blood pressure
- Abrupt sustained increase in P_{ETCO_2} (typically ≥40 mm Hg)
- Spontaneous arterial pressure waves with intra-arterial monitoring

Shock Energy
- **Biphasic:** Manufacturer recommendation (eg, initial dose of 120-200 J); if unknown, use maximum available. Second and subsequent doses should be equivalent, and higher doses may be considered.
- **Monophasic:** 360 J

Drug Therapy
- **Epinephrine IV/IO Dose:** 1 mg every 3-5 minutes
- **Vasopressin IV/IO Dose:** 40 units can replace first or second dose of epinephrine
- **Amiodarone IV/IO Dose:** First dose: 300 mg bolus. Second dose: 150 mg.

Advanced Airway
- Supraglottic advanced airway or endotracheal intubation
- Waveform capnography to confirm and monitor ET tube placement
- 8-10 breaths per minute with continuous chest compressions

Reversible Causes
- **H**ypovolemia
- **H**ypoxia
- **H**ydrogen ion (acidosis)
- **H**ypo-/hyperkalemia
- **H**ypothermia
- **T**ension pneumothorax
- **T**amponade, cardiac
- **T**oxins
- **T**hrombosis, pulmonary
- **T**hrombosis, coronary

Figure 43. The Cardiac Arrest Algorithm.

- Switch to the left side of the algorithm and perform steps according to the VF/VT sequence, starting with Number 5 or 7.
- Providers performing chest compressions should switch every 2 minutes, and CPR quality should be monitored (see Chapter 8, Part 1, Figure 42).

Coronary perfusion pressure (CPP) is aortic relaxation "diastolic" pressure minus right atrial relaxation "diastolic" pressure. During CPR, CPP correlates with both myocardial blood flow and ROSC (Figure 44). In one human study ROSC did not occur unless a CPP 15 mm Hg or higher was achieved during CPR.[1] A specific target arterial relaxation pressure that optimizes the chance of ROSC has not been established.

Pulseless Electrical Activity

As defined above, any organized rhythm without a pulse is called pulseless electrical activity. PEA is a heterogeneous group of rhythms that includes supraventricular rhythms without a detectable pulse or blood pressure. It should be noted that maintenance of an organized supraventricular rhythm without a pulse or blood pressure, such as sinus tachycardia, is usually short lived, and deterioration to other, more sinister rhythms usually develops in minutes.

Although electrical activity without a palpable pulse implies the absence of cardiac output, this characterization may not reflect the true cardiac condition. Research with cardiac ultrasonography and indwelling pressure catheters has confirmed that a pulseless patient with electrical activity may possess associated mechanical contractions at the onset of PEA. These contractions are too weak (or the ventricles might be empty) to produce the 45 to 60 mm Hg of pressure required for detection by manual palpation or sphygmomanometry.

It is critical that resuscitation providers understand that PEA may be associated with clinical states that are reversible if identified early and treated appropriately, because there may be some small but appreciable cardiac output. Unless a specific cause can be identified and an intervention performed to improve the condition, rhythm degeneration usually follows quickly. Degeneration of PEA into an agonal ventricular rhythm or asystole is most common.

Immediate assessment of blood flow by Doppler ultrasound may reveal an actively contracting heart and significant blood flow. But the blood pressure and flow may fall below the threshold of detection of simple arterial palpation, a condition originally termed *pseudo-electromechanical dissociation (EMD)*.[62] Patients with PEA and a Doppler-detectable blood flow are treated aggressively. Depending on the assessment of the probable cause, these patients may have peripheral vascular disease and/or may need volume expansion or vasopressor therapy (eg. epinephrine, vasopressin). They might benefit from early transcutaneous pacing (TCP) because the myocardium is healthy and only a temporarily disturbed cardiac conduction system stands between survival and death. Although in general PEA leads to poor outcomes, reversible causes should always be targeted and never missed when present. Look for, and treat, the H's and T's.

Frequency of, and Survival From, PEA

Because of imprecise and variable nomenclature, researchers have encountered difficulties obtaining definitive information about the frequency of PEA in out-of-hospital cardiac arrest. Published rates of survival to hospital discharge vary considerably, from 1% to more than 10% (Table 12). Given the wide range of causes of PEA arrest, such variation in frequency and survival would be expected.

Research and Reporting

Another source of imprecision in our understanding of PEA stems from researchers' use of inconsistent denominators. Table 12 demonstrates this problem and lists frequency and survival data from 9 studies. Notice that the authors of different studies used 3 markedly different denominators in calculating the frequency and survival rates: adult cardiac arrest due to nontraumatic causes (6 studies); adult cardiac arrest only, both traumatic and nontraumatic causes (1 study); and both adult and pediatric cardiac arrests due to both nontraumatic and traumatic causes (2 studies).

Note that with broader, less precise denominators in the studies, the frequency of PEA increases somewhat, but the survival rate decreases. This result would be expected because both traumatic cardiac arrests and pediatric cardiac arrests are more likely to be associated with non-VF arrest rhythms, primarily PEA. The rate of survival from non-VF arrest is much lower than the rate of survival from VF/pulseless VT arrest. Almost no one with blunt traumatic cardiac arrest and with very penetrating injuries as a cause survives. So when survival data from these 2 types of arrest are analyzed together, the overall survival rate is lower.

Standard reporting recommendations known as the *Utstein style* have been developed, and one of the major purposes of these guidelines is to help establish standardized nomenclature for reporting outcomes from cardiac arrest.[63-66] But for most of these published studies, researchers initiated data collection before publication and dissemination of the Utstein style guidelines. Subsequent research is helping to clarify the epidemiology of PEA.[67-73]

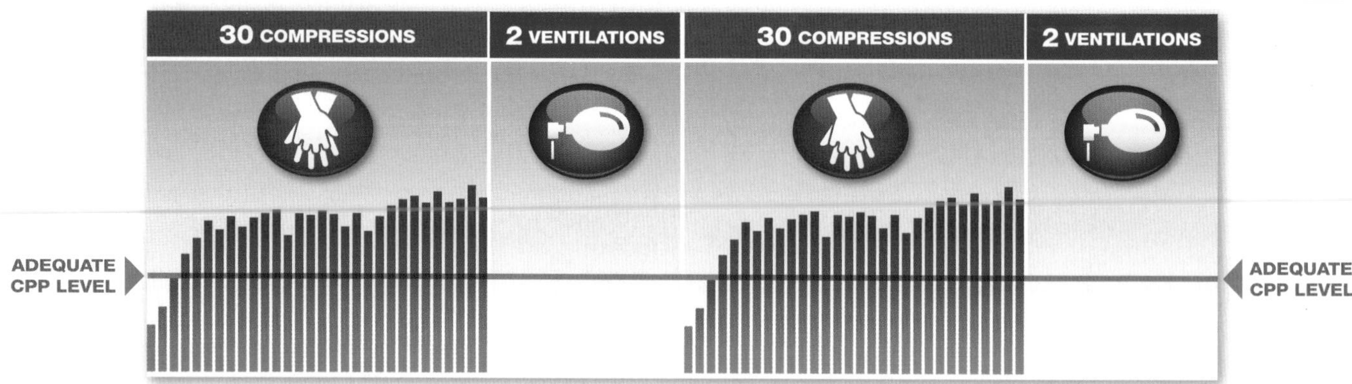

Figure 44. Relationship of quality CPR to CPP demonstrating the need for minimizing interruptions in compressions.

Table 12. Frequency of PEA and Survival to Hospital Discharge in 9 Studies*[3-11]

Location and Period of Study	Index Population	Number of Arrests	PEA Arrests	Survival to Hospital Admission	Survival to Hospital Discharge	Comment
Adults Only, Nontrauma Only						
Scotland; 1994	Adults only, nontrauma	258	4% (10/258) EMD 28% (72/258) bradycardia	–	10% (1/10)	Only arrests witnessed by EMS personnel
Houston, TX; 2 years	Adults only, nontrauma	2404	7% (168/2404) EMD 5% (120/2404) IVR 12% (288/2404) PEA	–	7% (12/168) EMD 5% (6/120) IVR 6% (18/288) PEA	2 tiers: EMT-Ds + paramedics
Helsinki, Finland; 1990	Adults only, nontrauma	489	21% (103/489)	26% (27/103)	6% (6/103)	2nd tier: doctors on ambulances
Seattle, WA; 1980-1986	Adults only, nontrauma	5145	4% (206/5145)	–	6% (12/206)	2 tiers: EMT-Ds + paramedics
Milwaukee, WI; 1980-1985	Adults only, nontrauma	503	503	19% (96/503)	4% (20/503)	50% of PEA arrests respiratory in origin
Tucson, AZ; 16 months	Adults only, nontrauma	298	27% (80/298)	20% (16/80)	4% (3/80)	2 tiers: EMT-Ds + paramedics
Adults Only, Trauma + Nontrauma						
Helsinki, Finland; 1996	Adults + trauma	344	21% (72/344)	28% (20/72)	3% (2/72)	2nd tier: doctors on ambulances
Adults + Children, Nontrauma + Trauma						
Göteborg, Sweden; 1980-1997	Adults + children + trauma	4662	23% (1069/4662)	15% (158/1069)	2% (26/1069)	1st tier: standard ambulance; 2nd tier: mobile CCU
Glamorgan, Scotland; 2.7 years	Adults + children + trauma	954	9% (86/954)	6% (5/86)	2% (2/86)	1st tier: standard ambulance; 2nd tier: MD response

Abbreviations: CCU, coronary care unit; EMS, emergency medical services; EMT-D, emergency medical technician-defibrillator; IVR, idioventricular rhythm; PEA, pulseless electrical activity.

*Studies are listed in order of decreasing magnitude of survival to hospital discharge.

Managing PEA: Diagnosing and Treating Underlying Causes

The survival rate from cardiac arrest with asystole or PEA is dismal. Often asystole represents "end-stage" VF as the final rhythm, following fine VF (Figure 45A). When CPR or defibrillation has been delayed, asystole and agonal rhythms often follow defibrillation (Figure 45B). This pattern is part of the rationale for a brief period of CPR before defibrillation in cases of delayed CPR and defibrillation, and for immediate resumption of CPR after defibrillation. In other cases an end-stage or critical comorbidity triggered cardiac arrest.

Reassess the monitored rhythm and note the rate and width of the QRS complexes. PEA with narrow complexes is more likely to have a noncardiac cause. In these situations, the only hope for resuscitation is the rapid identification and treatment of an immediately reversible cause.

Research with cardiac ultrasonography and indwelling pressure catheters has confirmed that many pulseless patients with electrical activity have associated mechanical contractions, but these contractions are too weak to produce a blood pressure detectable by palpation or non-invasive blood pressure monitoring. PEA is often caused by reversible conditions and can be treated if those conditions are identified and corrected. Therefore everyone on the resuscitation team must carry out the steps outlined in the algorithm and at the same time focus on the identification and treatment of the reversible causes of the arrest.

Rapid Identification of a Reversible Cause

In every cardiac arrest the potential cause of the arrest is an important consideration. In many patients who have ROSC, this etiology will become most important during the post–cardiac arrest period. For example, the leading cause of adult cardiac arrest is one of the acute coronary syndromes (ACS). In other cases an extracardiac cause may need to be treated during the arrest for optimal outcome.

ACLS providers must perform the BLS Survey and the ACLS EP Survey in an expeditious manner. A major component of the "critical thinking approach" is to constantly consider the ***D*** of the ACLS EP Survey***,*** ***D****ifferential* ***D****iagnoses*, and to think carefully about what could be causing the arrest. This is of paramount importance when dealing with asystolic and PEA cardiac arrest. The H's and T's is a memory aid that lists possible causes of the arrest.

A

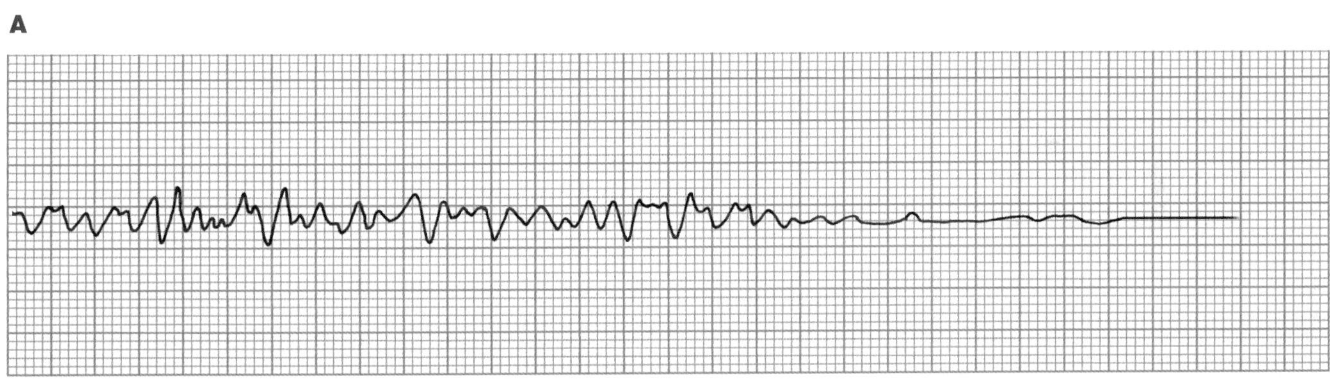

B

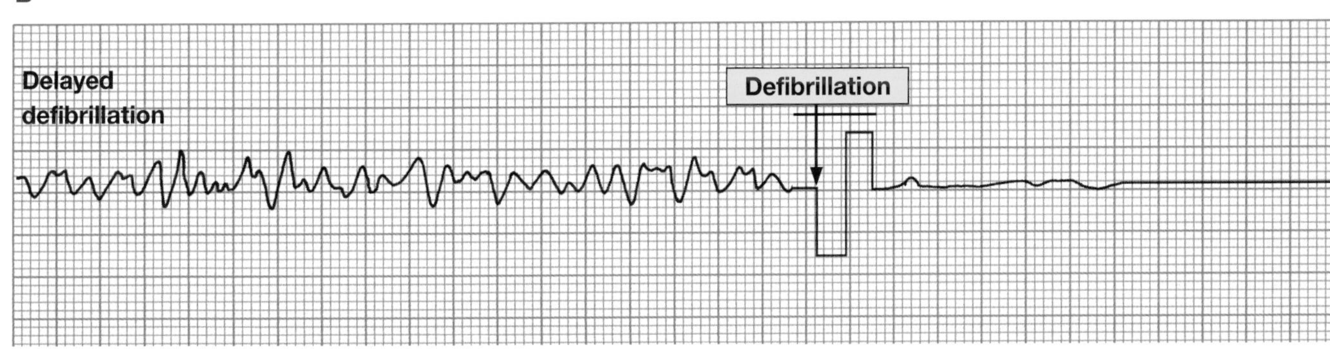

Figure 45. A, VF deteriorating to asystole over time. Effective chest compressions may delay the "decay" of VF into asystole until an AED or manual defibrillator arrives. **B,** VF resulting in asystole after delayed defibrillation. Prognosis is poor when this rhythm follows a shock.

H's	T's
Hypovolemia	**T**ension pneumothorax
Hypoxia	**T**amponade (cardiac)
Hydrogen ion (acidosis)	**T**oxins
Hyper-/hypokalemia	**T**hrombosis (pulmonary)
Hypothermia	**T**hrombosis (coronary)

This is an easy way to recall possible reversible causes of arrest, allowing a rapid review of the most likely diagnoses. The team leader should concurrently review and identify, if possible, any precipitating cause of cardiac arrest as part of the resuscitation protocol. Chapter 2 of this text, "The Expanded Systematic Approach," expanded further the **D** of the ACLS survey to include, in addition to the H's and T's, the memory aid SAMPLE (**S**igns and symptoms, **A**llergies, **M**edications, **P**ast medical history, **L**ast meal, and **E**vents), and perfusion assessments. Furthermore, the experienced provider considers special resuscitation situations, such as electrolyte abnormalities, toxic drug effects and overdoses, hypothermia, and pulmonary embolism, among others that are discussed in Chapters 14 to 23 of this text.

Hypovolemia

Hypovolemia, or low blood volume, is a common cause of PEA and initially produces the classic physiologic response of a rapid, narrow-complex tachycardia (sinus tachycardia) and typically produces increased diastolic and decreased systolic pressures. As loss of blood volume continues, blood pressure drops, eventually becoming undetectable, but the narrow QRS complexes and rapid rate continue (ie, PEA).

You should consider hypovolemia as a cause of hypotension, which can deteriorate to PEA. Providing prompt treatment to reverse the hypovolemia can reverse the pulseless state. Common nontraumatic causes of hypovolemia include occult internal hemorrhage and severe dehydration. Consider volume infusion for PEA associated with a narrow-complex tachycardia. A patient with PEA caused by severe volume loss or sepsis will potentially benefit from empirical administration of IV/IO fluids. For PEA caused by severe blood loss, a blood transfusion may be potentially beneficial.

Hypoxia

Hypoxia occurs when inadequate oxygen is reaching the body's tissues. As less oxygen reaches the heart, the heart rate slows and contractility becomes less effective. The extremities will show evidence of cyanosis. Given the potential association of PEA with hypoxemia, placement of an advanced airway is theoretically more important during PEA than VF/pulseless VT and might be necessary to achieve adequate oxygenation or ventilation.

Hydrogen Ion (Acidosis)

Acidosis is the accumulation of acid and hydrogen ions in the blood and body tissues. This may be marked by the depletion of the alkaline reserves in the blood, which results in a decreasing pH level. An ECG will show smaller-amplitude QRS complexes. Severe acidemia may reduce responsiveness to adrenergic medications.

Please refer to Chapter 15, "Life-Threatening Electrolyte and Acid-Base Abnormalities," for more information on acidosis.

Hyper-/Hypokalemia

Hyperkalemia, an abnormally high concentration of potassium ions in the blood, is one of the few potentially lethal electrolyte abnormalities. This is marked by tall, peaked T waves on the ECG along with P waves that get smaller. If hyperkalemia is left untreated, a sine-wave pattern, idioventricular rhythms, and asystolic cardiac arrest may develop. When cardiac arrest occurs secondary to hyperkalemia, it may be reasonable to administer adjuvant IV therapy as outlined for hyperkalemic cardiotoxicity in addition to standard ACLS (Class IIb, LOE C), in particular administration of calcium chloride (10%) 5 to 10 mL (500 to 1000 mg) IV over 2 to 5 minutes or calcium gluconate (10%) 15 to 30 mL IV over 2 to 5 minutes.

Hypokalemia or low blood potassium can produce ECG changes such as prominent U waves, T-wave flattening, and wide-complex tachycardia. It could also lead to ventricular arrhythmias, which, if left untreated, deteriorate to PEA or asystole.

Hyperkalemia, hypokalemia, and other electrolyte abnormalities are discussed in greater detail in Chapter 15.

Hypothermia

Hypothermia is defined as a decrease in core body temperature below 35°C or 95°F. This condition may present with J or Osborne waves on the ECG.

ACLS management of cardiac arrest due to hypothermia focuses on aggressive active core rewarming techniques as the primary treatment. Other therapeutic modalities are discussed in Chapter 21, "Cardiac Arrest in Accidental Hypothermia and Avalanche Victims."

Tension Pneumothorax

Tension pneumothorax may result from a wound in the chest that permits air to enter the pleural cavity but prevents it from escaping. This condition may be initially characterized by a narrow complex on the ECG and slow heart rate from hypoxia. The heart rate may also be fast because of hypovolemia and reduced preload. Tension pneumothorax is often associated with PEA, but VF and asystole may also result. There may be no pulse detected when performing CPR, and the patient is often difficult to ventilate with asymmetrical chest rise.

If tension pneumothorax (Figure 46) is clinically suspected as the cause of PEA, initial management includes needle decompression and chest tube placement.

Tamponade (Cardiac)

Cardiac tamponade is caused by an accumulation of fluid between the heart and the pericardium. Increasing fluid and pressure in the pericardium reduces atrial and ventricular filling. A rapid heart rate with a narrow complex is commonly seen on the ECG. As filling is reduced, stroke volume and cardiac output fall, with associated hypotension leading to cardiac arrest. Rapid diagnosis and drainage of the pericardial fluid are required to avoid cardiovascular collapse.

Pericardiocentesis guided by echocardiography is a safe and effective method of relieving tamponade in a nonarrest setting, especially when used in conjunction with a pericardial drain, and it may obviate the need for subsequent operating room treatment.[82-86] In the arrest setting and in the absence of echocardiography, emergency pericardiocentesis without imaging guidance can be beneficial (Class IIa, LOE C).

Emergency department thoracotomy may improve survival compared with pericardiocentesis in patients with pericardial tamponade that is secondary to trauma who are in cardiac arrest or who are prearrest,[87-89] especially if gross blood causes clotting that blocks a pericardiocentesis needle (Class IIb, LOE C).[90]

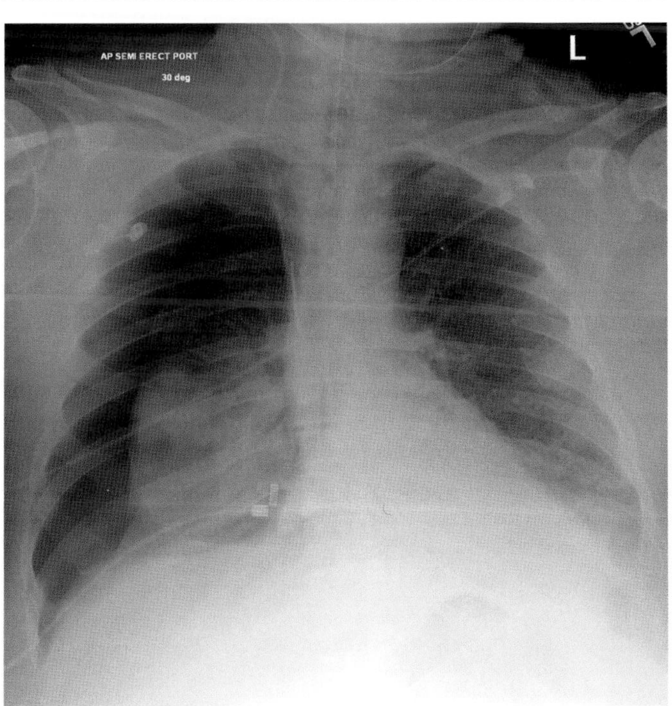

Figure 46. Tension pneumothorax (right lung).

Toxins

Certain drug overdoses and toxic exposures may cause PEA. Overdose and intoxication may lead to peripheral vascular dilatation and/or myocardial dysfunction with resultant hypotension. Toxins can have various effects on the ECG, including bradycardia and a prolonged QT interval. The diagnosis of drug overdose or toxic exposure may be best uncovered by a focused history.

The approach to poisoned patients should be aggressive because the toxic effects may progress rapidly and may be of limited duration. In these situations, myocardial dysfunction and arrhythmias may be reversible. Numerous case reports confirm the success of many specific limited interventions with one thing in common: they buy time.

Treatments that can provide this level of support include

- Prolonged basic CPR in special resuscitation situations
- Cardiopulmonary bypass
- Intra-aortic balloon pumping
- Renal dialysis
- Specific drug antidotes (eg, digoxin immune Fab, glucagon, bicarbonate, lipid emulsion)
- TCP
- Correction of severe electrolyte disturbances (potassium, magnesium, calcium, acidosis)
- Specific adjunctive agents (eg, naloxone)

More information can be found in Chapter 14, "Toxicologic Emergencies."

Thrombosis (Pulmonary)

A pulmonary thrombosis, or pulmonary embolism (PE), is a blood clot from a large vein that breaks off and travels to the pulmonary artery where it becomes lodged. This is characterized by a narrow QRS complex and rapid heart rate. Ultimately, a positive diagnosis can be made with an ultrasound, which can demonstrate preload issues caused by the thrombosis. A CT scan can also be used to reveal the thrombi.

Massive or saddle PE obstructs flow to the pulmonary vasculature and causes acute right heart failure. When PE is presumed or known to be the cause of cardiac arrest, empirical fibrinolytic therapy can be considered (Class IIa, LOE B). Despite the potential to increase the risk of severe bleeding, fibrinolytics may improve survival to discharge and long-term neurologic function in patients with presumed PE-induced cardiac arrest.[91-94]

In a small number of patients, percutaneous mechanical thromboembolectomy during CPR has been performed successfully.[95] Surgical embolectomy has also been used successfully in some patients with PE-induced cardiac arrest.[96-98] Survival after these procedures is independent of prior treatment with fibrinolysis.

Thrombosis (Coronary)

A coronary thrombosis will present on a 12-lead ECG with ST-segment changes as an ST-segment elevation myocardial infarction (STEMI) or non–ST-segment myocardial infarction (NSTEMI). Cardiac function is often impaired, but chest compressions are often very effective because the heart is adequately filled.

ACS involving a large amount of heart muscle can present as PEA. That is, occlusion of the left main or proximal left anterior descending coronary artery can present with cardiogenic shock rapidly progressing to cardiac arrest and PEA. However, fibrinolytic therapy should not be routinely used in cardiac arrest (Class III, LOE B). In patients with cardiac arrest and without known PE, routine fibrinolytic treatment given during CPR shows no benefit[38,99] and is not recommended (Class III, LOE A).

ACS is discussed in greater detail in Chapter 11, "Cardiovascular: ACS—STEMI, NSTEMI, Unstable Angina, and Heart Failure and Shock Complicating ACS."

Echocardiography

No studies specifically examined the impact of echocardiography on patient outcomes in cardiac arrest. However, a number of studies suggest[74-78] that transthoracic and transesophageal echocardiography have potential utility in diagnosing treatable causes of cardiac arrest such as cardiac tamponade, pulmonary embolism, ischemia, and aortic dissection. In addition, 3 prospective studies found that absence of cardiac motion on sonography during resuscitation of patients in cardiac arrest was highly predictive of inability to achieve ROSC.[79-81] Therefore, transthoracic or transesophageal echocardiography may be considered to diagnose treatable causes of cardiac arrest and guide treatment decisions.[11]

If available, echocardiography can be used to guide management of PEA because it provides useful information about intravascular volume status (assessing ventricular volume), cardiac tamponade, mass lesions (tumor, clot), left ventricular contractility, and regional wall motion.[100] Note that cardiac tamponade, tension pneumothorax, and massive PE cannot be treated unless recognized. Bedside ultrasound, when performed by a skilled provider, may aid in rapid identification of tamponade, PE, and even pneumothorax. Table 13 lists other potential assessment procedures and treatment modalities for the H's and T's.

QRS Rate and Width: Clues to the Cause of PEA

The rate and width of the QRS complexes can sometimes offer a clue to an underlying reversible cause of PEA arrest. Consider whether the QRS complex is wide versus narrow and fast versus slow. Most clinical studies have observed poor survival rates from PEA that presents with a wide QRS complex and a slow rate. These rhythms often indicate dysfunction of the myocardium or the cardiac conduction system, such as occurs with massive STEMI. These rhythms can represent the last electrical activity of a dying myocardium, or they may indicate specific critical rhythm disturbances. For example, severe hyperkalemia, hypothermia, hypoxia, preexisting acidosis, and a large variety of drug overdoses can produce wide-complex PEA. Overdoses of tricyclic antidepressants, β-blockers, calcium channel blockers, and digitalis will also produce a slow, wide-complex PEA.

In contrast, a fast, narrow-complex PEA indicates a relatively normal heart responding exactly as it should to severe hypovolemia, febrile infections, pulmonary emboli, or cardiac tamponade.

Table 14 summarizes some of the former nomenclature used for PEA and lists several causes of a PEA that is fast or slow and wide or narrow.

Asystole

The word *asystole* (from the Greek word *systole*, "contraction") means the total absence of ventricular contractile activity. Without contractions the surface ECG monitor, properly attached and calibrated, displays a "flat line," although agonal deflections may occasionally appear.

Clinicians have come to use the term *ventricular asystole* (Figure 47) when they see a total absence of electrical activity on the monitor. Attempts to distinguish among "slow PEA," "asystole," "fine VF," "coarse asystole," and "VF with an isoelectric vector that masquerades as asystole" are of little clinical use.

Correct Priorities: Access and Airway

Intravenous/intraosseous (IV/IO) access is a priority over advanced airway management unless bag-mask ventilation is ineffective or the arrest is caused by hypoxia. All resuscitation team members must simultaneously conduct a search for an underlying and treatable cause of the PEA in addition to performing their assigned roles.

Critical Concept **Common Reversible Causes of PEA**	• Hypovolemia and hypoxia are the 2 most common and easily reversible causes of PEA. • Be sure to look for evidence of these problems as you assess the patient.

Table 13. Potentially Reversible Causes of PEA and Asystole (H's and T's)

The H's: Causes (Examples)	Assessments	Actions/Treatments
Hypovolemia • Occult bleeding • Anaphylaxis • Supine position in late-term pregnancy • Sepsis	• History • Physical exam: flat neck veins • Hematocrit • ECG: narrow complex, rapid rate	• Administer volume • Administer blood if needed • Turn the pregnant patient to her left side: see Chapter 18
Hypoxia • Narcotic overdose • Drowning • Carbon monoxide poisoning • Methemoglobinemia	• History: airway problems • Physical exam: cyanosis, abnormal breath sounds • Pulse oximetry • Tube placement • Arterial blood gas • ECG: slow rate	• Oxygen • Ventilation • Advanced airway • Good CPR technique
Hydrogen ion (acidosis) • Respiratory or metabolic acidosis • DKA • Drug overdose, ingestion, exposure • Renal failure	• History: diabetes • Physical exam • Clinical setting • Arterial blood gas • Lab tests • ECG: smaller-amplitude QRS complexes	• See Chapter 15 • Optimize perfusion • Establish effective oxygenation and ventilation • Overdose: bicarbonate • Toxicologic causes, symptomatic and antidotal therapies: see Chapter 14
Hyper-/hypokalemia • Renal failure • Crush injury • Massive transfusion • Iatrogenic causes • Vomiting • Diarrhea	• History: diabetes, medications (diuretics) • Risk factors, eg, dialysis • Physical exam • ECG: both cause wide-complex QRS; flattened T waves, prominent U waves, prolonged QT, tachycardia may be seen in hypokalemia; peaked and tall T waves, small P waves, and sine wave may be seen in hyperkalemia	• Treat specific electrolyte imbalance: see Chapter 15 • Hyperkalemia: may use calcium, bicarbonate, insulin, glucose • Hypokalemia: potassium replacement
Hypothermia • Profound hypothermia	• History of exposure to cold • Physical exam: core body temperature • ECG: J or Osborne waves	• Hypothermia: see Chapter 21 • Active/passive, external/internal rewarming
The T's: Causes (Examples)	**Assessments**	**Actions/Treatments**
Tension pneumothorax • Asthma • Trauma • COPD • Ventilators plus positive pressures	• History • Risk factors • Physical exam: lung sounds diminished or unequal, tracheal deviation, neck-vein distention • No pulse felt with CPR • Difficult to ventilate patient • ECG: narrow complex, slow rate (hypoxia)	• Needle decompression • Chest tube thoracostomy
Tamponade (cardiac) • Trauma • Renal failure • Chest compressions • Carcinoma • Central-line perforations	• History: prearrest symptoms • Physical exam: neck vein distention • Risk factors • No pulse felt with CPR • Bedside ultrasonography, echocardiography • ECG: narrow complex, rapid rate	• Administer volume • Pericardiocentesis • Thoracotomy

(continued)

(continued)

The T's: Causes (Examples)	Assessments	Actions/Treatments
Toxins ***Drug overdose, ingestion, and exposure*** • Acetaminophen • Amphetamines • Anticholinergic drugs • Antihistamines • Barbiturates • Calcium channel antagonists • Cocaine • Cyclic antidepressants • Digoxin • Isoniazid • Local anesthetics • Opioid narcotics • Salicylates • SSRI, serotonin syndrome, NMS • Toxic alcohols • Theophylline/caffeine • Withdrawal states	• History • Risk factors • Physical exam: bradycardia, pupils, neurologic exam • Toxidrome • Clues like empty bottles at the scene • ECG: various effects, predominantly prolongation of QT interval	• Specific antidotes and more comprehensive list of therapies: see Chapter 14 • Possible volume therapy (titrate carefully) and vasopressors for hypotension • TCA overdose: bicarbonate • Calcium channel blocker or β-blocker overdose: glucagon, calcium • Cocaine overdose: benzodiazepines; do not give nonselective β-blockers • Local anesthetics: lipid emulsion • Prolonged CPR may be justified • Advanced airway management • Cardiopulmonary bypass
Thrombosis (coronary) • STEMI • Other ACS	• History: prearrest symptoms, chest pain • Physical exam • Serum cardiac markers • ECG: ST-segment changes, Q waves, T-wave inversions	• See Chapter 11 • Aspirin, oxygen, nitroglycerin, and morphine if no response to nitrates • Vasopressors • Emergent reperfusion (PCI or fibrinolytics) • IABP, CABG
Thrombosis (pulmonary) • PE	• History • Risk factors: prior positive test for deep vein thrombosis or pulmonary embolism • Physical exam: neck vein distention • Diagnostic imaging • ECG: narrow complex, rapid rate	• Administer volume • Dopamine • Heparin • Fibrinolytics • Consider rtPA • Surgical embolectomy

Abbreviations: ACS, acute coronary syndromes; CABG, coronary artery bypass graft; COPD, chronic obstructive pulmonary disease; CPR, cardiopulmonary resuscitation; DKA, diabetic ketoacidosis; ECG, electrocardiogram; IABP, intra-aortic balloon pump; NMS, neuroleptic malignant syndrome; PCI, percutaneous coronary intervention; PE, pulmonary embolism; PEA, pulseless electrical activity; rtPA, recombinant tissue plasminogen activator; SSRI, selective serotonin reuptake inhibitor; STEMI, ST-segment elevation myocardial infarction; TCA, tricyclic antidepressant.

Causes and Triggers of Asystole

In about 1 of every 8 patients who develop cardiac arrest, a progressively profound bradycardia that ends in asystole is observed after several minutes.[101] This is called a *bradyasystolic arrest.* Direct transition over several seconds from a rhythm that produces spontaneous circulation to asystolic cardiac arrest is uncommon. Typically the patient "passes through" other cardiac arrest rhythms, most commonly progressively slowing bradycardia, various types of heart block, PEA, "cardiac arrest," and then asystole. Case reports and case series of unexpected, sudden cardiac arrest due to asystole frequently identify some profound vasovagal stimulus as the precipitating cause.

Who Survives Asystole?

Patients in cardiac arrest whose first monitor display reveals "asystole" have a dismal rate of survival to hospital discharge. Studies reporting survival from out-of-hospital cardiac arrest seldom list survival greater than 1% for patients found to be in asystole on initial rhythm assessment. In fact, many experts think survival rates in the range of 1% for asystole represent misclassification caused by unconnected monitor/defibrillator electrodes or reduced gain control levels. But investigators from Göteborg, Sweden, in an excellent review of 16 years of data, observed an admission rate of 10% and a survival-to-discharge rate of 2% for all cardiac arrest victims with asystole as the first recorded

Table 14. Using QRS Rate and Width as Clues to the Cause of PEA

Rate of Complexes	Width of Complexes	
	Narrow More likely to have noncardiac cause; low volume, low vascular tone	**Wide** More often due to cardiac cause; also drug and electrolyte toxicities
Fast (>60/min)	Former nomenclature: • Sinus (P wave) EMD • Pseudo-EMD • PSVT Possible causes: • Hypovolemia • Shock • Cardiac tamponade • Massive PE	Former nomenclature: • VF • VT Possible causes: • Unstable VT • Unstable wide-complex tachycardia • Electrolyte abnormalities (potassium, calcium) • ACS
Slow (<60/min)	Former nomenclature: • EMD • Pseudo-EMD • Postdefibrillation rhythms • Idioventricular rhythms Possible causes: • Hypoxia • Acidosis	Former nomenclature: • Bradyasystolic rhythms • Idioventricular rhythms • Ventricular escape rhythms Possible causes: • Drug overdose, toxicities • Electrolyte abnormalities (potassium, calcium) • ACS

Abbreviations: ACS, acute coronary syndromes; EMD, electromechanical dissociation; PE, pulmonary embolus; PEA, pulseless electrical activity; PSVT, paroxysmal supraventricular tachycardia; VF, ventricular fibrillation; VT, ventricular tachycardia.

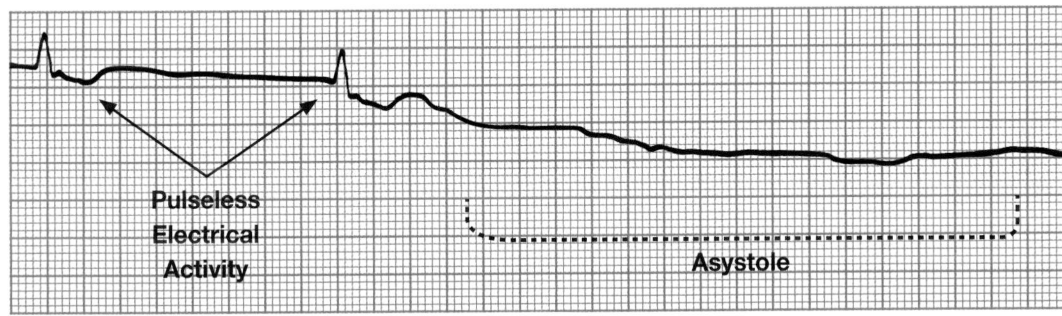

Figure 47. The "rhythm" of pulseless electrical activity and ventricular asystole. This patient is pulseless and unresponsive. Note the 2 QRS-like complexes at the start of this rhythm display. These complexes represent a minimum of electrical activity, probably ventricular escape beats. Ventricular electrical activity ceases after 2 beats, and asystole is present.

rhythm[67] (see "Relevant Research"). So when positive factors (eg, witnessed arrest, younger age, noncardiac cause, and short intervals from collapse to basic and advanced life support) are present, the survival rate can be much higher.

Confirmation of Asystole

ACLS providers should recognize that *asystole* is a specific diagnosis. A flat line is not. The term *flat line* is nonspecific; it could apply to several conditions, of which true asystole is only one.

Other Causes of a Flat Line

The following causes of a flat line are mainly technical and operational problems that must be identified and eliminated, if present:

- Power "OFF" to monitor or defibrillator
- Batteries dead
- Monitor gain too low
- Monitor cable not connected to patient, lead connector, or monitor

An Unplugged Defibrillator With a Dead Battery

A totally blank monitor screen means NO POWER. Surprisingly common errors are failure to plug the unit back into line power when it has been operating on batteries or inadvertently disconnecting the power cord. If the defibrillator/monitor is used for routine monitoring, the batteries will support display of the rhythm on the monitor while steadily discharging. A point can be reached where the rhythm displays normally but the batteries are too low to support multiple rapid charges and discharges of the defibrillator. Performing a routine checklist at appropriate intervals avoids this difficulty.

False or Occult Asystole

One cause of a flat line comes from the so-called "VF-has-a-vector" theory.[102] This frequently repeated theory remains viable despite the virtually total absence of confirmation in human studies. If VF moves through the myocardium with a sustained *direction* (or *vector*), then the monitor may display a flat line in any lead that records at 90 degrees to the direction of VF. This fact led to the practice of shocking asystole in case VF was masquerading as "occult" or

Relevant Research: "Can We Define Patients With No Chance and Those With Some Chance of Survival When Found in Asystole Out of Hospital?"

Investigators analyzed 16 years of data on out-of-hospital cardiac arrest in which asystole was the first arrhythmia recorded by emergency medical services (EMS) personnel. All arrests were included regardless of the age of victim or origin of arrest. Between 1981 and 1997 EMS personnel in Göteborg, Sweden, attended 4662 cardiac arrests. Asystole was the first-recorded arrhythmia for 1635 patients (35%). Of these patients, 10% (156) were admitted alive to the hospital and 2% (32) were discharged alive.

The following characteristics were associated with survival: younger age (median age 58 vs 68 years, P=0.01), witnessed arrest (78% vs 50%, P=0.03), shorter intervals from collapse to arrival of ambulance (3.5 vs 6 minutes) and mobile coronary care unit (5 vs 10 minutes, P<0.001), atropine given less often (P=0.05), noncardiac cause of arrest (48% vs 27%), and higher level of consciousness on arrival at the emergency department.

Fifty-five percent of patients discharged alive had no or small neurologic deficits (cerebral performance category 1 or 2). No patients older than 70 years with unwitnessed arrest (n=211) survived to discharge.

—*Condensed from Engdahl et al.*[67]

Shock for Asystole: Lack of Evidence

In 1984 Thompson et al from Milwaukee were the first to study Ewy's theory[102] that empiric shocks to asystole might "discover" people in occult VF and increase the dismal save rate for asystole. They entered 119 patients in initial asystole into the prospective study and observed that 10 patients showed a change in rhythm after a shock, and 6 of these people reached the hospital. None of the 6 survived to admission. Although the authors concluded that the result "justifies continuation of the study," no follow-up publication has ever appeared.

In 1985 Ornato and Gonzales published their data about whether electrical shock for asystole had any value. In a study of 24 patients they observed, without presenting specific figures, that "shock was more effective than epinephrine, atropine or calcium chloride in altering the rhythm from asystole." They concluded that "the rhythm diagnosed as asystole may actually be VF in many cases."[103]

In 1989 Losek et al published a retrospective review of initial shock of 49 children in asystole compared with 41 asystolic children who were not shocked. A change in rhythm occurred in 10 of the 49 (20%) children who received shocks; 3 of the 10 had ROSC, but none survived to hospital discharge. A change in rhythm occurred in 9 of the 41 (22%) children not shocked; 6 of the 9 had ROSC, and 1 survived. The authors concluded that immediate shock of asystole in children had no value and should not be recommended.[104]

In 1993 the Nine City High-Dose Epinephrine Study Group published an analysis of 77 asystolic patients who received initial shock compared with 117 who received standard therapy. In all outcomes studied, the shock group had a *worse* outcome than the no-shock group: ROSC occurred in 16% of the shock group and 23% of the no-shock group; survival to hospital discharge was 0% in the shock group and 2% in the no-shock group. Although no statistical significance was associated with these differences, the authors concluded that the no-shock group displayed a "tendency" to do better. The authors saw no justification for a study with a much larger sample size; they saw little reason to continue studying this question.[105]

In the past decade the only published advocacy for empiric shocks for asystole have been in letters to the editor and an occasional editorial expressing rational conjecture rather than empiric evidence. Based on the 4 studies noted above and the absence of any significant data subsequently, the American Heart Association does not recommend empiric shocks for asystole. Extrapolation of data from studies of the possible harm of electric shock supports a Class III recommendation (no benefit, possible harm) for this approach.

"false" asystole. In studies addressing this concept, there was no benefit from shock delivery for asystole. In fact, in all outcomes studied, including ROSC and survival, the group that received shocks showed a trend toward a *worse* outcome than the group that did not receive shocks. Thus, it is not useful to shock asystole (Class III, LOE B).

Pacing for Asystole?

Electric pacing is generally not effective in cardiac arrest, and no studies have observed a survival benefit from pacing in cardiac arrest. Existing evidence suggests that pacing by transcutaneous, transvenous, or transmyocardial means in cardiac arrest does not improve the likelihood of ROSC or survival outcome regardless of the timing of pacing administration, location of arrest, or primary cardiac rhythm targeted for treatment. Reports of success with TCP in the treatment of asystole are rare and anecdotal. A randomized, controlled trial of out-of-hospital TCP from King County, Washington, found no case of a pacing-dependent return of circulation in more than 120 cases of early TCP for primary or postshock asystole.[106] Because of the emphasis on continued and uninterrupted high-quality CPR in the *2010 American Heart Association Guidelines for Cardiopulmonary Resuscitation and Emergency Cardiovascular Care,* and a lack of evidence and potential for harm when chest compressions are interrupted, pacing is not recommended for asystole.

Drugs for PEA and Asystole

Vasopressors

Epinephrine or vasopressin is administered when asystole persists despite CPR. Epinephrine hydrochloride produces beneficial physiological effects in patients during cardiac arrest, primarily because of its α-adrenergic receptor–stimulating (ie, vasoconstrictor) properties.[13] The α-adrenergic effects of epinephrine can increase myocardial and cerebral perfusion pressure during CPR.[14] The value and safety of the β-adrenergic effects of epinephrine are controversial because the effects may increase myocardial work and reduce subendocardial perfusion.[15] Vasopressin is a nonadrenergic peripheral vasoconstrictor that also causes vasoconstriction but lacks β-adrenergic side effects.[16,17] Detailed descriptions of the receptors and mechanism of action of vasopressors are discussed in Part 1 of this chapter.

A prospective, nonrandomized, observational study evaluated the association between epinephrine use before hospital arrival and the short- and long-term mortality in patients with cardiac arrest. The study analyzed data from 417 188 out-of-hospital cardiac arrest patients in Japan. Patients were treated with or without epinephrine by EMS personnel on the scene and were transported to the hospital. Prehospital treatment with epinephrine was significantly ($P<0.001$) associated with increased chance of ROSC before hospital arrival. However, the prehospital administration of epinephrine was significantly ($P<0.001$) associated with decreased chance of survival and good functional outcomes (cerebral and neurologic performance) 1 month after the event.[26]

A vasopressor can be given as soon as feasible with the primary goal of increasing myocardial and cerebral blood flow during CPR and achieving ROSC. Providers should continue to search actively for reversible causes.

Epinephrine in Cardiac Arrest

Epinephrine is a natural catecholamine with both α- and β-adrenergic agonist activity. The beneficial effects of epinephrine during cardiac arrest come from its α-adrenergic effects. During resuscitation epinephrine increases peripheral vasoconstriction and improves coronary artery perfusion pressure. As a result, stimulation of α-adrenergic receptors during CPR increases myocardial and cerebral blood flow.[14] Stimulation of the β-adrenergic receptors results in increased heart rate, contractility, and conduction velocity.

Epinephrine is indicated in the following conditions:

- Cardiac arrest: VF and pulseless VT unresponsive to initial shocks (Part 1 of this chapter), asystole, and PEA
- Symptomatic bradycardia: After atropine has failed (see Chapter 9)
- Severe hypotension: Low blood pressure from shock, although its effects on myocardial oxygen demand may limit its usefulness in adults with coronary artery disease (see Chapter 11)
- Anaphylaxis, severe allergic reactions: Combine with large fluid volume administration, corticosteroids, and antihistamines (see Chapter 17)

It is reasonable to consider administering a dose of 1 mg epinephrine IV/IO every 3 to 5 minutes during adult cardiac arrest (Class IIb, LOE A). Initial or escalating high-dose epinephrine has occasionally improved initial ROSC and early

Critical Concept

The emphasis on treatment of asystole and PEA is

- High-quality CPR, primarily chest compressions
- The search for an immediately reversible cause

survival rates. But in 8 randomized clinical studies involving more than 9000 cardiac arrest patients, high-dose epinephrine produced no improvement in survival-to–hospital discharge rates or neurologic outcomes when compared with standard doses, even in subgroups initially given high-dose epinephrine.[2,4] Higher doses were previously used and advocated by some clinicians, but evidence has accumulated that higher doses have no incremental benefit.

In theory, higher doses may have the potential to cause harm. Careful laboratory studies corroborate both beneficial and harmful physiologic effects and outcomes. High-dose epinephrine may improve coronary perfusion and increase vascular resistance to promote initial ROSC during CPR. But these same effects may lead to increased myocardial dysfunction and occasionally a severely toxic hyperadrenergic state in the postresuscitation period. Higher doses may be indicated to treat specific problems, such as β-blocker or calcium channel blocker overdose, as discussed in Chapter 13 of this text. Higher doses can also be considered if guided by hemodynamic monitoring, such as arterial relaxation "diastolic" pressure or CPP. If IV/IO access is delayed or cannot be established, epinephrine may be given endotracheally at a dose of 2 to 2.5 mg.

Vasopressin in Cardiac Arrest

Vasopressin is a nonadrenergic peripheral vasoconstrictor that also causes coronary and renal vasoconstriction.[17,28] Two large randomized controlled human trials[29,30] failed to show an increase in rates of ROSC or survival when vasopressin (40 units, with the dose repeated in one study) was compared with epinephrine (1 mg, repeated) as the initial vasopressor for treatment of cardiac arrest. In the multicenter trial involving 1186 out-of-hospital cardiac arrests with all rhythms, a *post hoc* analysis of patients with asystole showed significant improvement in survival to hospital discharge but not neurologically intact survival when 40 units (repeated once if necessary) of vasopressin was used as the initial vasopressor compared with epinephrine (1 mg, repeated if necessary).[30]

Because the effects of vasopressin have not been shown to differ from those of epinephrine in cardiac arrest, 1 dose of vasopressin 40 units IV/IO may replace either the first or second dose of epinephrine in the treatment of pulseless arrest.

Arginine vasopressin is a naturally occurring hormone, also known as antidiuretic hormone. Endogenous vasopressin levels in patients undergoing CPR are significantly higher in patients who survive than in patients who have no ROSC. This finding stimulated interest in evaluation of vasopressin as a vasoconstrictor during cardiac arrest. It was hypothesized that vasopressin might be beneficial and avoid the harmful physiologic effects of epinephrine.

After a short duration of VF, vasopressin administration during CPR has been shown to increase

- CPP
- Vital organ blood flow
- Median frequency of VF
- Cerebral oxygen delivery

In higher doses than needed for its antidiuretic action, vasopressin is a nonadrenergic peripheral vasoconstrictor. Vasopressin causes vasoconstriction by directly stimulating smooth muscle V_1 receptors. A potential advantage is that vasopressin does not increase myocardial oxygen consumption during CPR because it has no β-adrenergic activity. The half-life of vasopressin in animal models with intact circulation is 10 to 20 minutes, which is longer than the half-life of epinephrine during CPR.

Special Considerations When Treating Asystole and PEA

Rapid Scene Survey

A common scenario, both in and out of hospital, occurs when providers respond to an emergency alarm and observe a person who appears far removed from life. A flat line on the monitor screen is often a confirmation of death. A rapid scene survey (also applies to VF and pulseless VT cardiac arrest) should be performed to determine if any reason exists not to initiate CPR:

- The patient has signs of *irreversible death,* such as rigor mortis, decapitation, or dependent lividity.
- Threat to safety of providers.

Evidence for DNAR (Do Not Attempt Resuscitation)?

Providers should observe and note any valid, signed, and dated DNAR order or advanced directive indicating that resuscitation is not desired. If yes, do not start or attempt resuscitation.

Critical Concept Atropine Use	• Available evidence suggests that the routine use of atropine during PEA or asystole is unlikely to have a therapeutic benefit. • Atropine has been removed from the Cardiac Arrest Algorithm.

Patient Self-Determination?

The concept of *patient self-determination, that a person has the right to make decisions about healthcare treatment at the end of life,* is now widely accepted internationally. In the United States it is a matter of both ethics and law.[15] EMS and hospital providers should be familiar with local policies, procedures, and practice. A few questions during the initial scene survey could provide guidance:

- Could DNAR be an appropriate approach for this patient?
- Are there any *objective* indicators of DNAR status, such as an alert bracelet or anklet?
- Written documents? Family statements? If yes, do not start or attempt resuscitation.

Family and Patient Wishes?

People call for emergency help for many reasons. Many families call 911 not to request resuscitation but to request help in coping with the dead. Physicians caring for terminally ill patients are now more aware that hospice programs frequently can address these issues; we encourage physicians to support the patient and family by referring them to these excellent programs. Making a terminally ill patient comfortable is more important than sustaining a few more moments of life for the patient and family. Legal barriers are often cited as reasons to withhold comfort measures and initiate resuscitation. Public knowledge and EMS planning are beginning to remove many of these concerns. People should be able to call for and receive emergency comfort and care, but they should not receive an unwanted attempt at resuscitation.

Calling the Code: When to Stop Resuscitative Efforts

In most resuscitation attempts this question seems to "sneak up" on the team. The question of whether the resuscitation attempt has reached the point where efforts should cease is best answered after consideration of the quality of the resuscitation attempt, the presence of atypical clinical events or features, and whether *cease-efforts protocols* are in place in the setting of the resuscitation.

The resuscitation team must make a conscientious and competent effort to give patients a trial of CPR and ACLS, provided that the patient has not expressed a decision to forgo resuscitative efforts. The final decision to stop efforts can never be as simple as an isolated time interval, but clinical judgment and respect for human dignity must enter into decision making. There are insufficient data to guide this decision, but the following considerations are important and can guide ACLS team leaders.

Consider Quality of Resuscitation

The resuscitation team leader should quickly review, in almost a checklist fashion, a series of questions similar to the following:

- Was there an adequate trial of BLS? ACLS?
- Has the team performed endotracheal intubation?
- Achieved effective ventilation?
- Shocked VF if present?
- Obtained IV/IO access?
- Given epinephrine IV/IO?
- Ruled out or corrected reversible causes?
- Documented continuous asystole after all of the above have been accomplished?

Atypical Features Present?

Even within the context of persistent asystole, exceptions and unusual circumstances can come into play. These exceptions are clinical features that in general would justify prolonging the resuscitation attempt beyond what would be appropriate for prolonged asystole:

- Young age?
- Asystole persists because of toxins or electrolyte abnormalities?
- Profound hypothermia?
- Therapeutic or illicit drug overdose?
- Nearby family or loved ones expressing opposition to stopping efforts?
- Victim of cold-water submersion?

A particularly challenging situation can arise when the person in cardiac arrest experiences effective circulation from the chest compressions of CPR. The blood flow can be sufficient to maintain higher brainstem functions such as gasping respirations, avoidance or protective movements, and even near consciousness. Although a rarely observed phenomenon, there are case reports, most often of young adults with drug overdoses, of CPR maintaining near consciousness for up to 6 hours.[72,73]

Terminating In-Hospital Resuscitative Efforts

The decision to terminate resuscitative efforts rests with the treating physician in the hospital and is based on consideration of many factors, including

- Time from collapse to CPR
- Time from collapse to first defibrillation attempt
- Comorbid disease
- Prearrest state
- Initial arrest rhythm
- Response to resuscitative measures

None of these factors alone or in combination is clearly predictive of outcome. Although prolonged duration of resuscitative efforts has been associated with poor outcome, a recent study[107] showed that patients who had cardiac arrests at hospitals with longer median resuscitation durations had higher rates of ROSC and survival to discharge than those who arrested in hospitals with shorter median resuscitation durations. This effect was most prominent in patients with PEA or asystolic cardiac arrests.

Terminating Out-Of-Hospital Resuscitative Efforts

Continue out-of-hospital resuscitative efforts until one of the following occurs:

- Restoration of effective, spontaneous circulation and ventilation
- Transfer of care to a senior emergency medical professional
- The presence of reliable criteria indicating irreversible death
- Rescuer unable to continue because of exhaustion or dangerous environmental hazards or because continued resuscitation would place the lives of others in jeopardy
- Presentation of a valid DNAR order
- Online authorization from the medical control physician or by prior medical protocol for termination of resuscitation

Duration of Resuscitative Efforts

Experts developed clinical rules to assist in decisions to terminate resuscitative efforts for in-hospital and out-of-hospital arrests. You should familiarize yourself with established policy or protocols for your hospital or EMS system.

It may also be appropriate to consider other issues, such as drug overdose and severe prearrest hypothermia (eg, submersion in icy water), when deciding whether to extend resuscitative efforts. Special resuscitation interventions and prolonged resuscitative efforts may be indicated for patients with hypothermia, drug overdose, or other potentially reversible causes of arrest. If ROSC of any duration occurs, it may be appropriate to consider extending the resuscitative effort.

In light of recent evidence of improved ROSC and survival rates,[107] it may be useful to develop efforts to systematically increase the duration of resuscitation for in-hospital cardiac arrest.

Here is a short list of considerations for cease-efforts protocols:

- Field protocols to cease resuscitative efforts or to pronounce death outside the hospital have been recommended for more than a decade. States should take all administrative, legislative, and regulatory steps necessary to allow rescuers to cease resuscitative efforts in the field.
- EMS systems directors should provide clear instructions to EMS personnel about leaving the body at the scene, what to do about death certification, and what to tell the family about arranging for the funeral home to pick up the deceased relative.
- EMS system directors should consider on-scene EMS-employed family advocates and a program involving local clergy members willing to assume on-call responsibility for 24/7 religious or nondenominational counseling.
- Larger EMS systems should consider having special-duty field officers respond to the site of an out-of-hospital death pronouncement to replace the departing field personnel and to provide more support and information to the family and loved ones. EMS personnel must be trained to deal sensitively with family members and others at the scene.
- Terminally ill patients in private homes, hospice programs, or nursing homes have the ethical and legal right to decline resuscitative attempts while maintaining access to emergency treatment for acute medical illness or traumatic injuries, comfort measures to relieve suffering, and transport by ambulance to a medical facility.
- Personal physicians are responsible for helping patients who are entering the terminal stages of an illness plan for death. Physicians must be familiar with local laws related to certification and pronouncement of death, the role of the coroner and police, and disposition of the body.
- Physicians have a responsibility to initiate frank discussions with patients and family members about comfort measures and hygiene, pain control and end-of-life support, when (and when not) to call the EMS system, use of a local hospice, when and how to contact the personal physician, funeral plans, disposition of the body, psychological concerns surrounding death and dying, and bereavement counseling and ministerial support.
- Most in-hospital DNAR orders are not transferable outside the hospital. An additional out-of-hospital DNAR form must be completed. Failure to address these issues may result in unnecessary confusion and inappropriate care.
- Many patients prefer to die at home surrounded by loved ones. The hospice movement and many societies for specific diseases provide excellent guidelines for planning an expected death at home.

Transport of Patients in Cardiac Arrest

Emergency medical response systems should not require field personnel to transport every patient in cardiac arrest back to a hospital or to an ED. Transportation with continuing CPR is justified if interventions available in the ED cannot be performed in the out-of-hospital setting and they are indicated for special circumstances (ie, cardiopulmonary bypass or extracorporeal circulation for patients with severe hypothermia).

After out-of-hospital cardiac arrest with ROSC, transport the patient to an appropriate hospital that has a comprehensive post–cardiac arrest treatment system of care that includes acute coronary interventions, neurologic care, goal-directed critical care, and hypothermia. Transport the in-hospital post–cardiac arrest patient to an appropriate critical care unit capable of providing comprehensive post–cardiac arrest care.

Providing Emotional Support to the Family During and After Resuscitation

In the absence of data documenting harm and in light of data suggesting that it may be helpful, offering select family members the opportunity to be present during a resuscitation is reasonable and desirable (assuming that the patient, if an adult, has not raised a prior objection) (Class IIa, LOE C for adults and Class I, LOE B for pediatric patients). Parents and other family members seldom ask if they can be present unless they are encouraged to do so by healthcare providers. Resuscitation team members should be sensitive to the presence of family members during resuscitative efforts, assigning a team member to remain with the family to answer questions, clarify information, and otherwise offer comfort.[108]

Notifying family members of the death of a loved one is also an important aspect of a resuscitation that should be performed compassionately, with care taken to consider the family's culture, religious beliefs, and preconceptions surrounding death and any guilt they may feel associated with the event or circumstances preceding the event.[109]

FAQ

Who has the best (but small) chance of survival from asystole?

Patients with a rapidly identified and correctable cause of arrest have the best chance of survival (2% to 10%) from asystole. Other factors associated with a better chance of ROSC include

- Witnessed arrest with short intervals from collapse to basic and advanced life support
- Younger age
- Noncardiac cause

Should we teach providers to shock patients with asystole in case fine VF or "occult" VF is present?

In studies addressing this question, there was no benefit from shock delivery for asystole. In all outcomes studied, including ROSC and survival, the group that received shocks showed a trend toward a *worse* outcome than the group that did not receive shocks.

Is pacing no longer recommended for asystole? Is this a change?

Because of the emphasis on continued and uninterrupted high-quality CPR in the *2005* and *2010 AHA Guidelines for CPR and ECC* and a lack of evidence and potential for harm when chest compressions are interrupted, pacing is no longer recommended.

References

1. Paradis NA, Martin GB, Rivers EP, Goetting MG, Appleton TJ, Feingold M, Nowak RM. Coronary perfusion pressure and the return of spontaneous circulation in human cardiopulmonary resuscitation. *JAMA*. 1990;263:1106-1113.
2. Vandycke C, Martens P. High dose versus standard dose epinephrine in cardiac arrest—a meta-analysis. *Resuscitation*. 2000;45:161-166.
3. Callaham M, Madsen CD, Barton CW, Saunders CE, Pointer J. A randomized clinical trial of high-dose epinephrine and norepinephrine vs standard-dose epinephrine in prehospital cardiac arrest. *JAMA*. 1992;268:2667-2672.
4. Gueugniaud PY, Mols P, Goldstein P, Pham E, Dubien PY, Deweerdt C, Vergnion M, Petit P, Carli P. A comparison of repeated high doses and repeated standard doses of epinephrine for cardiac arrest outside the hospital. European Epinephrine Study Group. *N Engl J Med*. 1998;339:1595-1601.
5. Choux C, Gueugniaud PY, Barbieux A, Pham E, Lae C, Dubien PY, Petit P. Standard doses versus repeated high doses of epinephrine in cardiac arrest outside the hospital. *Resuscitation*. 1995;29:3-9.
6. Brown CG, Martin DR, Pepe PE, Stueven H, Cummins RO, Gonzalez E, Jastremski M. A comparison of standard-dose and high-dose epinephrine in cardiac arrest outside the hospital. The Multicenter High-Dose Epinephrine Study Group. *N Engl J Med*. 1992;327:1051-1055.
7. Stiell IG, Hebert PC, Weitzman BN, Wells GA, Raman S, Stark RM, Higginson LA, Ahuja J, Dickinson GE. High-dose epinephrine in adult cardiac arrest. *N Engl J Med*. 1992;327:1045-1050.
8. Aung K, Htay T. Vasopressin for cardiac arrest: a systematic review and meta-analysis. *Arch Intern Med*. 2005;165:17-24.
9. Kudenchuk PJ, Cobb LA, Copass MK, Cummins RO, Doherty AM, Fahrenbruch CE, Hallstrom AP, Murray WA, Olsufka M, Walsh T. Amiodarone for resuscitation after out-of-hospital cardiac arrest due to ventricular fibrillation. *N Engl J Med*. 1999;341:871-878.
10. Dorian P, Cass D, Schwartz B, Cooper R, Gelaznikas R, Barr A. Amiodarone as compared with lidocaine for shock-resistant ventricular fibrillation. *N Engl J Med*. 2002;346:884-890.
11. Neumar RW, Otto CW, Link MS, Kronick SL, Shuster M, Callaway CW, Kudenchuk PJ, Ornato JP, McNally B, Silvers SM, Passman RS, White RD, Hess EP, Tang W, Davis D, Sinz E, Morrison LJ. Part 8: adult advanced cardiovascular life support: 2010 American Heart Association Guidelines for Cardiopulmonary Resuscitation and Emergency Cardiovascular Care. *Circulation*. 2010;122:S729-S767.
12. Olasveengen TM, Sunde K, Brunborg C, Thowsen J, Steen PA, Wik L. Intravenous drug administration during out-of-hospital cardiac arrest: a randomized trial. *JAMA*. 2009;302:2222-2229.
13. Yakaitis RW, Otto CW, Blitt CD. Relative importance of alpha and beta adrenergic receptors during resuscitation. *Crit Care Med*. 1979;7:293-296.
14. Michael JR, Guerci AD, Koehler RC, Shi AY, Tsitlik J, Chandra N, Niedermeyer E, Rogers MC, Traystman RJ, Weisfeldt ML. Mechanisms by which epinephrine augments cerebral and myocardial perfusion during cardiopulmonary resuscitation in dogs. *Circulation*. 1984;69:822-835.
15. Ditchey RV, Lindenfeld J. Failure of epinephrine to improve the balance between myocardial oxygen supply and demand during closed-chest resuscitation in dogs. *Circulation*. 1988;78:382-389.

16. Oyama H, Suzuki Y, Satoh S, Kajita Y, Takayasu M, Shibuya M, Sugita K. Role of nitric oxide in the cerebral vasodilatory responses to vasopressin and oxytocin in dogs. *J Cereb Blood Flow Metab*. 1993;13:285-290.
17. Lindner KH, Strohmenger HU, Ensinger H, Hetzel WD, Ahnefeld FW, Georgieff M. Stress hormone response during and after cardiopulmonary resuscitation. *Anesthesiology*. 1992;77:662-668.
18. Kern KB, Ewy GA, Voorhees WD, Babbs CF, Tacker WA. Myocardial perfusion pressure: a predictor of 24-hour survival during prolonged cardiac arrest in dogs. *Resuscitation*. 1988;16:241-250.
19. Shaffner DH, Eleff SM, Brambrink AM, Sugimoto H, Izuta M, Koehler RC, Traystman RJ. Effect of arrest time and cerebral perfusion pressure during cardiopulmonary resuscitation on cerebral blood flow, metabolism, adenosine triphosphate recovery, and pH in dogs. *Crit Care Med*. 1999;27:1335-1342.
20. Ahlquist RP. Development of the concept of alpha and beta adrenotropic receptors. *Ann N Y Acad Sci*. 1967;139:549-552.
21. Zaritsky AL. Catecholamines, inotropic medications, and vasopressor agents. In: Chernow B, ed. *The Pharmacologic Approach to the Critically Ill Patient*. Baltimore, MD: Williams & Wilkins; 1994:387-404.
22. Hornchen U, Lussi C, Schuttler J. Potential risks of high-dose epinephrine for resuscitation from ventricular fibrillation in a porcine model. *J Cardiothorac Vasc Anesth*. 1993;7:184-187.
23. Tang W, Weil MH, Sun S, Noc M, Yang L, Gazmuri RJ. Epinephrine increases the severity of postresuscitation myocardial dysfunction. *Circulation*. 1995;92:3089-3093.
24. Rivers EP, Wortsman J, Rady MY, Blake HC, McGeorge FT, Buderer NM. The effect of the total cumulative epinephrine dose administered during human CPR on hemodynamic, oxygen transport, and utilization variables in the postresuscitation period. *Chest*. 1994;106:1499-1507.
25. Cummins RO, Eisenberg MS, Hallstrom AP, Litwin PE. Survival of out-of-hospital cardiac arrest with early initiation of cardiopulmonary resuscitation. *Am J Emerg Med*. 1985;3:114-119.
26. Hagihara A, Hasegawa M, Abe T, Nagata T, Wakata Y, Miyazaki S. Prehospital epinephrine use and survival among patients with out-of-hospital cardiac arrest. *JAMA*. 2012;307:1161-1168.
27. Redding JS, Pearson JW. Resuscitation from ventricular fibrillation. Drug therapy. *JAMA*. 1968;203:255-260.
28. Lindner KH, Prengel AW, Pfenninger EG, Lindner IM, Strohmenger HU, Georgieff M, Lurie KG. Vasopressin improves vital organ blood flow during closed-chest cardiopulmonary resuscitation in pigs. *Circulation*. 1995;91:215-221.
29. Stiell IG, Hebert PC, Wells GA, Vandemheen KL, Tang AS, Higginson LA, Dreyer JF, Clement C, Battram E, Watpool I, Mason S, Klassen T, Weitzman BN. Vasopressin versus epinephrine for inhospital cardiac arrest: a randomised controlled trial. *Lancet*. 2001;358:105-109.
30. Wenzel V, Krismer AC, Arntz HR, Sitter H, Stadlbauer KH, Lindner KH. A comparison of vasopressin and epinephrine for out-of-hospital cardiopulmonary resuscitation. *N Engl J Med*. 2004;350:105-113.
31. Somberg JC, Bailin SJ, Haffajee CI, Paladino WP, Kerin NZ, Bridges D, Timar S, Molnar J. Intravenous lidocaine versus intravenous amiodarone (in a new aqueous formulation) for incessant ventricular tachycardia. *Am J Cardiol*. 2002;90:853-859.
32. Herlitz J, Ekstrom L, Wennerblom B, Axelsson A, Bang A, Lindkvist J, Persson NG, Holmberg S. Lidocaine in out-of-hospital ventricular fibrillation. Does it improve survival? *Resuscitation*. 1997;33:199-205.
33. Thel MC, Armstrong AL, McNulty SE, Califf RM, O'Connor CM. Randomised trial of magnesium in in-hospital cardiac arrest. Duke Internal Medicine Housestaff. *Lancet*. 1997;350:1272-1276.
34. Bar-Joseph G. Improved resuscitation outcome by EMS systems with earlier and greater use of sodium bicarbonate. *Acta Anaesthesiol Scand*. 2005;49:880.
35. Weaver WD, Fahrenbruch CE, Johnson DD, Hallstrom AP, Cobb LA, Copass MK. Effect of epinephrine and lidocaine therapy on outcome after cardiac arrest due to ventricular fibrillation. *Circulation*. 1990;82:2027-2034.
36. Stadlbauer KH, Krismer AC, Arntz HR, Mayr VD, Lienhart HG, Bottiger BW, Jahn B, Lindner KH, Wenzel V. Effects of thrombolysis during out-of-hospital cardiopulmonary resuscitation. *Am J Cardiol*. 2006;97:305-308.
37. Fatovich DM, Dobb GJ, Clugston RA. A pilot randomised trial of thrombolysis in cardiac arrest (the TICA trial). *Resuscitation*. 2004;61:309-313.
38. Bottiger BW, Arntz HR, Chamberlain DA, Bluhmki E, Belmans A, Danays T, Carli PA, Adgey JA, Bode C, Wenzel V. Thrombolysis during resuscitation for out-of-hospital cardiac arrest. *N Engl J Med*. 2008;359:2651-2662.
39. Skrifvars MB, Pettila V, Rosenberg PH, Castren M. A multiple logistic regression analysis of in-hospital factors related to survival at six months in patients resuscitated from out-of-hospital ventricular fibrillation. *Resuscitation*. 2003;59:319-328.
40. A comparison of antiarrhythmic-drug therapy with implantable defibrillators in patients resuscitated from near-fatal ventricular arrhythmias. The Antiarrhythmics versus Implantable Defibrillators (AVID) Investigators. *N Engl J Med*. 1997;337:1576-1583.
41. Buxton AE, Lee KL, Fisher JD, Josephson ME, Prystowsky EN, Hafley G. A randomized study of the prevention of sudden death in patients with coronary artery disease. Multicenter Unsustained Tachycardia Trial Investigators. *N Engl J Med*. 1999;341:1882-1890.
42. Connolly SJ, Gent M, Roberts RS, Dorian P, Roy D, Sheldon RS, Mitchell LB, Green MS, Klein GJ, O'Brien B. Canadian implantable defibrillator study (CIDS): a randomized trial of the implantable cardioverter defibrillator against amiodarone. *Circulation*. 2000;101:1297-1302.
43. Kuck KH, Cappato R, Siebels J, Ruppel R. Randomized comparison of antiarrhythmic drug therapy with implantable defibrillators in patients resuscitated from cardiac arrest: the Cardiac Arrest Study Hamburg (CASH). *Circulation*. 2000;102:748-754.
44. Wever EF, Hauer RN, van Capelle FL, Tijssen JG, Crijns HJ, Algra A, Wiesfeld AC, Bakker PF, Robles de Medina EO. Randomized study of implantable defibrillator as first-choice therapy versus conventional strategy in postinfarct sudden death survivors. *Circulation*. 1995;91:2195-2203.
45. Howard RF, Bingham RM. Endotracheal compared with intravenous administration of atropine. *Arch Dis Child*. 1990;65:449-450.
46. Lee PL, Chung YT, Lee BY, Yeh CY, Lin SY, Chao CC. The optimal dose of atropine via the endotracheal route. *Ma Zui Xue Za Zhi*. 1989;27:35-38.

47. Prengel AW, Lindner KH, Hahnel J, Ahnefeld FW. Endotracheal and endobronchial lidocaine administration: effects on plasma lidocaine concentration and blood gases. *Crit Care Med*. 1991;19:911-915.

48. Schmidbauer S, Kneifel HA, Hallfeldt KK. Endobronchial application of high dose epinephrine in out of hospital cardiopulmonary resuscitation. *Resuscitation*. 2000;47:89.

49. Raymondos K, Panning B, Leuwer M, Brechelt G, Korte T, Niehaus M, Tebbenjohanns J, Piepenbrock S. Absorption and hemodynamic effects of airway administration of adrenaline in patients with severe cardiac disease. *Ann Intern Med*. 2000;132:800-803.

50. Hahnel JH, Lindner KH, Schurmann C, Prengel A, Ahnefeld FW. Plasma lidocaine levels and PaO2 with endobronchial administration: dilution with normal saline or distilled water? *Ann Emerg Med*. 1990;19:1314-1317.

51. Brown LK, Diamond J. The efficacy of lidocaine in ventricular fibrillation due to coronary artery ligation: endotracheal vs intravenous use. *Proc West Pharmacol Soc*. 1982;25:43-45.

52. Jasani MS, Nadkarni VM, Finkelstein MS, Hofmann WT, Salzman SK. Inspiratory-cycle instillation of endotracheal epinephrine in porcine arrest. *Acad Emerg Med*. 1994;1:340-345.

53. Wenzel V, Lindner KH, Prengel AW, Lurie KG, Strohmenger HU. Endobronchial vasopressin improves survival during cardiopulmonary resuscitation in pigs. *Anesthesiology*. 1997;86:1375-1381.

54. Prengel AW, Rembecki M, Wenzel V, Steinbach G. A comparison of the endotracheal tube and the laryngeal mask airway as a route for endobronchial lidocaine administration. *Anesth Analg*. 2001;92:1505-1509.

55. Jasani MS, Nadkarni VM, Finkelstein MS, Mandell GA, Salzman SK, Norman ME. Effects of different techniques of endotracheal epinephrine administration in pediatric porcine hypoxic-hypercarbic cardiopulmonary arrest. *Crit Care Med*. 1994;22:1174-1180.

56. Johnston C. Endotracheal drug delivery. *Pediatr Emerg Care*. 1992;8:94-97.

57. Shy BD, Rea TD, Becker LJ, Eisenberg MS. Time to intubation and survival in prehospital cardiac arrest. *Prehosp Emerg Care*. 2004;8:394-399.

58. Wong ML, Carey S, Mader TJ, Wang HE. Time to invasive airway placement and resuscitation outcomes after inhospital cardiopulmonary arrest. *Resuscitation*. 2010;81:182-186.

59. Jennings PA, Cameron P, Walker T, Bernard S, Smith K. Out-of-hospital cardiac arrest in Victoria: rural and urban outcomes. *Med J Aust*. 2006;185:135-139.

60. Dumot JA, Burval DJ, Sprung J, Waters JH, Mraovic B, Karafa MT, Mascha EJ, Bourke DL. Outcome of adult cardiopulmonary resuscitations at a tertiary referral center including results of "limited" resuscitations. *Arch Intern Med*. 2001;161:1751-1758.

61. Bobrow BJ, Ewy GA, Clark L, Chikani V, Berg RA, Sanders AB, Vadeboncoeur TF, Hilwig RW, Kern KB. Passive oxygen insufflation is superior to bag-valve-mask ventilation for witnessed ventricular fibrillation out-of-hospital cardiac arrest. *Ann Emerg Med*. 2009;54:656-662.

62. Paradis NA, Martin GB, Goetting MG, Rivers EP, Feingold M, Nowak RM. Aortic pressure during human cardiac arrest. Identification of pseudo-electromechanical dissociation. *Chest*. 1992;101:123-128.

63. Cummins RO, Chamberlain DA. The Utstein Abbey and survival from cardiac arrest: what is the connection? *Ann Emerg Med*. 1991;20:918-919.

64. Cummins RO, Chamberlain D, Hazinski MF, Nadkarni V, Kloeck W, Kramer E, Becker L, Robertson C, Koster R, Zaritsky A, Bossaert L, Ornato JP, Callanan V, Allen M, Steen P, Connolly B, Sanders A, Idris A, Cobbe S. Recommended guidelines for reviewing, reporting, and conducting research on in-hospital resuscitation: the in-hospital 'Utstein style.' A statement for healthcare professionals from the American Heart Association, the European Resuscitation Council, the Heart and Stroke Foundation of Canada, the Australian Resuscitation Council, and the Resuscitation Councils of Southern Africa. *Resuscitation*. 1997;34:151-183.

65. Cummins RO, Chamberlain DA, Abramson NS, Allen M, Baskett PJ, Becker L, Bossaert L, Delooz HH, Dick WF, Eisenberg MS, et al. Recommended guidelines for uniform reporting of data from out-of-hospital cardiac arrest: the Utstein Style. A statement for health professionals from a task force of the American Heart Association, the European Resuscitation Council, the Heart and Stroke Foundation of Canada, and the Australian Resuscitation Council. *Circulation*. 1991;84:960-975.

66. Jacobs I, Nadkarni V, Bahr J, Berg RA, Billi JE, Bossaert L, Cassan P, Coovadia A, D'Este K, Finn J, Halperin H, Handley A, Herlitz J, Hickey R, Idris A, Kloeck W, Larkin GL, Mancini ME, Mason P, Mears G, Monsieurs K, Montgomery W, Morley P, Nichol G, Nolan J, Okada K, Perlman J, Shuster M, Steen PA, Sterz F, Tibballs J, Timerman S, Truitt T, Zideman D. Cardiac arrest and cardiopulmonary resuscitation outcome reports: update and simplification of the Utstein templates for resuscitation registries. A statement for healthcare professionals from a task force of the International Liaison Committee on Resuscitation (American Heart Association, European Resuscitation Council, Australian Resuscitation Council, New Zealand Resuscitation Council, Heart and Stroke Foundation of Canada, InterAmerican Heart Foundation, Resuscitation Council of Southern Africa). *Resuscitation*. 2004;63:233-249.

67. Engdahl J, Bang A, Lindqvist J, Herlitz J. Can we define patients with no and those with some chance of survival when found in asystole out of hospital? *Am J Cardiol*. 2000;86:610-614.

68. Engdahl J, Bang A, Lindqvist J, Herlitz J. Factors affecting short- and long-term prognosis among 1069 patients with out-of-hospital cardiac arrest and pulseless electrical activity. *Resuscitation*. 2001;51:17-25.

69. Herlitz J, Bang A, Gunnarsson J, Engdahl J, Karlson BW, Lindqvist J, Waagstein L. Factors associated with survival to hospital discharge among patients hospitalised alive after out of hospital cardiac arrest: change in outcome over 20 years in the community of Goteborg, Sweden. *Heart*. 2003;89:25-30.

70. Herlitz J, Engdahl J, Svensson L, Young M, Angquist KA, Holmberg S. Characteristics and outcome among children suffering from out of hospital cardiac arrest in Sweden. *Resuscitation*. 2005;64:37-40.

71. Wolf SM, Boyle P, Callahan D, Fins JJ, Jennings B, Nelson JL, Barondess JA, Brock DW, Dresser R, Emanuel L, et al. Sources of concern about the Patient Self-Determination Act. *N Engl J Med*. 1991;325:1666-1671.

72. Orzel JA. Tricyclic antidepressant poisoning and prolonged external cardiac massage during asystole. *Br Med J (Clin Res Ed)*. 1981;283:1399.

73. Orr DA, Bramble MG. Tricyclic antidepressant poisoning and prolonged external cardiac massage during asystole. *Br Med J (Clin Res Ed)*. 1981;283:1107-1108.

74. Memtsoudis SG, Rosenberger P, Loffler M, Eltzschig HK, Mizuguchi A, Shernan SK, Fox JA. The usefulness of transesophageal echocardiography during intraoperative cardiac arrest in noncardiac surgery. *Anesth Analg*. 2006;102:1653-1657.

75. van der Wouw PA, Koster RW, Delemarre BJ, de Vos R, Lampe-Schoenmaeckers AJ, Lie KI. Diagnostic accuracy of transesophageal echocardiography during cardiopulmonary resuscitation. *J Am Coll Cardiol*. 1997;30:780-783.

76. Comess KA, DeRook FA, Russell ML, Tognazzi-Evans TA, Beach KW. The incidence of pulmonary embolism in unexplained sudden cardiac arrest with pulseless electrical activity. *Am J Med*. 2000;109:351-356.

77. Niendorff DF, Rassias AJ, Palac R, Beach ML, Costa S, Greenberg M. Rapid cardiac ultrasound of inpatients suffering PEA arrest performed by nonexpert sonographers. *Resuscitation*. 2005;67:81-87.

78. Tayal VS, Kline JA. Emergency echocardiography to detect pericardial effusion in patients in PEA and near-PEA states. *Resuscitation*. 2003;59:315-318.

79. Salen P, O'Connor R, Sierzenski P, Passarello B, Pancu D, Melanson S, Arcona S, Reed J, Heller M. Can cardiac sonography and capnography be used independently and in combination to predict resuscitation outcomes? *Acad Emerg Med*. 2001;8:610-615.

80. Blaivas M, Fox JC. Outcome in cardiac arrest patients found to have cardiac standstill on the bedside emergency department echocardiogram. *Acad Emerg Med*. 2001;8:616-621.

81. Salen P, Melniker L, Chooljian C, Rose JS, Alteveer J, Reed J, Heller M. Does the presence or absence of sonographically identified cardiac activity predict resuscitation outcomes of cardiac arrest patients? *Am J Emerg Med*. 2005;23:459-462.

82. Maggiolini S, Bozzano A, Russo P, Vitale G, Osculati G, Cantu E, Achilli F, Valagussa F. Echocardiography-guided pericardiocentesis—with probe-mounted needle: report of 53 cases. *J Am Soc Echocardiogr*. 2001;14:821-824.

83. Salem K, Mulji A, Lonn E. Echocardiographically guided pericardiocentesis—the gold standard for the management of pericardial effusion and cardiac tamponade. *Can J Cardiol*. 1999;15:1251-1255.

84. Susini G, Pepi M, Sisillo E, Bortone F, Salvi L, Barbier P, Fiorentini C. Percutaneous pericardiocentesis versus sub-xiphoid pericardiotomy in cardiac tamponade due to post-operative pericardial effusion. *J Cardiothorac Vasc Anesth*. 1993;7:178-183.

85. Tsang TS, Barnes ME, Gersh BJ, Bailey KR, Seward JB. Outcomes of clinically significant idiopathic pericardial effusion requiring intervention. *Am J Cardiol*. 2003;91:704-707.

86. Tsang TS, Enriquez-Sarano M, Freeman WK, Barnes ME, Sinak LJ, Gersh BJ, Bailey KR, Seward JB. Consecutive 1127 therapeutic echocardiographically guided pericardiocenteses: clinical profile, practice patterns, and outcomes spanning 21 years. *Mayo Clin Proc*. 2002;77:429-436.

87. Coats TJ, Keogh S, Clark H, Neal M. Prehospital resuscitative thoracotomy for cardiac arrest after penetrating trauma: rationale and case series. *J Trauma*. 2001;50:670-673.

88. Powell DW, Moore EE, Cothren CC, Ciesla DJ, Burch JM, Moore JB, Johnson JL. Is emergency department resuscitative thoracotomy futile care for the critically injured patient requiring prehospital cardiopulmonary resuscitation? *J Am Coll Surg*. 2004;199:211-215.

89. Lewis G, Knottenbelt JD. Should emergency room thoracotomy be reserved for cases of cardiac tamponade? *Injury*. 1991;22:5-6.

90. Wang JC, Jiang P, Huang J, Qian GS. [The protective effects and mechanisms of peroxisome proliferator-activated receptor-gamma agonist in rats with acute lung injury]. *Zhonghua Jie He He Hu Xi Za Zhi*. 2008;31:425-430.

91. Lederer W, Lichtenberger C, Pechlaner C, Kinzl J, Kroesen G, Baubin M. Long-term survival and neurological outcome of patients who received recombinant tissue plasminogen activator during out-of-hospital cardiac arrest. *Resuscitation*. 2004;61:123-129.

92. Zahorec R. Rescue systemic thrombolysis during cardiopulmonary resuscitation. *Bratisl Lek Listy*. 2002;103:266-269.

93. Li X, Fu QL, Jing XL, Li YJ, Zhan H, Ma ZF, Liao XX. A meta-analysis of cardiopulmonary resuscitation with and without the administration of thrombolytic agents. *Resuscitation*. 2006;70:31-36.

94. Varriale P, Maldonado JM. Echocardiographic observations during in hospital cardiopulmonary resuscitation. *Crit Care Med*. 1997;25:1717-1720.

95. Fava M, Loyola S, Bertoni H, Dougnac A. Massive pulmonary embolism: percutaneous mechanical thrombectomy during cardiopulmonary resuscitation. *J Vasc Interv Radiol*. 2005;16:119-123.

96. Konstantinov IE, Saxena P, Koniuszko MD, Alvarez J, Newman MA. Acute massive pulmonary embolism with cardiopulmonary resuscitation: management and results. *Tex Heart Inst J*. 2007;34:41-45.

97. Schmid C, Zietlow S, Wagner TO, Laas J, Borst HG. Fulminant pulmonary embolism: symptoms, diagnostics, operative technique, and results. *Ann Thorac Surg*. 1991;52:1102-1105.

98. Dauphine C, Omari B. Pulmonary embolectomy for acute massive pulmonary embolism. *Ann Thorac Surg*. 2005;79:1240-1244.

99. Abu-Laban RB, Christenson JM, Innes GD, van Beek CA, Wanger KP, McKnight RD, MacPhail IA, Puskaric J, Sadowski RP, Singer J, Schechter MT, Wood VM. Tissue plasminogen activator in cardiac arrest with pulseless electrical activity. *N Engl J Med*. 2002;346:1522-1528.

100. Porter TR, Ornato JP, Guard CS, Roy VG, Burns CA, Nixon JV. Transesophageal echocardiography to assess mitral valve function and flow during cardiopulmonary resuscitation. *Am J Cardiol*. 1992;70:1056-1060.

101. Bayes de Luna A, Coumel P, Leclercq JF. Ambulatory sudden cardiac death: mechanisms of production of fatal arrhythmia on the basis of data from 157 cases. *Am Heart J*. 1989;117:151-159.

102. Ewy GA. Ventricular fibrillation masquerading as asystole. *Ann Emerg Med*. 1984;13:811-812.

103. Ornato JP, Gonzales ER, Morkunas AR, Coyne MR, Beck CL. Treatment of presumed asystole during pre-hospital cardiac arrest: superiority of electrical countershock. *Am J Emerg Med*. 1985;3:395-399.

104. Losek JD, Hennes H, Glaeser PW, Smith DS, Hendley G. Prehospital countershock treatment of pediatric asystole. *Am J Emerg Med*. 1989;7:571-575.

105. Martin DR, Gavin T, Bianco J, Brown CG, Stueven H, Pepe PE, Cummins RO, Gonzalez E, Jastremski M. Initial countershock in the treatment of asystole. *Resuscitation*. 1993;26:63-68.

106. Cummins RO, Graves JR, Larsen MP, Hallstrom AP, Hearne TR, Ciliberti J, Nicola RM, Horan S. Out-of-hospital transcutaneous pacing by emergency medical technicians in patients with asystolic cardiac arrest. *N Engl J Med*. 1993;328:1377-1382.

107. Goldberger ZD, Chan PS, Berg RA, Kronick SL, Cooke CR, Lu M, Banerjee M, Hayward RA, Krumholz HM, Nallamothu BK. Duration of resuscitation efforts and survival after in-hospital cardiac arrest: an observational study. *Lancet*. 2012; 380:1473-1481.

108. Eichhorn DJ, Meyers TA, Mitchell TG, Guzzetta CE. Opening the doors: family presence during resuscitation. *J Cardiovasc Nurs*. 1996;10:59-70.

109. Iserson KV. Notifying survivors about sudden, unexpected deaths. *West J Med*. 2000;173:261-265.

Chapter 9

Bradycardia

This Chapter

- Bradycardia and Symptoms
- Bradycardias: Refining the Diagnosis and Treatment
- Management of Symptomatic High-Degree AV Block of Uncertain Classification (Site of Block)
- Management of AV Block in ACS
- Emergency Cardiac Pacing

Overview

This chapter and the next highlight recommendations for management of patients with acute symptomatic arrhythmias. Electrocardiographic (ECG) and rhythm information should be interpreted within the context of total patient assessment. Errors in diagnosis and treatment are likely to occur if advanced cardiovascular life support (ACLS) providers base treatment decisions solely on rhythm interpretation and neglect clinical evaluation. Providers must use the Expanded Systematic Approach (Chapter 2) to evaluate the patient's symptoms and clinical signs, including ventilation, oxygenation, heart rate, blood pressure, level of consciousness, and signs of inadequate organ perfusion.

Unstable and *symptomatic* are terms typically used to describe the condition of patients with arrhythmias. Generally, *unstable* refers to the potentially dangerous condition in which vital organ function is acutely impaired because of circulatory compromise caused by the arrhythmia or because cardiac arrest is ongoing or imminent. An unstable condition can also result from the presence of serious symptoms, such as ischemic chest pain or acute heart failure. When an arrhythmia causes a patient to be unstable, immediate intervention is indicated. *Symptomatic* implies that an arrhythmia is causing subjective sensations, such as palpitations, lightheadedness, or dyspnea. Symptoms may be serious (suggestive of significant circulatory compromise and a potentially unstable condition) or merely bothersome but not life-threatening. In the latter circumstance, more time is available to decide on the most appropriate intervention in an otherwise stable patient. A circumstance may also arise in which a patient has an underlying arrhythmia for which there are no resulting symptoms (asymptomatic). For example, some patients with atrial fibrillation may not be aware of having an arrhythmia.

Introduction

A *bradyarrhythmia* is defined as a rhythm resulting in a heart rate less than 60/min. This term is commonly used interchangeably with the term *bradycardia* to describe a sinus bradycardia when the sinus rate has fallen below 60/min. This rate cutoff of 60 beats is arbitrary and does not necessarily imply that the rhythm is abnormal. For example, when bradycardia is abnormal and more likely to cause symptoms, the rate is generally much slower than 60 beats. Accordingly, a heart rate less than 50/min is the working definition used in this chapter for when bradycardia may become of clinical concern.

Definition

For purposes of the ACLS Experienced Provider Course and instructor teaching, the term *bradycardia* is used for bradyarrhythmia. In this context a bradycardia can be due to a sinus (automatic) mechanism (eg, sinus bradycardia) or atrioventricular (AV) block (eg, second- or third-degree AV block). In fact, the Bradycardia Algorithm (Figure 48) can be implemented without the delay that would be needed to initially identify the underlying rhythm disorder: Just the fact that the patient has a symptomatic bradycardia is enough to start. There are only 3 initial considerations:

1. A bradycardia is present.
2. Signs or symptoms are due to the bradycardia.
3. The patient's condition is judged to be stable or unstable.

The next consideration is identification of the rhythm disorder and then "tailoring" and "titrating" therapy to the arrhythmia and the patient.

Absolute and Relative Bradycardia

Clinicians must be able to distinguish an *absolute bradycardia* (defined as a heart rate less than 60/min) from a *relative bradycardia*. An absolute bradycardia is not necessarily abnormal. For example, a heart rate lower than 50/min may be physiologically normal and may produce effective systemic perfusion for many people, including trained athletes. Conversely, a heart rate greater than 60/min might be abnormally slow for a patient's specific condition.

A relative bradycardia is defined as a heart rate that is less than expected or required for the patient's condition. In a hypotensive and septic patient, a heart rate of 70/min is inappropriately slow for such a condition and would be referred to as a *relative bradycardia.* Under these clinical circumstances, a much higher rate, usually sinus tachycardia, would normally be expected as a compensatory response. It is important to note, however, that attempts to increase the heart rate using chronotropic agents and pacing are not indicated unless the patient is hemodynamically compromised by the slowness of the heart rate such that the rate itself results in an unstable condition.

Bradycardia and Symptoms

In managing patients with a bradycardia, the responsible clinician must first evaluate whether the slow heart rate is hemodynamically significant and is the actual cause of the presenting condition. Recall that heart rate is a major determinant of cardiac output: Cardiac Output = Heart Rate × Stroke Volume. Thus, unless compensated for by an increase in stroke volume, cardiac output (and blood pressure) will fall with a decline in heart rate, and patients may become symptomatic.

Alternatively, a low cardiac output (and blood pressure) may be principally due to a small stroke volume caused by hypovolemia, rather than to a slowly beating heart (↓Cardiac Output = Heart Rate × ↓Stroke Volume).

Clinicians are required to treat bradycardia only when the bradycardia itself is determined to be the principal cause of serious signs and symptoms.

Clinical *symptoms* that may be caused by bradycardia include

- Hypotension
- Acutely altered mental status
- Signs of shock
- Ischemic chest discomfort
- Acute heart failure

Rhythms for Bradycardia

- Sinus bradycardia
- First-degree AV block
- Second-degree AV block
  - Type I (Wenckebach/Mobitz I)
  - Type II (Mobitz II)
- Third-degree AV block

Sinus bradycardia is a slowing of the sinus impulse. Because of the normal one-to-one correspondence between atrial and ventricular rate, a slowing of the sinus rate will result in a corresponding slowing of the ventricular rate. However, if heart block (AV block) is present, the resulting ventricular rate may be slow (bradycardic) even when the rate of sinus rhythm is normal or rapid because of the loss of this one-to-one correspondence.

AV blocks are classified as first-, second-, and third-degree blocks. AV blocks may be caused by medications or electrolyte disturbances, as well as by structural problems resulting from acute myocardial infarction (AMI) or other myocardial diseases. You should know the major AV blocks because they are a common cause of bradycardia and because important treatment decisions are based on the type of block present.

Second- and third-degree (complete) AV blocks are generally the most important and clinically significant types of heart blocks. Additionally, a third-degree AV block is the type of block most likely to cause cardiovascular collapse and to require immediate pacing. *Recognition of a symptomatic bradycardia due to AV block is a primary goal of management,* whereas recognition of the type of AV block is a secondary goal.

Key Points

- If bradycardia produces signs and symptoms (eg, acute altered mental status, ongoing severe ischemic chest pain, congestive heart failure (CHF), hypotension, or other signs of shock that persist despite adequate airway and breathing), the initial treatment is atropine (Class IIa, LOE B),

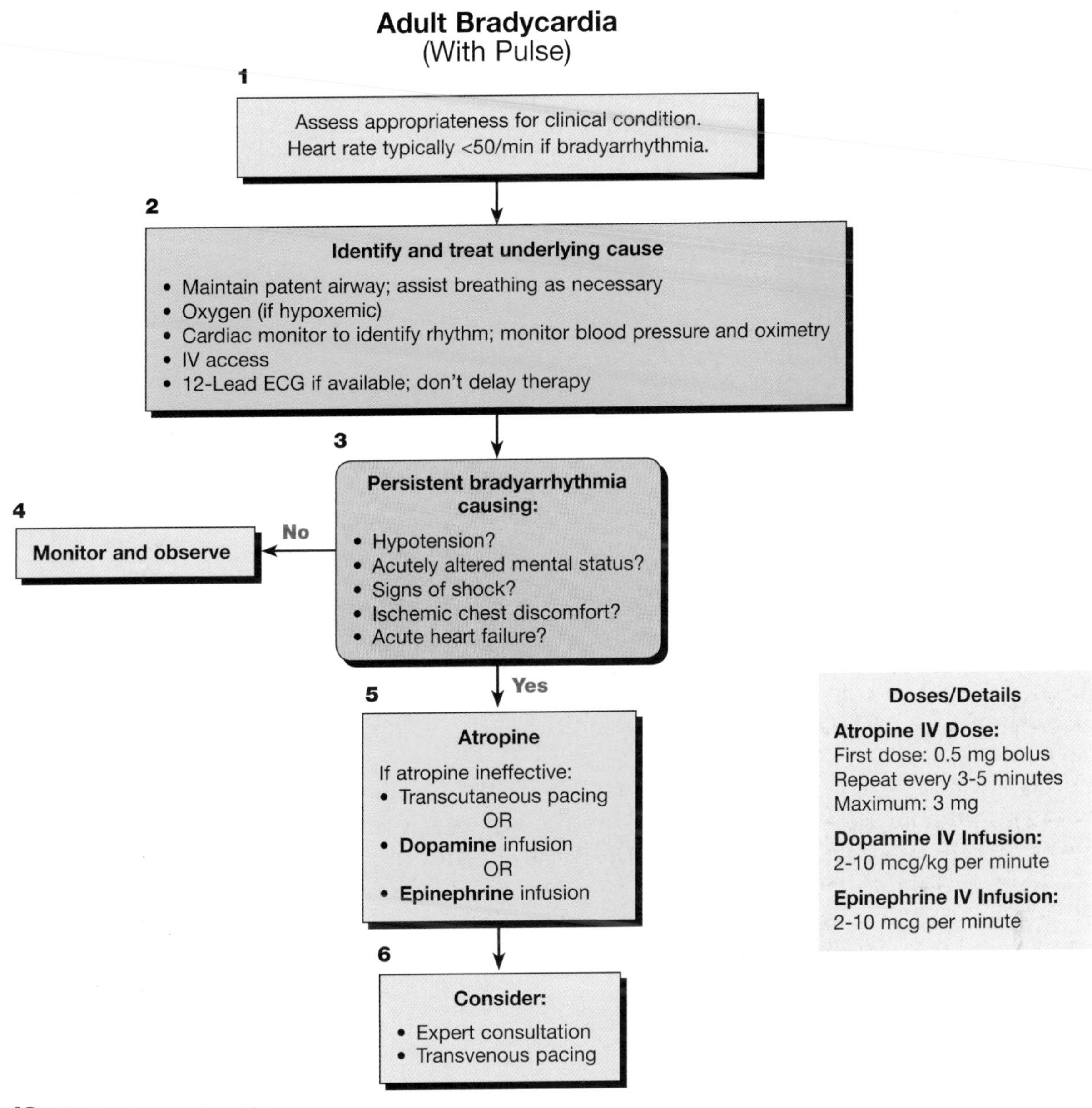

Adult Bradycardia
(With Pulse)
1
Assess appropriateness for clinical condition.
Heart rate typically <50/min if bradyarrhythmia.
2
Identify and treat underlying cause
• Maintain patent airway; assist breathing as necessary
• Oxygen (if hypoxemic)
• Cardiac monitor to identify rhythm; monitor blood pressure and oximetry
• IV access
• 12-Lead ECG if available; don't delay therapy
3
Persistent bradyarrhythmia causing:
• Hypotension?
• Acutely altered mental status?
• Signs of shock?
• Ischemic chest discomfort?
• Acute heart failure?
4
Monitor and observe
No
Yes
5
Atropine
If atropine ineffective:
• Transcutaneous pacing
OR
• Dopamine infusion
OR
• Epinephrine infusion
6
Consider:
• Expert consultation
• Transvenous pacing
Doses/Details
Atropine IV Dose:
First dose: 0.5 mg bolus
Repeat every 3-5 minutes
Maximum: 3 mg
Dopamine IV Infusion:
2-10 mcg/kg per minute
Epinephrine IV Infusion:
2-10 mcg per minute

Figure 48. The Bradycardia Algorithm.

- Atropine is the first-line drug for acute symptomatic bradycardia. In second-degree type I AV block (Wenckebach), where vagal activity is an etiologic factor, atropine administration may lessen the degree of block. Avoid relying on atropine in type II second-degree block and third-degree AV block or in patients with third-degree block with a new wide QRS complex where the location of block is likely to be in nonnodal tissue (such as in the bundle of His or more distal conduction system). These are not likely to respond to atropine and are preferably treated with transcutaneous pacing (TCP) or β-adrenergic agents.
- Atropine should be used cautiously in the presence of acute coronary ischemia or a myocardial infarction (MI) because their potential to accelerate heart rate may worsen ischemia or increase infarction size.
- TCP may be used for symptomatic bradycardia in unstable patients who do not respond to atropine.
- Although not first-line agents for treatment of symptomatic bradycardia, dopamine and epinephrine are alternatives when a bradycardia is unresponsive to or inappropriate for treatment with atropine. From a pharmacologic perspective, dobutamine and isoproterenol also have β_1-agonist effects, but these drugs have unwanted adverse effects such as hypotension and ventricular arrhythmias, respectively.
- When their ongoing use is required to maintain heart rate, TCP or pharmacologic therapies should be regarded as temporizing measures to use while the patient is prepared for transvenous pacing. If the patient does not respond to drugs or TCP, transvenous pacing is probably indicated (Class IIa, LOE C).

Intervention Sequence for Hemodynamically Significant Bradycardia at Rest

The Bradycardia Algorithm (Figure 48) lists interventions in a sequence assuming worsening clinical condition. When patients have signs and symptoms so severe as to be considered "pre–cardiac arrest," perform multiple interventions in rapid sequence. In such situations near-simultaneous provision of atropine, preparation for pacing, and intravenous (IV) catecholamine infusion (epinephrine or dopamine) are appropriate.

Atropine

The sinus and AV nodes are innervated by the vagus nerve, whose slowing effects on heart rate and conduction at these sites are mediated by local release of acetylcholine. Atropine works by blocking the effects of acetylcholine from vagal nerve discharges on the sinus and AV nodes. Areas of the heart not served by the vagus nerve may not respond to atropine. Atropine is useful in treating symptomatic sinus bradycardia and may be beneficial in the presence of AV block when the block occurs at the level of the AV node. In the absence of reversible causes, atropine remains the first-line drug for acute symptomatic bradycardia and should be considered a temporizing measure while awaiting a transcutaneous or transvenous pacemaker for patients with symptomatic sinus bradycardia, conduction block at the level of the AV node, or sinus arrest.[1] Atropine improves heart rate and signs and symptoms associated with bradycardia. In clinical studies an initial dose of 0.5 mg, repeated as needed to a total dose of 1.5 mg, was effective in both in-hospital and out-of-hospital treatment of symptomatic bradycardia.[1-3] The 2010 ACLS Guidelines recommend an IV atropine dose of 0.5 mg repeated every 3 to 5 minutes to a maximum total dose of 3 mg.[4] Doses of atropine sulfate of less than 0.5 mg may paradoxically result in further slowing of the heart rate.[5]

Avoid relying on atropine in type II second-degree or third-degree AV block or in patients with third-degree AV block with a new wide-QRS complex where the location of the block is likely to be in nonnodal tissue (such as in the bundle of His or more distal conduction system).

These bradyarrhythmias are not likely to be responsive to reversal of cholinergic effects by atropine and are preferably treated with TCP or β-adrenergic support as temporizing measures while the patient is prepared for transvenous pacing. Atropine administration should not delay implementation of external pacing or β-adrenergic infusion for patients with impending cardiac arrest.

Although not first-line agents for treatment of symptomatic bradycardia, a β-adrenergic infusion (ie, dopamine, epinephrine) is an alternative when a bradyarrhythmia is unresponsive to, or inappropriate for, treatment with atropine or as a temporizing measure while the patient is prepared for transvenous pacing. Alternative drugs may also be appropriate in special circumstances such as the overdose of a β-blocker or calcium channel blocker. Healthcare providers should not wait for a maximum dose of atropine if the patient is presenting with second-degree or third-degree block; rather, they may move to a second-line treatment after 2 to 3 doses of atropine.

Atropine and other pharmacologic therapies should be used cautiously in the presence of acute coronary syndromes (ACS) or infarction because excessive increases in heart rate may worsen ischemia or increase the zone of infarction. In rare cases, ventricular fibrillation (VF) and ventricular tachycardia (VT) have followed IV administration of atropine. A transplanted heart, lacking vagal innervation, typically does not respond to atropine and has a delayed response to catecholamines.[6] Paradoxical responses to atropine have also been reported with anesthesia after heart transplantation.[7-10]

Transcutaneous Pacing

TCP should be initiated quickly in patients who do not respond to atropine. Verify patient tolerance, electrical capture, and effective mechanical function. Pacing may fail to produce effective cardiac contractions, so the patient's pulse and systemic perfusion need to be monitored closely. The patient should be prepared for transvenous pacing, and expert consultation should be obtained. TCP can be painful, so use analgesia and sedation as needed and tolerated. Note that some sedatives may adversely affect the underlying rhythm.

Most recent-model defibrillator/monitors can perform TCP, making this intervention widely available. Unlike the skill required for insertion of *transvenous* pacemakers, TCP requires no invasive skills and can easily be mastered by most providers. As a bedside intervention, TCP has the advantages of speed and simplicity over transvenous pacing. Details and specifics of TCP are reviewed at the end of this chapter.

Alternative Chronotropic Drugs to Consider

Although not first-line agents for treatment of symptomatic bradycardia, β-adrenergic agents like dopamine and

Critical Concept **Atropine Administration**	Atropine administration should not delay implementation of external pacing or β-adrenergic infusion for patients with impending cardiac arrest.

epinephrine are alternatives when a bradyarrhythmia is unresponsive to or inappropriate for treatment with atropine, or as a temporizing measure while awaiting the availability of a pacemaker. These drugs may also be appropriate in special circumstances, such as an overdose of a β-blocker or calcium channel blocker.

Epinephrine and Dopamine

An epinephrine infusion of 2 to 10 mcg/min (eg, if 3 mg epinephrine is placed in 250 mL fluid bag [12 mcg/mL], this amounts to a drip rate of 10 to 50 mL/h) is titrated on the basis of heart rate, blood pressure, and systemic perfusion. Epinephrine infusion is also appropriate if the patient has symptomatic bradycardia unresponsive to atropine or dopamine. Use of vasoconstrictors requires that the recipient be assessed for adequate intravascular volume and volume status supported as needed.

Dopamine infusion may be used for patients with symptomatic bradycardia, particularly if associated with hypotension, in whom atropine may be inappropriate or after atropine fails (Class IIb, LOE B). Dopamine in doses of 2 to 10 mcg/kg per minute can be titrated to patient's response. This agent may cause splanchnic vasodilation and hypotension when given in low doses, complicating the clinical picture. For this reason it is necessary to assess that intravascular volume is adequate whenever you give dopamine in low doses.

Isoproterenol and Dobutamine

Isoproterenol is a β-adrenergic agent with β_1 and β_2 effects that result in an increase in heart rate and vasodilatation. The recommended adult dose is 2 to 10 mcg/min by IV infusion titrated according to heart rate and rhythm response. Isoproterenol can increase infarct size and cause life-threatening ventricular arrhythmias, so it requires careful titration.

Dobutamine is a β-adrenergic agent with primarily β_1 effects, which result in increased heart rate. The recommended adult dose is 2 to 20 mcg/kg per minute and should be titrated based on heart rate. Dobutamine has a smaller vasodilator effect than isoproterenol.

Bradycardias: Refining the Diagnosis and Treatment

Sinus Bradycardia

Sinus bradycardia (Figure 49) is a slow heart rate with regular P waves whose morphology on the 12-lead ECG is consistent with their origin from the sinoatrial node (P waves are upright in leads I, II, III, and aVF). Notably, sinus rhythm merely describes the kind of rhythm that is occurring in the atria; it makes no statement about AV conduction nor about the resulting ventricular response, which may be normal or abnormal. If AV conduction is normal, each P wave is followed at a consistent and normal interval by QRS complexes that are normal in configuration and width (Figure 49). Sinus bradycardia is often a manifestation of other conditions (eg, good physical conditioning, vagal impulses, or drug effects) rather than a primary arrhythmia that requires treatment. In ACS it is commonly seen in inferior MI.

Pathophysiology

- Sinus bradycardia is caused by a slow rate of spontaneous impulses originating at the sinoatrial node.
- Sinus bradycardia is typically a physical sign of other problems rather than a primary arrhythmia.

Defining ECG Criteria (*Figure 49*)

The key defining criteria of sinus bradycardia on the ECG are regular P waves consistent with their origin from the sinus node at a rate less than 60/min.

- **Rate:** Less than 60/min.
- **Rhythm:** Regular atrial (sinus) rhythm.
- **P waves:** Size and shape consistent with origin from the sinus node (typically upright in leads I, II, III, and aVF on the 12-lead ECG).
- **PR interval:** If AV and ventricular conduction are normal, each P wave is followed by a normal PR interval 0.12 to 0.20.
- **QRS complex:** If AV and ventricular conduction are normal, each P wave is followed by a normal-appearing

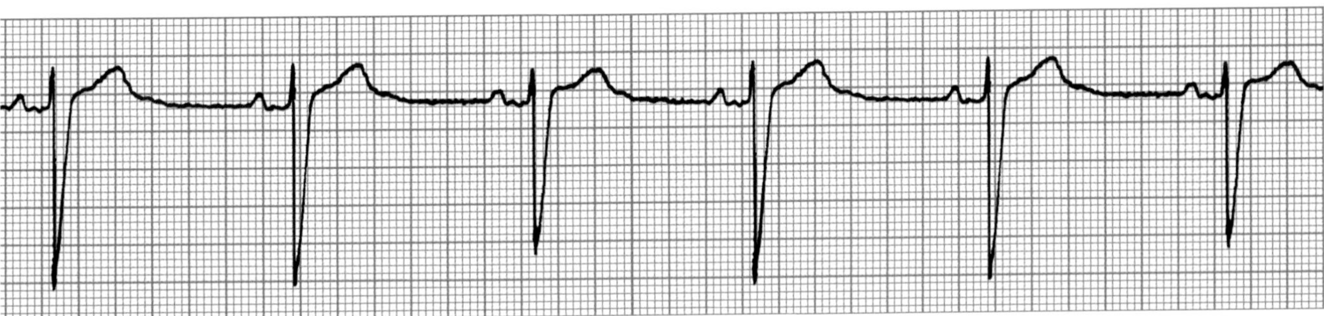

Figure 49. Sinus bradycardia. Sinus rate is 46/min and rhythm is regular.

QRS complex. The QRS complex is narrow: less than 0.12 second (often less than 0.11 second) in the absence of intraventricular conduction defects.

Clinical Manifestations

- Most people with sinus bradycardia are asymptomatic at rest.
- With increased activity, if the heart rate remains slow or does not rise sufficiently with exertion, a patient may become symptomatic.
- Common symptoms include fatigue, shortness of breath, dizziness or lightheadedness, and frank syncope. Common physical signs include hypotension, diaphoresis, pulmonary congestion, and frank pulmonary edema.
- The ECG can independently display acute ST-segment or T-wave deviations or ventricular arrhythmias. The QT interval normally lengthens as heart rate decreases, and its measurement requires correction for heart rate.

Common Etiologies

- Sinus bradycardia is often appropriate ("normal") for well-conditioned people. With age, resting heart rate also declines. It is not uncommon to observe significant sinus bradycardia during nighttime telemetry monitoring of patients.
- Sinus bradycardia can occur after an event that stimulates the vasovagal reflex or increases vagal tone, such as vomiting, a Valsalva maneuver, rectal stimuli, or inadvertent pressure on the carotid sinus in the elderly ("shaver's syncope").
- In most patients the blood supply of the sinoatrial node comes from the right coronary artery. For this reason ACS related to the right coronary artery can produce sinus node ischemia and sinus bradycardia.
- Sinus bradycardia can occur as a pharmacological or adverse clinical drug effect of a number of agents, including β-blockers, calcium channel blockers, digoxin, quinidine, amiodarone, and other agents that prolong the refractory period of the sinus node.

Recommended Therapy

- Unless extremely slow, sinus bradycardia rarely produces rate-related, serious signs and symptoms that merit emergent treatment.
- When sinus rhythm is judged to be hemodynamically significant, follow the intervention sequence listed in the Bradycardia Algorithm (atropine, TCP, dopamine, epinephrine).
- Try to determine the cause of bradycardia and treat it. For example, sinus bradycardia may be precipitated by inferior ST-segment elevation myocardial infarction (STEMI) or ischemia, or by hypoxia.
- Provide supportive measures for any potentially complicating factors (eg, oxygen supplementation for possible hypoxia).

AV Block

AV block is a delay or interruption in conduction between the atria and ventricles. The delay can occur at many levels in the conduction system and may occur insidiously or abruptly. To effectively anticipate progression in AV block, providers need to understand the conduction system, external influences on conduction tissue, and comorbidities that may precipitate high-degree AV block.

Common Etiologies

AV block may be caused by

- Pathological lesions along the conduction pathway (eg, calcium, fibrosis, necrosis).
- Enhanced vagal tone (inferior MI, carotid sinus sensitivity, visceral [gastrointestinal or urinary] stimulation).
- Increases in the refractory period or slowing of conduction in the conduction pathway (often caused by drugs).
- Physiologic block due to progressive slowing of AV node conduction with increasing atrial rates (sometimes referred to as *decremental conduction*). This intrinsic property of the AV node protects the ventricles from achieving excessive rates should a rapid atrial rhythm such as atrial flutter or atrial fibrillation occur. For example, in atrial flutter, the AV node may allow conduction at 150/min but not at 300/min. This conduction pattern becomes a "physiologic" 2:1 AV block. Physiologic AV block is distinguished from pathologic AV block by the underlying atrial rate when it is seen.
  - Physiologic AV block typically occurs with rapid atrial rates.
  - Pathologic AV block occurs at ordinary atrial (sinus) heart rates.

Classification of AV Block

AV block may be classified according to the *site* or *degree* of block. The AV node is anatomically a complicated network of fibers—not a discrete structure—and located inferiorly in the right atrium, anterior to the ostium of the coronary sinus, and in the vicinity of the tricuspid valve. The speed of conduction is normally slowed through the AV node, and the upper limit of normal of the PR interval is 0.20 second. These fibers converge at their lower margin to form a discrete bundle of fibers, the *bundle of His* (or *AV bundle*). This structure penetrates the annulus fibrosis and arrives at the upper margin of the muscular intraventricular septum. Here the infranodal structure of the conduction system beyond the AV node gives origin to the bundle branches (Figure 50).

Site of Block

- AV blocks occurring at the junction of AV node with atria (supranodal block) or within AV nodal tissue (intranodal block) are often grouped together and referred to as *nodal block.*

- AV blocks occurring distal to the AV node, anatomically at either the bundle of His or the bundle branches or beyond are referred to as *infranodal block.*

Degree of Block

- First-degree AV block.
- Second-degree AV block (type I or type II). In second-degree block there are more atrial than ventricular complexes; a second-degree block is further described by the ratio of atrial to ventricular beats, for example, 2:1 or 4:1 (expressed as "two-to-one" or "four-to-one") or greater.
- Third-degree or complete AV block.

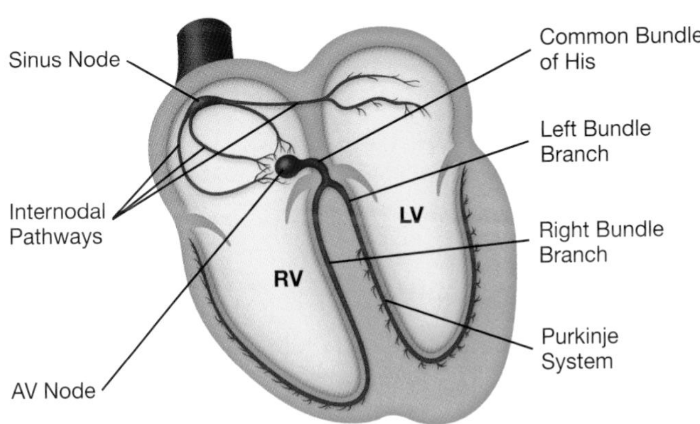

Figure 50. Relationship of the AV node to the anatomy of the conduction system. Although often portrayed as a "discrete structure," the AV node is a complicated network of fibers with different electrophysiologic properties.

The 3 degrees of block can generally be used to infer the anatomic site of block: at or within the AV node (nodal) and below the AV node (infranodal). The site of block is important because the pathogenesis, treatment, and prognosis vary with each site. There are exceptions to this classification, which may require electrophysiologic study for confirmation. Table 15 presents the major, general ECG features of first-degree, second-degree, and third-degree heart block.

First-Degree AV Block

First-degree AV block (Figure 51) is not a block per se, but rather a *delay* in passage of the electrical impulse from atria to ventricles. This delay manifests as prolongation of the PR interval. The specific site of delay can be anywhere from the AV node to the bundle branches, although typically it occurs in the AV node.

Pathophysiology

- In first-degree AV block conduction of the sinus impulse is slowed most commonly in the AV node. The duration of delay (eg, 0.22 second) is fixed, that is, remains the same from beat to beat.
- First-degree AV block can be a normal physiologic variant and does not necessarily imply the presence of serious pathology or need for treatment.
- In some clinical circumstances first-degree AV block is caused by a noncardiac condition (eg, excess vagal tone, drug effect).

Table 15. Major ECG Features of First-Degree, Second-Degree, and Third-Degree Heart Block

ECG Feature	First-Degree	Second-Degree	Third-Degree
Rate **Atrial** **Ventricular**	 Unaffected Same as atrial rate	 Unaffected Slower than atrial rate	 Unaffected Slower than atrial rate
Ventricular rhythm	Same as atrial rhythm or regular	**Type I:** Irregular (may be regularly irregular in a repetitive pattern) **Type II:** Regular or irregular	Ventricular escape beats are usually regular
P-QRS relationship	Consistent: 1:1	**Type I:** Variable PR intervals before the dropped QRS complex **Type II:** Fixed PR intervals before the dropped QRS complex	Absent (AV dissociation)
QRS duration	Unaffected	**Type I:** Narrow **Type II:** Most often wide; rarely narrow	Usually wide but can be narrow, depending on site of escape rhythm
Site of block	Anywhere from AV node to bundle branches, though typically in AV node	**Type I:** AV node **Type II:** Typically in or below the bundle of His	Anywhere from AV node to bundle branches

Abbreviations: AV, atrioventricular; ECG, electrocardiographic.

Defining ECG Criteria (Figure 51)

The key defining criterion on the ECG is a PR interval greater than 0.20 second.

- **Rate:** First-degree heart block can be seen at any sinus rate.
- **Rhythm:** Regular atrial (sinus) rhythm with each P wave followed by a QRS complex.
- **P waves:** Size and shape consistent with origin from the sinus node (typically upright in leads I, II, III, and aVF on the 12-lead ECG).
- **PR interval:** Prolonged (more than 0.20 second) and does not vary from beat to beat *(fixed)*.
- **QRS complex:** The QRS complex is narrow: less than 0.12 second (often less than 0.11 second) in the absence of intraventricular conduction defects.

Clinical Manifestations

The patient with first-degree AV block is usually asymptomatic.

Common Etiologies

- Many first-degree AV blocks are due to the adverse effects of drugs, most commonly drugs known to slow conduction through the AV node: β-blockers, calcium channel blockers, and digoxin. It can also be a manifestation of pathology in the conduction system associated with aging and with certain disease states.
- First-degree AV block can occur after an event that stimulates vagal activity, such as vomiting, a Valsalva maneuver, rectal stimuli, or inadvertent pressure on the carotid sinus (shaver's syncope).
- Acute coronary syndromes involving the right coronary artery often affect circulation to the AV node, thereby creating AV nodal ischemia and slowing AV nodal conduction.

Recommended Therapy

- Treatment of first-degree AV block is almost never necessary or indicated because few patients have significant signs or symptoms related to the first-degree AV block. If symptoms or signs are present, always search for and consider an alternative cause.
- When a patient develops new-onset first-degree AV block, be alert for progression of the block to second-degree AV block, either type I or type II, and consider a cause. Titrate oxygen administration to achieve oxygen saturation values of 94% or higher by pulse oximetry.
- Hemodynamically significant bradycardia is unlikely to occur from first-degree AV block. If first-degree AV block progresses to a more advanced form of symptomatic heart block, follow the intervention sequence listed in the Bradycardia Algorithm (atropine, TCP, dopamine, epinephrine).

Second-Degree AV Block (Mobitz 1 or Wenckebach)

In second-degree AV block some atrial impulses are conducted through the AV node and others are blocked—that is, "not every P wave is followed by a QRS complex."[11-13] Second-degree AV block is divided into 2 types:

- *Type I second-degree AV block* (also referred to as *Mobitz I* or *Wenckebach*) (see Table 16)
- *Type II second-degree AV block* (also referred to as *Mobitz II*)

Type I second-degree AV block almost always occurs at the level of the AV node and is characterized by a progressive prolongation of the PR interval from one beat to the next. Conduction velocity progressively slows through the AV node until an atrial (sinus) impulse is completely blocked. Usually only a single impulse is blocked, and the pattern is then repeated. The sequence of the block can be described by the ratio of the P waves to the QRS complexes. For example, 4:3 means that every fourth P wave is not followed by a QRS complex, or that for every 4 P waves there are only 3 QRS complexes (Figure 52).

Pathophysiology

Type I second-degree AV block (Mobitz I or Wenckebach) almost always occurs at the level of the AV node rather than at an *infranodal* level (ie, at the bundle of His or bundle branches). The AV node cells normally demonstrate a gradual and progressive conduction delay in response to rapid atrial impulses, such as in atrial flutter or fibrillation. This "physiologic" property of the AV node becomes

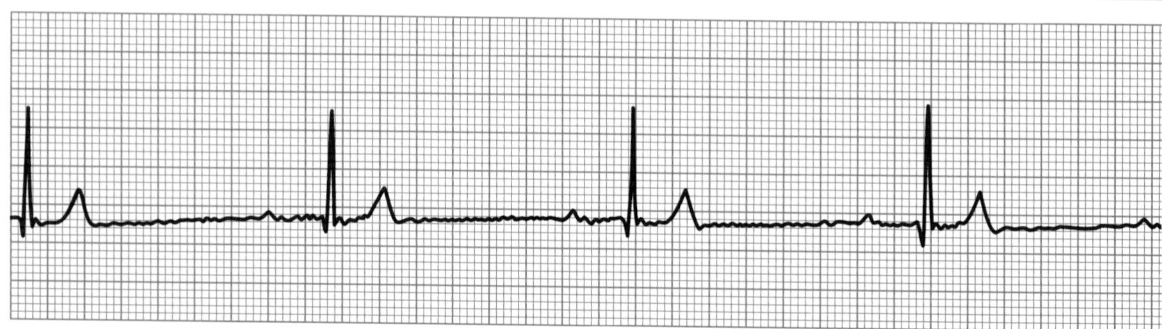

Figure 51. First-degree AV block. The PR interval in this instance is prolonged to about 0.34 second. Also present is sinus bradycardia.

pathologic and is called type I second-degree AV block when it occurs at normal heart rates. Type I second-degree AV block is generally considered the less ominous of the 2 types of second-degree AV block. This is because type I block occurs more proximally in the conduction system, typically at the AV nodal level. Should it worsen (resulting in more blocked P waves), the resulting ventricular escape rate is likely to be more rapid and life-sustaining.

It is important to remember that the hemodynamic significance of any heart block depends upon the severity of the heart block (how many QRS complexes are "dropped") and the characteristics of the escape pacemaker that compensates for the blocked QRS complexes by independently generating a ventricular rhythm. The escape pacemaker can be thought of as a "fail-safe system" of tissues in the heart that can spontaneously generate an impulse and provide a back-up rhythm should impulse generation or conduction fail somewhere above their location. When heart block results in an excessive slowing of ventricular rate, the escape pacemaker rhythm must originate distal to the site of block in order to effectively depolarize the ventricles. A general rule of thumb is that the rate and reliability of this escape rhythm progressively declines as its origin descends in the conduction system (eg, the rate will be slower and less reliable if the escape rhythm originates in the ventricle than in the AV node). The most common cause of type I second-degree block is increased parasympathetic tone, but it can also have pathologic causes, such as ischemia.

The typical footprint of type I second-degree AV block is slower and slower impulse conduction through the AV node. This slowed conduction is seen as gradual prolongation of the PR interval until one depolarization impulse from the atria is completely blocked, which is called a "dropped" QRS complex or "dropped beat."

- This pattern is repeated, resulting in "group beating" (eg, 3 conducted P waves with progressive lengthening in PR intervals and a fourth P wave that is not followed by a QRS complex). Such a "group" is referred to as *4:3 conduction.*
- The conduction ratio can change (eg, 4:3, 3:2, 2:1) or remain constant.
- Type I second-degree AV block is usually transient and does not necessarily imply underlying cardiac pathology, depending upon its precipitating cause.

Defining ECG Criteria (Figure 52)

The key defining criterion on the ECG is progressive lengthening of the PR interval until one P wave is not followed by a QRS complex. This represents the nonconducted P wave impulse or "dropped beat" (QRS complex).

- **Rate:** The atrial rate is unaffected. But the overall atrial rate is usually slightly faster than the overall ventricular rate because some atrial impulses are not conducted to the ventricles ("blocked P waves" or "dropped QRS complex beats).
- **Rhythm:** The atrial rhythm is usually regular. The ventricular rhythm is usually regularly irregular due to periodically dropped beats.
- **P waves:** Size and shape consistent with origin from the sinus node (typically upright in leads I, II, III, and aVF on the 12-lead ECG). An occasional P wave is blocked (not followed by a QRS complex).
- **PR interval:** The PR interval progressively lengthens from beat to beat and then one P wave is not followed by a QRS complex (the nonconducted P wave impulse or "dropped" QRS complex). In addition to the PR prolongation, there is also a telltale progressive shortening of the RR interval (the interval between successive QRS complexes) before the blocked P wave. The RR interval that brackets the nonconducted P wave is less than twice the atrial cycle length (the interval between successive P waves).
- **QRS complex:** The QRS complex is usually narrow: less than 0.12 second (often less than 0.11 second). A QRS complex does not follow every P wave.

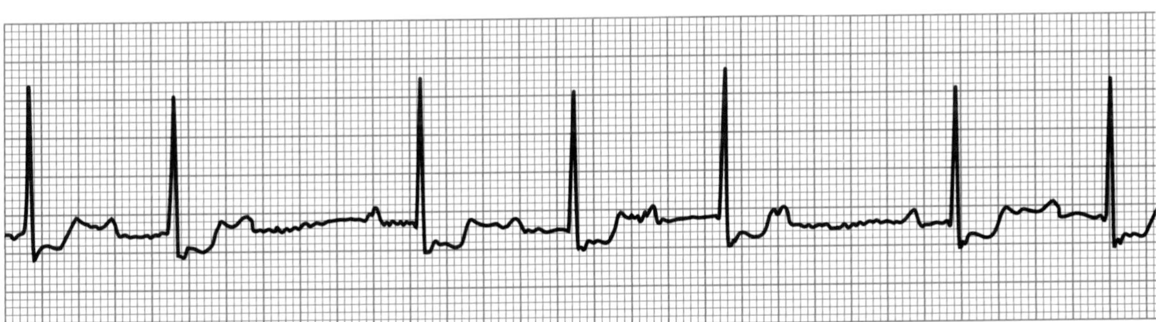

Figure 52. Type I second-degree AV block. Atrial rhythm is nearly regular. But there are pauses in ventricular rhythm because the depolarization impulse associated with every fourth P wave in this instance does not conduct into the ventricles. Note progressive prolongation of the PR interval, indicating increasing conduction delay in the AV node before an atrial (sinus) impulse fails to be conducted to the ventricles. In the center of the strip there are 4 P waves and 3 QRS complexes, representing a 4:3 cycle. The QRS complexes are normal.

Table 16. Major Features of Second-Degree AV Block Type I

	Second-Degree AV Block Type I (Mobitz I or Wenckebach)
Pathophysiology	• Site of pathology: AV node • AV node blood supply comes from branches of the right coronary artery • Impulse conduction is increasingly slowed at the AV node (causing increasing PR intervals) until one sinus impulse is completely blocked and a QRS complex fails to follow
Defining Criteria per ECG **Key:** There is progressive lengthening of the PR interval until one P wave is not followed by a QRS complex (the dropped beat)	• **Rate:** atrial rate just slightly faster than ventricular (because of dropped beats); usually normal range • **Rhythm:** regular for atrial beats; irregular for ventricular (because of dropped beats); can show regular P waves marching through irregular QRS • **P waves:** size and shape remain normal; occasional P wave not followed by a QRS complex (the "dropped beat") • **PR:** progressive lengthening of the PR interval occurs from cycle to cycle; then one P wave is not followed by a QRS complex (the "dropped beat") • **QRS complex:** $<$0.12 second most often, but a QRS "drops out" periodically
Clinical Manifestations—Rate-Related	**Due to bradycardia:** • **Symptoms:** chest pain, shortness of breath, decreased level of consciousness • **Signs:** hypotension, shock, pulmonary congestion, CHF, angina
Common Etiologies	• AV nodal blocking agents: β-blockers, calcium channel blockers, digoxin • Conditions that stimulate the parasympathetic system • An ACS that involves the *right* coronary artery

Recommended Therapy
Key: Treat only when patient has significant signs or symptoms that are due to the bradycardia
	Intervention sequence for type I second-degree AV block:
	• *Atropine* is first-line drug for symptomatic bradycardia
	• If unresponsive to atropine, treat with TCP or β-adrenergic support as temporizing measure while the patient is prepared for transvenous pacing
	• β-Adrenergic (catecholamine) infusion may be given as
	  – *Dopamine* 2 to 10 mcg/kg per minute
	  – *Epinephrine* 2 to 10 mcg/min
	• Consider expert consultation

Abbreviations: ACS, acute coronary syndrome; AV, atrioventricular; CHF, congestive heart failure; ECG, electrocardiogram; TCP, transcutaneous pacing.

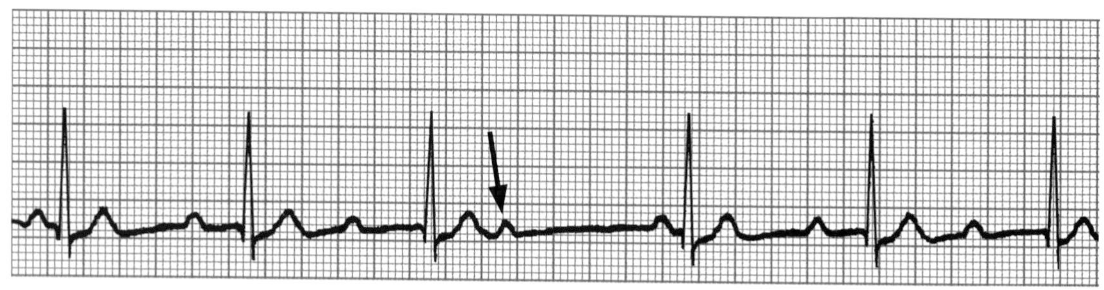

Type I second-degree AV block. Note progressive lengthening of PR interval until one P wave (arrow) is not followed by a QRS. This pattern then repeats itself.

Clinical Manifestations

In type I second-degree AV block the symptoms and signs are related to the severity of the bradycardia.

- **Symptoms:** With minimal exertion, patients may experience chest discomfort, shortness of breath, and decreased level of consciousness.
- **Signs:** Occasionally the bradycardia is slow enough to produce hypotension, shock, pulmonary congestion, CHF, and angina.

Common Etiologies

- The most frequent causes of type I second-degree AV block are drugs that slow conduction through the AV node: β-blockers, calcium channel blockers, and digoxin.

- The second most common cause of type I second-degree AV block is any condition that stimulates the parasympathetic system, increasing parasympathetic tone. Such conditions include any event that stimulates the vasovagal reflex, such as vomiting, a Valsalva maneuver, or rectal stimuli.
- Circulation to the AV node comes from the right coronary artery in most patients. For this reason acute coronary syndromes that affect the *right* coronary artery (or a dominant left circumflex coronary artery) can produce type I second-degree AV nodal block.

Recommended Therapy

Specific treatment is rarely needed unless severe signs and symptoms due to bradycardia are present. Clinicians should remain comfortable with *watchful waiting* and avoid unnecessary administration of atropine simply to treat the observed block.

- Place a high priority on identifying the underlying cause.
- If the bradycardia resulting from nonconducted P waves leads to serious signs and symptoms, initiate the Bradycardia Algorithm intervention sequence.
- If a vagal mechanism appears to be the cause of the type I block, administer atropine 0.5 mg IV. Further treatment is rarely necessary (see the Bradycardia Algorithm for additional therapies).

Second-Degree AV Block (Mobitz 2 or Infranodal)

Type II second-degree AV block (Figure 53) occurs below the level of the AV node (infranodal) typically at the bundle of His or bundle branches. A hallmark of this type of second-degree AV block is that the PR interval does not lengthen before a P wave fails to conduct to the ventricle; the block is an abrupt event. More than 1 blocked P wave impulse may occur in succession.

Pathophysiology

- In the type II form of second-degree AV block, the conduction pathology occurs *below* the level of the AV node at either the bundle of His (uncommon) or the bundle branches (more common).
- Unlike conduction through the AV node, which typically slows before an impulse is completely blocked, the signature of infranodal conduction block is that of abrupt block that is not forewarned by an increasing PR interval. Thus, with type II second-degree AV block, the PR interval does not lengthen before the nonconducted impulse.
- The bundle of His and Purkinje fibers are fast-response cells that tend to be depolarized as an "all or none" phenomenon. This explains why there is no progressive lengthening of the PR interval, but instead either a conduction or nonconduction of the impulse from the atria to the ventricles.
- Type II second-degree AV block is associated with a poorer prognosis. Often it progresses to complete heart block, and because the level of block is more distal, the escape rhythm is slower and less reliable.

Defining ECG Criteria (Figure 53)

- The hallmark of type II second-degree AV block is that the PR interval remains constant before an atrial impulse is blocked (not conducted to the ventricles), resulting in "a P wave not followed by a QRS complex." Unlike type I block, in type II block the PR interval does not lengthen before this nonconducted impulse.
- **Rate:** The atrial (sinus) rate is usually within the normal range. By definition the ventricular rate is slower than the atrial rate because some impulses are blocked between the atria and the ventricles so that ventricular activity (QRS) does not follow some P waves.
- **Rhythm:** The atrial rhythm is regular. The occasional nonconducted impulses render the ventricular rhythm irregular. However, if there is a constant conduction ratio between P and QRS (eg, every other P wave is blocked; 2:1), the ventricular rate is regular.
- **P waves:** Size and shape consistent with origin from the sinus node (typically upright in leads I, II, III, and aVF on the 12-lead ECG). An occasional P wave is blocked (not followed by a QRS complex).
- **PR interval:** The PR interval may be normal or prolonged, but it will remain constant from beat to beat. There is no progressive prolongation of the PR interval as is observed with type I second-degree block.
- **QRS complex:** The QRS complex is typically wide (0.12 second or more) because the block occurs below the AV node (infranodal). Infranodal block indicates the presence of distal conduction disease, which is often manifested in a wider-than-normal QRS complex

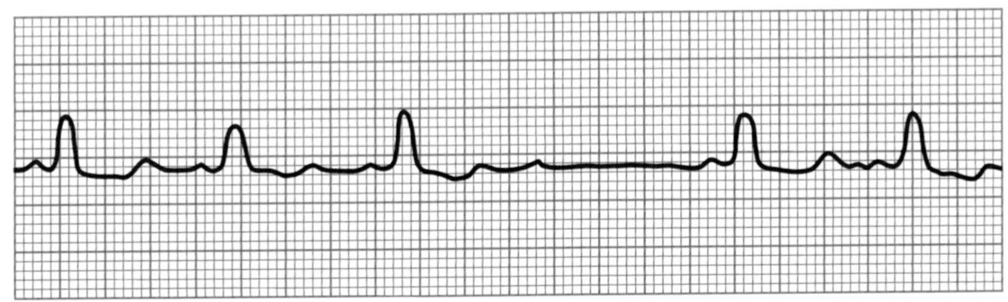

Figure 53. Type II second-degree AV block. In this example, the PR interval of the conducted P waves remains constant before the nonconducted P wave, and the QRS complex is wide.

and—should the number of blocked P waves increase—by a slower ventricular escape rhythm. The ventricular rhythm may be irregular when only occasional P waves are blocked. If every other P wave were blocked, the ventricular rhythm would be regular.

Clinical Manifestations

In type II second-degree AV block the following symptoms can result from the bradycardia:

- **Symptoms:** Chest discomfort, shortness of breath, and decreased level of consciousness
- **Signs:** Hypotension, shock, pulmonary congestion, congestive heart failure, angina, or acute ST-segment deviation

Common Etiologies

- Type II second-degree AV block is usually associated with a pathologic lesion in the conduction pathway.
- Unlike type I second-degree AV block, type II second-degree AV block is rarely the result of increased parasympathetic tone.
- New-onset type II second-degree block is most frequently caused by an ACS that involves the *left* coronary artery. More specifically, type II block develops with occlusion of one of the septal branches of the left anterior descending coronary artery. This occlusion can also produce bundle branch block.

Recommended Therapy

Note: In the presence of persistent signs and symptoms, the Bradycardia Algorithm suggests considering

- Obtaining expert consultation
- Preparing the patient for transvenous pacing

The intervention sequence for new-onset type II second-degree AV block with serious signs and symptoms is as follows:

- Atropine is the first-line drug for symptomatic bradycardia, but do not rely on atropine in Mobitz type II second-degree AV block. Atropine is unlikely to be effective because type II block occurs below the level of the AV node. Some experts discourage the use of

Table 17. Major Features of Second-Degree AV Block Type II

Second-Degree Heart Block Type II (Infranodal) (Mobitz II or Non-Wenckebach)	
Pathophysiology	• The pathology, ie, the site of the block, is most often *below* the AV node (infranodal); at the bundle of His (infrequent) or at the bundle branches
Defining Criteria per ECG	• **Atrial rate:** usually 60-100/min • **Ventricular rate:** by definition (due to the blocked impulses) slower than atrial rate • **Rhythm:** atrial = regular; ventricular = irregular (because of blocked impulses) • **P waves:** typical in size and shape; by definition some P waves will not be followed by a QRS complex • **PR:** constant and set; no progressive prolongation as with type I—a distinguishing characteristic • **QRS complex:** typically wide (0.12 second or more) because block is infranodal
Clinical Manifestations—Rate-Related	**Due to bradycardia:** • **Symptoms:** chest pain, shortness of breath, decreased level of consciousness • **Signs:** hypotension, shock, pulmonary congestions, CHF, AMI
Common Etiologies	• An ACS that involves branches of the *left* coronary artery

Recommended Therapy
Pearl: New-onset type II second-degree AV block in clinical context of ACS is indication for transvenous pacemaker insertion
	Intervention sequence for type II second-degree AV block:
	• *Atropine* is first-line drug for symptomatic bradycardia (do not rely on atropine in Mobitz type II second- or third-degree AV blocks or in patients with third-degree AV block with a new wide QRS complex)
	• If unresponsive to atropine, treat with TCP or β-adrenergic support as temporizing measure while the patient is prepared for transvenous pacing
	• β-Adrenergic (catecholamine) infusion may be given as
	  – *Dopamine* 2 to 10 mcg/kg per minute
	  – *Epinephrine* 2 to 10 mcg/min
	• Consider expert consultation

Abbreviations: ACS, acute coronary syndrome; AMI, acute myocardial infarction; AV, atrioventricular; CHF, congestive heart failure; ECG, electrocardiogram; TCP, transcutaneous pacing.

atropine in patients with suspected block in the distal conduction system because of a potential paradoxical effect, which can result in more nonconducted P waves and worsen the heart block. Atropine increases sinus node rate and AV nodal conduction—which in combination could result in more (and faster) impulses reaching the already compromised site of infranodal block—potentially resulting in even more conduction failure. If atropine is used, be prepared for TCP or β-adrenergic infusion in the event that conduction block worsens.

- Use β-adrenergic drugs or TCP if available as a bridge to transvenous pacing. With TCP, verify patient tolerance and electrical capture with effective systemic perfusion. Use sedation and analgesia as needed and tolerated.
- If TCP is undesirable, unavailable, or ineffective and there are delays to placement of a transvenous pacer, initiate a catecholamine infusion:
  - Dopamine 2 to 10 mcg/kg per minute
  - Epinephrine 2 to 10 mcg/min
- Immediately consult cardiology and begin preparations for a transvenous pacemaker.

Third-Degree AV Block

Third-degree AV block (Figure 54) results from injury or damage to the cardiac conduction system so that no impulses are conducted from the atria to the ventricles. The atrial rate is always faster than the ventricular rate when third-degree AV block is present. In third-degree AV block, there is no relationship between the atrial and ventricular complexes. *AV dissociation* is a broad term that describes an electrical "disconnect" between the atrial and ventricular electrical activity. This can occur in 2 settings:

- The first is third-degree AV block, which is characterized by atria that are beating faster and independently of the (slower-beating) ventricles.
- The second is when the ventricles beat faster and independently of the slower-beating atria because of a primary ventricular arrhythmia (eg, VT).

Pathophysiology

- Third-degree AV block (complete heart block) is caused by injury or damage to the cardiac conduction system such that no impulses *(complete)* can pass *(blocked)* in a forward fashion between atria and ventricles. Usually retrograde (backward) conduction from ventricles back to atria is also blocked. Atrial impulses are not conducted to the ventricles, and ventricular and atrial complexes have no relationship.
- By definition, third-degree AV block will result in ventricular standstill (asystole) unless an escape rhythm ensues.

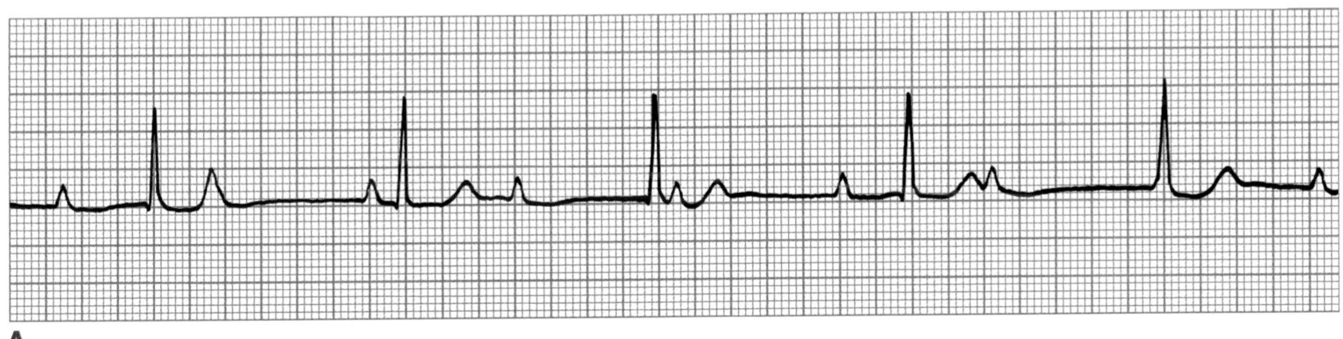

A

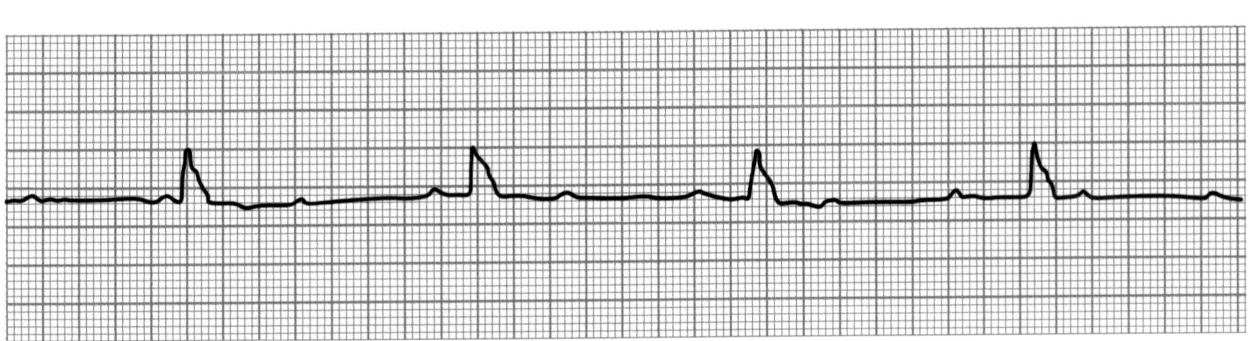

B

Figure 54. **A,** Third-degree AV block occurring at the level of the AV node (above bifurcation of the His bundle). Atrial rhythm is slightly irregular owing to the presence of sinus arrhythmia. Ventricular rhythm is regular at a slower rate (44/min). There is no consistent PR interval. QRS complexes are narrow, indicating that they originate above the bifurcation of the His bundle. **B,** Third-degree AV block occurring below the AV node (infranodal). There is no relation between the faster atrial and slower ventricular complexes, indicating AV dissociation. PR intervals are inconsistent from beat to beat. Ventricular rhythm is regular at a very slow rate (38/min). The QRS is wide because the block is in the more distal conduction system, and accordingly, the ventricular escape rhythm originates distal to that level.

The characteristic of this escape rhythm is often a clue to the anatomic site of the block. A more rapid, narrow complex escape implies block that is more proximal in the conduction system, whereas a slow, wide complex escape implies that heart block has occurred in the more distal conduction system.

- Complete heart block can occur at several different anatomic areas, and each anatomic level of block may be associated with a different pathogenesis, treatment, and prognosis:
  - AV nodal block (sometimes referred to as "high" or "supra," "junctional," or "nodal") block: At this anatomic site a junctional escape pacemaker frequently will initiate ventricular depolarization. This is usually a stable subsidiary pacemaker with a rate of 40 to 60/min.
    - Because this anatomic site is located above the bifurcation of the bundle of His, ventricular depolarization usually occurs in normal fashion, resulting in a normal QRS complex (less than 0.12 second). (Figure 54A).
    - Third-degree AV block with a junctional escape rhythm may be transient and associated with a favorable prognosis.
  - Low or infranodal block
    - Third-degree block at the level of the His bundle or lower (infranodal block) indicates the presence of extensive distal conduction system disease.
    - When this type of third-degree block is new in onset, it is usually associated with extensive anterior MI.
    - The only escape mechanism available to sustain a ventricular rhythm lies distal to the site of block. Such a ventricular escape pacemaker has an intrinsic rate that is slow (less than 40/min). Like any depolarization originating in a ventricle, the QRS complex will be wide (0.12 second or more) (Figure 54B). It is not a stable pacemaker, and episodes of ventricular asystole are common.
- Complete heart block can occur with any atrial rhythm, including sinus rhythm, or with atrial arrhythmias such as atrial fibrillation. However, for simplicity, in this discussion it will be assumed that the underlying rhythm is sinus.

Defining ECG Criteria (Figure 54)

The key defining criterion for third-degree block is that the atria and ventricles depolarize independently with no relationship to one another: there is *dissociation*.

- **Rate:** The atrial rate is usually 60 to 100/min. The atrial impulses are completely independent of *(dissociated* from) the ventricular impulses. The ventricular rate is determined by the rate of the ventricular escape pacemaker. With nodal complete heart block, the ventricular escape rate is slower than the atrial rate and may range from 40 to 50/min. With infranodal complete heart block, the ventricular rate is typically even slower, at 20 to 40/min.
- **Rhythm:** Both the atrial rhythm and the ventricular rhythm are regular, but each is independent of *(dissociated* from) the other.
- **P waves:** The P waves are consistent with sinus origin (unless there is an atrial arrhythmia).
- **PR interval:** By definition there is no consistent relationship between the P wave and QRS complex from beat to beat, resulting in widely variable PR intervals.
- **QRS complex:** The characteristics of the escape rhythm during complete heart block can provide a clue as to the site of block. A narrow (less than 0.12 second) QRS complex escape at a more rapid rate implies that block is occurring "higher" in the conduction system (ie, near the AV node); a wide (0.12 second or more) QRS complex at a slower rate implies low block within the more distal conduction system.

Clinical Manifestations

- **Symptoms:** Chest pain, shortness of breath, decreased level of consciousness, and syncope
- **Signs:** Hypotension, shock, pulmonary congestion, signs of CHF, angina, or AMI

Common Etiologies

- Third-degree AV block when presenting with a wide QRS complex escape rhythm is often due to an ACS that involves the *left* coronary artery. In particular the involvement is with the left anterior descending artery, the branches to the interventricular septum, and the corresponding bundle branches. Heart block in this instance occurs in the distal conduction system.
- When presenting with a narrow QRS complex escape rhythm, third-degree AV block is most likely occurring at the level of the AV node, with a resultant junctional escape rhythm. This type of AV block can result from increased parasympathetic tone, inferior infarction, or toxic drug effects (eg, digitalis, β-blockers) or from injury to the AV node and surrounding tissue. When the escape rhythm is wide (0.12 second or more) and slow

Critical Concept **Second- and Third-Degree AV Block Cautions**	• New-onset type II second-degree and third-degree AV block (particularly with a wide QRS complex escape) in the clinical context of an ACS is an indication for insertion of a transvenous pacemaker. • ***Do not administer lidocaine or amiodarone*** to patients with second-degree heart block (of any type) or third-degree AV block and a ventricular escape rhythm. These drugs may worsen the degree of heart block and/or suppress the ventricular escape rhythm, causing cardiac standstill.

Table 18. Major Features of Third-Degree AV Block and AV Dissociation

	Third-Degree AV Block and AV Dissociation
Pathophysiology **Pearl:** *AV dissociation* is the defining class; *third-degree* or *complete AV block* is one type of AV dissociation. By convention (outdated): if ventricular escape depolarization is faster than atrial rate, it is *"AV dissociation"*; if slower, it is "third-degree AV block."	Injury or damage to the cardiac conduction system so that no impulses *(complete block)* pass between atria and ventricles (neither antegrade nor retrograde) This complete block can occur at several different anatomic areas: • AV node ("high" or "supra" or "junctional" *nodal block)* • Bundle of His • Bundle branches ("low-nodal" or "infranodal" block)
Defining Criteria per ECG **Key:** The third-degree block (see Pathophysiology) causes the atria and ventricles to depolarize independently, with no relationship between the two (AV dissociation).	• **Atrial rate:** usually 60-100/min; impulses completely independent of *(dissociated* from) the ventricular impulses • **Ventricular rate:** depends on the rate of the ventricular escape beats that arise • **Rhythm:** both atrial rhythm and ventricular rhythm are regular but independent *(dissociated)* • **P waves:** consistent with sinus origin (unless there is an atrial arrhythmia) • **PR:** by definition there is no consistent relationship between P wave and QRS complex from beat to beat • **QRS complex:** narrow (<0.12 second) at a more rapid rate implies that block is occurring "higher" in the conduction system (ie, near the AV node); a wide (≥0.12 second) at a slower rate implies low block within the more distal conduction system
Clinical Manifestations—Rate-Related	**Due to bradycardia:** • **Symptoms:** chest pain, shortness of breath, decreased level of consciousness • **Signs:** hypotension, shock, pulmonary congestions, CHF, AMI
Common Etiologies	• An ACS that involves branches of the *left* coronary artery • An ACS that involves the *right* coronary artery
Recommended Therapy **Pearl:** New-onset third-degree AV block in clinical context of acute coronary syndrome is indication for transvenous pacemaker insertion **Pearl:** *Never treat third-degree AV block plus ventricular escape beats with lidocaine or amiodarone.*	**Intervention sequence for third-degree AV block:** • *Atropine* is first-line drug for symptomatic bradycardia (do not rely on atropine in Mobitz type II second- or third-degree AV blocks or in patients with third-degree AV block with a new wide QRS complex) • If unresponsive to atropine, treat with TCP or β-adrenergic support as temporizing measure while the patient is prepared for transvenous pacing • β-Adrenergic (catecholamine) infusion may be given as – *Dopamine* 2 to 10 mcg/kg per minute – *Epinephrine* 2 to 10 mcg/min • Consider expert consultation

Abbreviations: ACS, acute coronary syndromes; AMI, acute myocardial infarction; AV, atrioventricular; CHF, congestive heart failure; ECG, electrocardiogram; TCP, transcutaneous pacing.

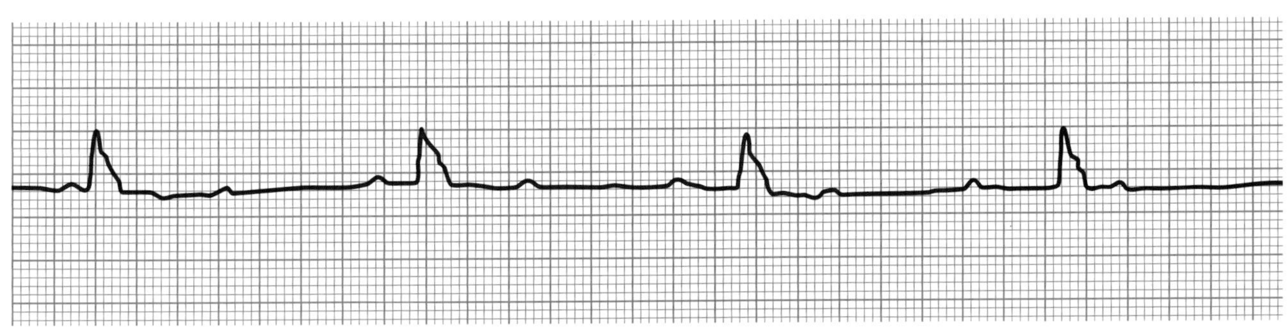

(20 to 40/min), the block is more ominous and should be presumed to be in the distal conduction system.

Recommended Therapy

Note: New-onset third-degree AV block (particularly with a wide QRS complex escape) is an indication for insertion of a transvenous pacemaker.

The intervention sequence for new-onset third-degree AV block with serious signs and symptoms is as follows (some may be initiated concurrently):

- Atropine (0.5 mg, may be repeated every 3 to 5 minutes to a maximum of 3 mg) remains the first-line drug for acute symptomatic bradycardia due to conduction block at the level of the AV node.
- If the location of the block is likely to be in nonnodal tissue (such as in the bundle of His or more distal conduction system), the bradycardia is unlikely to respond to reversal of cholinergic effects by atropine and is preferably treated with TCP or β-adrenergic support.
- TCP or β-adrenergic agents are indicated for symptomatic heart block that is unresponsive to or inappropriate for treatment with atropine.
- TCP or β-adrenergic agents should be regarded as temporizing measures while the patient is prepared for transvenous pacing.
- Immediate TCP should be considered in unstable patients with heart block if vascular access and pharmacologic therapies are not readily available.
- If severe signs and symptoms are unresponsive to atropine (if used) and TCP, and if there are delays to placement of a transvenous pacer, then initiate a β-adrenergic (catecholamine) infusion:
  - Dopamine 2 to 10 mcg/kg per minute
  - Epinephrine 2 to 10 mcg/min
- An expert consultation should be obtained while the patient is being prepared for transvenous pacing.

Other Terminology

The classification of AV blocks is simplified to allow providers to initiate emergency therapy for a large number of patients in circumstances where detailed consideration and differential rhythm diagnosis may not be possible. In some instances questions of a more advanced context may arise. Although such questions are beyond the scope of this chapter, a brief summary of the more common terminology is provided here to facilitate understanding.

2:1 AV Block

A 2:1 AV conduction ratio refers to conduction of every other P wave to the ventricles. It is often mistakenly classified as type II AV block because of the apparently "fixed" PR interval that follows conducted P waves. However, 2:1 AV block can be either type I or type II second-degree AV block. Distinguishing type I from type II second-degree AV block requires observing the PR interval associated with 2 *consecutively conducted* P waves. Unless this is observed, an assessment of the PR interval for progressive prolongation or a fixed interval cannot aid in the differential diagnosis. Certain "clues" can be used to suggest that a 2:1 AV block is more likely to be occurring at the AV nodal (type I) or infranodal (type II) level:

- If the PR interval of the conducted beat is prolonged and the QRS complex is narrow, the block is more likely type I second-degree AV block (see exception below).
- If there is a preexisting bundle branch block (a previously wide QRS when heart block was not present), it may not be possible to differentiate between type I and type II second-degree AV block.
- If the QRS is narrow and the patient has responded to atropine—given for an indicated reason—the block is likely in the AV nodal portion under vagal influence.
- If the QRS complex is wide, use of atropine is unlikely to be effective and treatment with TCP or β-adrenergic drugs may be required.

AV Dissociation

AV dissociation is a broad term that describes an electrical "disconnect" between the atria and ventricles such that electrical activity between the upper and lower chambers is no longer linked. Instead, the atria and ventricles beat completely independently of one another, just as though they were two different hearts. This can occur in 2 settings. The first is third-degree AV block, characterized by atria that are beating faster and independently of the (slower-beating) ventricles. The second setting is when the ventricles beat faster and independently of the (slower-beating) atria because of a primary ventricular arrhythmia (eg, VT) or a ventricular escape rhythm has occurred that is faster than the underlying atrial (sinus) rhythm.

- When sinus rhythm slows excessively, resulting in sinus bradycardia, a subsidiary escape pacemaker with a slightly faster rate may emerge. This escape rhythm will have a more rapid rate and a narrow QRS complex if originating near the AV node or a slower rate and wide QRS complex if coming from a more distal location (in the conduction system). This escape rhythm is sometimes referred to as an *accelerated junctional rhythm (AJR)* or *accelerated idioventricular rhythm (AIVR)* when the rate is faster than the sinus rhythm.
- In many patients who develop VT, the ventricular impulses do not conduct retrograde via the AV node back into the atria. Accordingly, amid the more rapid ventricular rate of the VT, the atria continue beating independently at a slower rate. This atrial activity may be seen "marching through" the VT. This is one of the "footprints" of VT, denoting independent atrial and ventricular activity (AV dissociation).

Critical Concept **AV Dissociation and AV Block**	• All patients with complete AV block have complete AV dissociation but not all patients with AV dissociation have AV block. The terms are not synonymous. • When the atrial rate is faster than the ventricular rate, AV dissociation is being caused by third-degree heart block. • When the ventricular rate is faster than the atrial rate, AV dissociation is being caused by a primary ventricular arrhythmia or accelerated escape rhythm, *not* by third-degree AV block.

High-Degree and Advanced AV Block

- High-degree (also called *advanced heart block)* is a more serious form of second-degree AV block, in which multiple successive P waves fail to conduct to the ventricle, although occasional P waves may still conduct. It indicates a more advanced stage of deranged conduction that, because of the greater number of "dropped" QRS complexes, more often results in symptoms and often leads to complete AV block.
- High-degree AV block is defined as the presence of 2 or more consecutive P waves that fail to conduct to the ventricle (Figure 55). As with ordinary type I or type II AV block, the appearance of the QRS complex may provide a clue as to the location of the heart block. If the QRS complex is wide (0.12 second or more), high-degree (advanced) heart block should be presumed to be occurring in the distal conduction system. A fixed versus progressively increasing PR interval on consecutively conducted P waves preceding the blocked P waves may help determine the site of block. However, regardless of the location of the heart block, because frequently blocked P waves are more likely to result in symptoms, advanced AV block should be considered an ominous sign and the patient expeditiously prepared for possible pacing.

Management of Symptomatic High-Degree AV Block of Uncertain Classification (Site of Block)

Recommended Therapy

The occurrence of high-degree AV blocks with or without symptoms must be taken seriously and in context of the setting in which it is occurring. When accompanied by a wide QRS complex (0.12 second or more), distal conduction block should be suspected, expert consultation obtained, vascular access established, and preparations made for transvenous pacing. Atropine is the first-line drug for symptomatic bradycardia, but do not rely on atropine in high-degree AV block. Immediate pacing might be considered in unstable patients with high-degree AV block when IV access is not available (Class IIb, LOE C). These measures should be considered temporizing and as a bridge to transvenous pacing while awaiting emergent cardiology consultation.

The intervention sequence for new-onset high-degree AV block of uncertain origin with serious signs and symptoms is identical to second- or third-degree AV block:

- **Do not delay—follow the Bradycardia Algorithm.**
- Give atropine 0.5 mg IV every 3 to 5 minutes to a maximum total dose of 3 mg for symptomatic sinus bradycardia.
- If severe signs and symptoms are unresponsive to atropine:
  - Use TCP when available as a bridge to transvenous pacing. Verify patient tolerance and electrical capture with effective systemic perfusion; use sedation and analgesia as needed and tolerated

    or
  - Initiate a catecholamine infusion:
    - Epinephrine 2 to 10 mcg/min (chronotropic infusion, titrated)
    - Dopamine 2 to 10 mcg/kg per minute (chronotropic infusion, titrated)

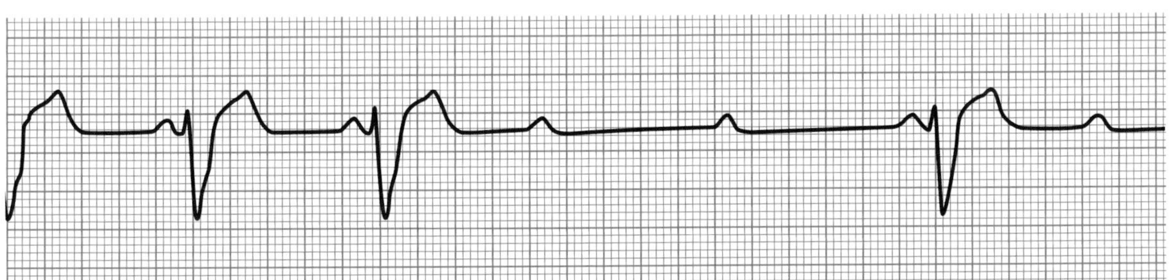

Figure 55. High-degree (or advanced) heart block is depicted. Note that 2 consecutive P waves fail to conduct to the ventricle. The wide QRS suggests that the level of advanced heart block is likely to be in the distal conduction system (infranodal), as does the failure of the PR interval to prolong before the blocked P waves.

- Arrange for a transvenous pacemaker and cardiac evaluation. Immediate pacing might be considered in unstable patients with high-degree AV block when IV access is not available (Class IIb, LOE C). If the patient does not respond to drugs or TCP, transvenous pacing is probably indicated (Class IIa, LOE C).

Management of AV Block in ACS

Sinus Bradycardia

Approximately 30% of patients with ACS attributable to AMI will develop sinus bradycardia. Patients with inferior wall infarcts secondary to occlusion of the right coronary artery often present with sinus bradycardia caused by ischemia of the sinus and/or AV node. Sinus bradycardia may also occur with reperfusion of the right coronary artery. Atropine-resistant bradycardia and AV block may occur, possibly from accumulation of adenosine in ischemic nodal tissue. Initial treatment with atropine is indicated only when serious signs and symptoms are related to the decreased rate.

Second-Degree or Third-Degree AV Block

Approximately 20% of patients with AMI will develop second-degree or third-degree AV block. Of those who develop AV block, 42% demonstrate the block on admission, and 66% demonstrate the block within the first 24 hours of presentation. In the majority of cases these abnormalities are the result of myocardial ischemia or infarction of muscle that encompasses the conduction system. Other factors responsible for the development of AV block include altered autonomic influence, systemic hypoxia, electrolyte disturbances, acid-base disorders, and complications of various medical therapies.

When promptly treated, AV block itself is rarely fatal; rather, it is associated with more extensive MI with cardiac dysfunction. Therefore, AV block is not an independent predictor of mortality but rather a marker for higher mortality as a result of worse ventricular function.

The prognosis for patients with AV block is related most consistently to the size and site of infarction (anterior or inferior). Treatment is influenced by the level of block in the conduction system, the presence and rate of escape rhythms, and the degree of hemodynamic compromise.

Use of Atropine

There are several caveats about the use of atropine for bradyarrhythmias associated with ACS:

- Use atropine cautiously in the presence of acute coronary ischemia or MI; increased heart rate may worsen ischemia or increase infarction size.
- In prehospital settings and emergency departments, use of atropine for hemodynamically significant bradyarrhythmias produces the same effects in patients with and without AMI.
- Atropine will likely be ineffective in patients who have undergone cardiac transplantation because the transplanted heart lacks vagal innervation.
- Do not rely on atropine for type II second-degree AV block with wide QRS. Theoretically, an atropine-induced increase in sinus rate may actually worsen AV block or precipitate third-degree AV block.
- Treatment of third-degree AV block:
  - Do not rely on atropine for treatment of third-degree AV block with a new wide QRS complex presumed to be due to AMI.
  - **Also do not administer lidocaine or amiodarone to these patients.** Lidocaine or amiodarone may suppress a slow ventricular escape rhythm and result in ventricular standstill.

Use of Pacing

TCP provides an emergency bridge to transvenous pacing for patients with appropriate indications who do not respond to atropine as first-line therapy, including hemodynamically unstable bradycardia and second- and third-degree AV blocks. Standby placement of a TCP device may also be considered in ACS patients who exhibit conduction abnormalities that potentially might lead to the need for emergent pacing, such as newly acquired left, right, or alternating bundle branch block (BBB) or bifascicular block. Management of transient and persistent conduction abnormalities in AMI is complicated and requires expert consultation. For more on this topic see the *American College of Cardiology/American Heart Association Guidelines for the Management of ST-Elevation Myocardial Infarction*,[14] available at http://www.acc.org/qualityandscience/clinical/guidelines/stemi/Guideline1/index.htm.

Cardiac Pacing

Since the first successful cardiac pacing in the 19th century, a variety of devices for pacing the heart have been developed. All cardiac pacemakers deliver an electrical stimulus through electrodes to the heart, causing myocardial depolarization and subsequent cardiac contraction. A TCP system delivers pacing impulses to the heart through the skin using cutaneous electrodes. Transvenous pacemakers use electrodes that have been passed through large central veins to the right chambers of the heart, or occasionally directly on the surface of the heart. Every pacing system requires a pulse generator. The pulse generator can be located outside the patient's body (external pacemakers) or surgically implanted inside the body (internal or permanent pacemakers). A temporary transvenous pacemaker typically consists of an electrode that has been passed through the large central veins into the right ventricle and is connected to a power source (external pacemaker generator) that sits outside the body. As implied by its name, temporary transvenous pacing is intended as a bridge from an unstable bradycardia to either placement of a permanent pacemaker or resolution of the bradycardia.

Table 19 summarizes the various types of pacemaker systems. Although this chapter focuses on temporary pacing, ACLS providers require knowledge about implantable pacemakers because these devices may produce a pacing artifact that can be confused with arrhythmias.

The introduction of new TCP systems during the 1980s led to more widespread use of pacing in emergency cardiac care, and these systems are summarized here.[14]

Indications for Emergency and "Standby" Pacing

Emergency Pacing

TCP may be useful in the treatment of symptomatic bradycardias. Because TCP is painful and not as reliable as transvenous pacing, it should be considered as an emergent bridge to transvenous pacing in patients with significant sinus bradycardia or AV block. It should also be considered as a precautionary (standby) measure in stable patients who manifest acute conduction abnormalities that might progress in severity and require pacing (eg, asymptomatic type II second-degree AV block or third-degree AV block with a narrow QRS complex junctional escape). It is not intended for protracted periods of pacing.

Should TCP be required, carefully assess the patient for clinical response after pacing is initiated. Because heart rate is a major determinant of myocardial oxygen consumption, set the pacing rate to the lowest effective rate based on clinical assessment and symptom resolution. Most patients will improve with a rate of 60 to 70/min if the symptoms are primarily due to bradycardia. If cardiovascular symptoms are not caused by the bradycardia, the patient may not improve despite effective pacing.

TCP is, at best, a temporizing measure. Because TCP results in skeletal muscle contraction with each impulse, it is painful in conscious patients and, whether effective (achieving consistent capture) or not, the patient should be prepared for transvenous pacing, and expert consultation should be obtained.

- TCP electrodes (patches) should be located in a manner that optimizes the likelihood of ventricular capture. Typically an anterior-posterior patch position is advised. Whether this is right posterior chest wall (scapular) and left anterior parasternal chest wall, or left posterior chest wall (scapular) to left anterior parasternal chest wall, or an alternate position, the important principle is to attempt to "sandwich" the heart between the patch electrodes. If one position fails to achieve ventricular capture at maximum pacing output, consider relocating one or the other patch to an alternative position.
- Following initiation of pacing, confirm electrical and mechanical capture. The stimulation artifact from TCP on the surface ECG can be misleading and suggest that ventricular capture (QRS complex) is occurring when it is not. If ventricular capture is occurring, the apparent QRS complex should be followed by a distinct T wave (repolarization wave). If a distinct T wave is not seen following each apparent QRS, ventricular capture is not

Table 19. Types of Cardiac Pacers

Type of Pacemaker	Electrode Location	Pulse Generator Location	Synonyms
Transcutaneous (TCP)	Skin (anterior chest wall and back)	External	External Noninvasive
Transvenous	Venous (catheter with tip in right ventricle, right atrium, or both)	External	Temporary transvenous Permanent transvenous
Transthoracic (no longer used)	Through anterior chest wall into heart	External	Transmyocardial
Transesophageal	Esophagus	External	Esophageal
Epicardial	Epicardium (electrodes placed on heart surface during surgery)	External or internal External generator may be used postoperatively with temporary wires. Permanent wires may also be placed at the time of surgery with later implantation of a permanent generator if needed.	Temporary or permanent epicardial
"Permanent"	Venous or epicardial	Internal	Implanted Internal

likely to be occurring. In such an instance the output from TCP should be increased, or consideration should be given to relocating the TCP electrodes.
- Assessment of a pulse to confirm mechanical capture can be challenging during TCP because electrical stimulation causes generalized muscular contraction (jerking) that may mimic the carotid pulse. A femoral pulse is occasionally more reliably palpated than a carotid pulse, given the femoral artery's greater distance away from the site of pacing and less surrounding muscle.
- Reassess the patient for symptomatic improvement and hemodynamic stability.
- Give analgesics and sedatives for pain control. Note that many of these drugs may further decrease blood pressure and affect the patient's mental status. Patients may also need to be intubated if the degree of sedation required for pain control compromises respiration.
- Try to identify and correct the cause of the bradycardia.

Most conscious patients will require and should be given sedation before pacing. If the patient is in cardiovascular collapse or rapidly deteriorating, it may be necessary to start pacing without prior sedation, particularly if drugs for sedation are not immediately available. The clinician must evaluate the need for sedation in light of the patient's condition and need for immediate pacing. The general approach could include the following:

- Give parenteral benzodiazepine for anxiety and muscle contractions.
- Give a parenteral narcotic for analgesia.
- Consider intubation in patients in whom sedation and pain control depress spontaneous respiration.
- Obtain expert consultation for transvenous pacing.

Standby Pacing

The indications for *standby pacing* (ie, placing TCP electrodes in anticipation of the potential future need for pacing) are multiple and most often occur in the setting of an ACS. These patients typically are clinically stable, yet the presence of a new conduction abnormality heightens concern for potential bradyarrhythmia decompensation in the near future. Often the conduction abnormality is a marker of a more ominous location and size of MI that is transpiring in these patients. That is, the development of the rhythm disorder is a secondary event and often portends impending mechanical failure. Accordingly, priority is given to reperfusion of such patients with suspected AMI, with precautionary placement of TCP or, if required, a temporary transvenous pacemaker.

Because of the wide availability and noninvasive nature of TCP, preparations for its use are appropriate whenever ACLS providers are concerned about the possibility of the development of high-degree symptomatic AV block.

Standby TCP has also been used successfully during surgery for high-risk patients who have chronic bifascicular or left bundle branch block with additional first-degree block,[15,16] in whom the risk of placing a temporary transvenous pacer is judged to be greater than the likelihood of their developing bradycardia due to heart block during the operative procedure. A transcutaneous pacemaker can be placed in standby mode for these and other at-risk patients. If then needed to treat hemodynamically significant bradycardia, the device provides a therapeutic bridge until a transvenous pacemaker can be placed under more controlled circumstances.

Pacing for Pulseless Bradyasystolic Cardiac Arrest

TCP has completely replaced transthoracic (transmyocardial) pacing in patients with bradyasystolic cardiac arrest. However, although less invasive, TCP has not proven to be any more successful in improving survival from bradyasystolic cardiac arrest than the older transthoracic modality. TCP has been studied extensively in the treatment of pulseless patients with bradycardia or asystole. Some studies had shown encouraging results in such patients when pacing was initiated within 10 minutes of cardiac arrest, but recent studies have documented no improvement in either short-term outcomes (admission to hospital) or long-term outcomes (survival to hospital discharge).[17-19] In addition, among patients with symptomatic bradycardia with a pulse, TCP has not proven to be better than pharmacologic interventions in improving survival.[2,20]

Prehospital studies of TCP for asystolic arrest or postshock asystole have also shown no benefit of pacing.[21] In a level 1, prospective, controlled trial of TCP for cardiac arrest, investigators observed no benefit even when CPR was combined with pacing, nor did they observe any benefit when the asystole was of only brief duration after a defibrillatory shock.[19]

Pacing for Drug-Induced Cardiac Arrest

An exception to the negative results of pacing for cardiac arrest is patients in drug overdose–induced cardiac arrest. Pacing may be successful for the treatment of profound bradycardia or pulseless electrical activity (PEA) under such circumstances.[22-26] Emergency pacing may also benefit patients with PEA due to acidosis or electrolyte abnormalities. Such patients often possess a normal myocardium with only temporary impairment of the conduction system.

While attempts are made to correct electrolyte abnormalities or profound acidosis, pacing can stimulate effective myocardial contractions. Similarly pacing can be life sustaining as the conduction system recovers from the cardiotoxic effects of a drug overdose or poisoning with other substances.[25]

Contraindications to Cardiac Pacing

Severe hypothermia is one of the few relative contraindications to cardiac pacing in patients with bradycardia. Bradycardia may be physiologic in these patients; the bradycardia is an appropriate response to a decreased metabolic rate associated with hypothermia. More important, the hypothermic ventricle is more prone to fibrillation with any sort of mechanical or electrical irritation, such as that of ventricular pacing. If the markedly hypothermic ventricle begins to fibrillate, it is believed to be more resistant to defibrillation. Thus the risk of pacing in such patients needs to be balanced against whether their bradyarrhythmia is itself judged to be life threatening.

As in adults, TCP has not been effective in improving the survival rate of children with out-of-hospital unwitnessed cardiac arrest. However, emergency TCP may be lifesaving in selected cases of bradycardia caused by congenital heart defects, complete heart block, abnormal sinus node function, complications following cardiovascular surgery, drug overdose, or a failing implanted pacemaker.[27] Therefore TCP use should not necessarily be withheld but instead deployed with tempered optimism.

Principles and Technique of TCP

In TCP the heart is stimulated with externally applied cutaneous electrodes that deliver an electrical impulse. This impulse is conducted through the intact chest wall to activate the myocardium.[28-30] TCP technique has been referred to as *external pacing, noninvasive pacing, external transthoracic pacing,* and *transchest pacing*. *Transcutaneous pacing* is the preferred term because it best conveys the concept of pacing the heart through electrodes attached to the skin surface.

Although TCP is appropriately termed "noninvasive" because it does not require vascular access or surgical placement, it is not without risk or discomfort. For example, electrical stimulation of the heart can precipitate ventricular arrhythmias.

If pacing is required, TCP is the initial pacing method of choice in emergency cardiac care because it can be instituted more rapidly than transvenous pacing and because it is the least invasive pacing technique available. Because no vascular puncture is required for electrode placement, this technique is preferred in patients who have received, or who may require, fibrinolytic therapy. Most manufacturers now produce external defibrillators with a built-in transcutaneous pacemaker, offering the rapid availability of pacing. Multifunction electrodes allow hands-off defibrillation, pacing, and ECG monitoring through a single pair of adhesive chest wall electrodes. Notably, while effective for defibrillation, the typical right anterior infraclavicular and anterior left apical chest wall electrode positions may not be effective for TCP. In such instances, relocating the right anterior electrode posteriorly may afford both defibrillation and improve TCP capability.

Limited experience suggests that TCP may also be useful in treating refractory tachyarrhythmias by overdrive pacing.[31-33] But overdrive pacing may also accelerate the tachycardia, so it is best deferred to expert consultation.

Equipment for TCP

Transcutaneous pacemakers should be available in all emergency departments and in many in-hospital and out-of-hospital care settings. The pacemakers introduced in the early 1980s were largely asynchronous devices with a limited selection of rate and output options. More recent units have demand-mode pacing with more output options. In newer units pacing is often combined with a defibrillator in a single unit.

Most transcutaneous pacemakers have similar basic features:

- **Operation mode:** Both a fixed-rate (nondemand or asynchronous) mode and a demand mode
- **Rate selection:** A range from 30 to 180/min
- **Current output:** Adjustable from 0 to 200 mA
- **Pulse duration:** Varies from 20 to 40 milliseconds but is not operator adjustable. (Rectangular pacing-pulse markers of 20 to 40 milliseconds are visible on the recorder.)
- **Monitor blanking:** A feature that prevents the large electrical spike from the pacemaker impulse from obscuring interpretation of the much smaller ECG complex. The majority of commercially available TCP units are integrated monitor/defibrillator/pacing devices that automatically blank the pacing complex. Without this feature large pacing artifacts can mask treatable VF or otherwise make rhythm interpretation difficult.

A preliminary trial of TCP should be undertaken to ensure that capture can be achieved and pacing is tolerated by the patient. If the patient is having difficulty tolerating the discomfort caused by TCP, administer medications such as diazepam (for treatment of anxiety and muscle contractions) and morphine (for analgesia).

TCP Step-by-Step Technique (Figure 56)

1. Attach the 2 pacing electrodes to the patient's chest.
   - a. Place the anterior electrode to the left of the sternum, centered as close as possible to the point of maximum cardiac impulse.
   - b. Place the posterior electrode on the back, between the shoulder blades, to the left or right of the thoracic spinal column. Consider relocation of the posterior electrode location if capture is unsuccessful at

maximum output of the device (eg, reposition a right posterior location to a left posterior position or vice versa).

c. Shaving may be required to ensure good contact on patients with excessive body hair; alternative pacing electrode positions may be needed.

2. Set the *pacing rate* (usually 60 to 80/min; see discussion above).
3. Set the *pacing current*. Start with the minimal setting and slowly increase the output until the *pacing spike* of the pacemaker appears on the monitor screen (Figure 56B). Continue increasing the output until *pacing capture* is achieved (see Number 4).
4. Monitor the ECG to assess *electrical* pacing capture. Pacing capture is present when each pacer spike is followed by a ventricular depolarization with a visible QRS complex *and* repolarization with a T wave (Figure 56C).
5. Each pacer spike that "captures" the ventricle will produce a wide QRS complex, a consistent ST segment, *and* a broad, slurred T wave that is often opposite in polarity (direction) from the QRS complex (Figure 56C), depending upon the monitored lead.
6. Do not mistake the mere presence of wide, slurred afterpotential following an external pacing spike for evidence of ventricular depolarization associated with electrical capture. Look specifically for T waves. If a T wave is not evident, it is unlikely that the ventricle has been captured by pacing.
7. Assess ventricular *function* and *cardiac output* (so-called *hemodynamic* or *mechanical capture*) during pacing by the patient's pulse and blood pressure.
8. Assessment of a pulse to confirm mechanical capture can be challenging during TCP because electrical stimulation causes generalized muscular contraction (jerking) that may mimic the carotid pulse. A femoral pulse is occasionally more reliably palpated than a carotid pulse, given the femoral artery's greater distance away from the site of pacing and less surrounding muscle.
9. Continue pacing at a pacemaker output level slightly higher (10%) than the threshold of initial electrical capture (the threshold is the minimal pacemaker output associated with consistent pacing capture) in order to ensure reliable capture while minimizing additional discomfort to the patient from an unnecessarily high output.

TCP Complications and Corrections

The following are the major complications or problems encountered during TCP and corrective measures to address them.

- **Failure to recognize the presence of underlying treatable VF.** Critically ill patients in need of emergency pacing are at risk for the development of sudden unstable VT or VF. The presence of VF/pulseless VT can be obscured by a large pacing artifact on an ECG monitor. The development of VF/pulseless VT is more likely to be obscured if the monitor lacks the feature of pacing stimulus filters that dampen or blank such artifacts. In some clinical situations a patient may be attached to a bedside or transport monitor when pacing is needed. If pacing is initiated without switching to a monitor with such filtering capabilities, the rhythm may be uninterpretable and the loss of ventricular capture or development of VF may be undetected.
  - **Correction.** Perform TCP with an integrated monitor constructed to display an interpretable rhythm during pacing stimuli. In addition, maintaining a hand on the femoral artery pulse during pacing assures that pacing is resulting in ventricular contraction. In the event that pulse is lost, consider a change in the underlying rhythm to VF or VT or the need to increase pacing output.
- **Failure to capture.** Failure to achieve myocardial (QRS) capture with pacing may result from inadequate pacing output or pacing pad configuration (location). In adults capture thresholds do not appear to be related to body weight. However, electrical current is particularly poorly conducted through air-filled cavities such as barrel-shaped chests (eg, severe emphysema) or through large amounts of intrathoracic air (eg, bullous emphysema, pneumothorax). The hearts of some patients may be refractory to capture at any output, such as with extreme electrolyte disorders (hyperkalemia). A large pericardial effusion or pleural fluid may also increase the output required for capture.
  - **Correction.** If increasing pacing output does not result in ventricular capture, consider relocating pacing pads. Often patients are semiconscious or so symptomatic that moving them to gain access to the back for pad placement is difficult. Although it is acceptable to use the same sternal-to-apex pacing route for pacing as for defibrillation, a posterior-anterior pacing pad position better encapsulates the heart within the path of current and is more likely to result in successful pacing capture. Boney structures, such as the left scapula and the thoracic column, may also reduce current flow between the pacing pads. Thus the optimal pad position often has to be located by trial and error. This remains one of the challenges with TCP and one of the reasons why it is at best regarded as a fragile bridge to transvenous pacing. If TCP is unsuccessful despite these efforts, use of alternate pharmacologic therapies (catecholamine infusion) is recommended.
- **Failure to recognize failure to capture.** This complication is primarily due to the size of the pacing artifact on the ECG screen, a technical problem inherent in systems without dampening circuitry. The rhythmic skeletal muscle contractions that occur during external pacing also can make it difficult to determine if capture occurs.

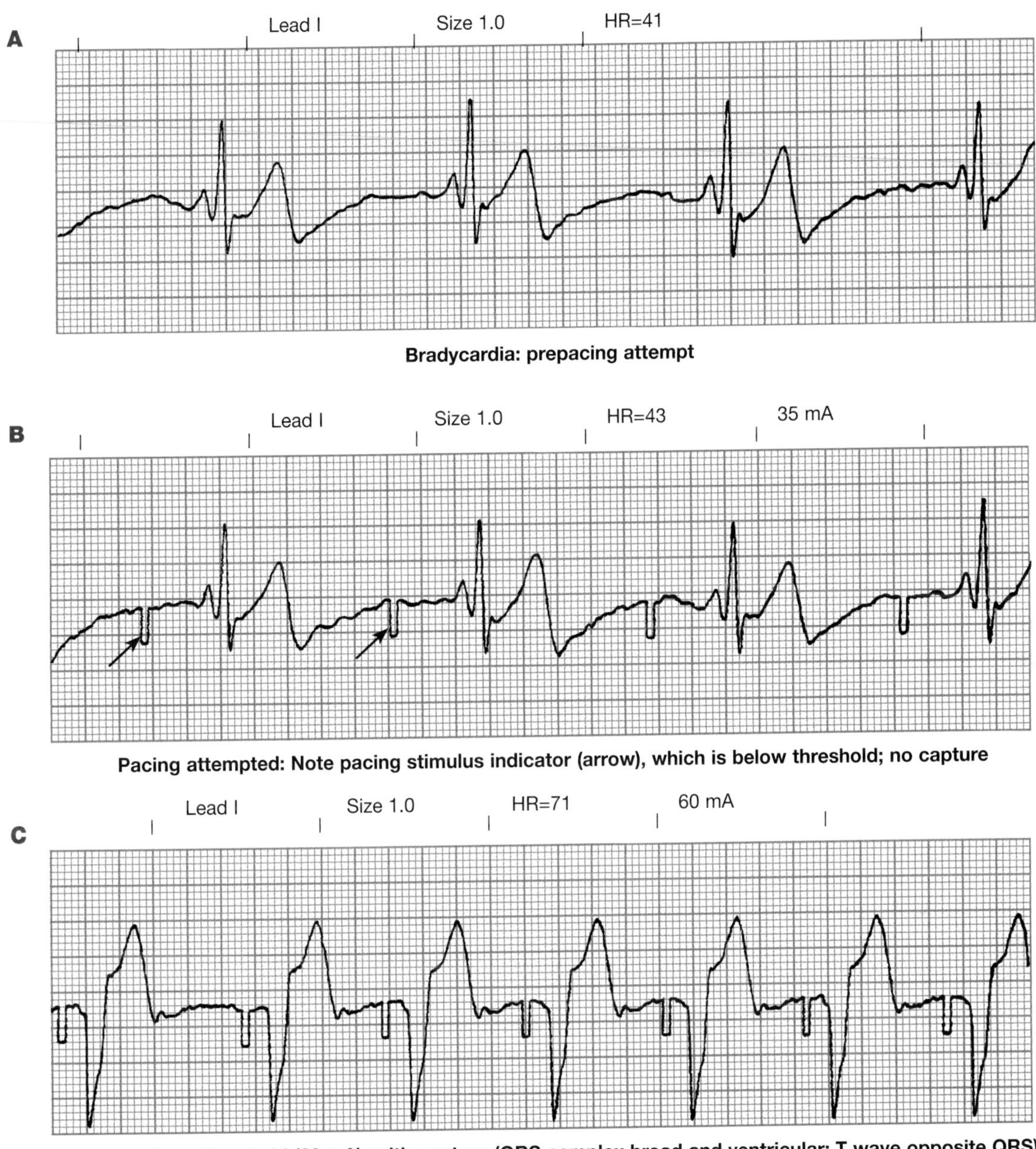

Figure 56. Transcutaneous pacing (TCP). **A,** Bradycardia, no pacing. Ventricular rate is 41/min. The underlying atrial rhythm is atrial fibrillation, which in the setting of the regular ventricular rhythm suggests the presence of third-degree AV block. Note that what appears to be a P wave ahead of each QRS has too short of a PR interval to be conducted and, accordingly, is actually part of the QRS complex, which is very wide (0.24 second). In this instance the patient was hypotensive and unresponsive to fluid administration. **B,** TCP initiated at low current (35 mA) and slow rate (50/min). The current is below the threshold needed to capture the myocardium. With TCP, monitor electrodes are attached in a modified lead II position. As current (in mA) is gradually increased, the monitor leads detect the pacing stimuli as squared-off, negative markers. Transcutaneous pacemakers incorporate standard ECG monitoring circuitry, but they also have filters to dampen the appearance of the artifact created by pacing stimuli. Without such filtering, the monitor may record this pacing artifact off the edge of the screen or paper (at the top and bottom borders) making the ECG uninterpretable. **C,** Pacing current is turned up above threshold (60 mA at 71/min), "capturing" the myocardium. The QRS that results from ventricular pacing is typically wide (0.12 second or more) because the heart is being depolarized outside the normal cardiac conduction system by direct electrical stimulation of the myocardium. For this reason a successful capture resembles a premature ventricular contraction with a wide QRS complex. Note that electrical capture of the ventricle (marked by the wide QRS complex) and mechanical contraction of the ventricle are not one in the same. Mechanical contraction implies the production of blood flow (usually assessed by a palpable pulse) and cannot be determined solely by the rhythm display. Thus, seeing ventricular capture (a wide QRS complex on the ECG) should prompt the provider to check for signs of circulation (a pulse) to ensure that the patient is not in PEA.

- **Correction.** Always look for the presence of a T wave to be assured that ventricular capture has occurred. In addition, checking for a pulse at a comparable rate as the paced rate provides reassurance that the ventricle is both being captured and mechanically contracting. Bedside ultrasound, looking at ventricular wall motion, has also been used to assess the effectiveness of TCP capture.

- **Failure to recognize "electrical" capture without effective myocardial function.** The ultimate objective of TCP is to produce hemodynamically effective cardiac contractions through effective depolarization of the ventricles. This requires effective excitation-mechanical coupling. Successful electrical capture with ventricular depolarization (wide QRS complexes each followed by a T wave) may occur without effective cardiac output, an example of true "electromechanical dissociation." This condition should be immediately recognized, CPR immediately instituted, and the asystole/PEA treatment algorithm instituted.
  - **Correction.** Provide chest compressions whenever pacing with electrical capture fails to result in a palpable pulse or other evidence of restored circulation (eg, an awakened patient). Several minutes of simultaneous pacing and chest compressions have sometimes reestablished "electromechanical association" in such patients. The amount of current used for TCP is unlikely to pose a contact risk for care providers, but gloved hands during the performance of chest compressions, particularly when pacing electrodes are both anteriorly located, will minimize the likelihood of "feeling" pacing current.

- **Pacing-induced arrhythmias or VF.** Pacing-induced arrhythmias are more of a theoretical than a frequently documented complication of pacing. Most observers consider VF associated with pacing to be coincidental and not cause and effect in critically ill patients. The current output required for TCP is, in fact, several factors lower than the current output required to induce fibrillation. However, a fortuitously timed paced QRS during an electrically vulnerable period of the cardiac cycle can sometimes precipitate VT/VF.
  - **Correction:** Monitor the rhythm and pulse continuously during TCP.

- **Pain and discomfort.** Most conscious patients who are paced for symptomatic bradycardias experience discomfort from the muscle contractions stimulated by pacing. Others find the pacing stimulus itself painful and

Table 20. TCP

A. Bradycardia: no pacing **B. Pacing stimulus below threshold: no capture** **C. Pacing stimulus above threshold: capture occurs**	
Rhythm Strip (Figure 56)	**Comments**
A. Bradycardia (third-degree AV block): no pacing (**Note:** Rates and intervals slightly altered due to monitor compensation for pacing stimulus).	• QRS rate = 41/min • P waves = 187/min • QRS = very wide, 0.24 second; ventricular escape beats • Patient: hypotensive and unresponsive to fluid administration
B. TCP initiated at low current (35 mA) and slow rate (50/min) Below the threshold current needed to stimulate the myocardium	• With TCP, monitor electrodes are attached in modified lead II position. • As current (in milliamperes) is gradually increased, the monitor leads detect the pacing stimuli as a squared off, negative marker. • Transcutaneous pacemakers incorporate standard ECG monitoring circuitry but incorporate filters to dampen the pacing stimuli. • A monitor without these filters records "border-to-border" tracings (off the edge of the screen or paper at the top and bottom borders) that cannot be interpreted.
C. Pacing current turned up above threshold (60 mA at 71/min) and "captures" the myocardium	• TCP stimulus does not work through the normal cardiac conduction system but by a direct electrical stimulus of the myocardium. • Therefore, a "capture," where TCP stimulus results in a myocardial contraction, will resemble a PVC. • Electrical capture is characterized by a wide QRS complex. • A "mechanically captured beat" will produce effective myocardial contraction with production of some blood flow (usually assessed by a palpable carotid pulse).

Abbreviations: ECG, electrocardiographic; PVC, premature ventricular complex; TCP, transcutaneous pacing.

intolerable. Pain from electrical skin and muscle stimulation was a significant complication of early devices.[33] While variable, some studies have found 1 of 3 patients rating the pain from TCP as severe or intolerable.

- **Correction.** If not contraindicated, analgesia with incremental doses of a narcotic, sedation with a benzodiazepine, or both can reduce the pain of TCP to an acceptable level. Some clinicians use procedural sedation protocols for patients needing emergency TCP. Occasionally intubation may be required when the level of sedation required for TCP compromises respiratory function.

Electrical Capture and Effective Myocardial Function: Excitation-Contraction Coupling

Myocardial depolarization and myocardial contraction involve a complex series of events that include the myocardial cells, electrolyte movement into and out of cells, calcium effects on actin and myosin filaments, and myocardial fiber shortening. These events are collectively referred to as *excitation-contraction coupling.* We know that electrical depolarization can occur without effective myocardial contraction or so-called *electromechanical dissociation* or *PEA.* This indicates ineffective excitation-contraction coupling. These patients have electrical depolarization but ineffective cardiac output.

During pacing, a pacer spike should be followed by myocardial depolarization (Figure 57A). A temporary pacemaker is typically placed in the right ventricle. However, permanently implanted pacemakers can be atrial, ventricular, or a combination (Figure 57B). Permanent pacemakers are outside the scope of this discussion, apart from the provider needing to recognize the general appearance of atrial, ventricular, and AV (dual-chamber) pacing when seen on a rhythm strip or ECG. As with temporary pacing, a wide QRS complex following a pacer spike merely reflects electrical capture of the heart and makes no statement about the effectiveness of myocardial contraction (fiber shortening) and stroke volume associated with this event. Clinical evaluation, such as echocardiography, or arterial catheterization is required to determine the hemodynamic response to a rhythm, whether paced or not. For this reason the clinician must frequently evaluate both pulse and systemic perfusion during pacing to ensure that electrical capture is associated with effective myocardial function.

FAQ

Will atropine increase the degree of high-degree AV block?

In type II second-degree AV block, in the region where the conduction abnormality lies distal to the AV node (infranodal), atropine usually has no conduction-enhancing effect. Theoretically, by increasing the rate of sinus node discharge and improving conduction through the AV node, atropine may result in more impulses bombarding the site of the block in the distal conduction system. This could result in even fewer impulses being conducted through the site of block, thus paradoxically worsening the degree of block and decreasing the ventricular rate. Thus, atropine should be deployed cautiously in such circumstances, with a readiness for pacing should the heart block worsen with treatment.

Can atropine be used for second-degree and third-degree AV block of uncertain level (AV nodal vs infranodal) while pacing is initiated?

- Atropine should be considered a temporizing measure while awaiting a transcutaneous or transvenous pacemaker for patients with symptomatic sinus bradycardia, conduction block at the level of the AV node, or sinus arrest.
- Atropine administration should not delay implementation of external pacing for patients with impending cardiac arrest.
- Avoid relying on atropine in type II second-degree or third-degree AV block or in patients with third-degree AV block with a new wide-QRS complex where the location of block is likely to be in nonnodal tissue (such as in the bundle of His or more distal conduction system). After 1 or 2 doses with no response, move to pacing or β-adrenergic support.
- These bradyarrhythmias are not likely to be responsive to reversal of cholinergic effects by atropine and are preferably treated with TCP or β-adrenergic support as temporizing measures while the patient is prepared for transvenous pacing.

Can atropine be used in patients with ACS?

Because all chronotropic drugs like atropine can accelerate sinus rate, caution is advised in its use in patients with ACS, in whom the resulting tachycardia might worsen myocardial ischemia.

Can atropine be used in patients who have undergone cardiac transplant?

- Atropine will likely be ineffective in this condition because the transplanted heart lacks vagal innervation. On occasion its use in the cardiac transplant patient has resulted in paradoxic worsening of bradycardia.

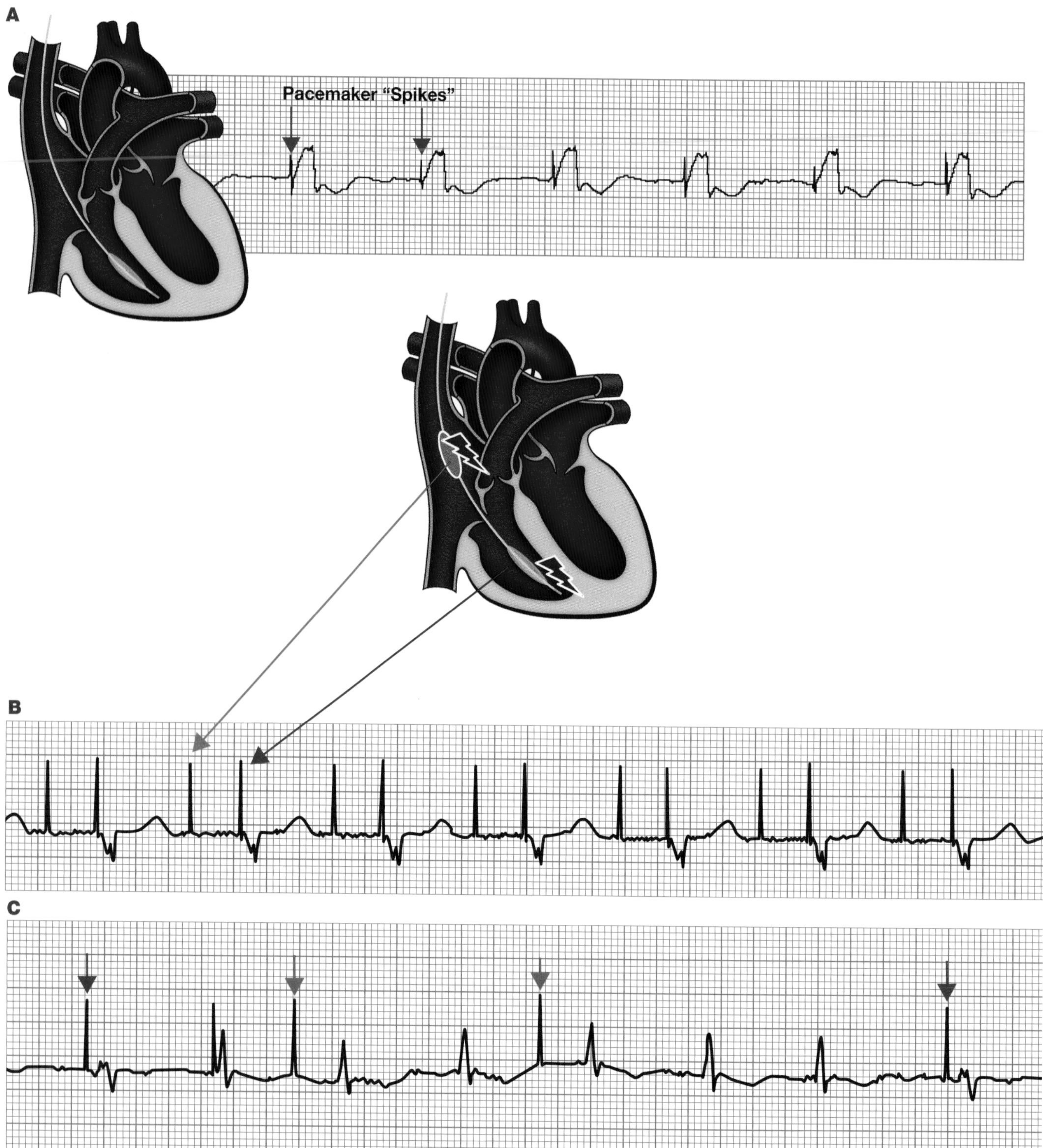

Figure 57. **A,** Single-chamber (ventricular) and **B,** dual-chamber (atrial and ventricular) pacing ("spikes"). Both rhythm strips are remarkable for a wide QRS complex. This can be mistaken for premature ventricular contractions and incorrectly interpreted as VT. But the rate is too slow. In each figure the wide QRS complex is preceded by pacemaker artifact (blue arrows), indicating that this wide complex is due to ventricular pacing. QRS conduction is wide because capture of the ventricles by the pacemaker occurs outside the normal conduction system. Pacing artifact from an atrial pacemaker is shown by the red arrow. P waves (as a result of atrial capture) are frequently small in amplitude (as in this example) and may be difficult to see without evaluating the tracing in a different ECG lead. In this example, although the ventricles are captured by pacing (each ventricular pacing spike is followed by a QRS), one could not be certain that the same is true with the atria (since P waves are not readily evident). **C,** Pacemaker artifacts that fail to capture (small green arrows). Note that the first and last spikes (small blue arrows) are followed by a captured beat. This is an example of intermittent capture or, alternatively, pacemaker malfunction with periods of failure to capture. Fortunately for this patient, the pacemaker is no longer needed because the patient's own rhythm has returned and is only transiently decreased below the preset pacer rate.

References

1. Chadda KD, Lichstein E, Gupta PK, Kourtesis P. Effects of atropine in patients with bradyarrhythmia complicating myocardial infarction. Usefulness of an optimum dose for overdrive. *Am J Med*. 1977;63:503-510.
2. Smith I, Monk TG, White PF. Comparison of transesophageal atrial pacing with anticholinergic drugs for the treatment of intraoperative bradycardia. *Anesth Analg*. 1994;78:245-252.
3. Brady WJ, Swart G, DeBehnke DJ, Ma OJ, Aufderheide TP. The efficacy of atropine in the treatment of hemodynamically unstable bradycardia and atrioventricular block: prehospital and emergency department considerations. *Resuscitation*. 1999;41:47-55.
4. Neumar RW, Otto CW, Link MS, Kronick SL, Shuster M, Callaway CW, Kudenchuk PJ, Ornato JP, McNally B, Silvers SM, Passman RS, White RD, Hess EP, Tang W, Davis D, Sinz E, Morrison LJ. Part 8: adult advanced cardiovascular life support: 2010 American Heart Association Guidelines for Cardiopulmonary Resuscitation and Emergency Cardiovascular Care. *Circulation*. 2010;122:S729-S767.
5. Dauchot P, Gravenstein JS. Effects of atropine on the electrocardiogram in different age groups. *Clin Pharmacol Ther*. 1971;12:274-280.
6. Ellenbogen KA, Thames MD, DiMarco JP, Sheehan H, Lerman BB. Electrophysiological effects of adenosine in the transplanted human heart. Evidence of supersensitivity. *Circulation*. 1990;81:821-828.
7. Errando CL, Peiro CM. An additional explanation for atrioventricular block after the administration of atropine. *Can J Anaesth*. 2004;51:88.
8. Maruyama K, Mochizuki N, Hara K. High-degree atrioventricular block after the administration of atropine for sinus arrest during anesthesia. *Can J Anaesth*. 2003;50:528-529.
9. Brunner-La Rocca HP, Kiowski W, Bracht C, Weilenmann D, Follath F. Atrioventricular block after administration of atropine in patients following cardiac transplantation. *Transplantation*. 1997;63:1838-1839.
10. Bernheim A, Fatio R, Kiowski W, Weilenmann D, Rickli H, Brunner-La Rocca HP. Atropine often results in complete atrioventricular block or sinus arrest after cardiac transplantation: an unpredictable and dose-independent phenomenon. *Transplantation*. 2004;77:1181-1185.
11. Mangrum JM, DiMarco JP. The evaluation and management of bradycardia. *N Engl J Med*. 2000;342:703-709.
12. Barold SS, Hayes DL. Second-degree atrioventricular block: a reappraisal. *Mayo Clin Proc*. 2001;76:44-57.
13. Barold SS. Lingering misconceptions about type I second-degree atrioventricular block. *Am J Cardiol*. 2001;88:1018-1020.
14. Antman EM, Anbe DT, Armstrong PW, Bates ER, Green LA, Hand M, Hochman JS, Krumholz HM, Kushner FG, Lamas GA, Mullany CJ, Ornato JP, Pearle DL, Sloan MA, Smith SC Jr, Alpert JS, Anderson JL, Faxon DP, Fuster V, Gibbons RJ, Gregoratos G, Halperin JL, Hiratzka LF, Hunt SA, Jacobs AK. ACC/AHA guidelines for the management of patients with ST-elevation myocardial infarction: a report of the American College of Cardiology/American Heart Association Task Force on Practice Guidelines (Committee to Revise the 1999 Guidelines for the Management of Patients with Acute Myocardial Infarction). *Circulation*. 2004;110:e82-e292.
15. Gauss A, Hubner C, Radermacher P, Georgieff M, Schutz W. Perioperative risk of bradyarrhythmias in patients with asymptomatic chronic bifascicular block or left bundle branch block: does an additional first-degree atrioventricular block make any difference? *Anesthesiology*. 1998;88:679-687.
16. Gauss A, Hubner C, Meierhenrich R, Rohm HJ, Georgieff M, Schutz W. Perioperative transcutaneous pacemaker in patients with chronic bifascicular block or left bundle branch block and additional first-degree atrioventricular block. *Acta Anaesthesiol Scand*. 1999;43:731-736.
17. Dalsey WC, Syverud SA, Hedges JR. Emergency department use of transcutaneous pacing for cardiac arrests. *Crit Care Med*. 1985;13:399-401.
18. Eitel DR, Guzzardi LJ, Stein SE, Drawbaugh RE, Hess DR, Walton SL. Noninvasive transcutaneous cardiac pacing in prehospital cardiac arrest. *Ann Emerg Med*. 1987;16:531-534.
19. Cummins RO, Graves JR, Larsen MP, Hallstrom AP, Hearne TR, Ciliberti J, Nicola RM, Horan S. Out-of-hospital transcutaneous pacing by emergency medical technicians in patients with asystolic cardiac arrest. *N Engl J Med*. 1993;328:1377-1382.
20. Morrison LJ, Long J, Vermeulen M, Schwartz B, Sawadsky B, Frank J, Cameron B, Burgess R, Shield J, Bagley P, Mausz V, Brewer JE, Dorian P. A randomized controlled feasibility trial comparing safety and effectiveness of prehospital pacing versus conventional treatment: 'PrePACE.' *Resuscitation*. 2008;76:341-349.
21. Paris PM, Stewart RD, Kaplan RM, Whipkey R. Transcutaneous pacing for bradyasystolic cardiac arrests in prehospital care. *Ann Emerg Med*. 1985;14:320-323.
22. Proano L, Chiang WK, Wang RY. Calcium channel blocker overdose. *Am J Emerg Med*. 1995;13:444-450.
23. Watson NA, FitzGerald CP. Management of massive verapamil overdose. *Med J Aust*. 1991;155:124-125.
24. Gotz D, Pohle S, Barckow D. Primary and secondary detoxification in severe flecainide intoxication. *Intensive Care Med*. 1991;17:181-184.
25. Cummins RO, Haulman J, Quan L, Graves JR, Peterson D, Horan S. Near-fatal yew berry intoxication treated with external cardiac pacing and digoxin-specific FAB antibody fragments. *Ann Emerg Med*. 1990;19:38-43.
26. Quan L, Graves JR, Kinder DR, Horan S, Cummins RO. Transcutaneous cardiac pacing in the treatment of out-of-hospital pediatric cardiac arrests. *Ann Emerg Med*. 1992;21:905-909.
27. Beland MJ, Hesslein PS, Finlay CD, Faerron-Angel JE, Williams WG, Rowe RD. Noninvasive transcutaneous cardiac pacing in children. *Pacing Clin Electrophysiol*. 1987;10:1262-1270.
28. Zoll PM. Development of electric control of cardiac rhythm. *JAMA*. 1973;226:881-886.
29. Zoll PM, Belgard AH, Weintraub MJ, Frank HA. External mechanical cardiac stimulation. *N Engl J Med*. 1976;294:1274-1275.
30. Syverud SA, Hedges JR, Dalsey WC, Gabel M, Thomson DP, Engel PJ. Hemodynamics of transcutaneous cardiac pacing. *Am J Emerg Med*. 1986;4:17-20.
31. Estes NA III, Deering TF, Manolis AS, Salem D, Zoll PM. External cardiac programmed stimulation for noninvasive termination of sustained supraventricular and ventricular tachycardia. *Am J Cardiol*. 1989;63:177-183.

32. Rosenthal ME, Stamato NJ, Marchlinski FE, Josephson ME. Noninvasive cardiac pacing for termination of sustained, uniform ventricular tachycardia. *Am J Cardiol*. 1986;58:561-562.

33. Sharkey SW, Chaffee V, Kapsner S. Prophylactic external pacing during cardioversion of atrial tachyarrhythmias. *Am J Cardiol*. 1985;55:1632-1634.

Chapter 10

Tachycardia

This Chapter

- When to Treat Fast Heart Rates in Stable Patients
- How to Use Vagal Maneuvers and Adenosine
- Do No Harm and Seek Expert Consultation When Initial Therapy Fails or a Wide-Complex Tachycardia Is Present
- What to Do if Patients Become Unstable

Introduction

This chapter reviews tachycardia with pulses for the ACLS provider. Tachycardia itself (eg, sinus tachycardia) is not necessarily abnormal. A tachyarrhythmia, however, is defined as a rhythm disorder with a heart rate faster than 100/min. These rhythms can be narrow-complex or wide-complex (QRS) tachycardias. The ACLS provider requires basic knowledge to initially differentiate sinus tachycardia, narrow-complex supraventricular tachycardia (SVT) and wide-complex tachycardia, and symptomatic from asymptomatic arrhythmias. Because ACLS providers may be unable to distinguish between supraventricular and ventricular rhythms, it is safest to presume that most wide-complex (broad-complex) tachycardias are ventricular in origin, particularly in persons with known heart disease. Irregularly irregular narrow-complex tachycardias (differing intervals between QRS complexes from beat to beat) are likely atrial fibrillation or multifocal atrial tachycardia; atrial flutter may be regular or irregular in rate.

Definition

The term *tachycardia* is used interchangeably with tachyarrhythmia. In this context a tachycardia can be sinus tachycardia or other SVT, such as atrial fibrillation or flutter, with a ventricular response rate faster than 100/min. The Tachycardia With a Pulse Algorithm (Figure 58), like the Bradycardia Algorithm, can be implemented without the delay to initially identify the underlying rhythm disorder. The same initial considerations apply:

1. Identification of a tachycardia
2. Determination that signs or symptoms are due to the tachycardia

The next consideration involves identification and differential diagnosis of the rhythm disorder and "tailoring" and "titration" of therapy to the arrhythmia and patient.

Tachycardia and Symptoms

Providers managing patients with a tachycardia must first evaluate whether the fast heart rate is symptomatic and hemodynamically significant. Does the tachycardia produce serious signs and symptoms that are the direct result of the heart's fast contractions or something else? Clinicians are required to emergently treat a tachycardia only when the rhythm disorder itself causes serious signs and symptoms.

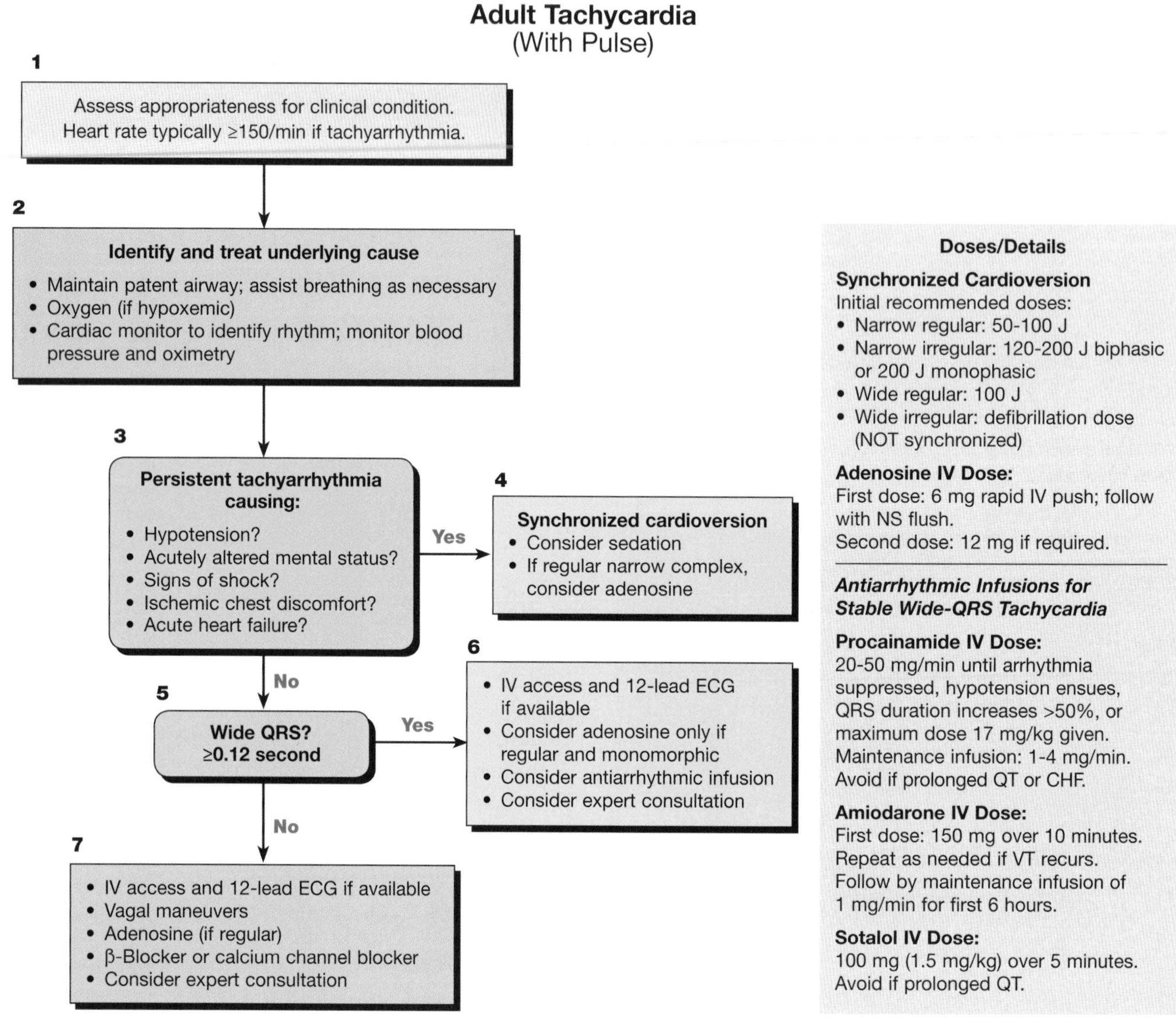

Adult Tachycardia
(With Pulse)
1
Assess appropriateness for clinical condition.
Heart rate typically ≥150/min if tachyarrhythmia.
2
Identify and treat underlying cause
• Maintain patent airway; assist breathing as necessary
• Oxygen (if hypoxemic)
• Cardiac monitor to identify rhythm; monitor blood pressure and oximetry
3
Persistent tachyarrhythmia causing:
• Hypotension?
• Acutely altered mental status?
• Signs of shock?
• Ischemic chest discomfort?
• Acute heart failure?
Yes
4
Synchronized cardioversion
• Consider sedation
• If regular narrow complex, consider adenosine
No
5
Wide QRS?
≥0.12 second
Yes
6
• IV access and 12-lead ECG if available
• Consider adenosine only if regular and monomorphic
• Consider antiarrhythmic infusion
• Consider expert consultation
No
7
• IV access and 12-lead ECG if available
• Vagal maneuvers
• Adenosine (if regular)
• β-Blocker or calcium channel blocker
• Consider expert consultation
Doses/Details
Synchronized Cardioversion
Initial recommended doses:
• Narrow regular: 50-100 J
• Narrow irregular: 120-200 J biphasic or 200 J monophasic
• Wide regular: 100 J
• Wide irregular: defibrillation dose (NOT synchronized)
Adenosine IV Dose:
First dose: 6 mg rapid IV push; follow with NS flush.
Second dose: 12 mg if required.
Antiarrhythmic Infusions for Stable Wide-QRS Tachycardia
Procainamide IV Dose:
20-50 mg/min until arrhythmia suppressed, hypotension ensues, QRS duration increases >50%, or maximum dose 17 mg/kg given.
Maintenance infusion: 1-4 mg/min.
Avoid if prolonged QT or CHF.
Amiodarone IV Dose:
First dose: 150 mg over 10 minutes.
Repeat as needed if VT recurs.
Follow by maintenance infusion of 1 mg/min for first 6 hours.
Sotalol IV Dose:
100 mg (1.5 mg/kg) over 5 minutes.
Avoid if prolonged QT.

Figure 58. The Tachycardia With a Pulse Algorithm.

Clinical *symptoms* that may be caused by tachycardia are similar to those caused by bradycardia and include

- Hypotension
- Acutely altered mental status
- Signs of shock
- Ischemic chest discomfort
- Acute heart failure

Classification of Tachyarrhythmias

Tachycardias can be classified in several ways, based on the appearance of the QRS complex, heart rate, and regularity.

- **Narrow–QRS-complex (SVT) tachycardias (QRS less than 0.12 second) include the following rhythms in order of frequency:**
  - Sinus tachycardia
  - Atrial fibrillation
  - Atrial flutter
  - Paroxysmal supraventricular tachycardia (PSVT)
    - Atrioventricular (AV) nodal reentry tachycardia (AVNRT)
    - Atrioventricular reentry tachycardia (AVRT), including accessory pathway–mediated AVRT
  - Atrial tachycardia (including automatic and reentry forms)
  - Multifocal atrial tachycardia
  - Junctional tachycardia (rare in adults)

- **Wide-QRS-complex tachycardias (QRS 0.12 second or more) include the following rhythms:**
  - Ventricular tachycardia (VT), including monomorphic and polymorphic VT
  - Ventricular fibrillation (VF)
  - Sinus tachycardia with aberrancy
  - SVT with aberrancy
  - Preexcited tachycardias (Wolff-Parkinson-White [WPW] syndrome)
  - Ventricular-paced rhythms

Key Points for Interventions

- Vagal maneuvers and adenosine are the preferred initial therapeutic choices for the termination of stable reentry SVT. Vagal maneuvers alone (Valsalva maneuver or carotid sinus massage, discussed below) will terminate about 20% to 25% of reentry SVT[1]; adenosine is required for the remainder.
- If a patient with tachycardia is unstable (ie, signs and symptoms are persistent despite airway management and provision of oxygen) and the instability is related to the tachycardia, immediate synchronized cardioversion is indicated.
- Management of hemodynamically stable wide-complex tachycardias is covered in the algorithm, but expert consultation is advised for these advanced arrhythmias.

Electrical Cardioversion for Stable and Unstable Tachycardias

Synchronized cardioversion is shock delivery that is timed (synchronized) to be given coincident with the QRS complex. This synchronization avoids shock delivery during the relative refractory period of the cardiac cycle (some call it the "vulnerable period"), when a shock could produce VF.[2] The energy (shock dose) required for organized QRS rhythms when using synchronized cardioversion is generally lower than the doses required for disorganized QRS rhythms (eg, VF), which require unsynchronized shocks. Low-energy shocks are just as painful and, if inappropriately timed, have as much or more potential to precipitate VF as high energy shocks, but potentially a lesser likelihood of resulting in bradyarrhythmias or tissue injury. Therefore, depending upon the rhythm, adjusted-energy synchronized cardioversion is preferred over high energy. However, for disorganized QRS rhythms when synchronization is not possible use high-energy unsynchronized shocks (defibrillation doses).

Synchronized cardioversion is recommended to treat arrhythmias caused by reentry when medications are ineffective or are not acceptable options because of patient instability. These rhythms include SVT, atrial fibrillation, atrial flutter, and monomorphic VT. Rhythms mediated by reentry are caused by an abnormal rhythm circuit that allows a wave of depolarization to travel in a circle, recirculating the same path over and over again. Delivery of a shock can stop these rhythms because the shock interrupts the circulating (reentry) pattern. Establish intravenous (IV) access before cardioversion and administer sedation if the patient is conscious. But do not delay cardioversion if the patient is unstable. Because attempted cardioversion can occasionally result in bradycardia or VF, the provider needs to be prepared to treat these possible complications in the aftermath of shock.

The terms *monophasic* and *biphasic waveform* refer to the characteristics of an administered shock. Monophasic waveforms deliver current of one polarity (direction of current flow), whereas biphasic waveforms change the polarity (direction of current flow) of the administered shock. Biphasic shock has largely displaced monophasic waveform shock in manufactured defibrillators. Definitive recommendations for the first and subsequent energy levels of biphasic shock are difficult to make because other characteristics of the shock waveform differ among manufacturers.

- In general, the recommended initial biphasic energy dose for cardioversion of adult atrial fibrillation is 120 to 200 J (Figure 59).
- With respect to either monophasic or biphasic shocks, limited available data make it difficult to give a dose equivalence or provide definitive recommendations about the selected energy for subsequent shocks if the initial energy is unsuccessful.
- On the basis of available evidence, it is recommended that subsequent energy levels be at least equivalent, and higher energy levels may be considered in stepwise fashion, if available.
- Cardioversion of adult atrial flutter and other SVTs generally requires less energy; an initial biphasic energy of 50 to 100 J is often sufficient.[3]
- If a monophasic waveform is used, adult cardioversion of atrial fibrillation should begin at 200 J; energy levels of 200 J may also be used for cardioversion of atrial flutter and other SVTs.

Cardioversion will not be effective for treatment of junctional tachycardia or ectopic or multifocal atrial tachycardia because these rhythms have an automatic focus, arising from cells that are spontaneously depolarizing at a rapid rate. Delivery of a shock cannot stop these rhythms. In fact, shock delivery to a heart with a rapid automatic focus may increase the rate of the tachyarrhythmia.

The amount of energy required for cardioversion of VT is determined by the morphologic characteristics and the rate of the VT.[3] If the patient with monomorphic VT (regular form and rate) is unstable but has a pulse, treat with synchronized cardioversion. To treat monomorphic VT using a monophasic or biphasic waveform, provide an initial shock of 100 J. If there is no response to the first shock, repeat or consider increasing the dose in a stepwise fashion (eg, 100 J, 200 J, 300 J, 360 J) (Figure 59).

If a patient has polymorphic VT and is unstable, treat the rhythm as VF and deliver high-energy (defibrillation dose) *unsynchronized* shocks. The recommended starting energy is 360 J for monophasic defibrillation. The characteristics of biphasic shock waveforms differ between defibrillator manufacturers, and have not been compared in humans with regard to efficacy. Therefore, for biphasic defibrillation, providers should use the manufacturer's recommended energy dose (usually 120 to 200 J). If the manufacturer's recommended dose is not known, providers may defibrillate at the maximum dose of the device. Although synchronized cardioversion is preferred for treatment of an organized ventricular rhythm, if synchronization is not possible or if there is any doubt about whether monomorphic or polymorphic VT is present in the *unstable* patient, do not delay shock delivery to perform detailed rhythm analysis: provide defibrillation doses of energy.

Electrical Cardioversion Algorithm

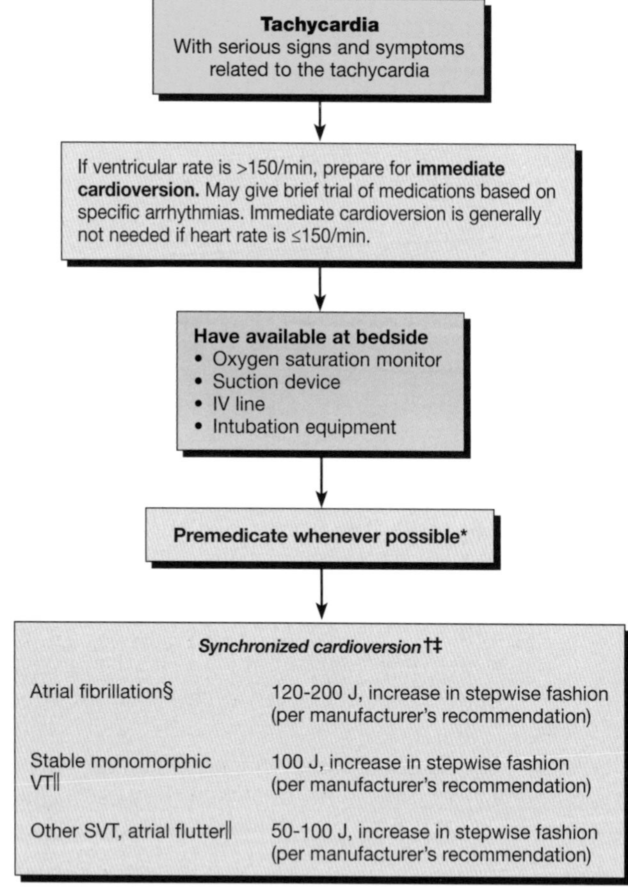

Tachycardia
With serious signs and symptoms related to the tachycardia
If ventricular rate is >150/min, prepare for **immediate cardioversion.** May give brief trial of medications based on specific arrhythmias. Immediate cardioversion is generally not needed if heart rate is ≤150/min.
Have available at bedside
• Oxygen saturation monitor
• Suction device
• IV line
• Intubation equipment
Premedicate whenever possible*
Synchronized cardioversion†‡
Atrial fibrillation§
120-200 J, increase in stepwise fashion (per manufacturer's recommendation)
Stable monomorphic VT||
100 J, increase in stepwise fashion (per manufacturer's recommendation)
Other SVT, atrial flutter||
50-100 J, increase in stepwise fashion (per manufacturer's recommendation)

Notes:

*Effective regimens have included a sedative **(eg, diazepam, midazolam, etomidate, methohexital, propofol)** with or without an analgesic agent **(eg, fentanyl, morphine)**. Many experts recommend anesthesia if service is readily available.

†Note possible need to resynchronize after each cardioversion.

‡If delays in synchronization occur and clinical condition is critical, go immediately to unsynchronized shocks.

§These doses are for biphasic waveforms. For monophasic waveforms, initial dose is 200 J for atrial fibrillation.

||Recommended biphasic and monophasic doses are equivalent.

Steps for Adult Defibrillation and Cardioversion

Using Manual Defibrillators (Monophasic or Biphasic)

Assess the rhythm. If VF or pulseless VT is present, continue chest compressions without interruptions during all steps until step 8.

Defibrillation (for VF and pulseless VT)

1. Turn on defibrillator. For biphasic defibrillators use manufacturer- specific energy if known. For monophasic defibrillators use 360 J. If unknown select the maximum energy available.
2. Set *lead select* switch to *paddles* (or *lead I, II,* or *III* if monitor leads are used).
3. Prepare adhesive pads (pads are preferred); if using paddles, apply appropriate conductive gel or paste. Be sure cables are attached to defibrillator.
4. Position defibrillation pads on patient's chest: one on the right anterior chest wall and one in the left axillary position. If paddles are used, apply firm pressure (about 15-25 pounds) when ready to deliver shock. If patient has an implanted pacemaker, position the pads so they are not directly over the device. Be sure that oxygen flow is not directed across the patient's chest.
5. Announce "Charging defibrillator!"
6. Press *charge* button on apex paddle or defibrillator controls.
7. When the defibrillator is fully charged, state firmly:
   "I am going to shock on three." Then count. "All clear!"
   (Chest compressions should continue until this announcement.)
8. After confirming all personnel are clear of the patient, press the *shock* button on the defibrillator or press the 2 paddle *discharge* buttons simultaneously.
9. Immediately after the shock is delivered, resume CPR beginning with compressions for 5 cycles (about 2 minutes), and then recheck rhythm. Interruption of CPR should be brief.

Cardioversion (for tachycardia with a pulse)

Assess the rhythm. If patient has a pulse but is unstable, proceed with cardioversion.

1-4. Follow steps for defibrillation above (except for energy dose).

5. Consider sedation.
6. Engage the ***synchronization*** mode by pressing the *sync control* button.
7. Look for markers on R waves indicating *sync* mode is operative. If necessary, adjust monitor gain until sync markers occur with each R wave.
8. Select appropriate energy level (see Electrical Cardioversion Algorithm on left).
9. Announce "Charging defibrillator!"
10. Press *charge* button on apex paddle or defibrillator controls.
11. When the defibrillator is fully charged, state firmly:
    "I am going to shock on three." Then count. "All clear!"
12. After confirming all personnel are clear of the patient, press the *discharge* buttons simultaneously on paddles or the *shock* button on the unit; hold paddles in place until shock is delivered.
13. Check the monitor. If tachycardia persists, increase the energy and prepare to cardiovert again.
14. Reset the ***sync*** mode after each synchronized cardioversion because most defibrillators default back to unsynchronized mode. This default allows an immediate shock if the cardioversion produces VF.

Figure 59. The ACLS Electrical Cardioversion Algorithm.

Critical Concept	Select and deliver the appropriate energy dose
Recommended Selected Energy Settings for Shock	**Monophasic shock** • Atrial fibrillation: 200 J synchronized • Monomorphic VT: 100 J synchronized • SVT/atrial flutter: 200 J synchronized • Polymorphic VT or VF: 360 J synchronized (defibrillation) **Biphasic shock*** • Atrial fibrillation: 120 to 200 J synchronized • Monomorphic VT: 100 J synchronized • SVT/atrial flutter: 50 to 100 J synchronized • Polymorphic VT or VF: 120 to 200 J* unsynchronized (defibrillation) *Consult the device manufacturer for specific recommendations.

Tachycardias: Refining the Diagnosis and Treatment

Premature Complexes

Patients often report "palpitations." Palpitations are caused by frequent premature complexes, and they may herald or initiate both supraventricular and ventricular paroxysmal or sustained tachycardia. By themselves palpitations are usually benign, but their presence should prompt the clinician to search for structural heart disease and exacerbating factors that may require treatment.

Premature Atrial Complexes

Premature atrial complexes (PACs) are very common. They are identified on the ECG by the occurrence of a premature P wave with a normal or occasionally prolonged PR interval (depending on the prematurity of the PAC). PACs are also identified by the differing appearance of the P wave as compared with sinus P waves, although this may not always be readily apparent. The normal regularity of rhythm and pulse is disrupted by the PAC, a situation that creates a regular rhythm that is occasionally irregular (sometimes referred to as a regularly irregular rhythm).

When a QRS does not appear to be preceded by a P wave, look closely at the preceding T wave for an abnormality that suggests the presence of a "hidden" premature P wave. When a P wave occurs very prematurely, it may find the conduction system still partially or completely refractory from the previously conducted impulse. This sometimes results in a blocked P wave or slowing/failure of impulse conduction to the ventricles. In this instance, there may be no QRS, or the QRS may be conducted with a longer-than-baseline preceding PR interval. In general, the shorter the RP interval (the interval from the preceding QRS [R] to the premature P wave [P]) the longer the PR interval (ie, the 2 intervals are inversely related). When the PR interval is prolonged or no QRS follows the P wave, confusion with pathologic AV block can occur.

Pathophysiology

A PAC occurs as a result of atrial depolarization from atrial muscle at a site other than the sinus node. This PAC can initiate paroxysmal SVT. But in and of themselves, PACs are usually benign, although they can create symptoms of palpitations.

Defining ECG Criteria

- The hallmark of a PAC is a P wave with the following characteristics:
  - Different morphology than a sinus-generated P wave.
  - Occurs prematurely, before the next sinus depolarization.
  - Is usually followed by a QRS complex that appears similar to others on the ECG (unless the PAC is aberrantly conducted to the ventricles: for example, with a bundle branch block).
  - If the PAC depolarizes the sinus node, it may reset the sinus cycle (eg, result in a brief pause before the next sinus P wave resumes).
- The PR interval of the PAC may be normal or prolonged compared with the patient's baseline PR intervals.
  - When the PR interval is prolonged, the P wave may be superimposed on the previous T wave.
  - A PAC may occasionally result in an unexpected pause in the ventricular rhythm when a very early P wave is completely blocked and no ventricular complex results.

Clinical Manifestations

Patients are seldom aware of any symptom other than "palpitations" or their heart "skipping a beat."

Common Etiologies

PACs may be secondary to endogenous factors such as fever, hypovolemia, or hyperthyroidism. More often they are secondary to exogenous factors such as medications and various stimulants, such as caffeine, ephedrine-based or phenylpropanolamine-based products, and methamphetamines.

Treatment

PACs require no specific treatment. Clinicians should take the same therapeutic approach as for sinus tachycardia (see "Sinus Tachycardia" later in this chapter), which is to identify the cause and treat the underlying condition.

Premature Ventricular Complex

A premature ventricular complex (PVC), also called a premature ventricular contraction, arises from a depolarization that occurs in either ventricle before the next expected conducted sinus impulse; hence the descriptor *premature* (Figure 60). Such impulses may originate from a focus of automaticity, a triggered impulse (unstable action potential), or from reentry. The following are general features and characteristics of PVCs:

- **QRS:** Abnormal in appearance, unusually broad, width 0.12 second or more.
- **Rhythm:** Regular until disrupted by the PVC, resulting in a regular rhythm that is occasionally irregular (regularly irregular).
- **P waves:** The underlying atrial (sinus) rhythm may be obscured by the components of the PVC (QRS deflections, ST segment, and T wave). Unless the PVC conducts retrograde back to the atria (ie, via the AV node or an accessory pathway, if present), it will not disturb the rate or regularity of the underlying sinus rhythm, which will often "march right through" the PVC(s).
  - Sinus P waves may be visible as a notching of the ST segment or T wave.
  - Retrograde P waves may be present if the PVC conducts back to the atria via the AV node. These P waves might be seen in the T wave of the PVC.

PVCs Wide and Bizarre

PVCs will alter the normal pattern of ventricular depolarization. Because the PVC bypasses the normal conduction pathways via the specialized His-Purkinje cells, conduction takes a different, slower course through the ventricles, resulting in a wide (0.12 second or more) and bizarre-looking QRS complex. Ventricular repolarization is also altered, often causing ST-segment deviation and T waves of different appearance than normal beats.

P Wave–PVC Relationships

Because PVCs occur in the ventricle, they occur independently of sinus node impulses. Accordingly, sinus node activity is not disturbed by events occurring below the level of the AV node (such as PVCs), allowing the underlying sinus rhythm to continue with regularity. Unless a retrograde impulse from the ventricles penetrates the AV node and conducts to the atria, sinus node impulses will continue completely undisturbed by ventricular events. That is, sinus P waves will continue to "march through" at their existing rate and regularity. Although there are other defining characteristics for PVCs, such as the presence or absence of a so-called compensatory pause or rules about the QRS configuration, there are enough exceptions to these "rules" that their use may not be useful for reliable diagnosis. Notably, aberrantly conducted supraventricular complexes, with a resulting wide QRS, can masquerade as PVCs. Rarely PVCs that originate in the fascicles of the His-Purkinje system may have a near-normal QRS width.

Compensatory Pause

The term *compensatory pause* is somewhat misleading because there is nothing truly "compensatory" about it. Rather, the pause is the result of the timing of the PVC, which prevents the next coincident sinus P wave from conducting to the ventricle and creates a pause between this nonconducted P wave and the next conducted sinus P wave. Whether there is such a pause at all after a PVC depends entirely upon its timing in relation to the underlying

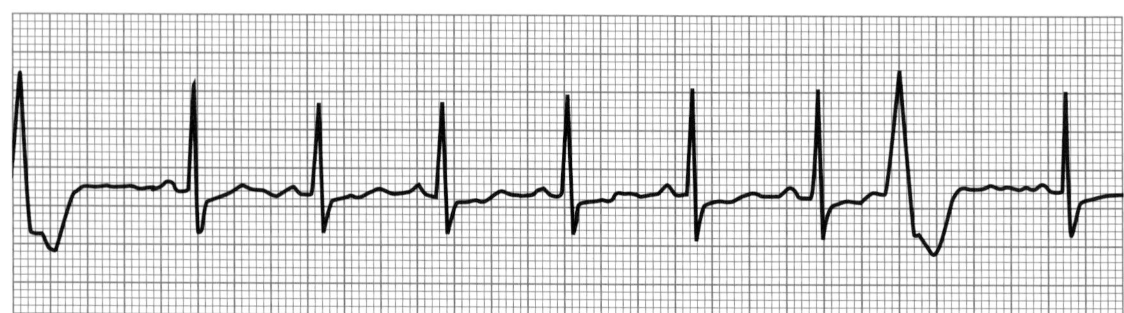

Figure 60. Premature ventricular complex (sometimes also called premature ventricular contraction).

sinus rhythm. For this reason, looking for a "compensatory pause" is not generally useful for diagnosis of PVCs.

Bigeminy and Trigeminy

Figure 61 displays a brief rhythm strip with several PVCs. Note that the morphology of each PVC is the same (uniform). These PVCs are sometimes called *unifocal*, a term that implies they originate from the identical location in the ventricle. Because every second ventricular complex in this strip is a PVC, this rhythm can be called *ventricular bigeminy.* If every third ventricular complex is a PVC, the term *ventricular trigeminy* is used; if every fourth ventricular complex is a PVC, *ventricular quadrigeminy* is present; and so on.

The Vulnerable Period and the R-on-T Phenomenon

The T wave represents the period when the ventricles are *repolarizing* in preparation for the next cardiac impulse. The peak of the T wave serves as a rough dividing point between the *absolute refractory period* of the cardiac cycle and the *relative refractory period*. The relative refractory period is known to be a particularly unstable and *vulnerable period* of ventricular repolarization.

Historically it was thought that if a PVC fell on the T wave during the relative refractory period of ventricular repolarization, it might precipitate VT or VF (Figure 62).[4] More recently it has been found that the timing of PVCs is of less importance, because even PVCs that occur at other times in the cardiac cycle can initiate spontaneous VT and VF[5] (Figure 63). Recent evidence suggests that conditions that cause a prolongation of the QT interval, such as drug overdoses and electrolyte abnormalities, can themselves trigger PVCs within the QT interval, which in turn, lead to unstable rhythms, VT, VF, and even death. For example, when these conditions are accompanied by bradycardia, an early PVC may be triggered by a long RR interval, resulting in a so-called "R-on-T," followed by polymorphic VT (torsades pointes).

Premature Junctional Complexes

Pathophysiology

A *premature junctional complex* (PJC) occurs when a premature impulse originates in the AV junction below the atria before the next expected sinus impulse (Figure 64). PJCs are the least common premature beats. From their site of origin between the atria and ventricles, conduction can occur both retrograde into the atria and antegrade into the ventricles. The retrograde P wave may occur after the QRS, be hidden within the QRS, or may precede the QRS if retrograde conduction to the atrium is more rapid than antegrade conduction to the ventricle. The retrograde P wave differs in appearance from the sinus P wave. If the retrograde P wave precedes the QRS, the PR interval is

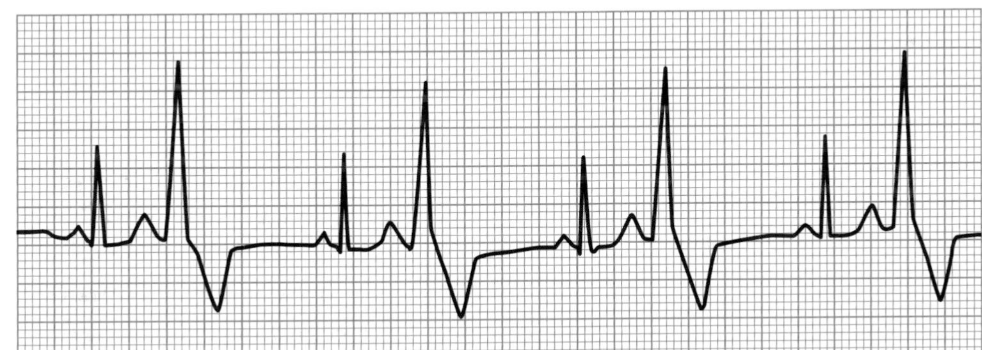

Figure 61. Ventricular bigeminy. Every second ventricular complex in this strip is a PVC.

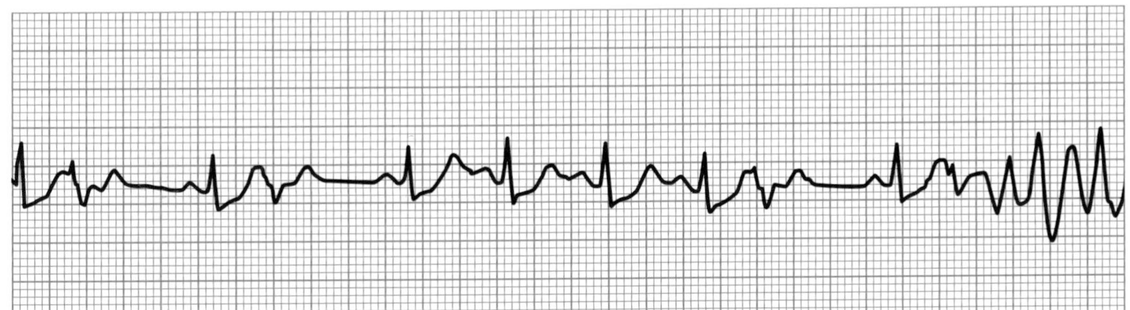

Figure 62. R-on-T phenomenon. Multiple PVCs are present. On the right a PVC is triggered by a long RR interval, falling on the T wave, followed by polymorphic VT and VF.

typically short (less than 0.12 second). The QRS is usually normal (narrow), unless a preexisting bundle branch block or distal conduction system disease is present and strained by the premature complex.

Defining ECG Criteria

- **Abnormal P waves:** A PJC often results in an abnormal P wave because of retrograde atrial depolarization (negative P wave in leads II, III, and aVF).
  - The retrograde P wave may precede, coincide with, or follow the QRS.
  - The relation of a retrograde P wave to the QRS complex depends on the relative conduction times from the site of origin of the premature impulse within the junction to the atria and ventricles.
  - An impulse arising in the higher portion of the AV junction or conducting more rapidly retrograde would result in a P wave that appears before or during the QRS complex, whereas one arising at a lower level or conducting more slowly retrograde would result in a P wave that appears within or after the QRS complex.
- **Normal QRS complexes:** The QRS complex is usually normal (narrow) because conduction from the AV junction to the ventricles usually occurs along normal conduction pathways.
  - The QRS complex can be wide if either a bundle branch block or aberrant conduction is present.
- **Variable rhythm:** A PJC may or may not "reset" the regularity of sinus rhythm, depending on whether retrograde conduction to the atrium occurs.

Narrow-Complex Supraventricular Tachycardias

Attempt to Establish a Specific Diagnosis

If the patient is stable, try to establish a definitive diagnosis of arrhythmia. The intent of this step is not to delay treatment but to give the patient a specific treatment for a specific diagnosis and to avoid therapy that may be ineffective or harmful.

Narrow-complex SVTs can be generally classified into 4 basic groups for purposes of initial assessment:

- Sinus tachycardia
- Reentry SVT
- Atrial fibrillation and atrial flutter
- Automatic atrial arrhythmias (not due to reentry), such as ectopic atrial tachycardia and multifocal atrial tachycardia

If the rhythm diagnosis is not immediately obvious, several features of the rhythm can be used to establish a specific diagnosis.

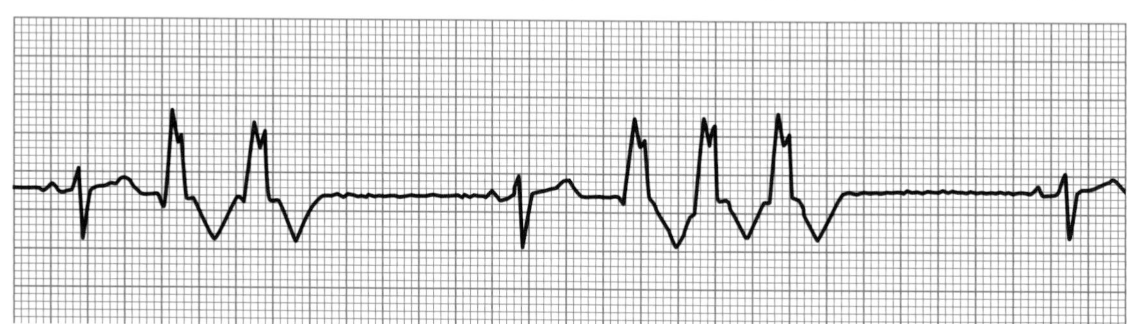

Figure 63. A brief run of VT occurs after a late-cycle PVC; the VT occurs well beyond the T wave.

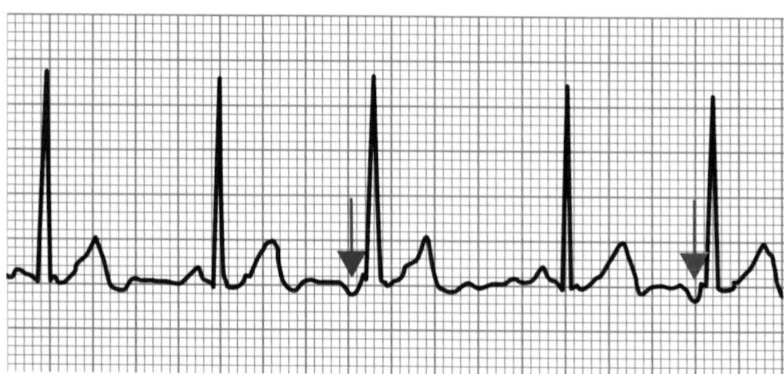

Figure 64. Premature junctional complexes. The third and fifth complexes occur early and are immediately preceded by inverted P waves (arrows). In lead II this pattern is consistent with retrograde atrial depolarization.

Assessment of Regularity, P Waves, and PR Intervals

In the case of narrow-complex QRS tachycardias (QRS less than 0.12, often 0.11 second or less), a rhythm diagnosis can be made by evaluation of the ECG for the features described below or by use of diagnostic maneuvers such as vagal stimulation or adenosine.

There are 3 important discriminating features of a narrow-complex tachycardia:

- Regularity of the rate
- Presence of P waves
- Appropriate PR interval preceding each QRS complex

A *regular* narrow-complex tachycardia is likely to be

- Sinus tachycardia or ectopic atrial tachycardia if each QRS is preceded by a P wave and a relatively normal PR interval
- Atrial flutter (with a fixed degree of AV block) if flutter waves precede each QRS
- Reentry SVT or (less commonly) junctional tachycardia if P waves are indiscernible before each QRS or the PR interval is short (less than 0.12 second)

An *irregular* narrow-complex tachycardia is most often due to

- Atrial fibrillation
- Atrial flutter (with variable AV block)
- Multifocal atrial tachycardia (not discussed in the ACLS Provider Course)

Assessment of Response to Vagal Stimulation and Adenosine

In addition to ECG characteristics, the clinical and rhythmic responses to vagal maneuvers or adenosine can help establish a specific diagnosis for a regular narrow-complex tachycardia. Vagal stimulation and adenosine induce a characteristic response for each of the different supraventricular arrhythmias:

- For PSVT the response can be abrupt termination of the tachycardia as a result of conduction block in the reentry circuit that creates it.
- For atrial flutter or atrial tachycardia the response can be a transient AV block with slowing of the ventricular rate but no alteration of the atrial arrhythmia. These responses may unmask the "flutter" waves of atrial flutter or the altered P waves of ectopic atrial tachycardia.
- For sinus tachycardia the response can be a transient slowing of the sinus mechanism, occasionally with transient AV block.
- For junctional tachycardia the response can be a temporary slowing of the rate.
- These diagnostic maneuvers are generally not necessary to determine the etiology of an irregularly irregular SVT, the cause of which (atrial flutter, atrial fibrillation, or MAT) can be discerned on the ECG.

Assessment of Wide Complexes

- A wide-complex tachycardia known to be of *supraventricular* origin (with aberrancy) is approached in the same manner as narrow-complex SVT.
- Wide-complex tachycardias known to be of *ventricular origin* are treated according to the Tachycardia With Pulses Algorithm. In most cases expert consultation is advised.
- Wide-complex tachycardias of *unknown etiology* require expert consultation to further assess diagnosis and appropriate intervention. Treating by trial and error with antiarrhythmic therapy could be dangerous because of the proarrhythmic effects of antiarrhythmics.

Sinus Tachycardia

Pathophysiology

Sinus tachycardia represents normal impulse formation and conduction at a rapid rate. It does not constitute a pathologic condition of and by itself. Sinus tachycardia is usually a physical sign of a problem or symptom. In rare cases inappropriate sinus tachycardia occurs in the absence of an obvious physiologic cause and in this context is regarded as a bona fide arrhythmia. The upper rate of sinus tachycardia is age-related (calculated as approximately 220/min, minus the patient's age in years) and may be useful in judging whether an apparent sinus tachycardia falls within the expected range for a patient's age.

Defining ECG Criteria

- **Rate:** By definition more than 100/min.
- **Rhythm:** Regular.
- **P waves:** Consistent with sinus node origin on the 12-lead ECG.
- **PR interval:** 0.12 to 0.20 second unless first-degree block is present.
- **QRS complex:** May be normal in width and configuration or abnormal if aberrant conduction to the ventricle is present (Figure 65).
- **Caution in diagnosis:** Clinicians will at times evaluate an unstable patient with an apparent rapid sinus tachycardia. The first question is whether the arrhythmia originates in the sinus node or represents an ectopic atrial tachycardia. Careful examination of the P-wave configuration on a 12-lead ECG can often answer this question. P waves that originate from the sinus node will have an appearance consistent with this origin (typically upright in leads I, II, III and aVF on the 12-lead ECG), whereas the P waves in ectopic atrial tachycardia will have a different appearance on the ECG.

Clinical Manifestations

Sinus tachycardia can cause a sensation of palpitations. In addition, the patient may develop symptoms secondary to the condition that is causing the tachycardia, such as fever, hypovolemia, or adrenergic stimulation.

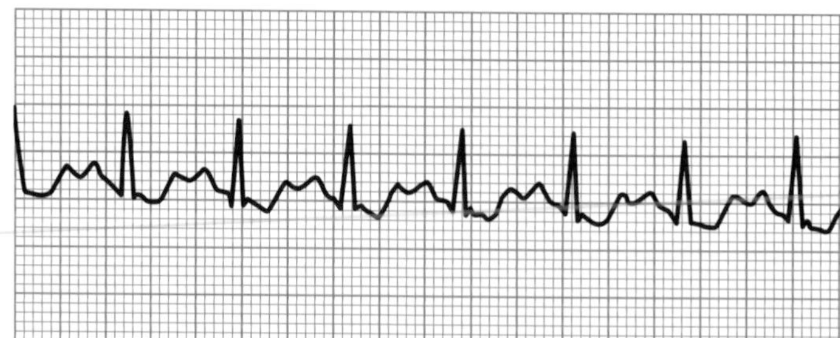

Figure 65. Sinus tachycardia. Note regular rhythm at the rate of 121/min. Each QRS is preceded by an upright P wave in lead II (also may be seen in leads I and aVF).

Common Etiologies

Some of the more common causes of sinus tachycardia are

- Normal exercise
- Fever
- Hypovolemia
- Adrenergic stimulation, anxiety
- Hyperthyroidism
- Anemia

Recommended Therapy

Treatment of sinus tachycardia involves several important principles:

- There is no specific treatment for sinus tachycardia. (*Note:* When sinus rhythm is inappropriately fast for the circumstances in which it occurs, this is called *inappropriate sinus tachycardia*. It may require treatment with β-blockers, calcium channel blockers, or elective radiofrequency catheter ablation.)
- Treat the cause of the sinus tachycardia rather than the tachycardia itself. When cardiac function is poor, cardiac output can depend on a rapid heart rate. In such compensatory tachycardias, stroke volume is limited, so "normalizing" the heart rate can be detrimental.
- Never attempt cardioversion or defibrillation for sinus tachycardia. The goal of electrical cardioversion is to produce sinus rhythm. A person who is already in sinus tachycardia cannot be helped by electrical therapy.

Reentry Supraventricular Tachycardia (Table 21)

Narrow-Complex Tachycardias: General Nomenclature Categories

The narrow-complex tachycardias bear a variety of rhythm labels based on anatomic site of origin, width of the QRS complex, characteristics of onset and termination, and mechanism of formation.[6,7]

- These tachycardias are called *narrow-complex tachycardias* because the QRS complexes are typically less than 0.12 second unless bundle branch block or aberrancy is present.
  - The rhythms are termed SVT because they originate in or above the level of the AV node. This term has displaced the now obsolete *paroxysmal atrial tachycardia (PAT)*. Applied to these arrhythmias, the term *paroxysmal (eg, PSVT)* refers to their *sudden onset, duration* of more than a few beats, and often equally sudden (within a single beat) *spontaneous termination* or abrupt interruption with treatment.
  - Some experts require documentation of the actual onset of the arrhythmia on an ECG monitor before applying the term *paroxysmal*.[8]
  - The most common narrow-complex tachycardia occurring in the paroxysmal manner described above involves reentry within the AV node and is more appropriately called AV nodal reentry tachycardia (AVNRT). PSVT may also result from a reentry circuit that includes the AV node and an accessory pathway (referred to as AV reentry tachycardia or AVRT). We now understand that both forms of PSVT originate in or above the AV node and require the AV node for initiation and maintenance. The majority of episodes of PSVT in adults are due to AV nodal reentry, in which the AV node provides both the antegrade and retrograde portions of the circuit (Figure 66).

The mechanism of reentry is similar in other cardiac tissues and involves these components:

- There are at least 2 conducting pathways between the site of origin of an impulse and its destination. In the case of the AV node (Figure 66) these are described as a fast and a slow conduction pathway.
- Each pathway has differing electrical properties. Typically, one pathway has a longer refractory period than the other, and one pathway has slower conduction properties than the other.
- An electrical impulse (often premature) that reaches the 2 pathways initiates the reentry process in the following manner:
  - The pathway with a longer refractory (recovery) period is initially unable to conduct the premature impulse in one direction (sometimes called one-way or unidirectional block) because it has not as yet completely recovered from having conducted the previous impulse.
  - The slow-conducting pathway permits passage of this impulse. This results in a transit time through it that is just long enough to allow the alternate pathway with the longer refractory period to recover.

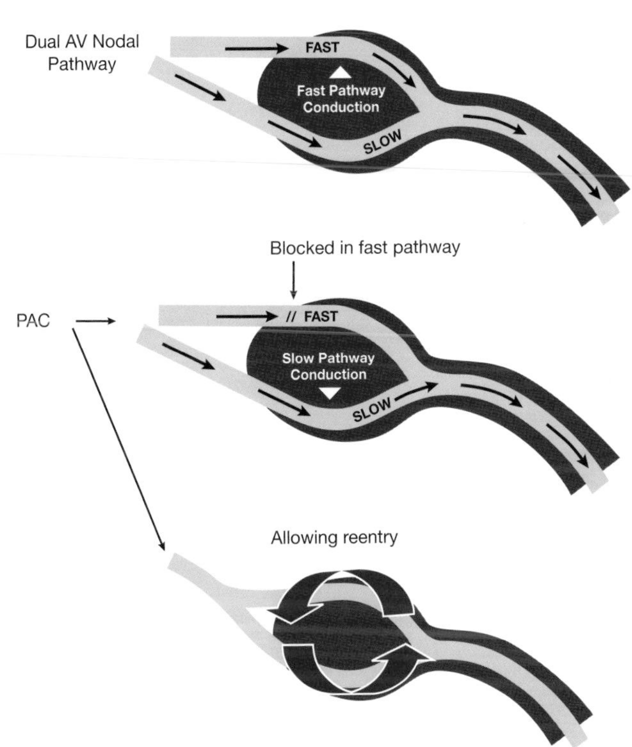

Figure 66. Basic components of reentry arrhythmias.

- The combination of these 2 pathways, one with a longer refractory period and one with slow conduction, allows just the right timing for the impulse to perpetually "spin" in the circuit without encountering refractory tissue. Each spin creates an impulse, and repetitive spins create a tachycardia. In the case that this "spin" occurs within the AV node, the resulting rhythm is AVRNT, typically a regular narrow-complex tachycardia.

Nomenclature Based on Tachycardia Mechanism

Most supraventricular, narrow-complex, AV tachycardias originate from 1 of 2 mechanisms:

- **Automaticity** tachycardias (due to enhanced automaticity). Major examples of this mechanism are sinus, ectopic atrial, junctional, and multifocal (ectopic) atrial tachycardias. These arrhythmias are not responsive to direct current (DC) cardioversion.
- **Reentry** tachycardias (due to reentry mechanism). Major examples of rhythms resulting from this mechanism include atrial fibrillation, atrial flutter, and PSVT. These tachycardias are typically responsive to DC cardioversion. There are 3 common anatomic sites for reentry (Figure 67):
  - The active reentry site is *atrial,* ie, occurring only in the atria. This commonly results in atrial fibrillation and atrial flutter.
  - The active reentry site involves the AV node, resulting in AVNRT.
  - The active reentry site involves both the AV node and an *accessory* or *bypass conduction* pathway, resulting in AVRT.

PSVT

This subgroup of reentry arrhythmias, due to either AVNRT or AVRT, is characterized by abrupt onset and termination and a regular rate that exceeds the typical upper limits of sinus tachycardia at rest (usually more than 150/min) and, in the case of an AVNRT, often presents without readily identifiable P waves on the ECG.

When PSVT is mediated by an accessory pathway, the AV node most commonly serves as the antegrade portion of the reentry circuit, and the accessory pathway serves as the retrograde portion (orthodromic reciprocating tachycardia). Conversely, when a reentry circuit circulates in the opposite direction (conducting antegrade down the accessory pathway and retrograde back to the atria via the AV node), a wide-complex (preexcited) PSVT (antidromic reciprocating tachycardia) results (Figure 68).

Recommended Therapy

Vagal maneuvers are the initial indicated intervention for PSVT. Adenosine markedly decreases both antegrade and retrograde conduction through the AV node, interrupting any reentrant circuit that depends on conduction through the AV node for its perpetuation, including AVNRT and AVRT.

Valsalva Maneuver

The Valsalva maneuver was named for Antonio Maria Valsalva (1666-1723), an Italian anatomist, surgeon, and pathologist who first described the procedure. The maneuver involves instructing a patient to exhale forcefully against a closed glottis so no air can escape.

Anatomy and Physiology

- The Valsalva maneuver produces an abrupt increase in intra-abdominal and intrathoracic pressure. The most common way to perform the Valsalva maneuver is to have the patient strain against a closed glottis during a held breath.
- The response to the Valsalva maneuver is complex:
  - First, the maneuver increases arterial pressure.
  - Second, the arterial pressure stimulates local baroreceptors.
  - Baroceptor signals travel to the brain where they connect with the parasympathetic and vagal nerve centers.
  - This response enhances vagal nerve output.
  - Vagal activation causes a reduction in heart rate in patients in sinus rhythm and slows AV node conduction.
  - The heightened vagal tone may terminate reentrant rhythms or cause a brief AV block in automatic rhythms, which can aid in diagnosis.

AV Reentry Tachycardia

Connection between atria and ventricle

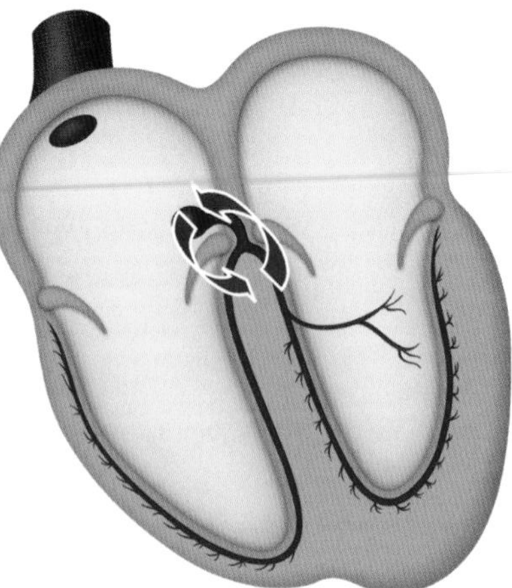

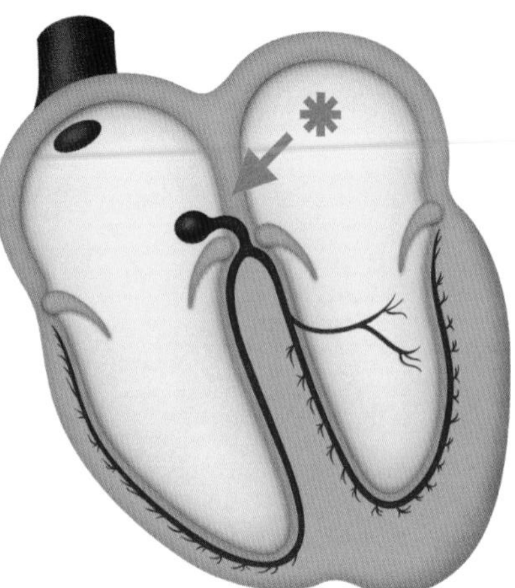

Figure 67. Example of 3 mechanisms for supraventricular arrhythmias. In AV reentry tachycardia there is an abnormal connection between the ventricles known as a bypass tract or accessory conduction pathway (eg, Wolff-Parkinson-White syndrome). In AV nodal reentry tachycardia there is a dual pathway within the AV node. In atrial tachycardia an automatic ectopic focus discharges.

AV Reentry Tachycardia

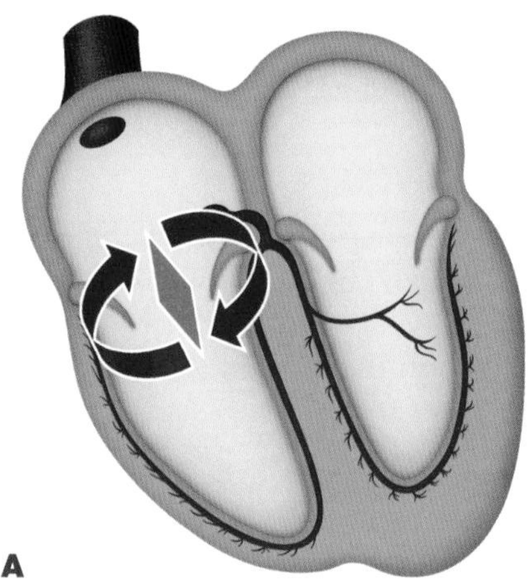

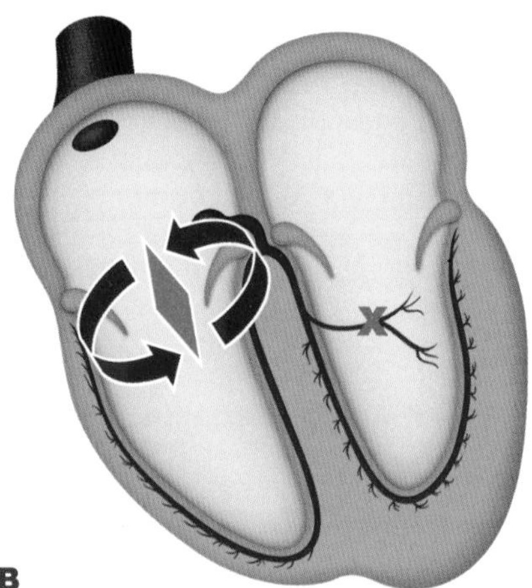

Figure 68. **A,** When PSVT is mediated by an accessory pathway, the AV node most commonly serves as the forward portion of the reentry circuit, and the accessory pathway serves as the retrograde portion. This is called orthodromic reciprocating tachycardia and results in a narrow QRS complex because the conduction pathway to the ventricles traverses the normal conduction system. **B,** When a reentry circuit circulates in the opposite direction (conducting antegrade down the accessory pathway and retrograde back to the atria via the AV node), a wide-complex (preexcited) PSVT (antidromic reciprocating tachycardia) results.

Table 21. Reentry Supraventricular Tachycardia

Reentry Supraventricular Tachycardia	
Pathophysiology	• **Reentry phenomenon:** Results from the presence of more than one conduction pathway (typically two) in tissue, each with differing electrical properties. With just the right timing, an impulse can perpetually "spin" in the circuit. If the "spin" occurs within the AV node, the resulting rhythm is AV nodal reentry tachycardia.
Defining Criteria and ECG Features **Key:** Regular, narrow-complex tachycardia without P waves, and sudden, *paroxysmal* onset or cessation, or both **Note:** To merit the diagnosis some experts require capture of the paroxysmal onset or cessation on a monitor strip	• **Rate:** exceeds upper limit of sinus tachycardia (>120 beats/min); seldom <150 beats/min; up to 250 beats/min • **Rhythm:** regular • **P waves:** seldom seen because rapid rate causes P wave loss in preceding T waves or because the origin is low in the atrium • **QRS complex:** narrow (<0.12 second usually)
Clinical Manifestations	• Palpitations felt by patient at the paroxysmal onset; becomes anxious, uncomfortable • Exercise tolerance low with very high rates • Symptoms of unstable tachycardia may occur
Common Etiologies	• Accessory conduction pathway in many PSVT patients • For such otherwise healthy people, many factors can provoke the paroxysm, such as caffeine, hypoxia, cigarettes, stress, anxiety, sleep deprivation, numerous medications • Also increased frequency of PSVT in unhealthy patients with CAD, COPD, CHF
Recommended Therapy If specific diagnosis unknown, attempt therapeutic/diagnostic maneuver with • Vagal stimulation • *Adenosine* . . . then	**Preserved heart function:** • AV nodal blockade – *β-Blocker* – *Calcium channel blocker* – *Digoxin* • DC cardioversion • Parenteral antiarrhythmics: – *Procainamide* – *Amiodarone* – *Sotalol* (not available in the United States) **Congestive heart failure:** • *DC cardioversion* • *Digoxin* • *Amiodarone*

Abbreviations: AV, atrioventricular; CAD, coronary artery disease; CHF, congestive heart failure; COPD, chronic obtrusive pulmonary disease; DC, direct current; PSVT, paroxysmal supraventricular tachycardia.

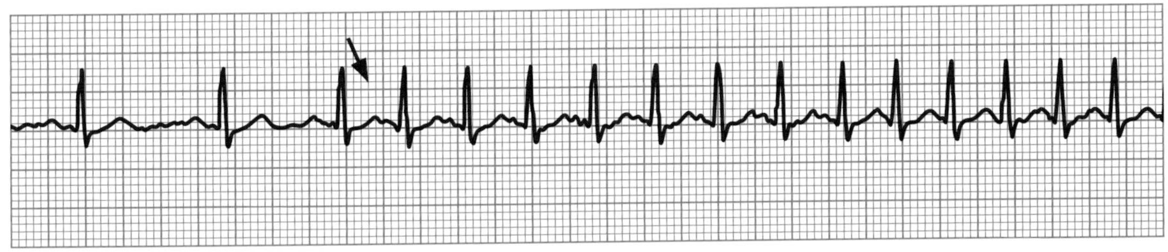

Sinus rhythm (3 complexes) with paroxysmal onset (arrow) of supraventricular tachycardia (PSVT)

- Variable success rates (from 6% to 18%) from vagal maneuvers have been reported in out-of-hospital settings and emergency departments.[1,9,10]
- Higher success rates have been achieved in electrophysiology laboratories for termination of induced PSVT.[11]
- Additional factors may decrease the conversion success rate of vagal maneuvers in PSVT.
  - The maneuver requires patient understanding and cooperation.
  - The response can be blunted in patients with common pathologic conditions (eg, CHF) and in patients with heightened adrenergic tone, including those receiving catecholamine infusions.
- The Valsalva maneuver can be used in conjunction with carotid sinus massage (see next section). These 2 vagal stimulation techniques are equally effective in terminating spontaneous SVT; one method may succeed after the alternative intervention fails.

Technique of Valsalva Maneuver

1. Position the patient in an erect or semierect position. As a precaution, consider placement of an IV catheter or have transcutaneous pacing readily available in case the maneuver provokes a symptomatic bradycardia requiring intervention.
   a. Explain the procedure to the patient.
   b. Instruct the patient to cough on command. The "vagolytic" effect of coughing can be helpful in terminating protracted bradyarrhythmias provoked by the Valsalva maneuver or carotid sinus massage.
2. Record baseline blood pressure and pulse, and obtain a rhythm strip.
3. Ask the patient to take a deep breath, hold it, and then bear down and strain. Alternatively the clinician can push firmly with 1 hand in the center of the patient's abdomen (short of causing discomfort) and then ask the patient to try to "push" the hand away with abdominal pressure.
4. The patient should hold the breath and strain for 15 to 30 seconds. If equipment is available, the patient can breathe into a small tube or syringe connected to a mercury manometer or spirometer. Have the patient maintain a pressure of 30 mm Hg for 15 to 30 seconds.
5. Record blood pressure and heart rate after 1 minute.
6. Obtain a rhythm strip after performing the maneuver. Obtain a 12-lead ECG if the rhythm converts.
7. Perform carotid sinus massage if the Valsalva maneuver fails.

Carotid Sinus Massage

Anatomy and Physiology

- The carotid sinus is a localized dilation in the common carotid artery at the branch point of the internal and external carotid arteries.
- The carotid sinus contains baroceptors that respond to pressure changes in the carotid artery.
- The carotid sinus contains nerve endings from the glossopharyngeal nerve; when stimulated, they convey impulses to the heart and vasomotor control centers in the brainstem.
  - These control centers, in turn, stimulate the efferent vagus nerve.
  - This increase in vagal tone inhibits impulse formation in the sinus node and slow conduction in the AV node.
  - Inhibition of the sinus node produces a marked slowing of heart rate and may transiently create AV nodal block.

This classic feedback loop is called the *vasovagal reflex* because it starts in the carotid artery (*vaso*), loops up to the brain and central nervous system, and then moves down the fibers of the vagus nerve (*vagal*) to the sinus and AV nodes. Of note, in addition to its nodal effects, vagal stimulation can cause peripheral vasodilation. Therefore hypotension can result from either the resulting slowing of heart rate, vasodilation, or both. For example, "vasovagal syncope" is a loss of consciousness (faint) provoked by vagal stimulation that is mediated by these mechanisms.

Preparation

Perform carotid sinus massage (CSM) after careful preparation. CSM should be limited to younger patients (those without suspected vascular disease, history of stroke, or transient ischemic attack) because of the potential risk of dislodging carotid artery plaque during massage.

1. Preparation for procedure:
   a. Functional IV line is in place.
   b. Atropine is available.
   c. ECG monitor accurately displays the rhythm.
   d. ECG is monitored continuously.
2. Obtain patient history. Exclude patients with a history of stroke or transient cerebral ischemia, recent myocardial infarction, or life-threatening ventricular arrhythmias. It may also be prudent to exclude elderly patients even in the absence of such a history because of the greater prevalence of vascular disease with increasing age.
3. Perform a physical examination. *Exclude patients with carotid bruits or history of carotid surgery*. As a precaution, consider placement of an IV catheter or have transcutaneous pacing readily available in case CSM provokes a bradycardia requiring intervention.

4. Explain the procedure to the patient.

Technique of Carotid Sinus Massage

Carotid sinus message is preferentially performed on the right carotid sinus principally as a safety precaution. An embolic event that might inadvertently result from CSM on the right side would affect the nondominant right cerebral hemisphere in most right-handed individuals, and potentially be less debilitating than might a dominant (left) hemispheric stroke resulting from left CSM.

1. Turn the patient's head to the left.
2. Continuously monitor cardiac rhythm (ideally, record on paper during the CSM maneuver).
3. Locate the right carotid sinus by palpating the carotid pulse immediately below the angle of the mandible and above the sternocleidomastoid muscle.
4. Using 2 fingers of the right hand, press down with some force and begin a firm, up-and-down massage for 5 to 10 seconds.
5. Massage the carotid sinus firmly in a longitudinal manner with posteromedial pressure, compressing the carotid sinus between your fingers and the cervical spine.
6. Repeat this massage 2 to 3 times, pausing 5 to 10 seconds between each attempt.
7. Monitor blood pressure and rhythm carefully; record a rhythm strip before and after CSM.
8. If unsuccessful, move to the opposite side (eg, the left carotid artery bifurcation near the angle of the jaw) once it is confirmed that vital signs are back at baseline levels.
9. Repeat CSM in the same manner as previously described.
10. It may take time and repetition before you can conclude that CSM has no effect. However, if a few attempts at CSM are unsuccessful in terminating tachyarrhythmia, move on to other therapies.
11. Never attempt simultaneous bilateral massage. This technique can compress the arteries and reduce blood flow to the brain
12. If CSM is successful, obtain a 12-lead ECG after conversion.
13. If CSM is ineffective, consider combining it with another vagal maneuver, such as the Valsalva maneuver.

Possible Complications

Numerous complications of CSM have been reported, but the incidence of side effects and complications is low when close attention is given to exclusion criteria and the technique is performed carefully (0.28% to 0.45% of patients, 0.7% to 0.17% of CSM episodes) even in older patients.[12-14]

Reported complications include the following:

- Cerebral emboli
- Stroke (embolic and occlusive)
- Syncope
- Sinus arrest
- Asystole
- Increased degree of AV block and paradoxical tachyarrhythmias in digoxin-toxic states

When CSM is properly performed in carefully selected patients (excluding those with known potential for complications), complications involving the central nervous system are rare (less than 1%). Complications are almost always transient, resolving in 24 hours. In rare cases CSM has induced VT.[15] Thus as with any rhythm-focused procedure, it is prudent to anticipate potential complications and have treatment in readiness (eg, establishing prior vascular access).

Adenosine

If reentry SVT does not respond to vagal maneuvers, adenosine can be given as a rapid 6-mg IV push over 1 to 3 seconds through a large (eg, antecubital) vein, followed by a 20-mL saline flush. This treatment achieves initially high levels of adenosine in the heart.[16,17] If the arrhythmia does not convert within 1 to 2 minutes, a 12-mg bolus can be given. This second dose can be followed by another 12-mg bolus if the arrhythmia again fails to convert within 1 to 2 minutes. **Adenosine should not be used for irregularly irregular tachyarrhythmias, especially when the QRS complex is widened.** Because of the possibility of initiating atrial fibrillation with very rapid ventricular rates in a patient with known preexcitation WPW, a defibrillator should be available when adenosine is administered to any patient in whom

Critical Concept

Right vs Left Carotid Sinus Massage

- Right (as opposed to left) carotid artery massage is preferred as the initial approach in a right-handed person (and conversely the left carotid artery in a left-handed person).
- This is because if CSM were to dislodge a plaque, resulting in stroke, the stroke would affect movement on the nondominant side of the body. The effects from such an untoward event would likely be less devastating than were the dominant side of the brain to be affected.

WPW is a consideration. Several trials have demonstrated that adenosine is safe and effective in terminating reentry SVT.[18-22] Although higher doses of adenosine are occasionally used (eg, 18 mg), in general if the initial and subsequent recommended doses are ineffective, further diagnosis and treatment require expert consultation.

Pharmacology

Although adenosine can be thought of as a potent "pharmacologic vagal maneuver," the drug has many cellular signaling effects. Adenosine acts on cardiac adenosine receptors to diminish automaticity and slow conduction in nodal tissue by opening inward potassium channels. These electrophysiologic effects can effectively terminate many episodes of PSVT. In the largest series reported in the literature, cumulative response rates after 6 mg of adenosine, followed by 12 mg if necessary, were 57% and 93%, respectively.[18] The effectiveness of adenosine is well established. It now stands as the drug of choice to terminate PSVT with AV nodal involvement. Adenosine has a very short half-life (10 to 30 seconds).

Diagnostic Value

In patients with atrial fibrillation or flutter without preexcitation, adenosine can provide valuable diagnostic information when it slows conduction through the AV node,[6,17] thereby revealing the underlying atrial rhythm. This is generally unnecessary when the ventricular rhythm is irregularly irregular, given the high likelihood of its representing atrial fibrillation. However, often atrial flutter can result in a regular SVT. In this instance, the atrial flutter waves are unaffected by adenosine, while the slowed conduction through the AV node increases the interval between successive QRS complexes, which affords a better display of atrial activity on the ECG monitor. As with vagal maneuvers and carotid sinus massage, administration of adenosine must be performed under continuous ECG monitoring, ideally with a paper recording the actual time of events and drug administration.

Caution

Adenosine is safe and effective for arrhythmias that might occur during pregnancy; effectively terminating reentry SVT with minimal effect on the fetus.[23-25] However, adenosine does have several important drug-drug interactions that alter its acute potency. Larger doses may be required for patients with a significant blood level of theophylline, caffeine, or theobromine, which antagonize the effects of adenosine. Conversely, the initial dose should be reduced to 3 mg in patients taking dipyridamole or carbamazepine, either of which enhances the effect of adenosine, or if given by central venous access (achieving higher acute concentrations in the heart than when given peripherally).[26] In such cases the bradycardia effects of adenosine may be more profound than expected, and prior precautions should be taken for rhythm support, including transcutaneous pacing. For different reasons, patients taking verapamil, diltiazem, or β-blockers may also require dose reduction because of the additive bradycardic effect these drugs can have on rhythm. Side effects with adenosine are common; transient flushing, dyspnea, and chest pain are the most frequently observed.[27] Because of risk of bronchoconstriction, adenosine should be avoided in patients with asthma as well as in patients with transplanted hearts, who might be hypersensitive to adenosine, and in whom such treatment can result in profound and protracted asystole.[28,29]

Calcium Channel Blockers and β-Blockers

If adenosine or vagal maneuvers fail to convert PSVT (Figure 58, Number 7), PSVT recurs after such treatment, or these treatments disclose a different form of SVT (such as atrial fibrillation or flutter), it is reasonable to use longer-acting AV nodal blocking agents, such as the non-dihydropyridine calcium channel blockers (verapamil and diltiazem) (Class IIa, LOE B) or β-blockers (Class IIa, LOE C). A wide variety of drugs are available for treatment and are listed in Table 22.

Pharmacology

Verapamil and diltiazem act primarily on nodal tissue either to terminate the reentry PSVTs that depend on conduction through the AV node or to slow the ventricular response to other SVTs by slowing conduction through the AV node. The alternate mechanism of action and longer duration of these drugs than adenosine may result in more sustained termination of PSVT or afford more sustained rate control of atrial arrhythmias (such as atrial fibrillation or flutter). A number of studies have established the effectiveness of verapamil and diltiazem in converting PSVT to normal sinus rhythm.[30]

β-Blockers (which include metoprolol, atenolol, propranolol, esmolol, and labetolol) exert their effect by antagonizing sympathetic tone in nodal tissue, resulting in slowing of conduction. Like calcium channel blockers, they also have negative inotropic effects and further reduce cardiac output in patients with heart failure.

Caution

Verapamil and diltiazem should be given *only* to patients with narrow-complex reentry SVT or arrhythmias known with certainty to be of supraventricular origin. Verapamil should not be given to patients with wide-complex tachycardias. It should not be given to patients with impaired ventricular function or heart failure.

β-Blockers should be used with caution in patients with obstructive pulmonary disease or congestive heart failure. Side effects of β-blockers can include bradycardias, AV conduction delays, and hypotension.

- Caution is advised when encountering preexcited atrial fibrillation or flutter that conducts to the ventricles via both the AV node and an accessory pathway. Treatment with an AV nodal blocking agent (including adenosine, calcium blockers, β-blockers, or digoxin) is unlikely to slow the ventricular rate and in some instances may accelerate the ventricular response. Expert consultation is advised before deploying these drugs in such patients.
- Caution is also advised to avoid giving AV nodal blocking agents that have a longer duration of action in combination. For example, both calcium channel and β-blockers have long half-lives; profound bradycardia can develop if they are given serially.

Table 22. **Intravenous Drugs Used for Tachycardia**

Drug	Characteristics	Indication(s)	Dosing	Side Effects	Precautions or Special Considerations
Intravenous Drugs Used to Treat Supraventricular Tachyarrhythmias					
Adenosine	Endogenous purine nucleoside; briefly depresses sinus node rate and AV node conduction; vasodilator	• Stable, narrow-complex regular tachycardias • Unstable narrow-complex regular tachycardias while preparations are made for electrical cardioversion • Stable, regular, monomorphic, wide-complex tachycardia as a therapeutic and diagnostic maneuver	6 mg IV as a rapid IV push followed by a 20 mL saline flush; repeat if required as 12 mg IV push	Hypotension, bronchospasm, chest discomfort	Contraindicated in patients with asthma; may precipitate atrial fibrillation, which may become very rapid in patients with unsuspected WPW; thus a defibrillator should be readily available. Reduce dose in patients taking dipyridamole or carbamazepine, and when administered via a central vein. Avoid use in post–cardiac transplant patients.
Diltiazem, Verapamil	Nondihydropyridine calcium channel blockers; slow AV node conduction and increase AV node refractoriness; vasodilators, negative inotropes	• Stable, narrow-complex tachycardias if rhythm remains uncontrolled or unconverted by adenosine or vagal maneuvers or if SVT is recurrent • Control ventricular rate in patients with atrial fibrillation or atrial flutter	**Diltiazem:** Initial dose 15 to 20 mg (0.25 mg/kg) IV over 2 minutes; additional 20 to 25 mg (0.35 mg/kg) IV in 15 minutes if needed; 5 to 15 mg/h IV maintenance infusion (titrated to atrial fibrillation heart rate if given for rate control) **Verapamil:** Initial dose 2.5 to 5 mg IV given over 2 minutes; may repeat as 5 to 10 mg every 15 to 30 minutes to total dose of 20 to 30 mg	Hypotension, bradycardia, precipitation of heart failure	Should only be given to patients with narrow-complex tachycardias (regular or irregular). Avoid in patients with heart failure and preexcited arial fibrillation or flutter or rhythms consistent with VT.

(continued)

(continued)

Drug	Characteristics	Indication(s)	Dosing	Side Effects	Precautions or Special Considerations
Atenolol, Esmolol, Metoprolol, Propranolol	β-Blockers; reduce effects of circulating catecholamines; reduce heart rate, AV node conduction and blood pressure; negative inotropes	• Stable, narrow-complex tachycardias if rhythm remains uncontrolled or unconverted by adenosine or vagal maneuvers, or if SVT is recurrent • Control ventricular rate in patients with atrial fibrillation or atrial flutter • Certain forms of polymorphic VT (associated with acute ischemia, familial LQTS, catecholaminergic)	**Atenolol (β_1 specific blocker):** 5 mg IV over 5 minutes; repeat 5 mg in 10 minutes if arrhythmia persists or recurs **Esmolol (β_1 specific blocker with 2- to 9-minute half-life):** IV loading dose 500 mcg/kg (0.5 mg/kg) over 1 minute, followed by an infusion of 50 mcg/kg per minute (0.05 mg/kg per minute); if response is inadequate, infuse second loading bolus of 0.5 mg/kg over 1 minute and increase maintenance infusion to 100 mcg/kg (0.1 mg/kg) per minute; increment; increase in this manner if required to maximum infusion rate of 300 mcg/kg (0.3 mg/kg) per minute **Metoprolol (β_1 specific blocker):** 5 mg over 1 to 2 minutes repeated as required every 5 minutes to maximum dose of 15 mg **Propranolol (nonselective β-blocker)**: 0.5 to 1 mg over 1minute, repeated up to a total dose of 0.1 mg/kg if required	Hypotension, bradycardia, precipitation of heart failure	Avoid in patients with asthma, obstructive airway disease, decompensated heart failure and pre-excited atrial fibrillation or flutter
Procainamide	Sodium and potassium channel blocker	• Preexcited atrial fibrillation	20 to 50 mg/min until arrhythmia suppressed, hypotension ensues, or QRS prolonged by 50%, or total cumulative dose of 17 mg/kg; or 100 mg every 5 minutes until arrhythmia is controlled or other conditions described above are met	Bradycardia, hypotension, torsades de pointes	Avoid in patients with QT prolongation and CHF. Avoid in patients who have been in atrial fibrillation or atrial flutter >48 hours, because of increased risk of stroke should procainamide terminate the arrhythmia.
Amiodarone	Multichannel blocker (sodium, potassium, calcium channel, and noncompetitive α/β-blocker)	• Stable irregular narrow-complex tachycardia (atrial fibrillation) • Stable regular narrow-complex tachycardia • To control rapid ventricular rate due to accessory pathway conduction in preexcited atrial arrhythmias	150 mg given over 10 minutes and repeated if necessary, followed by a 1 mg/min infusion for 6 hours, followed by 0.5 mg/min. Total dose over 24 hours should not exceed 2.2 g.	Bradycardia, hypotension, phlebitis	Because of the possible conversion of atrial fibrillation or flutter to sinus rhythm, use cautiously in patients who may have been in atrial fibrillation or flutter for >48 hours and not suitably anticoagulated.
Digoxin	Cardiac glycoside with positive inotropic effects; slows AV node conduction by enhancing parasympathetic tone; slow onset of action	• Stable, narrow-complex regular tachycardias if rhythm remains uncontrolled or unconverted by adenosine or vagal maneuvers or if SVT is recurrent • Control ventricular rate in patients with atrial fibrillation or atrial flutter	8 to 12 mcg/kg total loading dose, half of which is administered initially over 5 minutes, and remaining portion as 25% fractions at 4- to 8-hour intervals	Bradycardia	Slow onset of action and relative low potency renders it less useful for treatment of acute arrhythmias

(continued)

(continued)

Drug	Characteristics	Indication(s)	Dosing	Side Effects	Precautions or Special Considerations
Intravenous Drugs Used to Treat Ventricular Tachyarrhythmias					
Procainamide	Sodium and potassium channel blocker	• Hemodynamically stable monomorphic VT	20 to 50 mg/min until arrhythmia suppressed, hypotension ensues, or QRS prolonged by 50%, or total cumulative dose of 17 mg/kg; or 100 mg every 5 minutes until arrhythmia is controlled or other conditions described above are met	Bradycardia, hypotension, torsades de pointes	Avoid in patients with QT prolongation and CHF
Amiodarone	Multichannel blocker (sodium, potassium, calcium channel, α- and noncompetitive β-blocker)	• Hemodynamically stable monomorphic VT • Polymorphic VT with normal QT interval	150 mg given over 10 minutes and repeated if necessary, followed by a 1 mg/min infusion for 6 hours, followed by 0.5 mg/min. Total dose over 24 hours should not exceed 2.2 g.	Bradycardia, hypotension, phlebitis	
Sotalol (not available as IV formulation in the US)	Potassium channel blocker and nonselective β-blocker	• Hemodynamically stable monomorphic VT	In clinical studies 1.5 mg/kg infused over 5 minutes; however, US package labeling recommends any dose of the drug should be infused slowly over a period of 5 hours	Bradycardia, hypotension, torsades de pointes	Avoid in patients with QT prolongation and CHF
Lidocaine	Relatively weak sodium channel blocker	• Hemodynamically stable monomorphic VT	Initial dose range from 1 to 1.5 mg/kg IV; repeated if required at 0.5 to 0.75 mg/kg IV every 5 to 10 minutes up to maximum cumulative dose of 3 mg/kg; 1 to 4 mg/min (30 to 50 mcg/kg per minute) maintenance infusion	Slurred speech, seizures, altered consciousness, bradycardia	
Magnesium	Cofactor in variety of cellular processes including control of sodium and potassium transport	• Polymorphic VT associated with QT prolongation (torsades de pointes)	1 to 2 g IV over 15 minutes	Hypotension, CNS toxicity, respiratory depression	Follow magnesium levels if frequent or prolonged dosing required, particularly in patients with impaired renal function.

Abbreviations: AV, atrioventricular; CHF, congestive heart failure; CNS, central nervous system; IV, intravenous; LQTS, long QT syndrome; SVT, supraventricular tachycardia; VT, ventricular tachycardia.

Atrial Fibrillation: Rate and Rhythm Control

The treatment approach for atrial fibrillation and atrial flutter includes the following steps, *listed in order of priority:*

1. Urgent treatment of unstable patients with synchronized cardioversion
2. Control of the ventricular rate (rate control)
3. Appropriate anticoagulation measures before and after cardioversion in stable patients with atrial fibrillation or flutter of longer than 48 hours' duration (rhythm control)

Electrical or pharmacologic conversion of the rhythm should not be attempted in patients with atrial fibrillation or flutter of more than 48 hours' duration who have not first been suitably anticoagulated, unless the patient is unstable or without prior expert consultation. (Expert consultation may recommend cardioversion of such patients if first heparinized and the procedure is guided by transesophageal echocardiography.)

Pathophysiology

Atrial fibrillation is the most common sustained cardiac rhythm disturbance. The basic mechanism is thought to result in part from multiple reentrant wavelets that circulate chaotically throughout the atria and drive the ventricular rate in a typically rapid and *irregularly irregular* fashion. The atrial electrical activity occurs at multiple sites of reentry within the atria, resulting in very rapid atrial depolarizations (approximately 300 to 400/min or higher) that are too disorganized to result in effective atrial contraction. As a result, there is no contraction of the atria as a whole.

- Because there is no uniform atrial depolarization, no distinct P waves are visible on the ECG.
- The chaotic electrical activity produces a baseline deflection on the ECG, referred to as fibrillation waves.

Fibrillation waves vary in size and shape, and they are irregularly irregular in rhythm.

- Transmission of these multiple atrial impulses through the AV node is variable (ie, some impulses are conducted into, but not through the AV node), which results in an irregularly irregular ventricular rate. Atrial fibrillation impulses that are conducted into, but not through, the AV node constitute a form of "concealed conduction." Such nonconducted impulses contribute to an overall *refractoriness* of the AV node, and contribute to the degree of ventricular rate control that is seen in atrial fibrillation, although this typically must be augmented by use of AV nodal–blocking drugs.
- The typical ventricular response rate in patients with atrial fibrillation averages 120 to 160/min or higher.

Defining ECG Criteria

- **Key:** The key feature of atrial fibrillation is the presence of irregularly irregular atrial and ventricular rhythms. The irregular variations in both atrial and ventricular rates are observed as virtually constant, rapid atrial activity without clearly organized P waves. These fibrillation waves of variable amplitude create an undulating baseline between successive irregularly interspersed R waves (Figure 69).
- **Rate:** The atrial rate is irregular and as a rule too rapid to be counted. The frequency of the atrial "fibrillation" impulses is 300 to 400/min or higher. The ventricular response to these impulses varies widely from beat to beat.
- **Rhythm:** Both the atrial and ventricular rhythms are irregular. The ubiquitous clinical expression is *irregularly irregular* (Figure 70).
- **P waves:** Organized P waves as such are not seen. The chaotic atrial fibrillation waves create an undulating baseline.
- **PR interval:** The absence of discernible P waves and the presence of an undulating baseline precludes measurement of a PR interval.
- **QRS complex:** The QRS complexes are normal (narrow, less than 0.12 second) in duration unless widened by conduction defects through the ventricles (*aberrant* conduction).

Clinical Manifestations

- Patients will often perceive or describe the irregular rhythm of atrial fibrillation as "palpitations." With coexisting disease and advancing age, patients may complain of lightheadedness, weakness, or presyncope. Exertional dyspnea may be a prominent feature.
- Atrial fibrillation may be asymptomatic in some patients.
- Atrial fibrillation is associated with thromboembolic events, and the first presentation of atrial fibrillation might be a stroke. This risk is enhanced by conversion to sinus rhythm (either electrically or pharmacologically) when the rhythm has been present for more than 48 hours, unless anticoagulation precautions are first initiated.
- **Ventricular rate and function:** The major signs and symptoms of atrial fibrillation are a function of the resulting ventricular rate, the effect on cardiac output, and the patient's underlying ventricular function. The ventricular rate is determined by the number of atrial fibrillation waves that pass through the AV node and stimulate a ventricular response:
  - If AV conduction allows numerous impulses through, a *rapid ventricular response* can occur.
  - This response can lead to a *symptomatic tachycardia* with serious signs and symptoms due to the tachycardia, such as hypotension, shortness of breath, angina, and even frank acute pulmonary edema. In general,

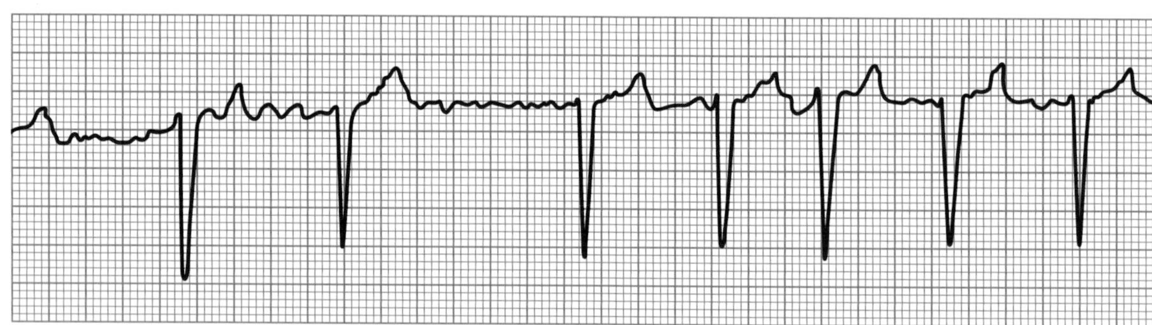

Figure 69. Atrial fibrillation with controlled ventricular response. Note irregular undulations of the baseline, which represent atrial electrical activity (fibrillation waves). The fibrillation waves vary in size and shape, and they are irregular in rhythm. Conduction through the AV node varies; hence the ventricular rhythm is irregular.

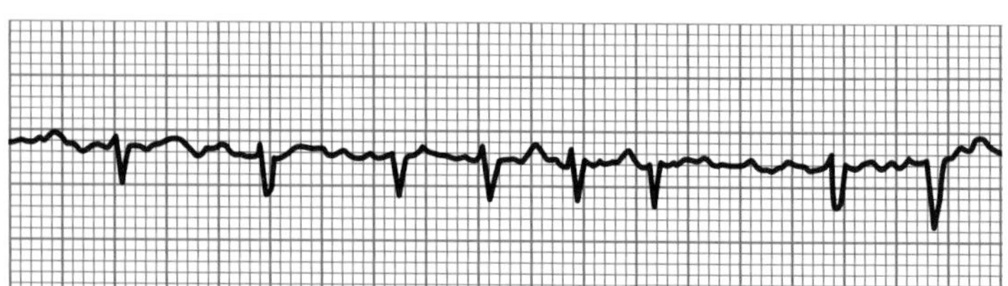

Figure 70. Atrial fibrillation with rapid ventricular response.

Critical Concept Caution—Drug Use in Atrial Fibrillation With Preexcitation	Treatment of preexcited atrial fibrillation with drugs that block conduction through the AV node (adenosine, calcium channel blockers, digoxin, or β-blockers) is contraindicated because such agents may paradoxically accelerate the ventricular rate.

rates exceeding 150/min are present when serious signs and symptoms are due to the ventricular rate unless another problem is present.

- **Loss of "atrial kick":** The absence of atrial contractions results in loss of the contribution of atrial contraction to ventricular filling. This "atrial kick" is responsible for approximately 25% of ventricular filling. Loss of the atrial kick can lead to a hemodynamically significant fall in stroke volume and cardiac output and a decrease in coronary perfusion.
- **Identification of coexistent Wolff-Parkinson-White (WPW) syndrome:** Atrial fibrillation or flutter occurring with preexcitation may be a medical emergency if rapid conduction occurs through an accessory pathway. Patients typically present with a very rapid, irregularly irregular wide-complex tachycardia that may be difficult to distinguish from VT unless there is a known history of WPW syndrome or there are discriminating features of the ECG (in the case of atrial fibrillation, varying degrees of QRS widening between successive irregularly irregular ventricular complexes).

Common Etiologies

- Although usually associated with some underlying form of heart disease, atrial fibrillation may be present in patients with no detectable heart disease (so-called lone atrial fibrillation).
- Atrial fibrillation can occur in these forms: paroxysmal (self-terminating), persistent (requiring treatment for termination), or permanent (unable to be terminated). When a patient has 2 or more episodes of atrial fibrillation, the arrhythmia is considered to be recurrent.
- Atrial fibrillation occurs most often in association with the following conditions:
  - Acute and chronic coronary syndromes, including coronary artery disease and congestive heart failure. Acute myocardial ischemia and infarction do not commonly cause atrial fibrillation, although atrial fibrillation frequently occurs in patients with chronic ischemic heart disease.
  - Structural heart disease, most commonly valvular, including disease at the mitral or tricuspid valve
  - Hyperthyroidism
  - Sick sinus syndrome
  - Acute pulmonary embolism
  - Hypoxia in general
  - Increased atrial pressure from multiple causes
  - Pericarditis
  - Drugs (alcohol, stimulants)

Reversible Causes

Reversible and underlying causes of atrial fibrillation should be identified and corrected if possible. The most commonly encountered reversible causes of atrial fibrillation are

- Hypoxemia
- Anemia
- Hypertension
- Congestive heart failure
- Mitral regurgitation
- Thyrotoxicosis
- Metabolic abnormalities (hypokalemia, hypomagnesemia)
- Drugs (alcohol, stimulants)

Recommended Therapy

Patients with atrial fibrillation who are stable require no additional therapy from an ACLS provider. Number 7 of the Tachycardia With a Pulse Algorithm (Figure 58) recommends seeking expert consultation. The algorithm recommends expert consultation because optimal treatment of atrial fibrillation with pharmacologic or drug therapy requires additional pharmacologic knowledge, appreciation of the proarrhythmic effects of agents, understanding of rate and rhythm-control strategies, and appreciation of ventricular function.

Selection of Therapy

Acute treatment of atrial fibrillation is directed by the answers to the following 4 questions:

1. Is this patient unstable and in need of urgent intervention?
2. Does this patient have significantly impaired ventricular function?
3. Is there evidence of preexcitation (WPW) syndrome?
4. Did this episode of atrial fibrillation or flutter start more than 48 hours ago?

Critical Concept Causes of Atrial Fibrillation	• Atrial fibrillation often occurs in the presence of structural heart disease. • Always search for a precipitating trigger or treatable comorbidity. For example, excess sympathetic tone may trigger the onset of atrial fibrillation in some patients, in whom treatment with β-blockers may be useful.

Table 23. Atrial Fibrillation/Atrial Flutter

Atrial Fibrillation/Atrial Flutter			
Pathophysiology	• Atrial impulses faster than SA node impulses • Atrial fibrillation → impulses take multiple, chaotic, random pathways through the atria • Atrial flutter → impulses take a circular course within the right atrium resulting in flutter waves • Mechanism of impulse formation: reentry		
Defining Criteria and ECG Features (Distinctions here between atrial fibrillation vs atrial flutter; all other characteristics are the same) **Atrial Fibrillation Key:** A classic clinical axiom: *"Irregularly irregular rhythm—with variation in both interval and amplitude from R wave to R wave—is always atrial fibrillation."* This one is dependable. **Atrial Flutter Key:** Flutter waves seen in classic "sawtooth" pattern		**Atrial Fibrillation**	**Atrial Flutter**
	Rate	• Wide-ranging ventricular response to atrial rate of 300-400 beats/min	• Atrial rate 220-350 beats/min • Ventricular response = a function of AV node block or conduction of atrial impulses • Ventricular response rarely >150-180 beats because of AV node conduction limits
	Rhythm	• Irregular (classic "irregularly irregular")	• Regular (unlike atrial fibrillation) • Ventricular rhythm often regular • Set ratio to atrial rhythm, eg, 2-to-1 or 3-to-1
	P waves	• Chaotic atrial fibrillatory waves only • Creates disturbed baseline	• No true P waves seen • Flutter waves in "sawtooth" pattern is classic
	PR	• Cannot be measured	
	QRS	• QRS may be normal (narrow) or wide if aberrancy is present	
Clinical Manifestations	• Signs and symptoms are function of the rate of ventricular response to atrial fibrillatory waves; *"atrial fibrillation with rapid ventricular response"* → dyspnea on exertion, shortness of breath, acute pulmonary edema • Loss of *"atrial kick"* may lead to drop in cardiac output and decreased coronary perfusion • Irregular rhythm often perceived as *"palpitations"* • Can be asymptomatic		
Common Etiologies	• Acute coronary syndromes; CAD; CHF • Disease at mitral or tricuspid valve • Hypoxia; acute pulmonary embolism • Drug-induced: *digoxin* or *quinidine* most common • Hyperthyroidism		

(continued)

(continued)

<table>
<tr><th colspan="4">Atrial Fibrillation/Atrial Flutter</th></tr>
<tr><td colspan="2">Recommended Therapy</td><td colspan="2">Control Rate</td></tr>
<tr><td>Evaluation Focus:</td><td>Treatment Focus:</td><td>Normal Heart</td><td>CHF</td></tr>
<tr><td rowspan="4">1. Patient clinically unstable?
2. Cardiac function impaired?
3. WPW present?
4. Duration ≤48 or >48 hours?</td><td rowspan="4">1. Treat unstable patients urgently
2. Control the rate
3. Convert the rhythm
4. Provide anticoagulation</td><td>• Diltiazem or another calcium channel blocker or metoprolol or another β-blocker</td><td>• Digoxin or amiodarone</td></tr>
<tr><td colspan="2">Convert Rhythm</td></tr>
<tr><td>Normal Heart</td><td>CHF</td></tr>
<tr><td>• If ≤48 hours:
– DC cardioversion or amiodarone or others
• If >48 hours:
– Anticoagulate × 3 wk, then
– DC cardioversion, then
– Anticoagulate × 4 wk
or
• IV heparin and TEE to rule out atrial clot, then
• DC cardioversion within 24 hours, then
• Anticoagulation × 4 more wk</td><td>• If ≤48 hours:
– DC cardioversion or amiodarone
• If >48 hours:
– Anticoagulate × 3 wk, then
– DC cardioversion, then
– Anticoagulate × 4 more wk</td></tr>
</table>

Abbreviations: AV, atrioventricular; CAD, coronary artery disease; CHF, congestive heart failure; DC, direct current; IV, intravenous; SA, sinoatrial; WPW, Wolff-Parkinson-White.

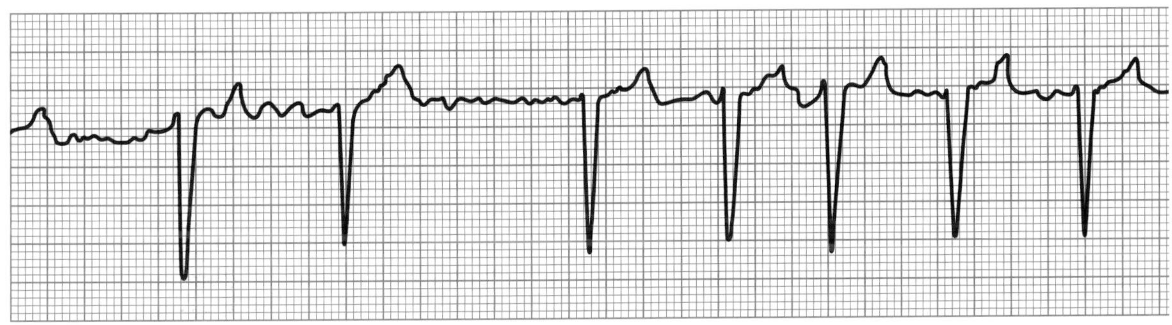

Atrial fibrillation

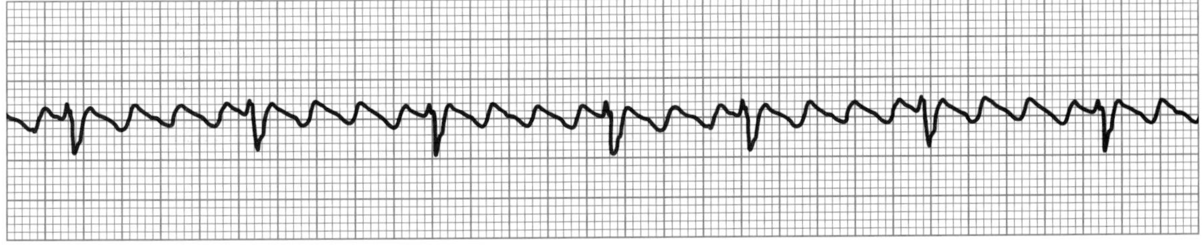

Atrial flutter

Clinically unstable patients require immediate cardioversion, whereas more stable patients may require ventricular rate control as directed by patient symptoms and hemodynamics. IV β-blockers and nondihydropyridine calcium channel blockers, such as diltiazem, are the drugs of choice for acute rate control in most individuals with atrial fibrillation and rapid ventricular response, in the absence of preexcitation (WPW syndrome). Drugs that block conduction through the AV node, such as adenosine, digoxin, calcium channel blockers, and β-blockers, pose a significant hazard for patients with WPW syndrome.

Finally, the 48-hour treatment window draws a sharp line between patients who need anticoagulation for several weeks before and after cardioversion or in whom cardioversion should be guided by findings on transesophageal echocardiography after acute heparinization, as compared with those who can safely undergo cardioversion without such precautions. A variety of agents have been shown to be effective in terminating atrial fibrillation (pharmacologic or chemical cardioversion), although success between them varies and not all are available as parenteral formulations. Expert consultation is recommended.

Atrial Flutter

Pathophysiology

- Unlike atrial fibrillation, which results from multiple reentry circuits, atrial flutter is typically the result of a single reentry circuit within the right atrium. As a result of the single reentry circuit, the impulse takes a circular course around the atria.
- Atrial flutter is characterized by flutter waves that occur rapidly with a characteristic "sawtooth" pattern. These "flutter waves" are best observed in leads II, III, and aVF.

Defining ECG Criteria

- **Key:** The key defining feature of atrial flutter is a classic "sawtooth" pattern visible in the flutter waves.
- **Atrial rate:** The flutter waves usually occur at a rate of 300/min. But the rate can range from 220 to 350/min.
- **Ventricular rate:** This rate is a function of how often the AV node conducts or blocks the atrial impulses. At an atrial rate of 300/min, the AV node succeeds in blocking about half the impulses, resulting in a 2:1 AV block and a regular VT of about 150/min (Figure 71). The ventricular rate may be faster or slower, and regular or irregular, depending on conduction through the AV node.
- **Rhythm:** The atrial rhythm is regular (unlike atrial fibrillation). The ventricular rhythm is regular if a constant degree of AV block is present, such as 2:1 or 4:1 (Figure 72). The ventricular rhythm can be grossly irregular if variable block is present (Figure 73).
- **P waves:** Flutter waves resemble a "sawtooth" or "picket fence" pattern. They are best seen in leads II, III, or aVF, as well as in V_1 and V_2. In the presence of 2:1 or 1:1 conduction ratios, it may be difficult to identify the flutter waves. In this instance carotid sinus massage (or IV adenosine used diagnostically) may produce a transient delay in AV nodal conduction, increasing the degree of AV block and slowing the ventricular response. This maneuver will "uncover" the flutter waves.
- **PR interval:** The PR interval is difficult to measure. It may be fixed or variable from beat-to-beat.
- **QRS complex:** The QRS complex appears normal with duration of less than 0.12 second unless aberrant ventricular conduction occurs.

Clinical Manifestations

The clinical manifestations of atrial flutter are similar to those of atrial fibrillation.

Common Etiologies

Atrial flutter typically occurs in association with organic heart disease. It is seen in association with mitral or tricuspid valvular heart disease, acute or chronic cor pulmonale, and coronary heart disease. Atrial flutter is rarely seen in the absence of organic heart disease.

Recommended Therapy

- Although acute atrial flutter differs somewhat in mechanism from atrial fibrillation, the initial management for rate control is the same.[31]
- Note that adenosine is not indicated for treatment of atrial fibrillation or flutter because of its ultrashort duration of action. But adenosine may be used diagnostically to induce brief AV block to search for atrial flutter waves. This step is seldom necessary and is not as helpful as ECG evaluation.

Polymorphic (Irregular) VT

Polymorphic (irregular) VT requires immediate defibrillation with the same strategy used for VF. Pharmacologic treatment to prevent recurrent polymorphic VT should be directed by the underlying cause of VT and the presence or absence of a long QT interval during sinus rhythm.

- If a long QT interval is observed during sinus rhythm (ie, the VT is torsades de pointes), the first step is to stop medications known to prolong the QT interval. Correct electrolyte imbalance and other acute precipitants (eg, drug overdose or poisoning: see Chapters 16-22 of this text). Polymorphic VT associated with familial long QT syndrome may be treated with IV magnesium, pacing, and/or β-blockers; isoproterenol should be avoided.
- Polymorphic VT associated with acquired long QT syndrome may be treated with IV magnesium. The addition of pacing or IV isoproterenol may be considered when polymorphic VT is accompanied by bradycardia or appears to be precipitated by pauses in rhythm.
- In the absence of a prolonged QT interval, the most common cause of polymorphic VT is myocardial ischemia. In this situation IV amiodarone and β-blockers may reduce the frequency of arrhythmia recurrence. Magnesium is unlikely to be effective in preventing polymorphic VT in these patients.

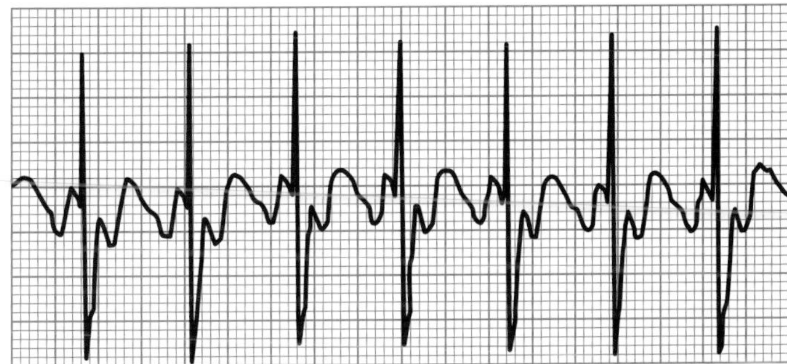

Figure 71. Atrial flutter. The atrial rate is 250/min, and the rhythm is regular. Every other flutter wave is conducted to ventricles (2:1 block), resulting in a regular ventricular rhythm at a rate of 125/min.

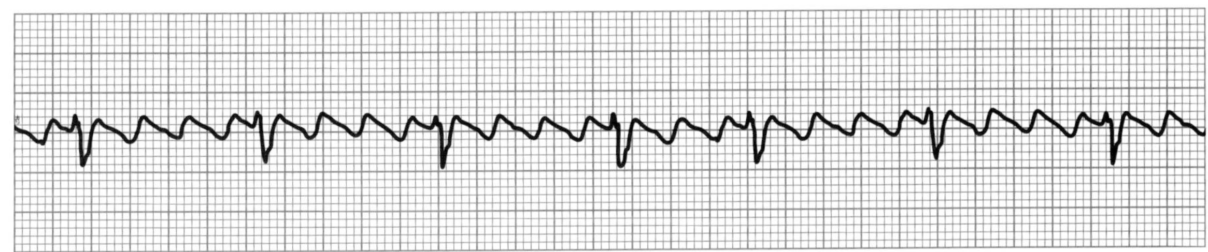

Figure 72. Atrial flutter with high-grade AV block. The atrial rhythm is regular (260/min), but only every fourth flutter wave is followed by a QRS (4:1 conduction).

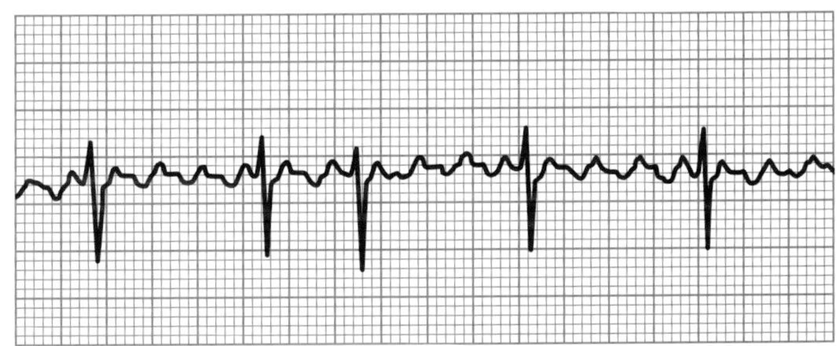

Figure 73. Atrial flutter with variable AV block. The atrial rhythm is regular, but variable AV block is present (2:1, 4:1 conduction ratios), which results in an irregular ventricular rhythm.

Stable Wide-Complex Tachycardia

A wide-complex tachycardia can be either ventricular or supraventricular in origin (Figure 74). The concept of aberrancy is not taught in the ACLS Provider Course. Basic providers should understand the following:

1. A wide-complex tachycardia is assumed to be ventricular until proven otherwise.
2. Unstable patients require immediate synchronized cardioversion if pulses are present.
3. Unstable pulseless patients are treated similarly to patients with VF.

Therapy for Regular Wide-Complex Tachycardias

In patients with stable undifferentiated wide-QRS complex tachycardia, a reasonable approach is to try to identify the wide-complex tachycardia as SVT or VT and treat based on the algorithm for that rhythm.

- If the etiology of the rhythm cannot be determined, the rate is regular, and the QRS is monomorphic, recent evidence suggests that IV adenosine is relatively safe for both treatment and diagnosis.[32] Typically, adenosine is administered in a manner similar to treatment of PSVT as discussed above.
- Verapamil is contraindicated for wide-complex tachycardias unless known to be of supraventricular origin. Profound hypotension was reported in patients known to have VT treated with verapamil.[33]

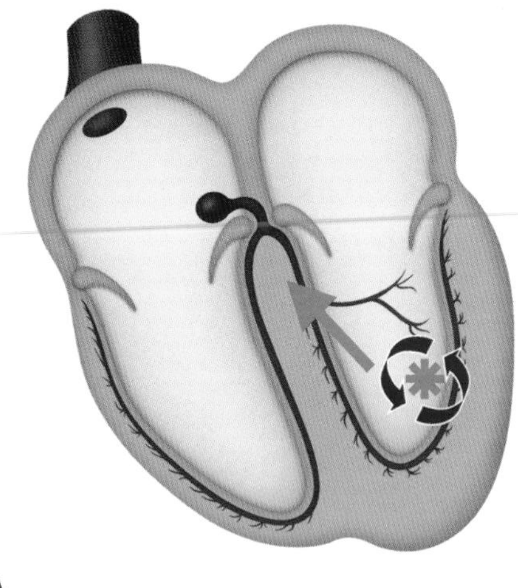

A

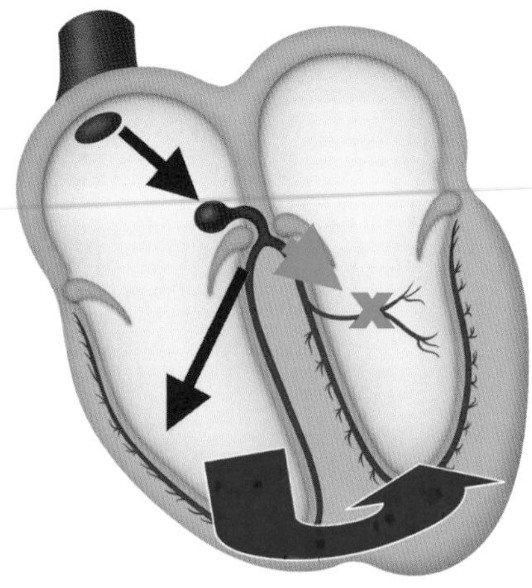

B

Figure 74. Wide-complex tachycardias can be ventricular or supraventricular (with aberrancy) in origin. **A,** An irritable ventricular focus excites the ventricular myocardium and spreads through the myocardium directly, a process that causes a wide QRS complex typical of a PVC. **B,** The electrical impulse normally originates in the sinus node and is conducted through the AV node but is blocked when it enters the left bundle after passing through the bundle of His. Conduction through the right bundle occurs normally, but the left ventricle is then activated by this pathway, slowing conduction through the myocardium. This results in a wide QRS complex called, in this case, a left bundle branch block pattern. If a rapid supraventricular tachycardia is conducted in this manner, it results in a wide-QRS (LBBB) tachycardia that can resemble VT.

Critical Concept Adenosine Therapy	Adenosine should **not** be given for unstable or for **irregular or polymorphic** wide-complex tachycardias, as it may cause degeneration of the arrhythmia to VF.

- For patients who are stable with likely VT, IV antiarrhythmic drugs or elective cardioversion is the preferred treatment strategy. If IV antiarrhythmics are administered, procainamide, amiodarone, or sotalol (not available in IV form in the United States) can be considered, and each is more effective than lidocaine in this setting. Procainamide and sotalol should be avoided in patients with prolonged QT.

FAQ

What are the initial assessments for the management of stable tachycardia?

Management of stable tachycardias can be challenging and the differential diagnosis uncertain. For the ACLS provider, initial assessment involves answering the following questions:

- Are symptoms present and due to the tachycardia?
- Is the patient stable or unstable?
- Is the QRS complex wide or narrow?
- Is the rhythm regular or irregular?

How do you treat a stable and symptomatic patient with a narrow-complex QRS?

- If the patient is stable and symptomatic with a narrow-complex QRS, you can use vagal maneuvers and adenosine to try to terminate the arrhythmia.
- If this strategy fails, expert consultation is advised.

How do you treat a patient with wide-complex tachycardia?

- If the wide-complex tachycardia is thought to be VT, search for triggers or exacerbating factors.
- If there is concern about deterioration of the VT or development of hemodynamic instability, you can give amiodarone 150 mg IV over 10 minutes (may be repeated once) while expert consultation is obtained.

References

1. Lim SH, Anantharaman V, Teo WS, Goh PP, Tan AT. Comparison of treatment of supraventricular tachycardia by Valsalva maneuver and carotid sinus massage. *Ann Emerg Med*. 1998;31:30-35.
2. Lown B. Electrical reversion of cardiac arrhythmias. *Br Heart J*. 1967;29:469-489.
3. Kerber RE, Kienzle MG, Olshansky B, Waldo AL, Wilber D, Carlson MD, Aschoff AM, Birger S, Fugatt L, Walsh S, et al. Ventricular tachycardia rate and morphology determine energy and current requirements for transthoracic cardioversion. *Circulation*. 1992;85:158-163.
4. El-Sherif N, Myerburg RJ, Scherlag BJ, Befeler B, Aranda JM, Castellanos A, Lazzara R. Electrocardiographic antecedents of primary ventricular fibrillation. Value of the R-on-T phenomenon in myocardial infarction. *Br Heart J*. 1976;38:415-422.
5. Kay GN, Plumb VJ, Arciniegas JG, Henthorn RW, Waldo AL. Torsade de pointes: the long-short initiating sequence and other clinical features: observations in 32 patients. *J Am Coll Cardiol*. 1983;2:806-817.

6. Ganz LI, Friedman PL. Supraventricular tachycardia. *N Engl J Med*. 1995;332:162-173.
7. Delacretaz E. Clinical practice. Supraventricular tachycardia. *N Engl J Med.* 2006;354:1039-1051.
8. Akhtar M, Jazayeri MR, Sra J, Blanck Z, Deshpande S, Dhala A. Atrioventricular nodal reentry. Clinical, electrophysiological, and therapeutic considerations. *Circulation*. 1993;88:282-295.
9. Ornato JP, Hallagan LF, Reese WA, Clark RF, Tayal VS, Garnett AR, Gonzalez ER. Treatment of paroxysmal supraventricular tachycardia in the emergency department by clinical decision analysis. *Am J Emerg Med*. 1988;6:555-560.
10. O'Toole KS, Heller MB, Menegazzi JJ, Paris PM. Intravenous verapamil in the prehospital treatment of paroxysmal supraventricular tachycardia. *Ann Emerg Med*. 1990;19:291-294.
11. Mehta D, Wafa S, Ward DE, Camm AJ. Relative efficacy of various physical manoeuvres in the termination of junctional tachycardia. *Lancet*. 1988;1:1181-1185.
12. Davies AJ, Kenny RA. Frequency of neurologic complications following carotid sinus massage. *Am J Cardiol*. 1998;81:1256-1257.
13. Munro NC, McIntosh S, Lawson J, Morley CA, Sutton R, Kenny RA. Incidence of complications after carotid sinus massage in older patients with syncope. *J Am Geriatr Soc*. 1994;42:1248-1251.
14. Richardson DA, Bexton R, Shaw FE, Steen N, Bond J, Kenny RA. Complications of carotid sinus massage—a prospective series of older patients. *Age Ageing*. 2000;29:413-417.
15. Schweitzer P, Teichholz LE. Carotid sinus massage. Its diagnostic and therapeutic value in arrhythmias. *Am J Med*. 1985;78:645-654.
16. DiMarco JP, Sellers TD, Berne RM, West GA, Belardinelli L. Adenosine: electrophysiologic effects and therapeutic use for terminating paroxysmal supraventricular tachycardia. *Circulation*. 1983;68:1254-1263.
17. diMarco JP, Sellers TD, Lerman BB, Greenberg ML, Berne RM, Belardinelli L. Diagnostic and therapeutic use of adenosine in patients with supraventricular tachyarrhythmias. *J Am Coll Cardiol*. 1985;6:417-425.
18. DiMarco JP, Miles W, Akhtar M, Milstein S, Sharma AD, Platia E, McGovern B, Scheinman MM, Govier WC. Adenosine for paroxysmal supraventricular tachycardia: dose ranging and comparison with verapamil. Assessment in placebo-controlled, multicenter trials. The Adenosine for PSVT Study Group. *Ann Intern Med*. 1990;113:104-110.
19. Brady WJ Jr, DeBehnke DJ, Wickman LL, Lindbeck G. Treatment of out-of-hospital supraventricular tachycardia: adenosine vs verapamil. *Acad Emerg Med*. 1996;3:574-585.
20. Furlong R, Gerhardt RT, Farber P, Schrank K, Willig R, Pittaluga J. Intravenous adenosine as first-line prehospital management of narrow-complex tachycardias by EMS personnel without direct physician control. *Am J Emerg Med*. 1995;13:383-388.
21. Madsen CD, Pointer JE, Lynch TG. A comparison of adenosine and verapamil for the treatment of supraventricular tachycardia in the prehospital setting. *Ann Emerg Med*. 1995;25:649-655.
22. Morrison LJ, Allan R, Vermeulen M, Dong SL, McCallum AL. Conversion rates for prehospital paroxysmal supraventricular tachycardia (PSVT) with the addition of adenosine: a before-and-after trial. *Prehosp Emerg Care*. 2001;5:353-359.
23. Harrison JK, Greenfield RA, Wharton JM. Acute termination of supraventricular tachycardia by adenosine during pregnancy. *Am Heart J*. 1992;123:1386-1388.
24. Podolsky SM, Varon J. Adenosine use during pregnancy. *Ann Emerg Med*. 1991;20:1027-1028.
25. Leffler S, Johnson DR. Adenosine use in pregnancy: lack of effect on fetal heart rate. *Am J Emerg Med*. 1992;10:548-549.
26. Chang M, Wrenn K. Adenosine dose should be less when administered through a central line. *J Emerg Med*. 2002;22:195-198.
27. Camm AJ, Garratt CJ. Adenosine and supraventricular tachycardia. *N Engl J Med*. 1991;325:1621-1629.
28. Ellenbogen KA, Thames MD, DiMarco JP, Sheehan H, Lerman BB. Electrophysiological effects of adenosine in the transplanted human heart. Evidence of supersensitivity. *Circulation*. 1990;81:821-828.
29. Anderson TJ, Ryan TJ Jr, Mudge GH, Selwyn AP, Ganz P, Yeung AC. Sinoatrial and atrioventricular block caused by intracoronary infusion of adenosine early after heart transplantation. *J Heart Lung Transplant*. 1993;12:522-524.
30. Lim SH, Anantharaman V, Teo WS. Slow-infusion of calcium channel blockers in the emergency management of supraventricular tachycardia. *Resuscitation*. 2002;52:167-174.
31. Waldo AL, Mackall JA, Biblo LA. Mechanisms and medical management of patients with atrial flutter. *Cardiol Clin*. 1997;15:661-676.
32. Staudinger T, Brugger S, Roggla M, Rintelen C, Atherton GL, Johnson JC, Frass M. [Comparison of the Combitube with the endotracheal tube in cardiopulmonary resuscitation in the prehospital phase]. *Wien Klin Wochenschr*. 1994;106:412-415.
33. Buxton AE, Marchlinski FE, Doherty JU, Flores B, Josephson ME. Hazards of intravenous verapamil for sustained ventricular tachycardia. *Am J Cardiol*. 1987;59:1107-1110.

Chapter 11

Cardiovascular: ACS—STEMI, NSTEMI, Unstable Angina, and Heart Failure and Shock Complicating ACS

This Chapter

- **Develop a Differential Diagnosis and Risk Assessment of Chest Discomfort**
- **Know Why STEMI Is a Rapid Reperfusion Emergency**
- **Know How to Identify Patients With STEMI on the Initial ECG**
- **List Initial Treatment Options and Indications for Heparin and Glycoprotein IIb/IIIa Inhibitor Therapy**
- **Weigh the Risks and Benefits of ACS Therapy**
- **Recognize Complications of STEMI**
- **Know the Initial Management of Shock and CHF**
- **Know the Difference Between Right vs Left Heart Failure and Shock**

Key Points

The initial 12-lead electrocardiogram (ECG) is used in all acute coronary syndrome (ACS) cases to classify patients into 1 of 3 ECG categories (Figure 75), each with different strategies of care and management needs. These 3 ECG categories are ST-segment elevation suggesting acute injury, ST-segment depression suggesting ischemia, and nondiagnostic or normal ECG. These are all outlined in the Acute Coronary Syndromes Algorithm, but ST-segment elevation myocardial infarction (STEMI) with time-sensitive reperfusion strategies is the focus of this chapter.

STEMI patients need rapid identification by experienced providers and interventions aimed at rapid reperfusion performed in a comprehensive system of care. Patients with unstable angina or non–ST-segment elevation myocardial infarction (NSTEMI) may have a similar underlying pathophysiologic process, but their management requires additional assessment for risk stratification and treatment. Complications of ACS include shock, pulmonary edema, and hypotension, with cardiogenic shock being the leading cause of death in patients with acute myocardial infarction (AMI).

Priorities for management of patients with ACS are

- Rapidly identify chest discomfort that could be ischemic in origin.
- Perform and immediately interpret the 12-lead ECG for acute ischemic syndromes.
- Use the ECG interpretation to place patients into 1 of 3 possible acute ischemic symptom categories: STEMI, NSTEMI, and normal or nondiagnostic ECG. Further risk-stratify patients with NSTEMI and high-risk unstable angina (UA).
- Quickly evaluate patients with STEMI and those with new or presumably new left bundle branch block (LBBB) on the basis of their eligibility and options for reperfusion therapy. Treat eligible patients with fibrinolytic therapy within 30 minutes or with percutaneous coronary intervention (PCI) within 90 minutes or less of arrival at the hospital. For inpatients with STEMI, the time from onset of ischemia to intervention should be as short as possible.[1]
- Know how to use drugs for relief of discomfort and as aids to reperfusion therapy.

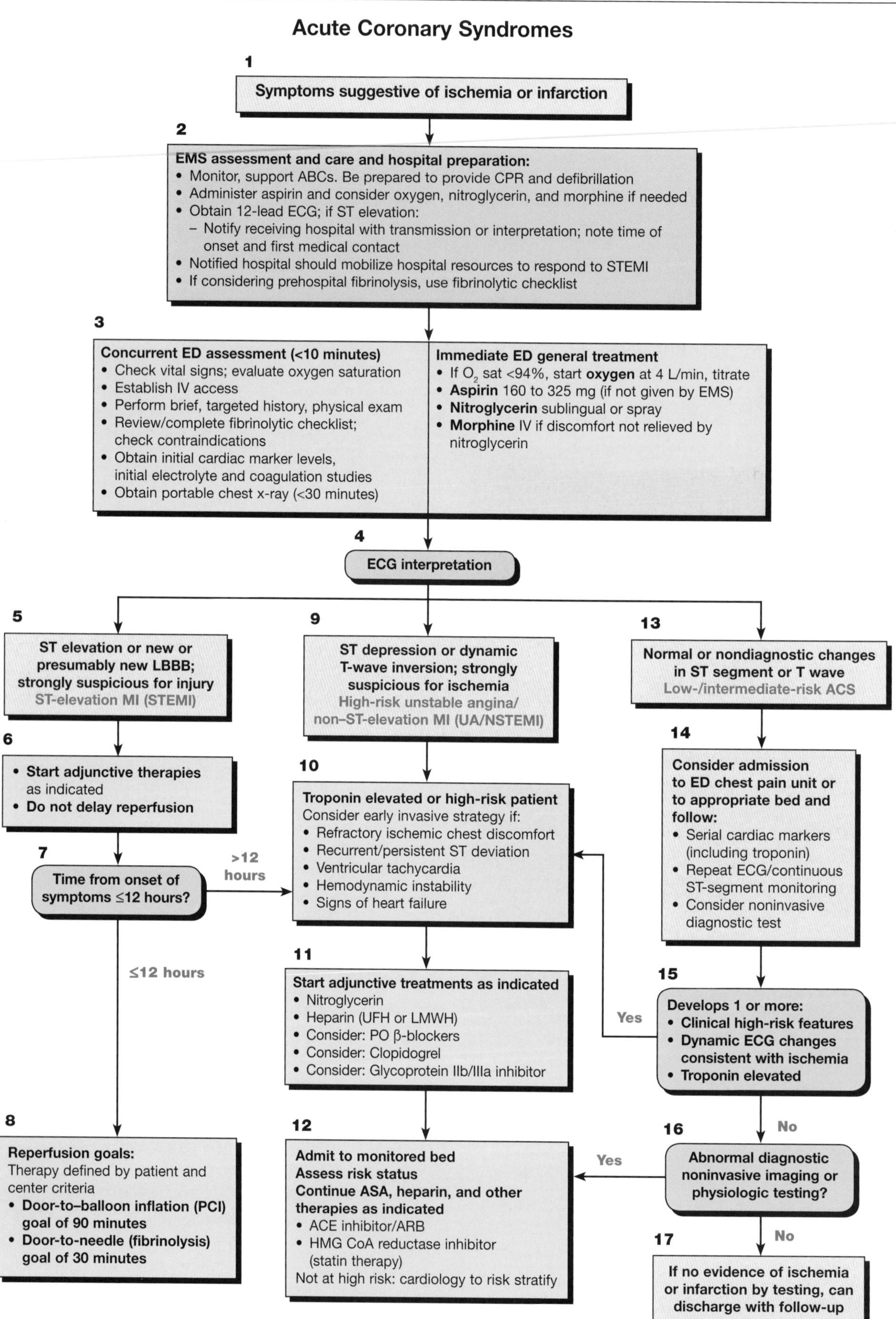

Acute Coronary Syndromes
1
Symptoms suggestive of ischemia or infarction
2
EMS assessment and care and hospital preparation:
• Monitor, support ABCs. Be prepared to provide CPR and defibrillation
• Administer aspirin and consider oxygen, nitroglycerin, and morphine if needed
• Obtain 12-lead ECG; if ST elevation:
– Notify receiving hospital with transmission or interpretation; note time of onset and first medical contact
• Notified hospital should mobilize hospital resources to respond to STEMI
• If considering prehospital fibrinolysis, use fibrinolytic checklist
3
Concurrent ED assessment (<10 minutes)
• Check vital signs; evaluate oxygen saturation
• Establish IV access
• Perform brief, targeted history, physical exam
• Review/complete fibrinolytic checklist; check contraindications
• Obtain initial cardiac marker levels, initial electrolyte and coagulation studies
• Obtain portable chest x-ray (<30 minutes)
Immediate ED general treatment
• If O_2 sat <94%, start oxygen at 4 L/min, titrate
• Aspirin 160 to 325 mg (if not given by EMS)
• Nitroglycerin sublingual or spray
• Morphine IV if discomfort not relieved by nitroglycerin
4
ECG interpretation
5
ST elevation or new or presumably new LBBB; strongly suspicious for injury
ST-elevation MI (STEMI)
6
• Start adjunctive therapies as indicated
• Do not delay reperfusion
7
Time from onset of symptoms ≤12 hours?
>12 hours
≤12 hours
8
Reperfusion goals:
Therapy defined by patient and center criteria
• Door-to–balloon inflation (PCI) goal of 90 minutes
• Door-to-needle (fibrinolysis) goal of 30 minutes
9
ST depression or dynamic T-wave inversion; strongly suspicious for ischemia
High-risk unstable angina/ non–ST-elevation MI (UA/NSTEMI)
10
Troponin elevated or high-risk patient
Consider early invasive strategy if:
• Refractory ischemic chest discomfort
• Recurrent/persistent ST deviation
• Ventricular tachycardia
• Hemodynamic instability
• Signs of heart failure
11
Start adjunctive treatments as indicated
• Nitroglycerin
• Heparin (UFH or LMWH)
• Consider: PO β-blockers
• Consider: Clopidogrel
• Consider: Glycoprotein IIb/IIIa inhibitor
12
Admit to monitored bed
Assess risk status
Continue ASA, heparin, and other therapies as indicated
• ACE inhibitor/ARB
• HMG CoA reductase inhibitor (statin therapy)
Not at high risk: cardiology to risk stratify
13
Normal or nondiagnostic changes in ST segment or T wave
Low-/intermediate-risk ACS
14
Consider admission to ED chest pain unit or to appropriate bed and follow:
• Serial cardiac markers (including troponin)
• Repeat ECG/continuous ST-segment monitoring
• Consider noninvasive diagnostic test
15
Develops 1 or more:
• Clinical high-risk features
• Dynamic ECG changes consistent with ischemia
• Troponin elevated
Yes
16
No
Abnormal diagnostic noninvasive imaging or physiologic testing?
Yes
17
No
If no evidence of ischemia or infarction by testing, can discharge with follow-up

Figure 75. The Acute Coronary Syndromes Algorithm.

- Patients with cardiogenic shock and STEMI should be primarily transported or secondarily transferred (with a door-to-departure time of 30 minutes or less) to facilities capable of invasive strategies, such as PCI, insertion of an intra-aortic balloon pump (IABP), and coronary artery bypass grafting (CABG).

Introduction to ACS: STEMI, NSTEMI, and UA

This chapter reviews the evaluation of patients with possible ischemic chest discomfort with an emphasis on rapid identification of patients with STEMI. These patients require fast reperfusion to save heart muscle and reduce the complications of myocardial infarction (MI). This chapter also provides a detailed review of the initial management of these patients.

Patient-based delay in recognition of ACS and activation of the emergency medical services (EMS) system often constitutes the longest period of delay to treatment.[2] With respect to the prehospital recognition of ACS, numerous issues have been identified as independent factors for prehospital treatment delay (ie, symptom-to-door time), including older age,[3] racial and ethnic minorities,[4,5] female gender,[6] lower socioeconomic status,[7,8] and solitary living arrangements.[4,9] Hospital-based delays in ACS recognition range from nonclassical patient presentations and other confounding diagnostic issues to provider misinterpretation of patient data and inefficient in-hospital systems of care.[6,10-13]

The major recommendations for the care of patients with ACS include

- Aspirin:
  - EMS dispatch should encourage the caller to provide aspirin 160 to 325 mg to the patient to chew while awaiting EMS arrival, unless contraindicated.[14,15]
  - Hospital nurses should follow protocol to provide aspirin, unless contraindicated.
- Early acquisition of a 12-lead ECG:
  - Hospital nurses should obtain a 12-lead ECG without delay.
  - Prehospital care providers should obtain a 12-lead ECG within the first 10 minutes of arrival at the patient's side and transmit the ECG to or contact the receiving facility for rapid reperfusion identification and team activation.
- Rapidly triage STEMI patients to reperfusion strategy and risk stratification.
- Reperfusion should occur as soon as possible after symptoms begin. Several prospective studies[16-18] have documented reduced time to administration of fibrinolytics and decreased mortality rates when out-of-hospital fibrinolytics were administered to patients with STEMI. Reperfusion goals include a door-to-needle (fibrinolytic) time of less than 30 minutes and a door-to-balloon (angioplasty or stent) time of less than 90 minutes.
  - In some EMS systems, patients are transferred directly to the catheterization lab from the field to shorten the time interval further.
  - Inpatients who develop STEMI should move to definitive therapy as rapidly as possible.
- Appropriate facility:
  - If PCI is the chosen method of reperfusion for the prehospital STEMI patient, transport patients directly to the nearest PCI facility.
  - Transfer goal to another facility for PCI or cardiogenic shock is less than 30 minutes. Hospital and ED protocols should be developed.
- Adjunctive medications:
  - Use clopidogrel, prasugrel, or ticagrelor as adjunctive therapy for fibrinolytic strategy or for patients who are ineligible for fibrinolytics.

Differential Diagnosis of Chest Discomfort

Patients who present with chest discomfort are rapidly screened for life-threatening causes. The initial ECG and focused clinical assessment will identify patients with ST-segment deviation eligible for reperfusion or aggressive antiplatelet and antithrombin therapy. In other patients, a noncardiac cause of chest discomfort is identified early, and appropriate additional diagnostic tests and treatment are initiated. For many patients, the question of whether the chest discomfort is ischemic persists, particularly when the initial ECG is nondiagnostic or normal. Many of these patients will be found to be at low risk for major adverse cardiac events (MACE) and to have noncardiac causes of chest discomfort. The initial evaluation of the patient with chest discomfort begins with this question: *What is the likelihood that the presenting symptoms represent ischemia caused by underlying coronary artery disease?*

ACS: A Spectrum

Atherosclerosis is the formation and accumulation of lipid and oxidative byproducts in an arterial wall. When this plaque deposit involves the coronary arteries, physicians call this *coronary atherosclerosis*. This process is gradual (Figure 76), but once the coronary artery lumen becomes sufficiently narrowed, the condition can cause exertional symptoms. Sometimes small disruptions in the plaque deposit resolve spontaneously but produce mild symptoms called *angina pectoris*. On the other hand, an abrupt change in an atherosclerotic plaque of a diseased coronary arterial wall can cause a much more serious spectrum of clinical conditions referred to as *ACS*. The 3 components of ACS are *UA, NSTEMI,* and *STEMI.* Sudden cardiac death can complicate any of these clinical conditions and may be the first, only, or last presentation of the disease.

Angina Pectoris

Angina is a *symptom* often associated with chronic and gradual coronary artery narrowing. There are other causes of angina, and symptoms may occur in the absence of coronary artery narrowing as a result of other conditions. Typically discomfort is located in the *center of the lower chest (substernal)* and is described as *squeezing, heavy,* or *tight.* Two more features are characteristic of angina. First, the discomfort is *precipitated by exertion or emotion;* second, it is *relieved by rest or nitroglycerin.*

When an ACS occurs, these symptoms can occur at rest or with minimal exertion. More recently, descriptions of angina use the term chest (or neck, or arm) *discomfort* to describe symptoms. When angina or discomfort is caused by ACS, it is referred to as *ischemic discomfort* to distinguish the cause as cardiac and due to ischemia. See page 203 for a detailed discussion on angina.

ACS: The ECG

The ECG is central to the diagnosis and triage of patients with possible acute ischemic symptoms (Figure 77 and 78). The ECG allows initial placement of patients into 3 categories that have diagnostic and treatment implications. When the patient presents with symptoms of a possible ACS, a clinician proficient in ECG interpretation rapidly reviews the ECG and places the patient into 1 of 3 categories:

1. ***STEMI*** is characterized by ST-segment elevation in 2 or more contiguous leads or new LBBB. Threshold values for ST-segment elevation consistent with STEMI are J-point elevation of 2 mm (0.2 mV) in leads V_2 and V_3 and 1 mm (0.1 mV) in all other leads or by new or

Chronology of Atherosclerotic Vascular Disease Process

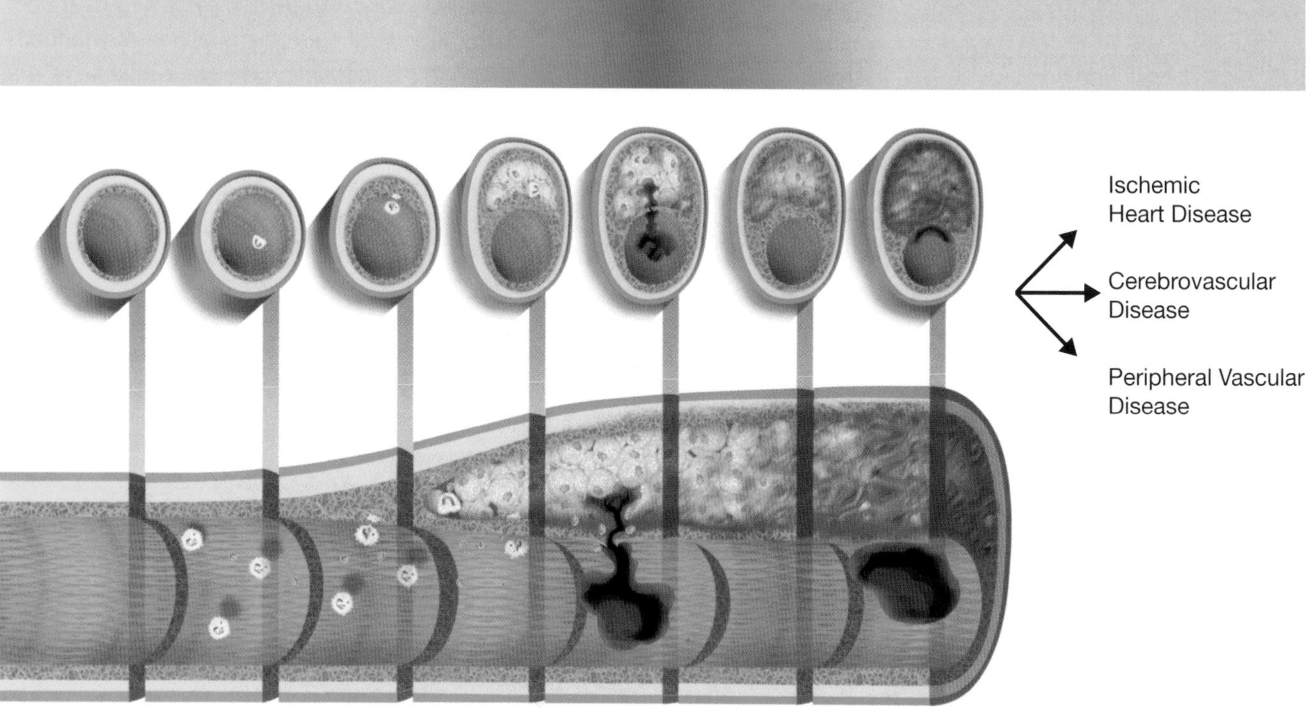

Figure 76. Timeline of atherosclerosis and ACS. Slices through the coronary artery, each of which represents a decade of life, depict the development of coronary atherosclerosis. Gradual narrowing of the artery can cause the development of angina when a critical or "significant" narrowing develops, usually 90% cross-sectional narrowing of the artery. If plaque rupture or erosion occurs, an ACS can develop and result in STEMI, NSTEMI, or unstable angina. Sudden cardiac death can complicate any of these syndromes and can be the first, last, and only symptom. When this process occurs in other vascular beds, stroke or peripheral vascular disease may occur. Modified from Libby.[19]

presumed new LBBB in men 40 years old or older. In men younger than 40 years old, the threshold values are J-point elevation of 2.5 mm (0.25 mV) in leads V_2 and V_3 and 1 mm (0.1 mV) in all other leads. In women the threshold values are J-point elevation of 1.5 mm (0.15 mV) in leads V_2 and V_3 and 1 mm (0.1 mV) in all other leads.[19,20]

2. ***High-risk UA/NSTEMI*** is characterized by ischemic ST-segment depression 0.5 mm (0.05 mV) or higher or dynamic T-wave inversion with pain or discomfort. Nonpersistent or transient ST elevation 0.5 mm or higher for less than 20 minutes is also included in this category. Threshold values for ST-segment depression consistent with ischemia are J-point depression of −0.5 mm (0.05 mV) in leads V_2 and V_3 and −1 mm (−0.1 mV) in all other leads (men and women).[20]

3. ***Intermediate or low-risk ACS*** is characterized by normal or nondiagnostic changes in the ST segment or T wave that are inconclusive and require further risk stratification. This classification includes patients with normal ECGs and those with ST-segment deviation in either direction of less than 0.5 mm (0.05 mV) or T-wave inversion less than or equal to 2 mm (0.2 mV). Serial cardiac studies and functional testing are appropriate. Note that additional information (troponin) may place the patient into a higher risk classification after initial classification.

Figures 77 and 78 show characteristic ECG findings and images for ACS.

If STEMI is present, immediately assess for reperfusion therapy and arrange for fibrinolytic therapy or primary PCI if the patient has no contraindications. Patients with ST-segment depression do not receive fibrinolytics (except for true posterior MI); these agents may increase mortality and morbidity despite the magnitude and extent of ST-segment depression. Antiplatelets and antithrombins are indicated for patients with ST-segment depression. These patients do not receive fibrinolytics (except for true posterior MI) because these agents may increase mortality and morbidity despite the magnitude and extent of ST-segment depression. Although the largest group of patients with acute ischemic symptoms will have nonspecific or normal ECGs, only a very few will have an ACS. Serial studies and risk stratification are appropriate if coronary artery disease (CAD) is thought to be of intermediate or high probability. Aspirin is indicated for all ACS if no contraindications are present.

STEMI

With prolonged ischemia or significant coronary artery occlusion, myocytes die and the ST segment of the ECG elevates. The majority of these patients will develop an MI. ST-segment elevation is an early ECG finding that identifies patients who may benefit from rapid reperfusion of the coronary artery. Confirmation of MI by detection of cardiac markers is variable, and elevation begins approximately 4 to 6 hours later. If the infarction process is not interrupted, Q waves, a later ECG finding consistent with a scar, will develop in many patients, and cardiac markers are necessary to distinguish UA from MI. Older terminology for this type of infarction included *transmural* or *Q-wave* MI. MI was previously classified as *Q wave* or *non–Q wave*, but these terms are pathological terms and are not helpful for risk stratification at the time of the patient's initial presentation. Q waves generally are a late finding.

How to Measure ST-Segment Deviation

ST-segment deviation (either elevation or depression) must be measured precisely and uniformly (Figure 79):

1. Draw the baseline ("zero ST deviation") from the *end* of the T wave to the *beginning* of the P wave (the TP segment).
   - The conventional baseline for measurement of ST deviation has been the PR segment, but a baseline drawn from the end of the T wave to the beginning of the P wave is considered to be *a more accurate baseline* for evaluation of ST deviation than the PR segment. The TP baseline is particularly helpful in ECGs with coved or concave ST segments or hyperacute T waves.
   - If the TP segment cannot be identified because of a rapid heart rate or artifact, use the PR *junction* as the baseline reference point. The PR junction is the intersection of the PR segment with the QRS complex.
2. Locate the J point, the position of juncture (angle change) between the QRS complex and the ST segment.
3. Locate 0.04 second (1 mm) after the J point. Measure the vertical deviation from this point (1 mm after the J point) either up or down to the baseline. This distance is the amount of ST deviation.

Critical Concept **12-Lead ECG**	
	• The 12-lead ECG is at the center of the decision pathway in the management of ischemic chest discomfort and is the only means to identify STEMI. • Obtain an ECG as soon as possible (within 10 minutes of ED arrival if not already done by EMS or by protocol for inpatients).

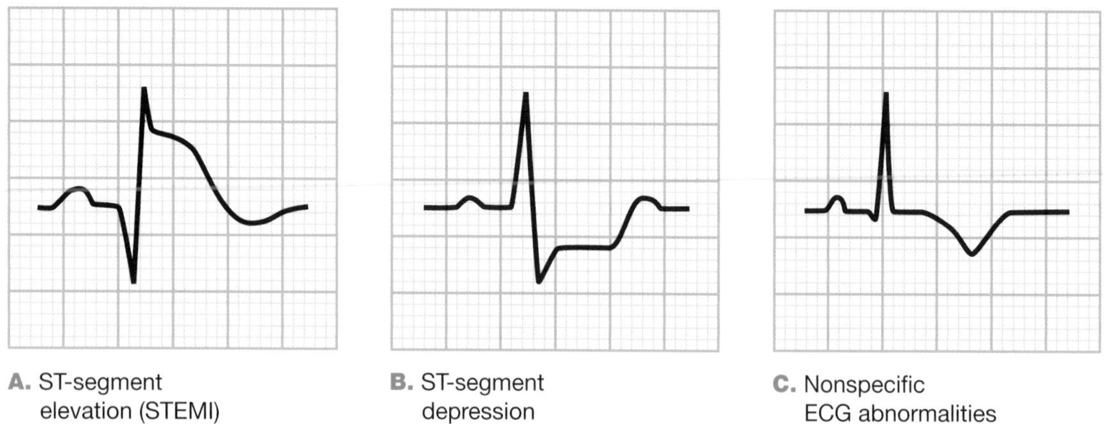

Figure 77. ECG findings of the spectrum of ACS. **A,** This tracing shows >1 mm of ST-segment elevation, measured 0.04 second after the J point (STEMI). **B,** This tracing shows ≥0.5 mm of ST-segment depression, measured 0.04 second after the J point. **C,** The nonspecific ST-segment and T-wave changes on this tracing are consistent with either NSTEMI or unstable angina. Cardiac markers could be positive with any of these ECG tracings.

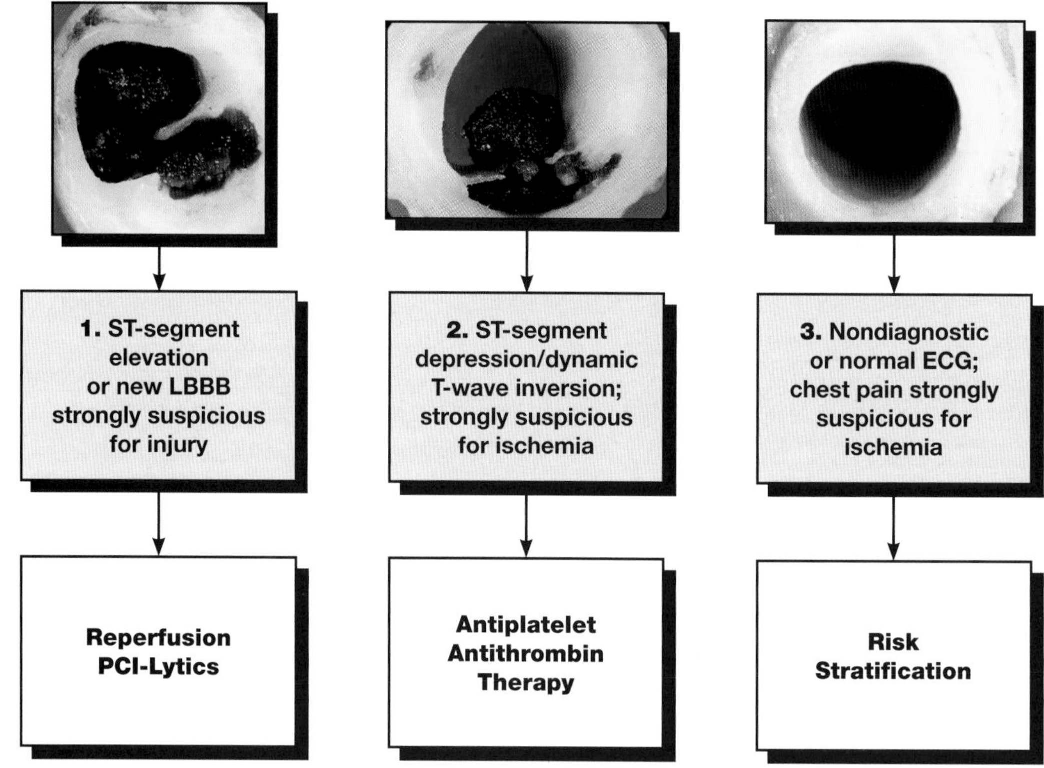

Figure 78. The 12-lead ECG is used to initially sort patients into 1 of 3 categories based on the presence or absence of ST-segment deviation and new or presumably new LBBB. Patients with ST-segment elevation or new LBBB (**1**) are evaluated for rapid reperfusion. Those with high-risk NSTEMI and an ACS (**2**) are treated with aggressive antiplatelet and antithrombin therapy. Patients with a low probability of ACS events (**3**) receive aspirin and undergo further risk stratification. Figures courtesy of Professor Michael Davies, Guy's Hospital, London, England. First and second figures reproduced from Field JM. Pathophysiology and initial triage of acute coronary syndromes. In: Field JM, ed. *The Textbook of Emergency Cardiovascular Care and CPR.* Philadelphia, PA: Lippincott Williams & Wilkins; 2009:1-10; and Davies MJ. The pathophysiology of acute coronary syndromes. *Heart.* 2000;83:361-366, with permission from BMJ Publishing Group Ltd.

Other Causes of ST Elevation

Evaluation of the patient with acute chest discomfort includes a short list of emergency differential diagnoses and a long list of other non–life-threatening causes. Initial triage involves a determination of the likelihood of these causes. It may not be possible to rule out some of these causes, and the risk-benefit assessment involves an estimation of which additional causes are unlikely. This process requires

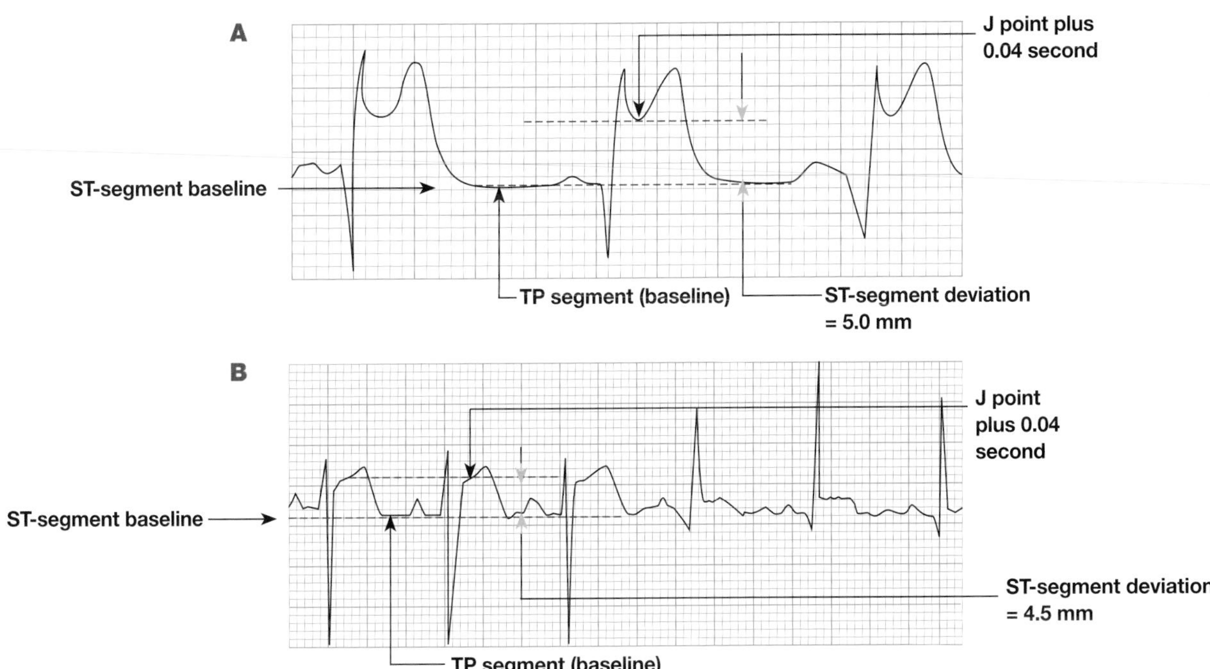

Figure 79. ECG findings of STEMI showing ST-segment elevation, measured 0.04 second after the J point. **A,** Inferior MI. ST segment has no low point (it is coved or concave). **B,** Anterior MI.

integration of clinical and ECG data, because time is crucial if early reperfusion is to be achieved. In general, reperfusion is not delayed to obtain diagnostic tests for these other conditions. Clinical judgment will be needed to determine whether delays in door-to-drug/balloon time for imaging studies such as a spiral computed tomography (CT) scan or an echocardiogram are warranted for a given clinical case. These other conditions may cause or be associated with ST elevation on the initial ECG and can be difficult to discriminate from acute injury. Healthcare providers must be aware that conditions other than acute ischemic injury can cause ST elevation[21,22] (Table 24), such as

- Old LBBB
- Left ventricular (LV) hypertrophy
- Early repolarization
- Neurological injury

NSTEMI

When ischemia is prolonged but the coronary artery is incompletely occluded, cardiac markers may increase, but the ECG may demonstrate elevated, normal, or depressed ST-segment changes. Detection of elevated cardiac markers in this setting defines NSTEMI (discussed below).

Evolution of the 12-Lead ECG in ACS

The ECG changes and "evolves" during a process that initially involves ischemia, then injury, and finally necrosis of cardiac muscle cells. Not all phases may be noted in every patient, and the findings vary on the basis of patient characteristics (eg, coronary anatomy), ECG sensitivity, and location of the infarct. Early in STEMI, T waves may be tented or "peaked"; these changes are referred to as hyperacute changes. Other ECGs may show changes that are nonspecific or nondiagnostic. Finally, Q waves generally represent necrosis and are a late finding, although they may be observed early in STEMI and may decrease or resolve contrary to the usual evolutionary pattern (Figure 80).

Sudden Cardiac Death

Acute ischemia or MI can cause electrical instability or catastrophic hemodynamic impairment. Sudden cardiac death results and is the major cause of out-of-hospital adult cardiac arrest in the hours after onset of symptoms. If an arrhythmia occurs as a primary event (not caused by cardiogenic shock), *ventricular fibrillation* (VF) is a common presentation. Defibrillation success depends on many factors, including high-quality CPR, early defibrillation, and the underlying acute coronary syndrome. Resuscitation is more successful when VF occurs in the absence of an ACS, such as during cardiac rehabilitation or exercise stress testing.

ACS: Pathophysiology

Stable and Unstable Plaques

Coronary atherosclerosis is a diffuse process with segmental lesions called *coronary plaques* that gradually enlarge and extend, which causes variable degrees of coronary

Table 24. Conditions That Can Elevate the ST Segment of the ECG but Are Not STEMI

Condition	Features
Normal variant (so-called *male pattern*)	• Seen in approximately 90% of healthy young men; therefore, normal • Elevation of 1 to 3 mm • Most marked in V_2 • Concave ST segment
Early repolarization	• Most marked in V_4, with notching at J point • Tall, upright T waves • Reciprocal ST depression in aVR, not in aVL, when limb leads are involved
ST elevation of normal variant	• Seen in V_3 through V_5 with inverted T waves • Short QT, high QRS voltage
Left ventricular hypertrophy	• Concave • Other features of left ventricular hypertrophy
Left bundle branch block	• Concave • ST-segment deviation discordant from the QRS
Acute pericarditis	• Diffuse ST-segment elevation • Reciprocal ST-segment depression in aVR, not in aVL • Elevation seldom >5 mm • PR-segment depression
Hyperkalemia	Other features of hyperkalemia present: • Widened QRS and tall, peaked, tented T waves • Low-amplitude or absent P waves • ST segment usually downsloping
Brugada syndrome	• rSR′ in V_1 and V_2 • ST-segment elevation in V_1 and V_2, typically downsloping
Pulmonary embolism	• Changes simulating myocardial infarction seen often in both inferior and anteroseptal leads
Cardioversion	• Striking ST-segment elevation, often >10 mm, but lasting only a minute or 2 immediately after direct-current shock
Prinzmetal's angina	• Same as ST-segment elevation in infarction but transient
Neurologic injury	• Neurologic injury may cause ST elevation, depression, or any variant of ST/T-wave changes

Adapted from Wang et al,[21] copyright © 2003 Massachusetts Medical Society. With permission from Massachusetts Medical Society.

artery occlusion. Intravascular ultrasound of the coronary arteries has shown that the majority of the atheroma burden is subluminal and not visible by coronary angiography. Coronary arteries are usually closed approximately 70% by angiography (90% closed when viewed by a pathologist) before they cause symptoms and are considered for stenting or surgery.

Most plaques do not cause symptoms and are nonocclusive, but nonocclusive plaques are the ones most prone to cause ACS. They have little hemodynamic effect before rupture, and stress testing and angiography cannot predict which ones will rupture and cause an ACS. Plaques can be classified as *stable* or *vulnerable* on the basis of their lipid content, the thickness of the cap that covers and separates them from the arterial lumen, and the degree of inflammation in the plaque itself.

1. A *stable* intracoronary plaque (Figure 81A) has a lipid core separated from the arterial lumen by a thick fibrous cap. Stable plaques have less lipid, and the thick cap makes them resistant to fissuring and formation of thrombi. Over time the lumen of the vessel becomes progressively narrower, which leads to flow limitations, supply-demand imbalance, and exertional angina.
2. A *vulnerable* intracoronary plaque (Figure 81B) has a lipid-rich core combined with an active inflammatory process, which makes the plaque soft and prone to

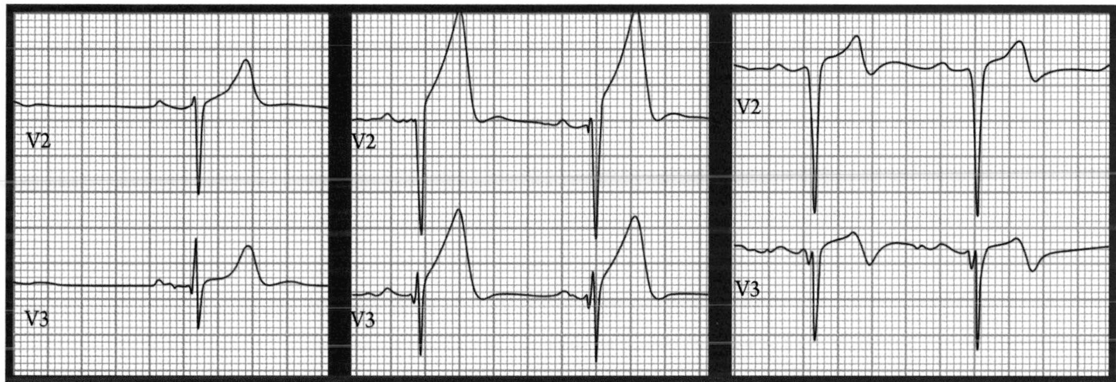

Figure 80. This figure from left to right demonstrates the ST-segment changes of STEMI. The left panel shows minimal ST-segment elevation that is downwardly concave, possibly because of early repolarization in the baseline tracing. This patient, however, was having symptoms of ischemic chest discomfort, and the ECG was repeated 10 minutes later. Clearly seen in the middle panel are tented and peaked ST segments. In the right panel, evolution of the ST-segment and T-wave changes are seen in a tracing obtained 1 hour later, immediately after to PCI. The ST segments are elevated but returning to normal, and the T waves are biphasic. In addition, there is a QS complex in lead V_2 and further loss of R wave in V_3.

rupture. These plaques infrequently restrict blood flow enough to cause clinical angina, and functional studies (eg, stress tests) often yield negative results. Imaging techniques such as cardiac CT and magnetic resonance imaging are being investigated as tools to identify unstable and inflamed plaques and may be helpful in the future.

3. Inflammation is often found in the plaque (Figure 81C). Inflammatory processes are concentrated in the leading edge impacted by coronary blood flow. It is here that most plaque ruptures occur. A plaque that is inflamed and prone to rupture is called *unstable*.

STEMI: Goals of Therapy

The primary goals of reperfusion therapy in patients with STEMI are to

- Limit infarct size
- Prevent or treat serious or fatal cardiac arrhythmias
- Avoid or manage congestive heart failure (CHF)
- Treat life-threatening complications such as myocardial rupture and acute valvular dysfunction

Complete occlusion of an epicardial coronary artery (ie, coronary arteries that run on the surface of the heart) eventually produces elevation of the ST segment of the ECG in most patients. Myocardial cell death begins and proceeds rapidly from subendocardium to epicardium unless flow is reestablished (Figure 82). In a minority of patients, the clot resolves spontaneously. In all others, fibrinolytic therapy or mechanical reperfusion with PCI with balloons and stents is necessary to limit myocardial damage. Loss of heart muscle is time dependent—*time is muscle.* The majority of myocyte necrosis (MI) occurs within the first several hours. Reperfusion has been shown to reduce mortality, preserve LV function, and reduce or limit the development of CHF.

STEMI: Initial Management *(Figure 83)*

Community and Out-of-Hospital Management

Half of the patients who die of AMI do so before reaching the hospital. VF or pulseless ventricular tachycardia (VT) is the precipitating rhythm in most of these deaths,[24-26] and sudden cardiac death is most likely to develop during the first 4 hours after onset of symptoms.[27-30] Communities should develop programs to respond to out-of-hospital cardiac arrest that include prompt recognition of symptoms of ACS, early activation of the EMS system, and if needed, early CPR and early defibrillation.

The major community and EMS issues in the management of ACS are

- Patient delay
- Potential need for early defibrillation
- Out-of-hospital 12-lead ECGs
- EMS notification of receiving facility
- EMS triage to appropriate facility

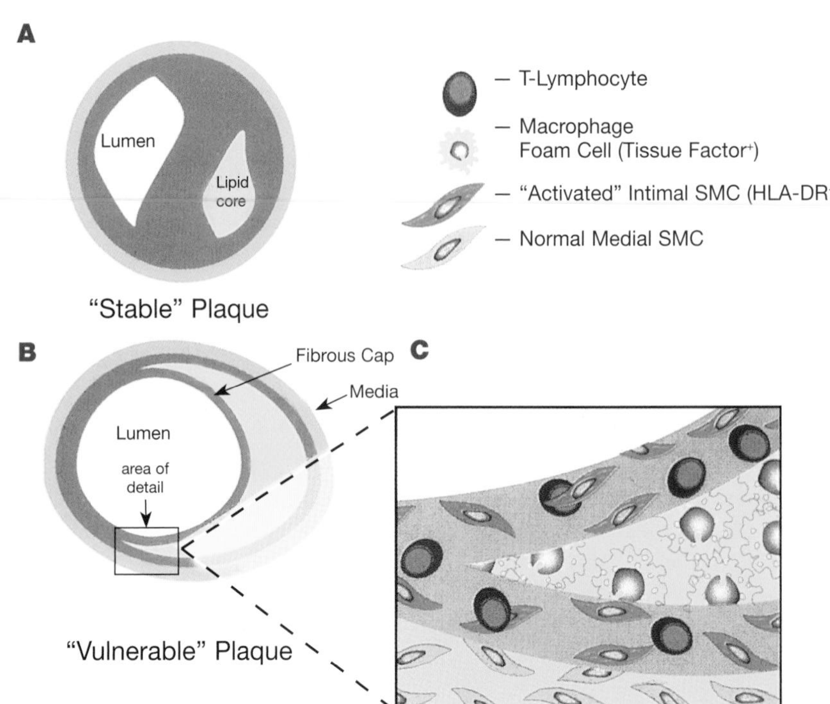

Figure 81. Stable and vulnerable plaques. **A,** Stable plaque. **B,** Vulnerable plaque. **C,** Area of detail of vulnerable plaque showing infiltration of inflammatory cells. SMC stands for smooth muscle cell. Reproduced from Libby.[23]

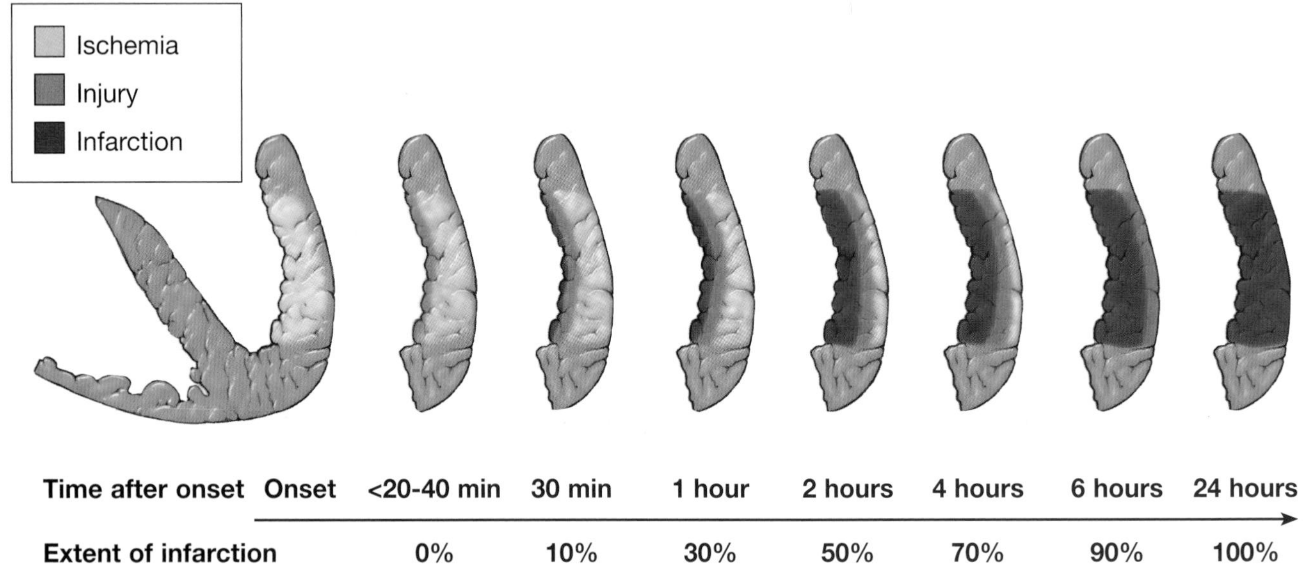

Figure 82. After occlusion of a coronary artery, progressive cell death occurs. Note that the majority of myocardial infarction occurs by 4 hours after the onset of symptoms. After 6 hours the infarct is nearly complete. The extent and degree of myocardial infarction depends on several factors: the coronary artery involved, the amount of myocardium downstream, the degree and duration of occlusion, and the presence or absence of collateral supply.

The Problem of Delay

Any delay in coronary reperfusion reduces the effectiveness of fibrinolytic-based or catheter-based therapy, increases mortality, and decreases myocardial salvage. Because the potential for myocardial salvage decreases with time and most benefit occurs in the first few hours, patients, family members, EMS personnel, and healthcare providers should operate with a sense of urgency—*time is muscle!*

There are 3 major time intervals from the onset of ACS symptoms to the delivery of reperfusion therapy that provide opportunity for delay in treatment:

Patient delay, the interval from the onset of symptoms to the patient's recognition of them, accounts for 60% to 70% of the delay to definitive therapy.[31] EMS transport accounts for the least amount of delay, and prehospital notification of ACS patients can speed the diagnosis and reduce the time to reperfusion. Unfortunately, the majority of patients still arrive by private vehicle and not EMS. Physicians and healthcare providers should encourage patients, especially those with known coronary disease, to use their nitroglycerin and activate EMS if symptoms persist or worsen 5 minutes after they use the first nitroglycerin dose. The interval from ED arrival to treatment accounts for 25% to 33% of the delay. Over the past decade, many EDs have reduced the average time to fibrinolytic therapy through education, improved patient triage, and development of multidisciplinary protocols, including prehospital administration of fibrinolytics. In some areas, bypassing the ED altogether and traveling directly to the cath lab has improved the time from symptom onset to PCI.

Chest discomfort is the major symptom in most patients (both men and women) with ACS, but patients frequently deny or misinterpret this and other symptoms. The elderly, women, diabetic patients, and hypertensive patients are most likely to delay, in part because they are more likely to have atypical symptoms or presentations. In the US Rapid Early Action for Coronary Treatment (REACT) trial, the median out-of-hospital delay was 2 hours or longer in non-Hispanic blacks, the elderly and disabled, homemakers, and Medicaid recipients.[32] The decision to use an ambulance was an important variable that reduced out-of-hospital delay; this reduction persisted after correction for variables associated with severity of symptoms. Other factors that can affect the interval between symptom onset and presentation to hospital include time of day, location (eg, work or home), and presence of a family member.

Reducing Patient Delay

Education of patients with known CAD appears to be the only effective primary intervention to reduce denial or misinterpretation of symptoms. Public educational programs have had only transient effects. The physician and family members of patients with known coronary disease should reinforce the need to seek medical attention when symptoms recur, because these patients paradoxically present later than patients with no known disease.

Recognition of Possible Ischemic Discomfort (Number 1, Figure 83)

Chest discomfort of ischemic origin is usually substernal and is often described as crushing, heavy, constricting, or oppressive. Symptoms suggestive of ACS include

- Uncomfortable pressure, fullness, squeezing, or discomfort in the center of the chest lasting several minutes (usually more than a few minutes)
- Chest discomfort that spreads to the shoulders, neck, one or both arms, or jaw
- Chest discomfort that spreads in the back or between the shoulder blades
- Chest discomfort with lightheadedness, dizziness, fainting, sweating, nausea, or vomiting
- Unexplained sudden shortness of breath with or without chest discomfort
- Less commonly the discomfort occurs in the epigastrium and is described as indigestion. Just as a response to nitroglycerin is *not diagnostic* of cardiac ischemic discomfort, relief of discomfort with antacids in these patients is *not diagnostic* of a gastrointestinal cause.

In one large study only 54% of patients with typical ischemic symptoms developed an ACS.[33] On the other hand, of all patients who developed an ACS, 43% had burning or indigestion, 32% had a chest ache, 20% had sharp or stabbing pain, and 42% could not describe their pain. The pain was *partially* pleuritic in 12%. In patients without a history of coronary disease, chest pain that was sharp or stabbing *and* pleuritic, positional, or reproducible with chest palpation was almost never caused by ischemic syndromes.

Critical Concept **Patient Use of Nitroglycerin for Acute Chest Discomfort**	Guidelines recommend that healthcare providers instruct patients and family to activate EMS if symptoms persist or worsen ***5 minutes after the first nitroglycerin dose.*** These patients may have STEMI or prolonged ischemia and are at risk for sudden cardiac death.

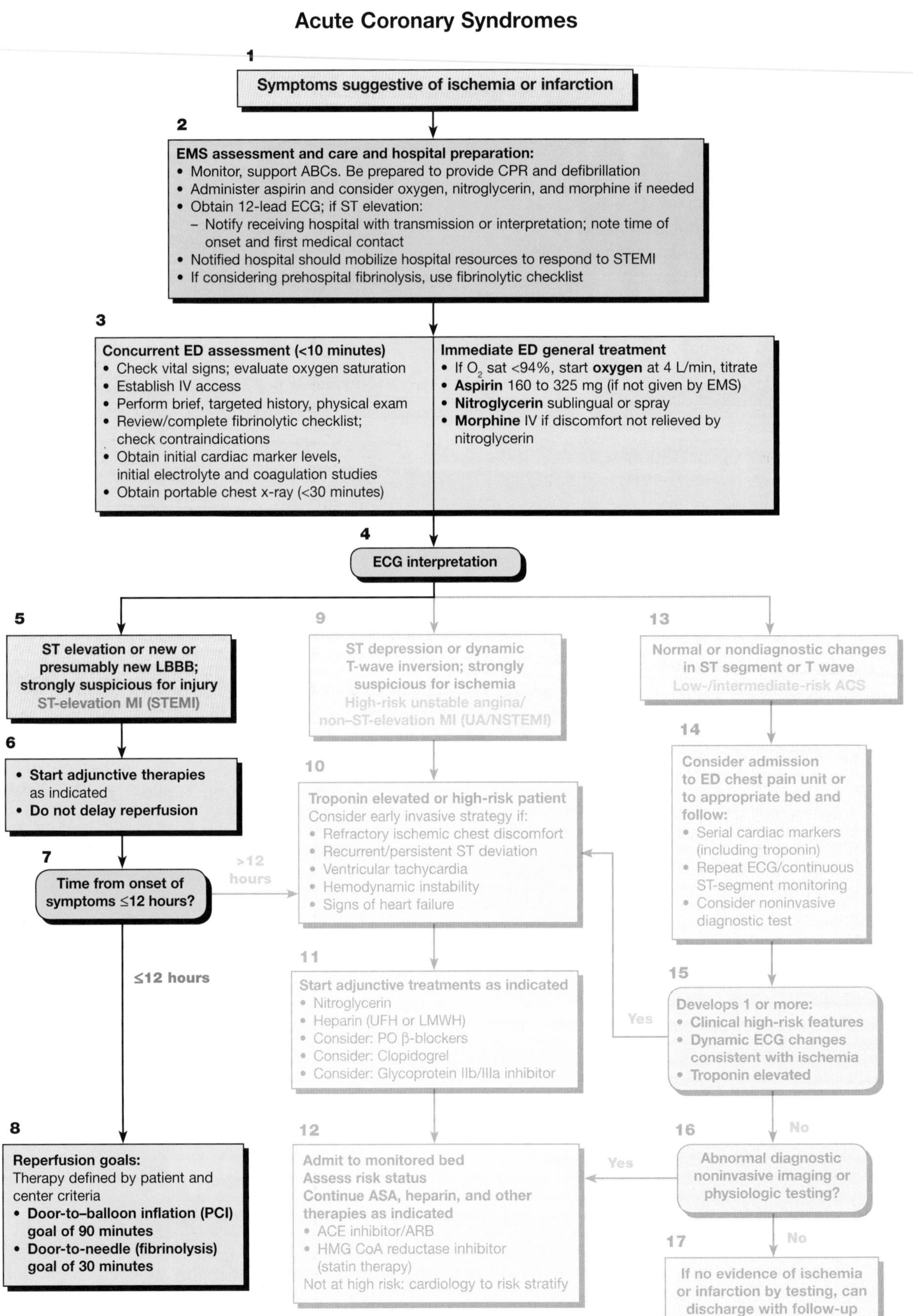

Acute Coronary Syndromes
1
Symptoms suggestive of ischemia or infarction
2
EMS assessment and care and hospital preparation:
• Monitor, support ABCs. Be prepared to provide CPR and defibrillation
• Administer aspirin and consider oxygen, nitroglycerin, and morphine if needed
• Obtain 12-lead ECG; if ST elevation:
– Notify receiving hospital with transmission or interpretation; note time of onset and first medical contact
• Notified hospital should mobilize hospital resources to respond to STEMI
• If considering prehospital fibrinolysis, use fibrinolytic checklist
3
Concurrent ED assessment (<10 minutes)
• Check vital signs; evaluate oxygen saturation
• Establish IV access
• Perform brief, targeted history, physical exam
• Review/complete fibrinolytic checklist; check contraindications
• Obtain initial cardiac marker levels, initial electrolyte and coagulation studies
• Obtain portable chest x-ray (<30 minutes)
Immediate ED general treatment
• If O_2 sat <94%, start oxygen at 4 L/min, titrate
• Aspirin 160 to 325 mg (if not given by EMS)
• Nitroglycerin sublingual or spray
• Morphine IV if discomfort not relieved by nitroglycerin
4
ECG interpretation
5
ST elevation or new or presumably new LBBB; strongly suspicious for injury
ST-elevation MI (STEMI)
6
• Start adjunctive therapies as indicated
• Do not delay reperfusion
7
Time from onset of symptoms ≤12 hours?
>12 hours
≤12 hours
8
Reperfusion goals:
Therapy defined by patient and center criteria
• Door-to-balloon inflation (PCI) goal of 90 minutes
• Door-to-needle (fibrinolysis) goal of 30 minutes
9
ST depression or dynamic T-wave inversion; strongly suspicious for ischemia
High-risk unstable angina/ non–ST-elevation MI (UA/NSTEMI)
10
Troponin elevated or high-risk patient
Consider early invasive strategy if:
• Refractory ischemic chest discomfort
• Recurrent/persistent ST deviation
• Ventricular tachycardia
• Hemodynamic instability
• Signs of heart failure
11
Start adjunctive treatments as indicated
• Nitroglycerin
• Heparin (UFH or LMWH)
• Consider: PO β-blockers
• Consider: Clopidogrel
• Consider: Glycoprotein IIb/IIIa inhibitor
12
Admit to monitored bed
Assess risk status
Continue ASA, heparin, and other therapies as indicated
• ACE inhibitor/ARB
• HMG CoA reductase inhibitor (statin therapy)
Not at high risk: cardiology to risk stratify
13
Normal or nondiagnostic changes in ST segment or T wave
Low-/intermediate-risk ACS
14
Consider admission to ED chest pain unit or to appropriate bed and follow:
• Serial cardiac markers (including troponin)
• Repeat ECG/continuous ST-segment monitoring
• Consider noninvasive diagnostic test
15
Develops 1 or more:
• Clinical high-risk features
• Dynamic ECG changes consistent with ischemia
• Troponin elevated
Yes
16
No
Abnormal diagnostic noninvasive imaging or physiologic testing?
Yes
17
No
If no evidence of ischemia or infarction by testing, can discharge with follow-up

Figure 83. The Acute Coronary Syndromes Algorithm—STEMI treatment pathway for reperfusion therapy.

Initial EMS Care for Patients With STEMI

Major Emergency Assessments and Treatments (Number 2, Figure 83)

Dispatchers and emergency providers for both out-of-hospital and in-hospital settings must be trained to recognize symptoms of ACS and activate the STEMI Chain of Survival (Figure 84). The following assessments and actions may be performed during the stabilization, triage, and transport of the patient to an appropriate facility or service:

- Identify patients with acute ischemic chest discomfort.
- Monitor and support ABCs.
  - Monitor vital signs and cardiac rhythm.
  - Be prepared to provide CPR.
  - Use a defibrillator if needed.
- Obtain an initial 12-lead ECG, provide prearrival notification to the receiving hospital, and transmit the ECG or their interpretation of the ECG.
- Obtain a targeted history with a fibrinolytic checklist to help determine eligibility for fibrinolytic therapy as appropriate.
- Establish vascular access and measure vital signs and oxygen saturation.
- Document initial rhythms and prepare for treatment of ischemic arrhythmias, in particular VF/VT.
- Place transcutaneous patches for transcutaneous pacing if symptomatic sinus bradycardia or advanced atrioventricular block occurs.
- Start initial medical treatment:
  - Administer oxygen if O_2 saturation is less than 94%.
  - Give aspirin.
  - Give 1 sublingual nitroglycerin tablet (or spray "dose") every 3 to 5 minutes for ongoing symptoms if permitted by medical control and no contraindications exist. Healthcare providers may repeat the dose twice (total of 3 doses).
  - Give morphine if chest discomfort is unresponsive to nitrates.
- Morphine should be used with caution in UA/NSTEMI because of an association with increased mortality in a large registry.[34]

Out-of-Hospital ECGs

Out-of-hospital 12-lead ECGs and advance notification to the receiving facility speed diagnosis, shorten time to fibrinolysis, and may be associated with lower in-hospital mortality.[36-39] The reduction in door-to–reperfusion therapy interval in most studies ranges from 10 to 60 minutes. EMS providers can efficiently acquire and transmit diagnostic-quality ECGs to the ED[40,41] with a minimal increase in the on-scene time interval (0.2 to 5.6 minutes).[36,40-44] Implementation of 12-lead ECG diagnostic programs with concurrent medically directed quality assurance is recommended.

Qualified and specially trained paramedics and prehospital nurses can accurately identify typical ST elevation in the 12-lead ECG with a specificity of 91% to 100% and a sensitivity of 71% to 97% compared with emergency medicine physicians or cardiologists[27,28] and can provide advance notification by radio or cell phone to the receiving hospital.[29] If providers are not trained to interpret the 12-lead ECG, field transmission of the ECG or a computer report to the receiving hospital is recommended.

If EMS providers identify STEMI on the ECG, it is reasonable for them to begin assessment of the patient for fibrinolytic therapy (ie, the Fibrinolytic Checklist; Figure 85).

Early Interventions for Hospital Inpatients

There is some evidence that hospitalized patients with STEMI often have longer time to intervention than patients who are managed via the EMS system. In some cases this is due to the increased complexity of the patient population; however, in many hospitals, the system of care for this type of emergency is either poorly defined or unknown. It is likely that many of the systems that have worked well in the out-of-hospital setting can be adapted and applied to inpatients. Rapid Response Teams and Medical Emergency Teams have sometimes strengthened the links in the chain. Hospitals that review their data on such cases can identify and implement improvements that will reduce the time between the onset of signs and symptoms and definitive therapy for inpatients with STEMI.

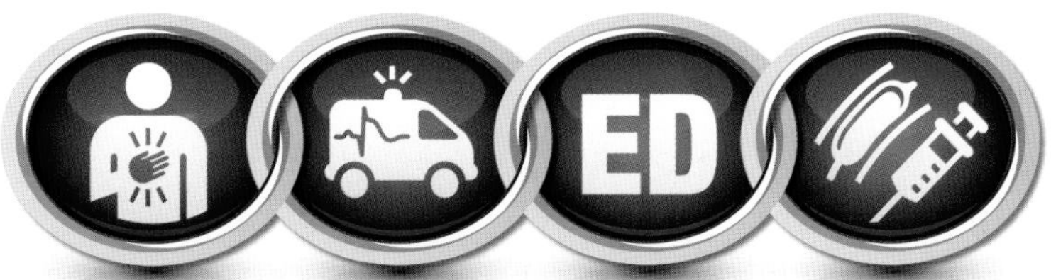

Figure 84. The STEMI Chain of Survival displays the 4 links essential for survival of patients who present with STEMI.

Critical Concept **Community EMS Priority**	• VF or pulseless VT is the precipitating rhythm that causes death in ACS.[24-26] • VF is most likely to develop during the first 4 hours after symptom onset.[27-30] • Communities should develop programs to respond to out-of-hospital cardiac arrest that include recognition of ACS symptoms, activation of the EMS system, and availability of high-quality CPR and an AED.[35]

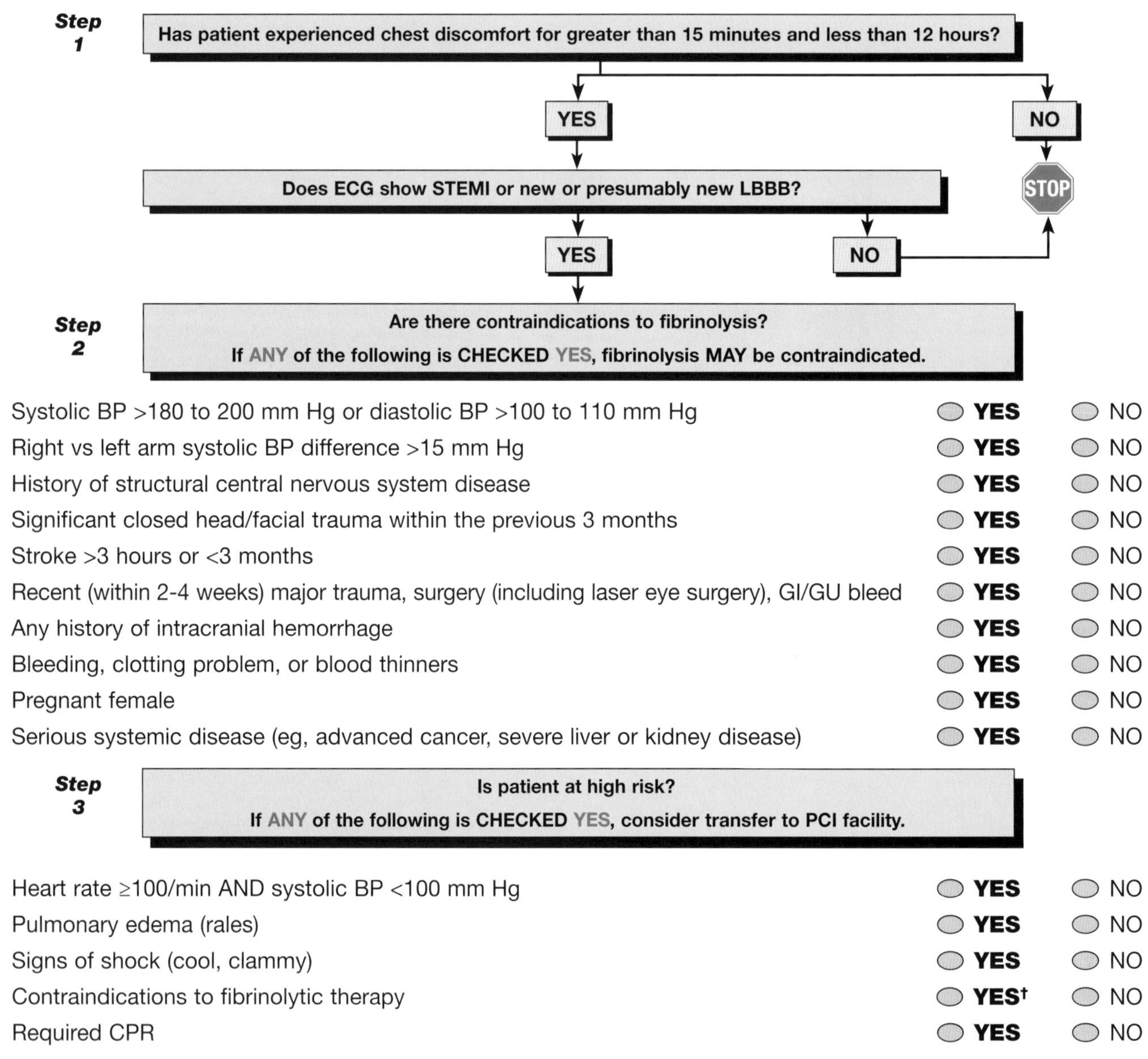

Prehospital Fibrinolytic Checklist*

Step 1

Has patient experienced chest discomfort for greater than 15 minutes and less than 12 hours?

YES → Does ECG show STEMI or new or presumably new LBBB?

NO → STOP

Does ECG show STEMI or new or presumably new LBBB?

YES → Step 2

NO → STOP

Step 2

Are there contraindications to fibrinolysis?
If ANY of the following is CHECKED YES, fibrinolysis MAY be contraindicated.

Systolic BP >180 to 200 mm Hg or diastolic BP >100 to 110 mm Hg	◯ **YES**	◯ NO
Right vs left arm systolic BP difference >15 mm Hg	◯ **YES**	◯ NO
History of structural central nervous system disease	◯ **YES**	◯ NO
Significant closed head/facial trauma within the previous 3 months	◯ **YES**	◯ NO
Stroke >3 hours or <3 months	◯ **YES**	◯ NO
Recent (within 2-4 weeks) major trauma, surgery (including laser eye surgery), GI/GU bleed	◯ **YES**	◯ NO
Any history of intracranial hemorrhage	◯ **YES**	◯ NO
Bleeding, clotting problem, or blood thinners	◯ **YES**	◯ NO
Pregnant female	◯ **YES**	◯ NO
Serious systemic disease (eg, advanced cancer, severe liver or kidney disease)	◯ **YES**	◯ NO

Step 3

Is patient at high risk?
If ANY of the following is CHECKED YES, consider transfer to PCI facility.

Heart rate ≥100/min AND systolic BP <100 mm Hg	◯ **YES**	◯ NO
Pulmonary edema (rales)	◯ **YES**	◯ NO
Signs of shock (cool, clammy)	◯ **YES**	◯ NO
Contraindications to fibrinolytic therapy	◯ **YES**†	◯ NO
Required CPR	◯ **YES**	◯ NO

*Contraindications for fibrinolytic use in STEMI are viewed as advisory for clinical decison making and may not be all-inclusive or definitive. These contraindications are consistent with the 2004 ACC/AHA Guidelines for the Management of Patients With ST-Elevation Myocardial Infarction.

†Consider transport to primary PCI facility as destination hospital.

Figure 85. Fibrinolytic Checklist.[15]

Immediate General Treatment

Four agents are routinely recommended for immediate general treatment of patients with possible ischemic-type chest discomfort unless allergies or other contraindications exist:

- **Oxygen (If Spo_2 is less than 94% or patient is dyspneic)**
- **Aspirin** 160 to 325 mg
- **Nitroglycerin** sublingual or spray
- **Morphine** IV 2 to 4 mg if chest discomfort is unrelieved by nitrates

Immediate Discomfort Relief

Healthcare professionals must place a high priority on alleviating acute ischemic discomfort. Ischemic discomfort produces complex neurohumoral activation, which in turn induces a heightened catecholamine state. As a result, ischemic discomfort increases myocardial oxygen demand by accelerating heart rate, raising systolic blood pressure (SBP), and increasing contractility. This increased myocardial oxygen demand worsens existing ischemia and can lead to hemodynamic compromise.

Acute relief of discomfort will

- Reduce myocardial oxygen demand (morphine, nitrates, β-blockers)
- Attenuate the hyperactive catecholamine state (β-blockers)
- Reduce anxiety (morphine)

Oxygen

Many patients with AMI (up to 70% in the first 24 hours[30]) demonstrate hypoxemia because of either ventilation-perfusion mismatch or subclinical pulmonary edema from LV dysfunction. Experimental studies have shown that oxygen administration can reduce ST elevation in anterior infarction.[31,32] The effects of hypoxemia and respiratory insufficiency on a heart already compromised by coronary occlusion can be profound. Increased demand on a heart with marginal blood flow and oxygen supply–demand can lead to increased infarct size and cardiovascular collapse. It is difficult, however, to document the effects of oxygen on morbidity or mortality. A small, double-blind clinical trial in which investigators randomly assigned 200 patients to room air or oxygen by mask found no difference in mortality, incidence of arrhythmias, or use of pain medications. No clinical studies, including one prospective randomized controlled trial and a recent clinical trial evaluating hyperbaric oxygen, have shown a reduction in morbidity, mortality, or complications caused by arrhythmias with routine use of supplemental oxygen.

Oxygen should be administered to patients with breathlessness, signs of heart failure, shock, or an arterial oxyhemoglobin saturation less than 94%, or if the O_2 saturation is unknown. Providers should titrate therapy to 94% or higher based on noninvasive monitoring of oxyhemoglobin saturation. There is insufficient evidence to support the routine use of oxygen in uncomplicated ACS without signs of hypoxemia, heart failure, or both.

Aspirin

Administration of aspirin has been associated with reduced mortality in clinical trials, and multiple trials support the safety and efficacy of aspirin.[45-48] Unless a true aspirin allergy or a recent history of gastrointestinal bleeding is present, aspirin should be given to all patients with possible ACS.

A dose of 160 to 325 mg of non–enteric-coated aspirin causes immediate and near-total inhibition of thromboxane A_2 production by inhibiting platelet cyclooxygenase (COX-1). Platelets are one of the principal and earliest participants in thrombus formation. This rapid inhibition also reduces coronary reocclusion and other recurrent events independently and after fibrinolytic therapy. Platelet inhibitors are central to the prevention of acute stent thrombosis after placement in a coronary artery. Aspirin is absorbed better when chewed than when swallowed whole, particularly if morphine has been given. Use rectal suppositories (300 mg) for patients unable to chew or swallow oral aspirin and for patients with nausea or vomiting or with active peptic ulcer disease or other disorders of the upper gastrointestinal tract.

The importance of aspirin was demonstrated in early fibrinolytic trials. Aspirin alone reduced death caused by MI in the Second International Study of Infarct Survival (ISIS-2), and its effect was additive to the effect of streptokinase.[46] Clot lysis by fibrinolytics exposes free thrombin, a known platelet activator. Thus, an antiplatelet effect is needed when fibrinolytic agents are administered. Patients can develop a paradoxical procoagulable state with fibrinolytic therapy

Critical Concept **Discomfort Relief and STEMI**	Relief of discomfort is an important early goal for patients with STEMI or another ACS. Surges of catecholamines have been implicated in • Plaque fissuring • Thrombus propagation • Reduction in VF threshold

unless platelet aggregation is reduced. In a review of 145 trials involving aspirin, investigators from the Antiplatelet Trialists' Collaboration reported a reduction in vascular events from 14% to 10% in patients with AMI. In high-risk patients, aspirin reduced the incidence of nonfatal AMI by 30% and vascular death by 17%.[49]

Aspirin is contraindicated if patients have a history of true aspirin allergy, such as urticaria (hives) or systemic anaphylactic reaction. Patients with significant allergies or asthma may have an aspirin allergy—remember to ask!

Many patients will say they are allergic to aspirin when in fact they have had aspirin intolerance or a "side effect" in the past. That is, they may have had indigestion, nausea, or gastrointestinal upset. Although this may preclude aspirin use on a chronic basis or require the addition of another medicine to aspirin for gastrointestinal prophylaxis, it does not preclude the use of aspirin in this life-threatening situation. Carefully review the history and weigh the risks and benefits. In patients with a true aspirin allergy, substitute a 300 mg oral dose of clopidogrel for aspirin.

Oral aspirin is relatively contraindicated for

- Patients with nausea, vomiting, active peptic ulcer disease, or other disorders of the upper gastrointestinal tract
- Patients with a true aspirin allergy or recent GI bleeding
- Patients with bleeding disorders or severe hepatic disease

Nonsteroidal anti-inflammatory drugs (NSAIDs), except aspirin, both nonselective as well as COX-2–selective agents, are contraindicated and should not be administered during hospitalization for STEMI because of the increased risk of mortality, reinfarction, hypertension, heart failure, and myocardial rupture associated with their use.[50-52]

Nitroglycerin (or Glyceryl Trinitrate)

Nitroglycerin effectively reduces ischemic chest discomfort, and it has beneficial hemodynamic effects. The physiologic effects of nitrates cause reduction in left and right ventricular preload through peripheral arterial and venous dilation. Nitroglycerin is an endothelium-independent vasodilator of the coronary arteries (particularly in the region of plaque disruption), the peripheral arterial bed, and venous capacitance vessels. Nitroglycerin sublingual or spray is the initial drug of choice for ischemic chest discomfort.

Nitroglycerin has limited outcome benefits, and no conclusive evidence supports routine use of intravenous, oral, or topical nitrate therapy in patients with AMI.[53] Carefully consider use of these agents, especially when low blood pressure precludes the use of other agents shown to be effective in reducing morbidity and mortality (eg, angiotensin-converting enzyme [ACE] inhibitors).

- Use nitroglycerin as the first drug (before morphine) to help relieve ischemic chest discomfort.
- Use 1 tablet (0.3 to 0.4 mg) sublingually or spray 1 metered dose (0.4 mg) under or onto the tongue; repeat 2 times at 5-minute intervals for ongoing symptoms if permitted by medical control and no contraindications exist. Monitor clinical effects and blood pressure.
- In patients with recurrent ischemia, nitrates are indicated in the first 24 to 48 hours.
- **Recent phosphodiesterase inhibitor use.** Avoid the use of nitroglycerin if it is suspected or known that the patient has taken sildenafil or vardenafil within the previous 24 hours or tadalafil within 48 hours. Nitrates may cause severe hypotension refractory to vasopressor agents.
- **Hypotension, bradycardia, or tachycardia.** Avoid use of nitroglycerin in patients with hypotension (SBP less than 90 mm Hg), marked bradycardia (heart rate less than 50/min), or tachycardia in the absence of heart failure (heart rate more than 100/min).
- **Right ventricular (RV) infarction.** Use nitroglycerin with caution in patients with inferior wall MI with possible RV involvement. Patients with RV dysfunction and acute infarction are very dependent on maintenance of RV filling pressures to maintain cardiac output and blood pressure. If right-sided precordial leads or clinical findings by an experienced provider confirm the presence of RV infarction, nitroglycerin and other vasodilators (morphine) or volume-depleting drugs (diuretics) are contraindicated. Until a 12-lead ECG confirms ST elevation or new LBBB ACS, it is prudent to avoid the use of nitroglycerin in patients with borderline low blood pressure (SBP 100 mm Hg or less) or borderline sinus bradycardia (heart rate less than 60/min). Patients with excess vagal tone are unable to compensate when venodilation decreases blood pressure. Remember, cardiac output is the result of stroke volume and heart rate. If stroke volume falls because of decreased ventricular preload (caused by vasodilation), heart rate will be unable to compensate by increasing. Patients with a tachycardia may already be compensating (compensatory tachycardia) and unable to increase rate further. They also may become hypotensive.

Cardiac Output = Heart Rate × Stroke Volume

- Topical nitrates are acceptable alternatives for patients who require anti-anginal therapy but who are hemodynamically stable and do not have ongoing refractory ischemic symptoms. Avoid long-acting oral preparations, especially in patients who may become hemodynamically unstable. The topical nitrate preparation is absorbed into the dermal skin layers and may not be completely removed by wiping to stop action.

IV Nitroglycerin

IV nitroglycerin is not used *routinely* in patients with STEMI. A pooled analysis of more than 80 000 patients showed only a possible small effect of nitrates on mortality (odds reduction 7.7% to 7.4%). Do not administer IV nitroglycerin when it precludes the use of agents shown to have a greater treatment effect for STEMI (β-blockers, ACE inhibitors).

STEMI Indications for IV Nitrates

- Ongoing (after sublingual or spray) or recurrent ischemic discomfort
- Preferred agent for hypertension and ACS
- Adjunct to treat pulmonary congestion (CHF)

The same cautions and contraindications exist for intravenous and oral nitrates. When intravenous nitrates are given, take care to frequently assess the patient and titrate the dose to avoid complications of therapy in the setting of ACS. Drug-induced hypotension decreases coronary perfusion and microvascular flow and has the potential to increase ischemia.

- Check vital signs and heart rate for contraindications before starting and before each increase in dose.
- IV bolus: Use 12.5 to 25 mcg bolus (if no sublingual tablet or spray given).
- Infusion: Begin at 10 mcg/min. Titrate to response; increase by 10 mcg/min every 3 to 5 minutes until desired effect is achieved. A ceiling dose of 200 mcg/min is commonly used. This is the route of choice for emergencies.
- SBP generally should not be reduced to below 110 mm Hg in previously normotensive patients or 25% below the starting SBP in hypertensive patients.

Morphine Sulfate

Morphine is indicated in STEMI when chest discomfort is unresponsive to nitrates (Class I, LOE C). Morphine is an important treatment, particularly for STEMI, because complete coronary occlusion is often associated with a hyperadrenergic state. Surges of catecholamines have been implicated with plaque fissuring, thrombus propagation, and a reduction in VF threshold. Morphine has the following effects:

- Produces central nervous system analgesia, which reduces the harmful effects of neurohumoral activation, catecholamine release, and heightened myocardial oxygen demand
- Produces venodilation, which reduces LV preload and oxygen requirements
- Decreases systemic vascular resistance, thereby reducing LV afterload
- Helps redistribute blood volume in patients with acute pulmonary edema

Similar to nitroglycerin, morphine is a vasodilator and is not to be used in patients with suspected hypovolemia or inadequate right or left ventricular preload.

Dosing Recommendation

- STEMI: Give 2 to 4 mg IV; may give additional doses of 2 to 8 mg IV at 5-minute to 15-minute intervals.
- UA/NSTEMI: Give 1 to 5 mg IV only if symptoms are not relieved by nitrates or if symptoms recur.
- Avoid morphine in patients who are hypotensive and in patients with suspected hypovolemia.
- Morphine-induced hypotension is secondary to its vasodilatory properties; it most often develops in volume-depleted patients.
- If hypotension develops in a supine patient in the absence of pulmonary congestion, elevate the patient's legs and administer a normal saline bolus of 200 to 500 mL IV. Assess the patient frequently.
- The respiratory depression associated with morphine seldom presents a significant problem because the increased adrenergic state associated with infarction or pulmonary edema maintains respiratory drive.
  - If significant respiratory depression does occur, administer naloxone 0.4 to 4 mg IV at 3-minute intervals; titrate to reverse morphine-induced respiratory depression while maintaining pain control. If hypoventilation persists, consider other causes.

Prehospital Fibrinolysis

Clinical trials have shown that the greatest potential for myocardial salvage comes from initiation of fibrinolysis as soon as possible after the onset of ischemic-type chest discomfort. To reduce the time to treatment, a number of researchers have proposed and evaluated out-of-hospital administration of fibrinolytics. Physicians in the Grampian Region Early Anistreplase Trial (GREAT) administered fibrinolytic therapy to patients at home 130 minutes earlier than to patients at the hospital and reported both a 50% reduction in hospital mortality and greater 1-year and 5-year survival in those treated earlier.[18,54] A meta-analysis of multiple out-of-hospital fibrinolytic trials found a 17% relative improvement in outcome associated with out-of-hospital fibrinolytic therapy.[55] The greatest improvement was observed when therapy was initiated 60 to 90 minutes earlier than in the hospital. More recently, a meta-analysis evaluated time to therapy and impact of prehospital

Critical Concept **Morphine**	Use morphine with caution in patients with UA/NSTEMI because of its association with increased mortality.

fibrinolysis on all-cause mortality.[16] Analysis of pooled results from 6 randomized trials with more than 6000 patients showed a significant 58-minute reduction in time to drug administration. This time reduction was associated with decreased all-cause hospital mortality. These studies concluded that out-of-hospital–initiated fibrinolytic therapy can definitely shorten the time to fibrinolytic treatment. However, *these time savings can be offset whenever effective ED triage results in a door-to-needle time of 30 minutes or less, which obviates the need for implementation of special training and a rigorous out-of-hospital protocol*.

However, persistent delay to fibrinolysis (2½ to 3 hours) after symptom onset has led to a reexamination of prehospital bolus fibrinolytic therapy. More recent trials have continued to show a reduction in treatment time when fibrinolytics are administered before arrival at the hospital. The Assessment of the Safety and Efficacy of a New Thrombolytic Regimen trial (ASSENT III Plus) showed reduced treatment delay (40 to 45 minutes) but increased cerebral hemorrhage (in patients older than 75 years of age).[56] The Early Retavase–Thrombolysis in Myocardial Infarction (ER-TIMI 19) trial and the Comparison of Angioplasty and Prehospital Thrombolysis in Acute Myocardial Infarction (CAPTIM) trial evaluated prehospital fibrinolysis and demonstrated a consistent decrease in time to treatment.[57,58] In the CAPTIM trial, prehospital fibrinolysis was not inferior to primary angioplasty in patients who presented within 6 hours of onset of MI.

When prehospital personnel identify a patient with STEMI, it is appropriate for them to begin a fibrinolytic checklist when clinically indicated by protocol (Figure 85). If fibrinolysis is chosen for reperfusion, the goal is a door-to-needle time of less than 30 minutes, with effort focused on shortening the time to therapy. Patients treated within the first 70 minutes of onset of symptoms have a more than 50% reduction in infarct size and a 75% reduction in mortality rates.[59] It is also estimated that 65 lives will be saved per 1000 patients treated if fibrinolytics are provided in the first hour of onset of symptoms and a pooled total of 131 lives saved per 1000 patients treated if fibrinolytics are provided within the first 3 hours of onset of symptoms.[60]

Patients with STEMI who present at later times in the evolution of MI are much less likely to benefit from fibrinolysis. Fibrinolytic therapy is generally not recommended for patients presenting between 12 and 24 hours after onset of symptoms based on the results unless continuing ischemic discomfort is present with continuing ST-segment elevation. Fibrinolytic therapy should not be administered to patients who present more than 24 hours after the onset of symptoms.

Prehospital Fibrinolysis Program

It is strongly recommended that systems that administer fibrinolytics in the prehospital setting include the following features: (1) protocols that use fibrinolytic checklists, (2) 12-lead ECG acquisition and interpretation, (3) experience in advanced life support, (4) communication with the receiving institution, (5) medical director with training and experience in STEMI management, and (6) continuous quality improvement.

Reperfusion Therapies

Acute reperfusion therapy with primary PCI (PPCI) or fibrinolytic (mechanical or pharmacologic) therapy in patients with STEMI restores flow in the infarct-related artery, limits infarct size, and translates into an early mortality benefit that is sustained over the next decade. While optimal fibrinolysis restores normal coronary flow in 50% to 60% of patients, PPCI is able to achieve restored flow in more than 90% of patients (Figure 86). The patency rates achieved with PPCI translate into reduced mortality and reinfarction rates than with fibrinolytic therapy. This benefit is even greater in patients who present with cardiogenic shock. PPCI also results in a decreased risk of intracerebral hemorrhage (ICH) and stroke, which makes it the reperfusion strategy of choice in the elderly and those at risk for bleeding complications.

If PCI cannot be accomplished within 90 minutes of first medical contact, independent of the need for emergent transfer, then fibrinolysis is recommended, provided the patient lacks contraindications to such therapy. For those patients with a contraindication to fibrinolysis, PCI is recommended despite the delay. For those STEMI patients who present in shock, PCI is the preferred reperfusion treatment.

Destination Protocols

Prehospital Triage and Interfacility Transfer

Every community should have a written protocol that guides EMS system personnel as to where to take patients with

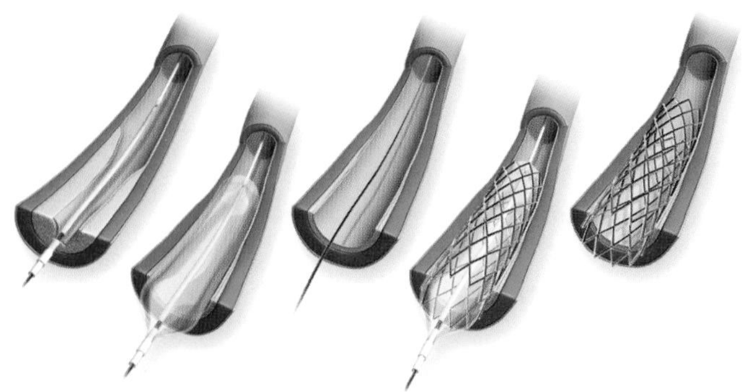

Figure 86. Progression of primary percutaneous coronary intervention with a stent placed in the artery.

possible STEMI. EMS transport directly to a PCI-capable hospital for primary PCI is the recommended triage strategy for patients with STEMI, ideally with a system goal of 90 minutes or less from first medical contact until PCI (Class I, LOE B).[61] In a large, historically controlled clinical trial, the mortality rate was significantly reduced (8.9% versus 1.9%) when transport time was *less than 30 minutes*.

Patients in cardiogenic shock or with a large MI with a high risk of dying should be taken primarily or transferred secondarily to a PCI facility. The goal for interfacility transfer is a door-to-departure time of 30 minutes or less.

Special Considerations

Patients in cardiogenic shock benefit from aggressive therapy, including intra-aortic balloon pump and percutaneous or surgical revascularization, when this can be accomplished within 36 hours of onset of MI and 18 hours from onset of shock.

Systems of Care

A well-organized approach to STEMI care requires integration of community, EMS, physician, and hospital resources. The most appropriate STEMI system of care starts "on the phone" with activation of EMS. Hospital-based components include ED protocols, activation of the cardiac catheterization laboratory, and admission to the coronary intensive care unit. In PCI-capable hospitals, an established "STEMI Alert" activation plan is critical. Continuous review and quality improvement with the involvement of EMS and prehospital care providers are important to achieve ongoing optimal reperfusion time.

Immediate ED Assessment and Treatment (Number 3, Figure 83)

Early evaluation and management in the ED emphasizes efficient, focused evaluation of the patient with ischemic chest discomfort. Ideally, within 10 minutes of ED arrival, providers should

- Obtain a targeted history and perform a physical exam while a monitor is attached to the patient
- Obtain a 12-lead ECG and establish IV access (if not done in the prehospital setting)
- Check vital signs and evaluate oxygen saturation
- Complete the fibrinolytic checklist and check for contraindications
- Obtain a blood sample to evaluate initial cardiac marker levels, electrolytes, and coagulation
- Obtain and review portable chest x-ray (less than 30 minutes after patient's arrival in ED), without delaying fibrinolytic therapy for STEMI

Unless allergies or contraindications exist, consider oxygen, aspirin, nitroglycerin, and morphine for treatment of patients with ischemic-type chest discomfort. Administer initial or supplemental doses as indicated, because these agents may have been given out-of-hospital.

The 4 D's of STEMI Survival

Time is muscle. Limitation of infarct size historically relied on early reperfusion therapy with fibrinolytic drugs. Goals were developed on the basis of the open artery hypothesis: open the infarct-related artery, restore perfusion to the myocardium, limit infarct size, and reduce death and complications of MI (eg, CHF). The 4 D's represent benchmarks and time goals in the reperfusion strategy: **D**oor, **D**ata, **D**ecision, and **D**rug. Potential delays during the in-hospital evaluation period may occur from door to data (ECG), data to decision, or decision to drug (or PCI). The door-to–drug administration goal is 30 minutes.[62] As PCI became available, the door-to-balloon goal became 90 minutes. According to the current ACC/AHA STEMI guidelines, primary PCI is the recommended method of reperfusion when it can be performed in a timely fashion by experienced operators (Class I, LOE A). In the absence of contraindications, fibrinolytic therapy should be given to patients with STEMI and onset of ischemic symptoms within the previous 12 hours when it is anticipated that primary PCI cannot be performed within 120 minutes of first medical contact (Class I, LOE A).[61]

Initial Risk Stratification

Part of the decision process is weighing the potential benefits of therapy against the risks (Table 25). In patients receiving fibrinolytic therapy, the major risk is ICH. There is an early hazard of fibrinolysis, and the mortality rate in patients treated with fibrinolysis is paradoxically higher during the first 24 hours after treatment. Although the risk of ICH is minimal with PCI, there are attendant risks associated with PCI, including hemorrhage and distal emboli.

Patients with ACS may receive a variety of treatments and evaluation strategies. In every case the physician must make a decision, weighing the risk versus the benefit for that patient. Evidence-based medicine can provide general data and recommendations for groups or types of patients, but the knowledgeable healthcare provider must in the end apply

Critical Concept Fibrinolytic Therapy	Results of cardiac markers, chest x-ray, and laboratory studies should not delay reperfusion therapy unless clinically necessary, eg, suspicion of aortic dissection or coagulopathy.

Critical Concept Routine Consultation	Routine consultation with a cardiologist is not necessary except in equivocal or uncertain cases because it delays therapy and is associated with increased hospital mortality rates.

these data at the bedside to a single patient. Some decisions are easy, such as the use of aspirin in ACS. Others require a careful evaluation of the benefits, risks, and potential complications of therapy. Patients may meet eligibility criteria for a therapy, but the benefit may be small compared with the risk. For example, a patient with a small inferior STEMI who presents relatively late may be within the treatment time window for fibrinolytics, but an increased risk of ICH may favor conservative therapy or transfer for primary PCI.

Pinto and colleagues have performed an analysis of the "PCI versus fibrinolysis" consideration in the STEMI patient.[63] Their report provides the emergency physician with a recommendation for the total elapsed time that he or she should wait for PCI, at which point the survival benefit of the invasive strategy decreases and the patient should receive a fibrinolytic agent. These times include the following:

- For patients presenting within 2 hours of symptom onset: 94 minutes
- For patients presenting beyond 2 hours of symptom onset: 190 minutes
- For patients less than 65 years of age: 71 minutes
- For patients more than 65 years of age: 155 minutes
- Anterior STEMI: 115 minutes
- Nonanterior STEMI: 112 minutes

Further analysis combined commonly encountered clinical variables in typical STEMI presentations, as follows:

- Patient presentation within 2 hours of symptom onset and
  - Anterior STEMI with age less than 65 years: 40 minutes
  - Anterior STEMI with age more than 65 years: 107 minutes
  - Nonanterior STEMI with age less than 65 years: 58 minutes
  - Nonanterior STEMI with age more than 65 years: 168 minutes
- Patient presentation beyond 2 hours of symptom onset and
  - Anterior STEMI with age less than 65 years: 43 minutes
  - Anterior STEMI with age more than 65 years: 148 minutes
  - Nonanterior STEMI with age less than 65 years: 103 minutes
  - Nonanterior STEMI with age more than 65 years: 179 minutes

Basic ECG Measurements

Healthcare providers who may evaluate acute chest discomfort should be familiar with the basic concepts of ECG measurements and intervals from rhythm analysis. The ST segment is the cornerstone of decision making in the initial triage of patients into the 3 treatment categories. STEMI is emphasized in the ACLS Provider Course because of the urgency of timely intervention. The majority of patients with ST-segment elevation will develop transmural or Q-wave MI unless an intervention or spontaneous reperfusion reopens the coronary artery.

Table 25. **ST-Segment Elevation or New or Presumably New LBBB: Evaluation for Reperfusion**

Step 1: Assess time and risk
Time since onset of symptoms Risk of STEMI Risk of fibrinolysis Time required to transport to skilled PCI catheterization suite
Step 2: Select reperfusion (fibrinolysis or invasive) strategy

If presentation <3 hours and no delay for PCI, then no preference for either strategy.
Fibrinolysis is generally preferred if
• Early presentation (≤3 hours from symptom onset)
• Invasive strategy is not an option (eg, lack of access to skilled PCI facility or difficult vascular access) or would be delayed
  – Medical contact-to-balloon or door-to-balloon time >90 minutes
  – (Door-to-balloon) minus (door-to-needle) is >1 hour
• No contraindications to fibrinolysis
An invasive strategy is generally preferred if
• Late presentation (symptom onset >3 hours ago)
• Skilled PCI facility available with surgical backup
• Medical contact-to-balloon or door-to-balloon time <90 minutes
• (Door-to-balloon) minus (door-to-needle) is <1 hour
• Contraindications to fibrinolysis, including increased risk of bleeding and ICH
• High risk from STEMI (CHF, Killip class ≥3)
• Diagnosis of STEMI is in doubt

Abbreviations: CHF, congestive heart failure; ICH, intracerebral hemorrhage; LBBB, left bundle branch block; PCI, percutaneous coronary intervention; STEMI, ST-segment elevation myocardial infarction.

Figures 87 and 88 demonstrate ST elevation.

Serial, Repeat, or Continuous 12-Lead ECGs?

If the initial ECG is nondiagnostic, serial ECGs are recommended. The clinician must determine the frequency of repeat ECGs but should perform at least 1 repeat ECG approximately 1 hour after the first. If the initial ECG is nondiagnostic but the patient is symptomatic and there is a high clinical suspicion for STEMI, obtain repeat ECGs at 5- to 10-minute intervals or initiate continuous 12-lead ST-segment monitoring.

Dynamic ECG Changes

Repeat or serial ECGs often show *dynamic 12-lead changes,* which means that the ST changes on the initial ECG normalize or a nondiagnostic initial ECG becomes abnormal. For example, ST elevation shown on an initial 12-lead ECG obtained in a satellite clinic or by EMS personnel in the field may be resolved minutes later on the ED ECG. One should base further management on the initial abnormal recording rather than on the normalized ECG.

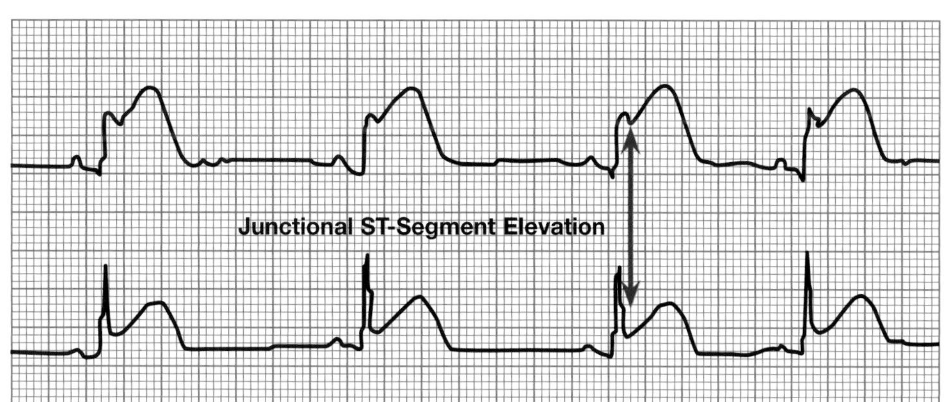

Figure 87. Leads III (top) and aVF (bottom) demonstrate significant ST-segment elevation typical of STEMI. In this instance, leads III and aVF are contiguous inferior leads. A 12-lead ECG is required to confirm an inferior MI.

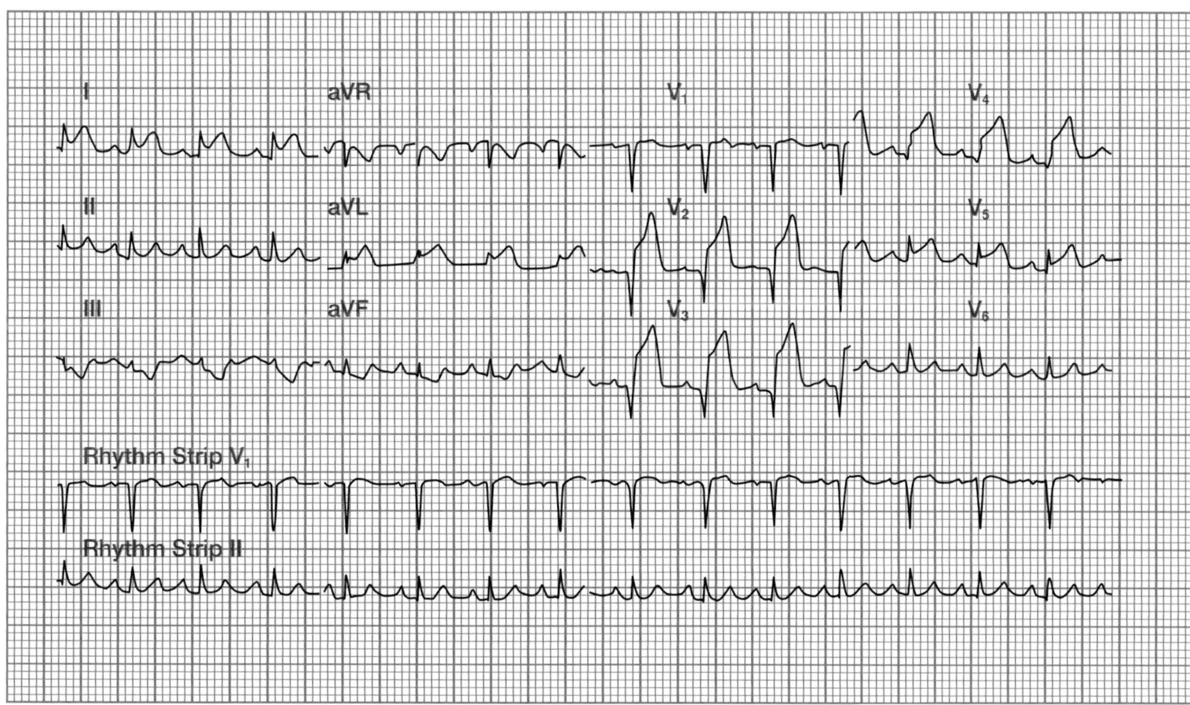

Figure 88. A 12-lead ECG demonstrating ST-segment elevation in anterior leads V_1 through V_5 and leads I and aVL, consistent with a large anterior wall MI. Note the "reciprocal" ST-segment depression in the inferior leads III and aVF.

New or Presumably New LBBB?

A *new* LBBB in the context of ischemic-like chest discomfort is an ominous event that indicates an occlusion in the left coronary artery system, usually above the septal branch of the left anterior descending artery. When an LBBB is present, the delayed LV depolarization of LBBB distorts the ST segment, which prevents accurate identification of ST elevation. Thus, the clinician operates without the ability to identify ST elevation. Because ST elevation has become the essential criterion for the use of fibrinolytics, its secondary repolarization change in patients with LBBB has posed difficulties in the many clinical trials of fibrinolytic therapy. In an excellent recent review of this problem, Kontos et al[64] observed that the fibrinolytic mega-trials were inconsistent and contradictory in regard to "new BBB." The trials used highly variable inclusion and exclusion criteria for chest discomfort patients presenting with "bundle branch block," "left bundle branch block," or "right bundle branch block."

Fibrinolytic trials have defined some changes in ECG morphology that increase the likelihood of MI in the presence of LBBB. However, in most cases, an experienced electrocardiographer is needed.

Determination of "New or Presumably New" Bundle Branch Block

This determination requires copies or reports of previous ECGs that may be difficult or impossible to obtain. This inability to determine whether the bundle branch block (BBB) is old or new forces the clinician to resort to unassisted clinical judgment and consideration of the benefits versus the risks of fibrinolytic therapy. In this clinical situation, most clinicians let the patient's account of symptom onset and the degree of severity weigh heavily in the final decision about therapy. The more the discomfort and associated signs and symptoms match with an acute ischemic event, the more likely the patient has a new BBB. In a recent, thoughtful decision analysis, Gallagher[65] compared outcomes from a treatment strategy based on criteria identified by Sgarbossa et al[66-68] with outcomes from a treatment strategy of simply giving fibrinolytics to all symptomatic patients with LBBB. The analysis intentionally ignored the question of "new versus old" BBB and concluded that fibrinolytic administration was appropriate for all patients with BBB and ischemic-like chest discomfort.[65]

New or Presumably New RBBB?

A new right bundle branch block (RBBB) is also associated with increased mortality when associated with AMI. Acute ST-segment changes are more readily identified with RBBB and should not be overlooked. RBBB obscures the terminal portion of the QRS complex; significant or new Q waves can also be identified. However, any BBB that obscures ST-segment evaluation in the setting of a high clinical suspicion of AMI may be an indication for reperfusion therapy. If fibrinolytic therapy is contraindicated, consider coronary angiography if suspicion remains high.

Cardiac Biomarkers in STEMI

Previously called "cardiac enzymes," cardiac biomarkers released from myocytes when they undergo necrosis are not used to identify patients with STEMI who are candidates for reperfusion therapy. In many patients, cardiac biomarkers are not elevated within the first several hours after onset of chest discomfort. They may take 6 to 8 hours to reach detectable levels. The clinical markers used today are mainly the creatine kinase subform found predominantly in the heart (CK-MB) and the cardiac-specific troponins (cTn; Figure 89).

Clinicians should take into account the timing of symptom onset and the sensitivity, precision, and institutional norms of the assay, as well as the release kinetics and clearance of the measured biomarker. If biomarkers are initially negative within 6 hours of symptom onset, it is recommended that their levels be measured again 6 to 12 hours after symptom onset.

There is insufficient evidence to support the use of troponin point-of-care testing (POCT) either in or out of hospital. There is also insufficient evidence to support the use of myoglobin, β-natriuretic peptide (BNP), N-terminal prohormone of brain natriuretic peptide (NT-proBNP), D-dimer, C-reactive protein, ischemia-modified albumin, pregnancy-associated plasma protein A (PAPP-A), or interleukin-6 in isolation.

STEMI: Adjunctive Therapy

Additional drug therapy may be appropriate after initial management and stabilization. Although adjunctive therapy applies generally to many patients, the selection of drugs—and sometimes doses—is individualized on the basis of management strategies, local protocols, and the clinician's patient and data assessments. The following is an overview and is not to be viewed as routine recommendations for patients with ACS or STEMI. In addition, this area is fluid, and clinical trials continue to evolve. There is no substitute for a knowledgeable physician applying these data to individual patients at the bedside.

Clopidogrel

Clopidogrel is an oral thienopyridine prodrug that irreversibly inhibits the adenosine diphosphate (ADP) receptor on the platelet, which results in a reduction in platelet aggregation through a different mechanism than aspirin. Several important clopidogrel studies have been published that document its efficacy for patients with both NSTEMI and STEMI. Approval was based on results of the Clopidogrel

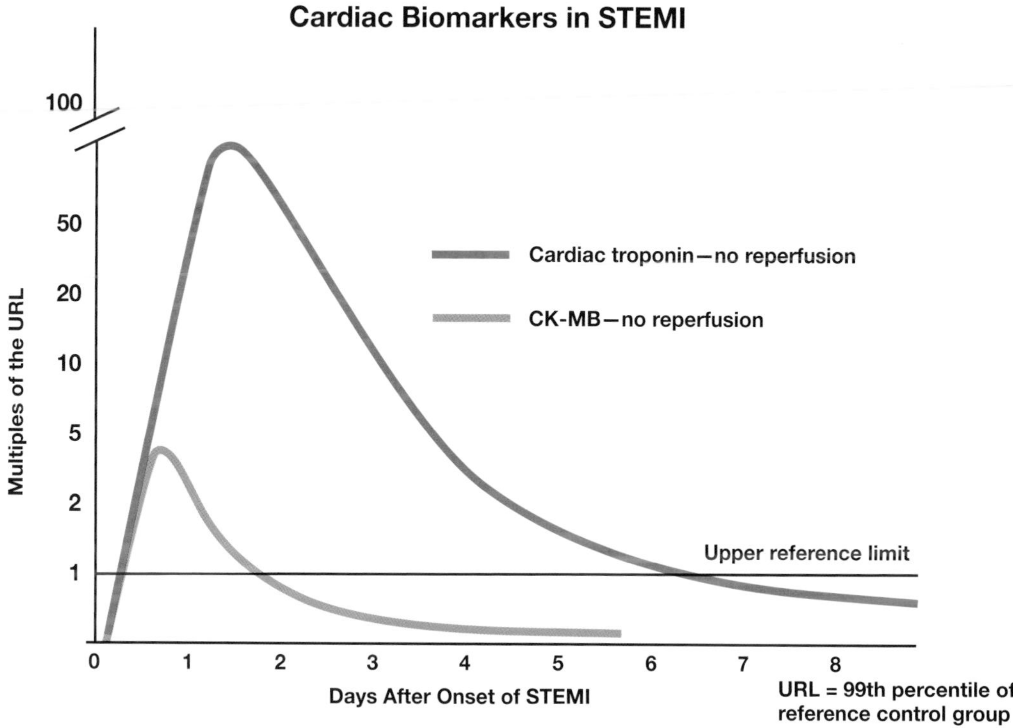

Figure 89. Cardiac biomarkers in STEMI. Typical cardiac biomarkers that are used to evaluate patients with STEMI include the MB isoenzyme of CK (CK-MB) and cardiac-specific troponins. The horizontal line depicts the upper reference limit (URL) for the cardiac biomarker in the clinical chemistry laboratory. The URL is that value that represents the 99th percentile of a reference control group without STEMI. The kinetics of release of CK-MB and cardiac troponin in patients who do not undergo reperfusion are shown. Adapted from Wu et al,[70] with permission of American Association for Clinical Chemistry, Inc. Permission conveyed through Copyright Clearance Center, Inc.

as Adjunctive Reperfusion Therapy (CLARITY-TIMI 28) and Clopidogrel in Unstable Angina to Prevent Recurrent Ischemic Events (CURE) trials, which demonstrated increased efficacy of dual therapy with aspirin with no increase in ICH.[71,72]

- Patients with ACS and a rise in cardiac biomarkers or ECG changes consistent with ischemia had reduced stroke and MACE if clopidogrel was added to aspirin and heparin within 4 hours of hospital presentation. Moreover, clopidogrel given 6 hours or more before elective PCI for patients with ACS without ST elevation reduced adverse ischemic events at 28 days.
- In patients up to 75 years of age with STEMI managed by fibrinolysis, a consistent improvement in combined event rate (cardiovascular mortality, nonfatal infarction, and nonfatal stroke) and/or mortality was observed when clopidogrel, in a 300 mg loading dose, was administered in addition to aspirin and heparin (low-molecular-weight heparin [LMWH] or unfractionated heparin [UFH]) at the time of initial management (followed by a 75 mg daily dose for up to 8 days in hospital). A small increase in major bleeding was also observed.
- In patients with STEMI managed with PCI, a reduction in combined event rate and/or mortality with a resultant small increase in major bleeding was observed when clopidogrel was administered by ED, hospital, or prehospital providers.
- The CURE trial documented an increased rate of bleeding (but not intracranial hemorrhage) in the 2072 patients undergoing CABG within 5 to 7 days of administration.[72] Although a post hoc analysis of this trial reported a trend toward life-threatening bleeding[73] and a prospective study failed to show increased bleeding in 1366 patients undergoing CABG,[74] a subsequent risk-to-benefit ratio analysis concluded that the bleeding risk with clopidogrel in patients undergoing CABG was modest. The use of clopidogrel in ACS patients with a high likelihood of needing CABG requires that the risk of bleeding if given be weighed against the potential for perioperative ACS events if withheld. The current ACC/AHA guidelines recommend withholding clopidogrel for 5 days in patients for whom CABG is anticipated.[61]

Dosing and Recommendation

- For patients with moderate- to-high-risk NSTEMI ACS and STEMI, providers should administer a loading dose of clopidogrel in addition to providing standard care (aspirin, anticoagulants, and reperfusion) (Class I, LOE A).
  - For patients less than 75 years of age, the loading dose is 300 to 600 mg, regardless of approach to management.
  - For ED patients up to 75 years of age with STEMI who receive aspirin, heparin, and fibrinolysis, administer a 300 mg oral dose.

Critical Concept Out-of-Hospital Administration of Clopidogrel	Providers should refrain from administration of clopidogrel out-of-hospital unless and until a treatment strategy and reperfusion status have been determined by an experienced physician, planned protocol, or PCI team. • Patients requiring urgent surgical intervention for complications of MI and left main or 3-vessel disease in shock should not receive clopidogrel. • Patients 75 years of age and older **should not** receive a loading dose (300 or 600 mg) of clopidogrel.

- The ideal dose of clopidogrel in patients over 75 years of age has yet to be delineated.

- A 300 mg oral dose of clopidogrel is reasonable for ED patients with suspected ACS (without ECG or cardiac marker changes) who are unable to take aspirin because of hypersensitivity or major gastrointestinal intolerance.

Prasugrel

Prasugrel is an oral thienopyridine prodrug that irreversibly binds to the ADP receptor to inhibit platelet aggregation. Prasugrel may be associated with a reduction in combined event rate (cardiovascular mortality, nonfatal infarction, and nonfatal stroke) with no benefit in mortality compared with clopidogrel but with an overall resultant increase in major bleeding (compared with clopidogrel) when administered after angiography to patients with NSTEMI undergoing PCI.[76-80]

- Risk factors associated with a higher rate of bleeding with prasugrel use are age 75 years, previous stroke or transient ischemic attack (TIA), and body weight less than 60 kg.
- Small improvements in combined event rate (cardiovascular mortality, nonfatal infarction, and nonfatal stroke) and/or mortality are observed when prasugrel (compared with clopidogrel) is administered before or after angiography to patients with NSTEMI and STEMI managed with PCI.[76-78,81,82]

Recommendations

- Prasugrel (60 mg oral loading dose followed by 10 mg maintenance dose) may be substituted for clopidogrel after angiography in patients who have been determined to have non–ST-segment elevation ACS or STEMI more than 12 hours after symptom onset before planned PCI.
- In patients who are not at high risk for bleeding, administration of prasugrel (60 mg oral loading dose) before angiography may be substituted for administration of clopidogrel in patients determined to have STEMI within 12 hours of onset of symptoms.
- Prasugrel is not recommended in STEMI patients managed with fibrinolysis or in NSTEMI patients before angiography.
- There is no direct evidence for the use of prasugrel in the ED or prehospital settings.

Ticagrelor

Ticagrelor is an alternative to clopidogrel for patients found to have NSTEMI or STEMI who are managed with an early invasive strategy.

β-Adrenergic Receptor Blockers

In-hospital administration of β-blockers may reduce the size of the infarct, the incidence of cardiac rupture, and mortality in patients who do not receive fibrinolytic therapy.[83-87] These data were largely observed during clinical trials before the "reperfusion era." β-Blockers also reduce the incidence of ventricular ectopy and fibrillation.[88] In patients who receive fibrinolytic agents, IV β-blockers decrease postinfarction ischemia and nonfatal AMI. A small but significant decrease in death and nonfatal infarction has been observed in patients treated with β-blockers very soon after the onset of symptoms.[89]

IV β-blockers may also be beneficial for NSTEMI; however, β-blockers increase the incidence of cardiogenic shock. Recent evidence shows no particular benefit to the IV administration of β-blockers on mortality, infarct size, prevention of arrhythmias, or reinfarction. There may be a short-term benefit to 6-week mortality when IV β-blockers are given to low-risk (ie, Killip class I) patients.[90] IV β-blockers are often administered in the ED on the basis of the results from the Metoprolol in Acute Myocardial Infarction (MIAMI) trial, but they are not "routine," and they require risk stratification. In the reperfusion era, early administration of β-blockers decreased recurrent ischemia but did not appear to confer a mortality benefit. IV β-blocker therapy is reasonable in specific situations, such as severe hypertension or tachyarrhythmias in patients without contraindications.

Oral β-blockers should be administered in the ED for ACS of all types unless contraindications are present. They should be given irrespective of the need for revascularization therapies. To assess modern use, the Clopidogrel and Metoprolol in Myocardial Infarction Trial (COMMIT CCS2) trial used the MIAMI dosing schedule, with 3 doses of metoprolol 5 mg IV administered over 15 minutes.[91] In this large trial, there was no benefit of early administration of IV β-blockers. An analysis of prespecified subgroups showed that approximately 10 lives per 1000 were saved by a reduction in VF, but this benefit was offset by an increase in patient death caused by cardiogenic shock. Lives lost because of cardiogenic shock increased with increasing Killip class, likely as a result of an increase in death from heart failure because LV dysfunction increases with infarct size. For this reason, careful attention should be given to treatment of patients with CHF. Tachycardia in these patients may be a compensatory response for impaired and decreased stroke volume caused by infarction (Figure 90).

Recommendations

- Initiate oral β-blockade within the first 24 hours in STEMI in the absence of
  - Signs of heart failure
  - Evidence of low-output state
  - Increased risk for cardiogenic shock
  - Other relative contraindications

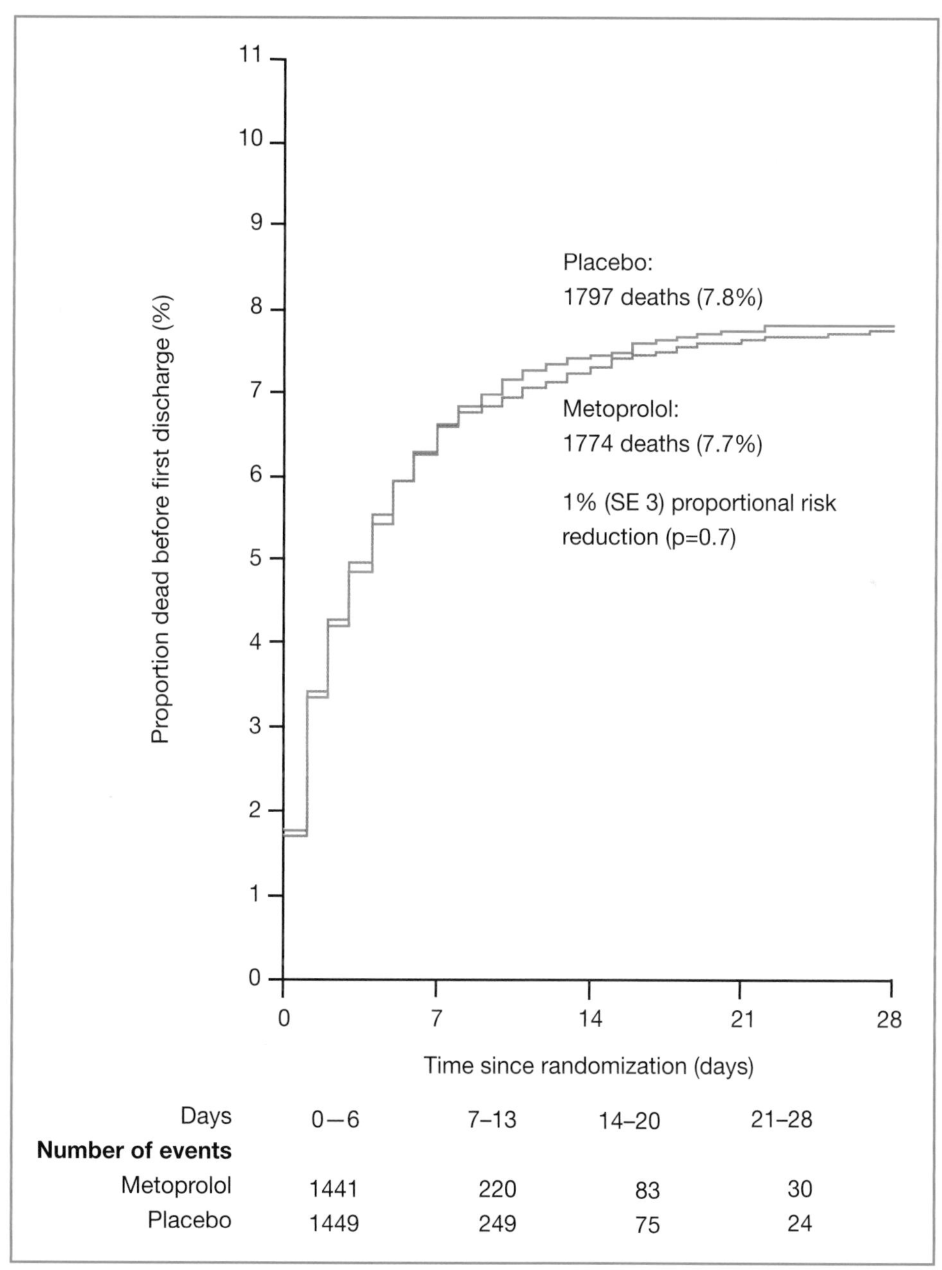

Days	0–6	7–13	14–20	21–28
Number of events				
Metoprolol	1441	220	83	30
Placebo	1449	249	75	24

Figure 90. Effects of metoprolol allocation on death before first discharge from hospital in the COMMIT CCS2 Trial. Reproduced from Chen et al,[91] with permission from Elsevier.

- Patients with early contraindication to β-blockade should be reevaluated for candidacy for secondary prevention before discharge.
- Patients with moderate to severe heart failure should receive β-blockade as secondary prevention with a gradual titration scheme.
- It is reasonable to administer IV β-blockade to patients who are *hypertensive* and who ***do not*** have
  - Signs of heart failure
  - Evidence of low-output state
  - Increased risk for cardiogenic shock
  - Other relative contraindications, such as PR interval more than 0.24 second or higher AV block, active asthma, or reactive airway disease
- There is little evidence that calcium channel blocking agents can be safely used as an alternative or additional therapy to β-blockers when the latter are contraindicated or their maximum dose has been achieved.

Contraindications to use of β-blockers are moderate to severe LV failure and pulmonary edema, bradycardia (heart rate less than 60/min), hypotension (SBP less than 100 mm Hg), signs of poor peripheral perfusion, second- or third-degree AV block, or reactive airway disease. In the presence of moderate or severe heart failure, oral β-blockers are preferred. They may need to be given in low and titrated doses after the patient is stabilized. This approach permits earlier administration of ACE inhibitors, which are documented to reduce 30-day mortality rates (see below).

Heparins

Heparin is an indirect inhibitor of thrombin that has been widely used in ACS as adjunctive therapy for fibrinolysis and in combination with aspirin and other platelet inhibitors for the treatment of non–ST-segment elevation ACS.

Unfractionated Heparin

UFH is a heterogeneous mixture of sulfated glycosaminoglycans with varying chain lengths. UFH has several disadvantages, including an unpredictable anticoagulant response in individual patients, the need for IV administration, and the requirement for frequent monitoring of the activated partial thromboplastin time (aPTT). Heparin can also stimulate platelet activation, causing thrombocytopenia. One benefit is that UFH can be readily reversed with protamine, a consideration in patients with a high risk for bleeding.

When UFH is used as adjunctive therapy with fibrin-specific thrombolytics in STEMI, the current recommendations call for a bolus dose of 60 units/kg followed by infusion at a rate of 12 units/kg per hour (a maximum bolus of 4000 units and infusion of 1000 units per hour). An aPTT of 50 to 70 seconds is considered optimal.

The duration of therapy is 48 hours. The available data do not suggest a benefit from prolonging an infusion of heparin beyond this time in the absence of continuing indications for anticoagulation.

Low-Molecular-Weight Heparin

LMWHs have been found to be superior to UFH in patients with STEMI in terms of overall grade of flow (Thrombolysis in Myocardial Infarction [TIMI] grade)[92,93] and reduction of the frequency of ischemic complications,[94] with a trend to a 14% reduction in mortality rates in a meta-analysis.[95] No superiority was found in studies in which an invasive strategy (PCI) was used.

Two randomized controlled trials have compared UFH with LMWH as ancillary treatment to fibrinolysis in the out-of-hospital setting.[56,96] Administration of LMWH for patients with STEMI showed superiority in composite end points compared with UFH, but this benefit must be balanced against the *increase in intracranial hemorrhage in patients more than 75 years of age* who received LMWH (enoxaparin).[56] Patients initially treated with enoxaparin should not be switched to UFH and vice versa to avoid increased risk of bleeding.

Treatment Recommendations

- There is insufficient evidence to provide a recommendation on bivalirudin for use in STEMI patients undergoing fibrinolysis.
- An LMWH, such as *enoxaparin*, is an acceptable alternative to UFH in the ED setting. Patients *less than 75 years of age* who are receiving fibrinolytic therapy may be treated with an initial bolus IV dose of 30 mg of enoxaparin followed by 1 mg/kg subcutaneously every 12 hours (first subcutaneous dose shortly after the IV bolus).
- Patients 75 years of age or older may be treated with enoxaparin 0.75 mg/kg subcutaneously every 12 hours without an initial IV bolus. Patients with impaired renal function (creatinine clearance less than 30 mL/min) may be given enoxaparin 1 mg/kg subcutaneously once daily. Patients with known impaired renal function may alternatively be managed with UFH.
- For patients with STEMI who are not receiving fibrinolysis or revascularization, LMWH (specifically enoxaparin) may be considered an acceptable alternative to UFH in the ED setting.
- For patients with STEMI undergoing PCI (ie, additional broad use of glycoprotein [GP] IIb/IIIa inhibitors and a thienopyridine), enoxaparin may be considered a safe and effective alternative to UFH.
- Although it is not an LMWH, hospital personnel may consider administering fondaparinux (initially 2.5 mg IV followed by 2.5 mg subcutaneously once daily) to patients treated specifically with non–fibrin-specific thrombolytics (ie, streptokinase), provided the creatinine is less than 3 mg/dL. Fondaparinux may be considered as an alternative to UFH for patients with STEMI undergoing PCI; however, there is an increased risk of catheter thrombi.

The use of heparin in ACS and as an adjunct to other treatments can increase major bleeding and cause mortality. Healthcare providers administering heparin should be familiar with its use in different ACS settings and strategies. The administration of heparin and other therapies should preferably be protocol driven. Providers need to be aware of recent trials and new guidelines and recommendations as they emerge. Table 26, reproduced from the *ECC Handbook,* can serve as a general reference.

ACE Inhibitor Therapy

In general, ACLS providers will not initiate ACE inhibitor therapy. ACE inhibitor therapy is usually started in the hospital when the patient is hemodynamically stable and after reperfusion therapy. Oral ACE inhibitors reduce fatal and nonfatal major cardiovascular events in STEMI patients. Their protective effects have been demonstrated independent of the use of other pharmacotherapies (eg, fibrinolytics, aspirin, and β-blockers).[97] Proof of an early benefit (within the first 24 hours) supports the prompt use of these agents in patients without exisiting contraindications (hypotension, shock, bilateral renal artery stenosis or history of worsening of renal function with ACE inhibitor/ ARB exposure, renal failure, or drug allergy.) The 2012 ACC/AHA STEMI guidelines recommend that ACE inhibitor be administered within the first 24 hours to all patients with STEMI with anterior location, heart failure, or ejection fraction less than or equal to 0.40, unless contraindicated (Class I, LOE A). ACE inhibitors are also reasonable for all other patients with STEMI and no contraindications to their use (Class IIa, LOE A).[61]

Table 26. Use of Heparin in ACS

Drug Therapy	Indications/Precautions	Adult Dosage
Heparin, Unfractionated (UFH) Concentrations range from 1000 to 40 000 units/mL	**Indications** • Adjuvant therapy in AMI. • Begin heparin with fibrin-specific lytics (eg, alteplase, reteplase, tenecteplase). **Precautions/Contraindications** • Same contraindications as for fibrinolytic therapy: active bleeding; recent intracranial, intraspinal, or eye surgery; severe hypertension; bleeding disorders; gastrointestinal bleeding. • Doses and laboratory targets appropriate when used with fibrinolytic therapy. • Do not use if platelet count is or falls below <100 000 or with history of heparin-induced thrombocytopenia. For these patients consider direct antithrombins. See bivalirudin on the next page.	**UFH IV Infusion—STEMI** • Initial bolus 60 units/kg (maximum bolus: 4000 units). • Continue 12 units/kg per hour, round to the nearest 50 units (maximum initial rate: 1000 units per hour). • Adjust to maintain aPTT 1.5 to 2 times the control values (50 to 70 seconds) for 48 hours or until angiography. • Check initial aPTT at 3 hours, then every 6 hours until stable, then daily. • Follow institutional heparin protocol. • Platelet count daily. **UFH IV Infusion—UA/NSTEMI** • Initial bolus 60 units/kg. Maximum: 4000 units. • 12 units/kg per hour. Maximum initial rate: 1000 units per hour. • Follow institutional protocol (see Heparin in ACS section).
Heparin, Low Molecular Weight (LMWH)	**Indications** For use in ACS, specifically patients with UA/NSTEMI. These drugs inhibit thrombin generation by factor Xa inhibition and also inhibit thrombin indirectly by formation of a complex with antithrombin III. These drugs are **not** neutralized by heparin-binding proteins. **Precautions** • Hemorrhage may complicate any therapy with LMWH. Contraindicated in presence of hypersensitivity to heparin or pork products or history of sensitivity to drug. Use **enoxaparin** with extreme caution in patients with type II heparin-induced thrombocytopenia. • Adjust dose for renal insufficiency. • Contraindicated if platelet count <100 000. For these patients consider direct antithrombins. **Heparin Reversal** ICH or life-threatening bleed: Administer protamine; refer to package insert.	**STEMI Protocol** • Enoxaparin — Age <75 years, normal creatinine clearance: initial bolus 30 mg IV with second bolus 15 minutes later of 1 mg/kg subcutaneously, repeat every 12 hours (maximum 100 mg/dose for first 2 doses). — Age ≥75 years: Eliminate initial IV bolus, give 0.75 mg/kg subcutaneously every 12 hours (maximum 75 mg/dose for first 2 doses). — If creatinine clearance <30 mL per minute, give 1 mg/kg subcutaneously every 24 hours. **UA/NSTEMI Protocol** • Enoxaparin: Loading dose 30 mg IV bolus. Maintenance dose 1 mg/kg subcutaneously every 12 hours. If creatinine clearance <30 mL per minute, give every 24 hours. • Bivalirudin: Bolus with 0.1 mg/kg IV; then begin infusion of 0.25 mg/kg per hour.

Abbreviations: ACS, acute coronary syndromes; AMI, acute myocardial infarction; aPTT, activated partial thromboplastin time; ICH, intracerebral hemorrhage; IV, intravenous; NSTEMI, non–ST-segment elevation myocardial infarction; STEMI, ST-segment elevation myocardial infarction; UA, unstable angina.

HMG-Coenzyme A Reductase Inhibitors (Statins)

A variety of studies document consistent reduction in incidence of MACE (reinfarction, recurrent angina, rehospitalization, stroke) when patients receive statin treatment within a few days after onset of an ACS.[98-101] There are few data to suggest that this therapy should be initiated in the ED, but early initiation of statin therapy (within 24 hours of presentation) is safe and feasible in patients with an ACS or AMI. If patients are already undergoing statin therapy, it should be continued. Healthcare providers should not discontinue statins during the index hospitalization unless contraindicated, to avoid short-term mortality and increased incidence of MACE.

Glucose-Insulin-Potassium

Although glucose-insulin-potassium (GIK) therapy was formerly thought to reduce the chance of mortality during AMI by several mechanisms, recent clinical trials found that GIK did not show any benefit in STEMI.[102] In a randomized controlled trial of 20 201 patients worldwide with STEMI who presented within 12 hours of symptoms, patients received either GIK intravenous infusion for 24 hours plus usual care or usual care alone. High-dose GIK infusion had a neutral effect on mortality, cardiac arrest, and cardiogenic shock in patients with acute STEMI. At this time there is little evidence to suggest that this intervention is helpful.

Therapy for Cardiac Arrhythmias

Treatment of ventricular arrhythmias during and after AMI has been a controversial topic for 2 decades. Primary VF accounts for the majority of early deaths during AMI. The incidence of primary VF is highest during the first 4 hours after onset of symptoms, but it remains an important contributor to mortality during the first 24 hours. Secondary VF that occurs in the setting of CHF or cardiogenic shock can also contribute to death caused by AMI. VF is a less common cause of death in the hospital with the early use of fibrinolytics in conjunction with β-blockers.

Although prophylaxis with lidocaine reduces the incidence of VF, an analysis of data from ISIS-3 and a meta-analysis suggests that lidocaine increased all-cause mortality rates.[68] For this reason the practice of prophylactic administration of lidocaine has been largely abandoned. Routine administration of magnesium to patients with MI has no significant clinical mortality benefit, particularly in patients receiving fibrinolytic therapy. The definitive studies on the subject are ISIS-4 and Magnesium in Coronaries (MAGIC).[53,103]

There are no conclusive data to support the use of amiodarone, lidocaine, or any particular strategy for prevention of VF recurrence after an episode of VF. Further management of ventricular rhythm disturbances is discussed in Chapters 8, 9, and 10 of this text.

Overview of UA/NSTEMI

This section discusses the patient with possible ischemic chest discomfort, UA/NSTEMI. Even though the underlying pathophysiologic process is usually similar to that of STEMI, these patients are managed differently. Initially the patient who presents with chest discomfort is rapidly evaluated for life-threatening causes of chest discomfort. This evaluation plus the 12-lead ECG is used for initial assessment of the probability of ACS and other life-threatening causes of chest discomfort. If the clinical probability of other causes of chest discomfort is low, then the ECG is used to place the patient into an initial diagnostic and treatment category. This category may change or develop with time as additional tests and serial patient assessments are made (Figures 77 and 78).

Chest Discomfort Suggestive of Ischemia

Clinicians should perform a targeted history and physical examination to aid in the diagnosis of ACS or to identify other causes of the patient's symptoms. Although the use of clinical signs and symptoms may increase suspicion of ACS, no single sign or combination of clinical signs and symptoms alone can confirm the diagnosis prospectively.[104-107]

The "Rule Out" Process

During evaluation of a patient with chest discomfort, the responsible clinician attempts to assess and estimate the probability of life-threatening problems in the differential diagnosis, but none of these life threats can be "ruled out" with absolute confidence during initial triage and evaluation. This fact underscores an important point: *Healthcare providers should focus on both risk stratification and continuing assessment and diagnosis during initial patient evaluation.* As the evaluation proceeds and an initial strategy is defined, the risks and benefits of testing and treatment are balanced against the probability and risk assessment of disease by use of clinical judgment and prudent assessment.

Healthcare providers initially use symptoms to estimate the likelihood of ACS and to assess the probability of other life-threatening causes of chest discomfort. A differential diagnosis is developed, and the probability of ACS and other life-threatening causes of chest discomfort is prioritized (Table 27).

Table 27. **Immediate Life-Threatening Causes of Chest Discomfort**

1. ACS
2. Aortic dissection
3. Pulmonary embolism
4. Pericardial effusion with acute tamponade
5. Tension pneumothorax

Definition of Angina and UA

Stable angina is a clinical syndrome usually characterized by deep, poorly localized chest discomfort. Stable angina is *reproducibly* associated with physical exertion or emotional stress and is *predictably* and promptly (within 5 minutes) relieved with rest or sublingual nitroglycerin. Patients learn through experience how much physical exertion they can perform before the symptoms of angina begin. They also learn how soon and to what degree rest or nitroglycerin relieves the discomfort.

UA is an acute process of myocardial ischemia of insufficient severity and duration to cause myocardial necrosis. Patients with UA are at risk for serious complications of ACS called major adverse cardiac events, or *MACE.* MACE usually includes death, nonfatal MI, or the need for urgent coronary intervention, such as PCI (angioplasty and/or stent) or surgical revascularization (CABG). In general these symptoms are caused by a change in a segment of an artery significantly involved with coronary arteriosclerosis, usually plaque rupture or erosion. Patients with UA typically do not present with ST-segment elevation on the ECG and do not release cardiac-specific biomarkers. Various terminology has been used in the past, originally when a change occurred in the predictable pattern of stable angina. These definitions have evolved over time, and UA now indicates a period (usually over days or hours) of increasing symptoms precipitated by less exertion or prolonged episodes with minimal or no exertion. There are 3 principal presentations of UA:

- **Rest angina:** Angina that occurs at rest, usually lasting less than 15 to 20 minutes.
- **Nocturnal angina:** Chest discomfort that awakens a patient at night.
- **Accelerating angina:** Angina that is distinctly more frequent, longer in duration, or lower in threshold. *Threshold* is the level of activity (or class of angina) that induces discomfort.

Angina and Myocardial Infarction

Angina—either stable or unstable—does not cause permanent myocardial damage, but if the reduction in blood flow is prolonged or complete, heart cells (called myocytes) die, which produces necrosis. When this happens, myocyte cellular membrane lysis releases internal cellular contents, which can be detected via serum cardiac markers. This process usually takes 20 to 30 minutes or longer. Cardiac markers of necrosis that are often measured clinically are CK-MB and cardiac troponins. In contrast to more nonspecific changes of ischemia, infarction usually causes characteristic ECG changes. Confirmation of the diagnosis of MI caused by ACS requires a positive biomarker and either clinical symptoms or pathological confirmation.

Classes of Angina

Angina can be graded according to the amount of physical activity that causes the pain[108]:

- **Class I:** Ordinary physical activity does not cause the angina. Pain requires strenuous, rapid, or prolonged exercise.
- **Class II:** Slight limitation of ordinary activity. Pain occurs on (1) walking or climbing stairs rapidly, walking uphill, climbing stairs after meals, or walking in the wind or cold, or (2) walking more than 2 blocks or climbing more than 1 flight of stairs at a normal pace.
- **Class III:** Marked limitation of ordinary physical activity. Pain occurs after walking 1 or 2 blocks on the level or climbing 1 or 2 flights of stairs at a normal pace.
- **Class IV:** Inability to perform any physical exertion.

Symptom Clues and Limitations

Approximately three quarters of patients with ACS—men and women—will present with chest discomfort. However, some presentations are "atypical," and patients do not have chest discomfort as the presenting symptom.

To aid in the assessment of chest discomfort and link the presentation to adverse events, Braunwald classified patients *without* STEMI into 3 risk groups based on the likelihood that their symptoms were ischemic in origin (Table 28).[108,109] Note that patients with an intermediate or

Critical Concept

Unstable Angina—Pattern for MACE

Unstable angina with a high likelihood of a MACE is best defined by an accelerating tempo of symptoms over a period of 24 to 48 hours:

- Symptoms increase in frequency or severity.
- Symptoms occur with less and less exertion.
- Symptoms occur at rest or awaken the patient at night.

high likelihood that symptoms are ischemic in origin have chest discomfort or left arm pain as a *chief* symptom. In high-risk patients, this pain reproduces prior anginal pain. Age older than 70 years, male sex, or diabetes mellitus also places a patient at intermediate risk. In men, premature coronary disease by definition occurs by age 55 (65 in women). Physical findings largely involve evidence of LV dysfunction (high risk) or evidence of other vascular disease, such as bruits (intermediate risk). ECG findings are grouped into degrees of ST-segment deviation (see "ST-Segment Deviation and Risk Stratification" later in this chapter).

Patients with atypical symptoms can be challenging, but adherence to an organized, evidence-based protocol makes the likelihood of a MACE very low. Clinical observation and research have identified several groups of patients who tend to experience an ACS in an "atypical" manner with "atypical" symptoms.

Women,[111-113] the elderly,[114] and insulin-dependent diabetics who develop ACS often do not present with the classic pattern of severe, crushing substernal chest pain or discomfort, nausea, diaphoresis, and pain radiating into the jaw, neck, or lateral aspect of the left arm (Table 29). In fact, many middle-aged men with ACS do not present with this pattern. For this reason the "typical" ACS symptom *complex* is not a particularly sensitive indicator for ACS. In a large study of all patients who presented to an ED with "typical" ischemic symptoms, only 54% developed an ACS. In addition, the patients who did develop an ACS described a variety of symptoms: 43% had burning or indigestion, 32% had a "chest ache," and 20% had "sharp" or "stabbing" pain; 42% could not provide specific descriptors of their pain. The pain was partially pleuritic in 12%.

The ACS symptom complex for women, the elderly, and diabetics may vary greatly. Chest discomfort or ache in itself may be minor. These patients may describe an ache or discomfort that may or may not be felt in the center of the chest but that seems to spread up to and across the shoulders, neck, arms, jaw, or back; between the shoulder blades; or into the epigastrium (upper left or right quadrant). The discomfort in the chest is less troublesome to the patient than the discomfort in the areas of radiation. This pattern of symptom localization *outside* the chest was found to be the most common atypical symptom of women evaluated in the Women's Ischemia Syndrome Evaluation (WISE) study. The patient may be bothered more by associated lightheadedness, fainting, sweating, nausea, or shortness of breath. This is another example of the dominance of symptoms outside the chest. A global feeling of distress, anxiety ("something is wrong" or "something is just not right"), or impending doom may be present.

Symptoms in Women

Women presenting with MI typically present approximately 1 hour later than men, in part because of the nature of the presenting symptoms in women, which include epigastric

Table 28. **Likelihood That Signs and Symptoms Represent ACS Secondary to Coronary Artery Disease**

Feature	**High Likelihood** *Any of the following:*	**Intermediate Likelihood** *Absence of high-likelihood features and presence of the following:*	**Low Likelihood** *Absence of high- or intermediate-likelihood features but may have the following:*
History	Chest or left arm pain or discomfort as chief symptom reproducing prior documented angina; known history of CAD including MI	Chest or left arm pain or discomfort as chief symptom; age >70 years; male sex; diabetes mellitus	Probable ischemic symptoms in absence of any intermediate-likelihood characteristics; recent cocaine use
Examination	Transient MR murmur, hypotension, diaphoresis, pulmonary edema, or rales	Extracardiac vascular disease	Chest discomfort reproduced by palpation
ECG	New or presumably new transient ST-segment deviation (≥1 mm) or T-wave inversion in multiple precordial leads	Fixed Q waves ST depression 0.5 to 1 mm or T-wave inversion >1 mm	T-wave flattening or inversion <1 mm in leads with dominant R waves; normal ECG
Cardiac Markers	Elevated cardiac TnI, TnT, or CK-MB	Normal	Normal

Abbreviations: CAD, coronary artery disease; CK-MB, MB fraction of creatine kinase; ECG, electrocardiogram; MI, myocardial infarction; MR, mitral regurgitation; TnI, troponin I; TnT, troponin T.

Modified from Braunwald et al.[110]

Table 29. Angina in Women and Men

	Women	Men
Presentation of CAD	Angina (65%)	ACS (63%)
Most common cause of angina	Noncardiac	CAD
Significant CAD	≤50%	80%
Follow-up	Increases with age	Plateau (55-65 y)

Abbreviations: ACS, acute coronary syndromes; CAD, coronary artery disease.

discomfort, shortness of breath, nausea, and fatigue. Several factors complicate evaluation of chest discomfort in women. Premenopausal women have a low likelihood of CAD and commonly present with typical angina. The low incidence of positive angiograms in these women has led to a perception that their chest discomfort is benign and *nonischemic*. This misperception leads to underassessment of women with chest discomfort, so women with chest discomfort are less likely than men to be tested and treated for CAD. There is also a misperception that the course of CAD in women is more benign than it is in men, but the prognosis of women with CAD is similar to that of men, and women often have more angina and disability than men. Atypical symptoms in women often include the following:

- More angina at rest, at night, or precipitated by mental rather than physical stress
- Shortness of breath, fatigue, palpitations, pre-syncope, sweating, nausea, or vomiting
- Atypical angina (in women with or without CAD)

Symptoms in Diabetic Patients

Diabetic patients may present without chest discomfort but with complaints of weakness, fatigue, or severe prostration. Anginal equivalents such as shortness of breath, syncope, and lightheadedness may be their only symptoms. In diabetics with neuropathy, these presentations have often been attributed to altered discomfort and neural perception.

Anginal Equivalents

Patients with ACS present with signs and symptoms that have been termed *ischemic equivalents* or *anginal equivalents*. It is important to note that these patients are *not* having atypical chest discomfort as described above. These patients seldom offer complaints of "discomfort" in the chest, below the sternum, or elsewhere, and the healthcare provider may not be able to elicit a report of such discomfort. Instead they may present with a symptom or sign that reflects the effects of the ischemia on LV function or electrical stability. Diabetic patients and the elderly are most likely to present with these symptoms. With advancing age, the elderly are more likely to present with diaphoresis. Some of the more common chest discomfort equivalent symptoms experienced by these ACS patients are

- Ischemic LV dysfunction: shortness of breath, dyspnea on exertion
- Ischemic arrhythmias: palpitations, lightheadedness or near-syncope with exercise, syncope

The most common signs of anginal equivalents are acute pulmonary edema or pulmonary congestion, cardiomegaly, and a third heart sound. Ventricular arrhythmias can cause symptoms in these patients. Ventricular extrasystoles, nonsustained VT, and symptomatic VT or VF have been documented. Ventricular ectopy that *increases* with activity (most benign ventricular premature contractions become suppressed at increased sinus rates) is suggestive of ischemia. Atrial fibrillation is uncommonly an ischemic presentation. In most cases an anginal equivalent is diagnosed retrospectively when some objective evidence of ischemia has been linked to the patient's symptom complex. For example, left arm discomfort alone may raise suspicion of ACS in the appropriate clinical setting, but it is ischemic in origin only when definitely associated with ACS or reproduced with functional testing.

Differential Diagnosis of Nonischemic Life-Threatening Chest Discomfort

The ACLS provider may encounter patients who present with many of the typical chest discomfort signs and symptoms reported by ACS patients but who are in fact experiencing another problem altogether. Some of these "ACS mimics" are relatively benign (eg, costochondritis or gastroesophageal reflux disease), but several are severe and life-threatening, and the ACLS provider must be able to identify them. There are numerous non-ACS causes of chest discomfort.

Aortic Dissection

Signs and Symptoms

Aortic dissection is rare compared with ACS. The incidence of aortic dissection has been estimated at 5 to 30 per 1 million people per year; approximately 4400 MIs occur per 1 million people per year.[115] Severe discomfort is the most common presenting symptom of aortic dissection. Untreated aortic dissection is a lethal disease; 25% of patients die in the first 24 hours and 75% in 2 weeks.

Risk factors for aortic dissection include hypertension (70% to 90% of patients), chest trauma, male sex, advancing age (usually sixth or seventh decade), bicuspid aortic valve, Marfan syndrome, aortitis, and cocaine use. Cardiac catheterization is the most common cause of iatrogenic aortic dissection.

The typical patient is a man in his 70s with a history of hypertension, a predisposing factor in 70% to 90% of patients. Although hypertension is a predisposing factor, it does not help in the differential diagnosis because many more patients with ACS have hypertension. Chest discomfort is the most frequent initial complaint caused by aortic dissection. The onset of the discomfort of aortic dissection is abrupt, and the discomfort is most severe at onset. Think *aortic dissection* when patients report sudden or abrupt discomfort that is most severe at the start, but remember that such discomfort neither confirms dissection nor rules out ACS.

The discomfort of aortic dissection may be migratory or may change in severity and location with time. The initial location of pain provides a valuable clue about the origin and extension of the dissection. This discomfort may be similar to that of ACS. In ascending and transverse aortic dissection, anterior chest discomfort is typical. Anterior chest discomfort also occurs in descending aortic dissection, but these patients also have more back and abdominal discomfort.

More often, though, the discomfort is described as sharp. Classically the discomfort of aortic dissection is described as "ripping" or "tearing" and migratory (as the dissection plane advances). The International Registry of Aortic Dissection has found a classic symptom complex in only a minority of patients. Tearing or ripping pain occurred in 50% of patients. Thirty-two percent of patients had a murmur of aortic regurgitation, and 15% had a pulse deficit.[116] Table 30 lists signs and symptoms of patients with acute aortic dissection.

12-Lead ECG in Aortic Dissection

The majority of patients will have nondiagnostic ECGs with nonspecific changes. Approximately 25% of patients will have LV hypertrophy on their ECG caused by a history of hypertension. ST-segment and T-wave changes that suggest ischemia are often secondary repolarization changes caused by LV hypertrophy as well, although ischemia with associated CAD cannot be excluded. In rare cases a patient will have ST-segment elevation. This elevation may be caused by compression of the origin of a coronary artery in the proximal aortic root, most often the right coronary artery. For this reason the ECG has little value in differentiating these 2 causes of chest discomfort. If the acute aortic dissection occludes a coronary artery, it will produce ECG changes that closely mimic the ECG changes of ACS.

Pulmonary Embolism

Pulmonary embolism (PE) is a life-threatening complication of venous thrombosis, usually of the lower extremities. PE occurs when microthrombi manage to evade the body's intrinsic fibrinolytic system, enlarge, eventually break loose, and travel to the right heart and into the pulmonary artery. Depending on the size and fragmentation of the thrombus, the patient can be asymptomatic or in cardiac arrest caused by acute right heart failure. An interruption in pulmonary blood flow produces effects both downstream (ventilation-perfusion mismatch, atelectasis, pain) and upstream (cor pulmonale, RV failure caused by pulmonary hypertension).[117] An international cooperative registry of PE, ICOPER (International Cooperative Pulmonary Embolism Registry), documented the serious nature of pulmonary thromboembolism, showing a 3-month mortality rate of 15%.[118] Among symptomatic patients with PE, the initial clinical presentation is sudden death in 25%.[119] Massive PE is rare, occurring in less than 5% of patients with PE, but 30-day mortality exceeds 50%.[120]

Signs and Symptoms

The symptoms and manifestations of PE are often nonspecific, and the differential diagnosis is extensive. The diagnosis is difficult, and both underdiagnosis and overdiagnosis occur. As with aortic dissection, the classic triad of PE (hemoptysis, shortness of breath, and pleuritic chest discomfort) has limited diagnostic value, because it occurs in fewer than 20% of confirmed cases. This symptom complex is usually observed with smaller emboli that migrate to the lung periphery and cause pulmonary infarction and pleuritis. A small effusion may be present on chest x-ray. Dyspnea is the most common presenting symptom, and tachypnea is the most frequent presenting sign. In the ICOPER study, 89% of patients were symptomatic and hemodynamically stable, and only 4% were unstable.[118] The only consistent finding in the majority of patients with PE is tachypnea, present in 96%. The most common signs and symptoms of PE are shortness of breath (82%), chest discomfort (49%), cough (20%), and hemoptysis (7%).

12-Lead ECG in PE

The ECG is nonspecific or nondiagnostic in patients with PE. It is useful in the sense that it may suggest alternative diagnoses. Tachycardia and nonspecific ST-T-wave changes are the most common finding. Because of RV pressure overload and acute failure, RBBB and atrial fibrillation were present in approximately 15% of patients in ICOPER.

Table 30. Presenting Symptoms and Physical Examination of Patients With Acute Aortic Dissection (N = 464)

Category	Present, No. Reported (%)	Type A,* No. (%)	Type B,* No. (%)	*P* Value, Type A vs B
Presenting symptoms				
Any pain reported	443/464 (95.5)	271 (93.8)	172 (98.3)	.02
Abrupt onset	379/447 (84.8)	234 (85.4)	145 (83.8)	.65
Chest pain	331/455 (72.7)	221 (78.9)	110 (62.9)	<.001
Anterior chest pain	262/430 (60.9)	191 (71.0)	71 (44.1)	<.001
Posterior chest pain	149/415 (35.9)	85 (32.8)	64 (41)	.09
Back pain	240/451 (53.2)	129 (46.6)	111 (63.8)	<.001
Abdominal pain	133/449 (29.6)	60 (21.6)	73 (42.7)	<.001
Severity of pain: severe or worst ever	346/382 (90.6)	211 (90.1)	135 (90)	NA
Quality of pain: sharp	174/270 (64.4)	103 (62)	71 (68.3)	NA
Quality of pain: tearing or ripping	135/267 (50.6)	78 (49.4)	57 (52.3)	NA
Radiating	127/449 (28.3)	75 (27.2)	52 (30.1)	.51
Migrating	74/446 (16.6)	41 (14.9)	33 (19.3)	.22
Syncope	42/447 (9.4)	35 (12.7)	7 (4.1)	.002
Physical examination findings				
Hemodynamics (n = 451)†				
Hypertensive (SBP ≥150 mm Hg)	221 (49.0)	99 (35.7)	122 (70.1)	<.001
Normotensive (SBP 100-149 mm Hg)	156 (34.6)	110 (39.7)	46 (26.4)	
Hypotensive (SBP <100 mm Hg)	36 (8.0)	32 (11.6)	4 (2.3)	
Shock or tamponade (SBP ≤80 mm Hg)	38 (8.4)	36 (13.0)	2 (1.5)	
Auscultated murmur of aortic insufficiency	137/434 (31.6)	117 (44)	20 (12)	<.001
Pulse deficit	69/457 (15.1)	53 (18.7)	16 (9.2)	.006
Cerebrovascular accident	21/447 (4.7)	17 (6.1)	4 (2.3)	.07
Congestive heart failure	29/440 (6.6)	24 (8.8)	5 (3.0)	.02

Abbreviations: NA, not applicable; SBP, systolic blood pressure.

*Type A dissections involve the aorta; type B dissections occur distal to the left subclavian artery.

†Systolic blood pressure is reported for 277 patients with type A and 174 patients with type B acute aortic dissection.

Reprinted from Hagan et al.[116]

Why Are Troponins Positive in Some Patients With PE?

During the course of evaluation for ACS, patients have been identified with elevated cardiac markers but negative coronary angiograms. Investigation has found that troponins and occasionally CK-MB (the MB isoenzyme of creatine kinase) will elevate with PE. This finding correlates with a large PE and RV dysfunction. The acute increase in RV afterload imposed by submassive and massive PE causes right heart ischemia that can lead to subendocardial infarction.

Primary fibrinolytic therapy with tissue plasminogen activator for massive PE in a patient who presents with arterial hypotension is approved by the FDA. However, this therapy remains controversial because there are few randomized trials and because

- The risk of intracranial hemorrhage may be as high as 3%.[121]
- Although the therapy may be lifesaving, the extent of clinical benefit (risk-benefit) remains unclear.[120]

What Can Early Recognition and Triage by ACLS Providers Do to Improve Outcome Beyond Traditional Therapy (Heparin)?

Risk stratification with echocardiography has now been introduced for patients with PE. Clinically, approximately 5% of patients with PE present in shock and are candidates for fibrinolytic therapy or mechanical fragmentation techniques where available. Approximately 40% of patients with PE have RV dysfunction demonstrated by transthoracic echocardiography. This RV dysfunction is manifest as RV hypokinesis of variable degrees and normal arterial pressure. Some studies have shown that fibrinolytic therapy can rapidly improve RV function and lower the incidence of recurrent PE. Treatment of these patients is currently controversial, but most experts will seriously weigh the risks and benefits of the treatment options if hemodynamics are borderline or tenuous cardiopulmonary comorbidity exists. At the very least, the finding of RV dysfunction alerts the provider to pay close attention to anticoagulation parameters and adjunctive therapy.

For a complete discussion of the diagnosis and management of deep venous thrombosis and PE, see "Acute Pulmonary Embolism," parts I and II, in *Circulation.*[122,123]

Pericarditis With Acute Tamponade

This disease complex is often confused with ACS because it produces discomfort and ECG abnormalities that can be similar to those caused by ACS.[124] It is important to differentiate pericarditis from ACS because administration of fibrinolytics to patients with pericarditis can produce fatal hemorrhage because of the ease with which the inflamed pericardium can bleed. Heparin is also contraindicated except in a special form of postinfarction focal pericarditis. Cardiac tamponade refers to the hemodynamic effects of fluid accumulation in the pericardial sac. The most common causes of pericardial effusions with tamponade are pericarditis, malignancy, uremia associated with renal failure, aortic dissection, and tuberculosis (in areas where it is endemic).[125] Hemopericardium is increasing in frequency, and tuberculous effusions are rare in developed countries.

The pericardial complex around the heart comprises the outer fibrous pericardium and a thin serous layer that adheres to the surface of the heart. Because of the close proximity of the serous pericardium to the heart, most instances of pericarditis are actually myopericarditis. This can further confuse the diagnosis because the myopericarditis may produce elevation of cardiac markers. A potential space exists between the fibrous and serous pericardial layers. Normally the space contains approximately 20 mL of plasma-like fluid. It can accommodate roughly 120 mL before pericardial pressure increases. If fluid accumulation continues, the pericardial pressure can rise sharply. This increased pressure results in a significant decrease in cardiac output and blood pressure. However, it is the *rate* of accumulation rather than the absolute *volume* that is most important. Acute effusions, including hemopericardium from penetrating trauma, occur rapidly and can produce rapid decompensation. Cardiac rupture of the LV after AMI also causes immediate fatal hemopericardium. The patient usually presents with a sudden onset of pulseless electrical activity. Survival is rare even with immediate pericardiocentesis and cardiac surgery.

RV perforation can occur after temporary pacer placement, pulmonary artery catheter insertion, and RV biopsy. RV pressures are lower than LV pressures, so survival after RV perforation is possible with prompt recognition and drainage. Previously, idiopathic pericarditis was considered the primary cause of pericardial effusion and tamponade, but with the recent increase in the number of cardiology interventions performed, the provider who is monitoring these in-hospital patients must be able to detect and treat pericardial effusion as a potential complication of cardiac catheterization. Small guidewires are used to track angioplasty balloons for dilation and stent placement. Microperforation of a coronary artery or dissection of the vessel may present with delayed tamponade after patients leave the catheterization suite, particularly if platelet inhibitors are administered after the procedure.

Signs and Symptoms

Chest discomfort is the most frequent symptom of acute pericarditis.[126] Patients may describe pericarditis with the same terms used to describe ACS. Patients will describe the discomfort as sharp or stabbing. The pain is localized in the middle of the chest or below the sternum. Onset may be sudden or gradual. The discomfort may radiate to the back, neck, left arm, or left shoulder. Inspiration or movement can aggravate the discomfort. This is called a respirophasic component. A unique feature of pericardial discomfort is that it typically increases when the patient lies supine and decreases when the patient sits and leans forward. This is believed to occur because the diaphragmatic surface of the pericardium is richly innervated. When the patient lies supine, the diaphragmatic surface of the heart comes into contact with this pericardial segment,

Critical Concept **Troponin and PE**	Consider the possibility of PE if the patient has normal coronary angiograms and elevated levels of troponin.

which creates more discomfort. Patients often have fever (low-grade or intermittent), shortness of breath, cough, or painful swallowing. Patients with tuberculous pericarditis commonly have the fever, night sweats, and weight loss of tuberculosis infection.

A *pericardial friction rub* is present in approximately half of all patients with pericarditis. The character of the rub often changes from one hour to the next, from heartbeat to heartbeat, and with changes in position. Many clinicians describe it as sounding like footsteps in crunchy snow or sandpaper rubbed together. It is loudest along the lower left border of the sternum and at the apex of the heart. The rub is best heard when the patient sits and leans forward or assumes the "hands-and-knees" position, bringing the anterior epicardium into contact with the inflamed pericardial segment. Patients may have occasional premature atrial or ventricular beats, tachypnea and dyspnea, ascites, or hepatomegaly.

Cardiac Tamponade

As fluid accumulates in the pericardial sac, the patient may develop dyspnea, easy fatigue, anxiety, and other signs of hemodynamic compromise. The volume of fluid, the rate of fluid accumulation, and the compliance of the pericardial sac all affect the onset and severity of clinical consequences. Rapid or substantial fluid accumulation or a constrictive pericardium will produce more acute cardiovascular deterioration than gradual fluid accumulation in the presence of a distensible pericardial sac.

Very few patients with pericardial tamponade demonstrate the 3 symptoms associated with tamponade that are known as *Beck's triad:* jugular venous distention, hypotension, and muffled or distant heart sounds. The finding of clear lungs, hypotension, and jugular venous distention alerts trauma teams to the possible presence of traumatic hemopericardium with effusion.

Pulsus paradoxus is commonly present with tamponade. Pulsus paradoxus is a fall in SBP of 8 to 10 mm Hg or more during spontaneous inspiration. A fall in SBP of more than 10 mm Hg is significant.[126] However, providers need to know that acute airway disorders—rather than tamponade—are the most common causes of pulsus paradoxus. The name itself, *paradoxus,* is a misnomer. The pulse is actually not a paradox but an accentuation of the normal fall in SBP with inspiration. The difference is that the normal fall is not more than 10 mm Hg.

12-Lead ECG in Pericardial Tamponade

The 12-lead ECG can yield pathognomonic findings in both pericarditis and ACS. Four stages of ECG findings have been reported to occur in pericarditis, but all 4 stages occur in only approximately half of involved patients. The clinical clue involves the finding of ST-segment elevation in multiple leads, in contrast to the regional elevation observed in acute coronary artery occlusion in STEMI. When combined with depression of the PR interval, the ECG is highly suggestive of acute pericarditis. It is important to remember that pericarditis and pericardial effusion may present with nonspecific ECG changes. Echocardiography can be a useful bedside tool to aid in the diagnosis, especially in the ED. In addition, ACS can mimic pericarditis and vice versa. Electrical alternans is an ECG finding that can alert the physician to a diagnosis of pericardial effusion. The 4 stages of pericarditis are

- Stage 1: ST-segment elevation with ST segments that are upwardly concave. This stage occurs within hours of the onset of pericarditis-associated chest discomfort. The elevation is frequently noted in all leads except V_1. ST-segment elevation may last several days.
- Stage 2: T waves flatten as the ST elevation returns to baseline.
- Stage 3: T waves become inverted, but Q waves do not form.
- Stage 4: The ECG gradually returns to normal.

The amplitude (voltage) of each ECG complex (the P wave, QRS, and T wave) alternates from complex to complex. This pattern is caused by motion of the heart toward and away from the precordial leads. The motion is exacerbated by the large effusion. The heart "bobs" in the fluid, similar to a boat bobbing on the water.

Tension Pneumothorax

An injury to the lung parenchyma or a bronchus that produces an air leak can cause a tension pneumothorax (Figure 91). When a tension pneumothorax develops, air accumulates in the chest and pressure in the pleural space increases, which compresses the lung on the involved side and pushes the heart and mediastinum to the opposite side. The mediastinum can compress the opposite lung, which causes collapse and worsening hypoxia. The pneumothorax compresses the heart and great vessels, which impedes venous return and cardiac output. Hypotension and hypoxia can combine to produce hemodynamic collapse, shock, and death.

A pneumothorax can be primary or secondary. A primary pneumothorax is also called a spontaneous pneumothorax; it rarely causes tension pneumothorax, although it can cause acute chest discomfort.

Clinical circumstances raise suspicion of a tension pneumothorax in certain patient groups. These include patients with a recently inserted central venous catheter; those who have had any recent diagnostic procedure in the chest, lower

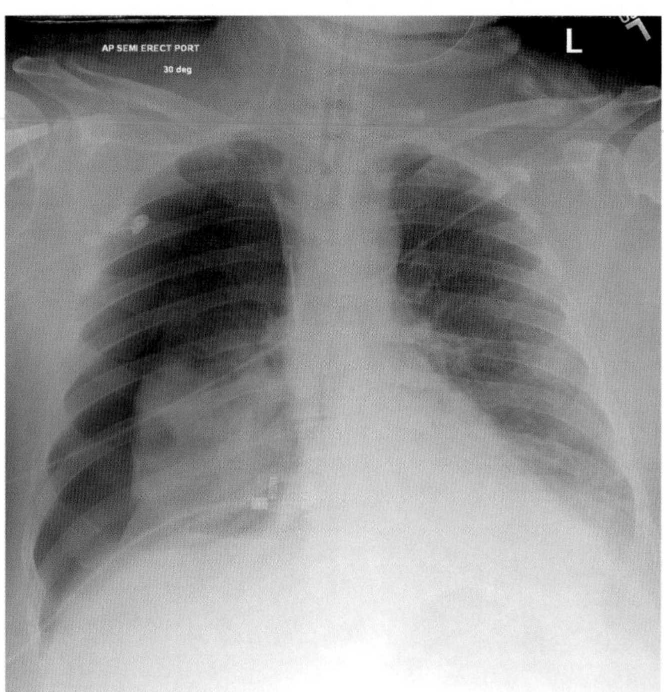

Figure 91. Tension pneumothorax (right lung).

neck, or upper abdomen; ventilated patients with underlying pulmonary disease or high peak inspiratory airway pressures; and patients with chest or multisystem trauma. Tension pneumothorax may also follow removal of chest tubes.

Signs and Symptoms

Shortness of breath, which may progress in some patients to acute respiratory distress, is the most common presenting symptom. The classic signs of tension pneumothorax are

- Decreased breath sounds, decreased chest expansion, and hyperresonance on the involved side
- Hypoxemia

The diagnosis of a tension pneumothorax is a clinical, not a radiographic, diagnosis. The ACLS provider should not wait to obtain a chest radiograph to make the diagnosis. The following clinical signs and symptoms of extreme compromise in cardiopulmonary function indicate the need for empiric needle decompression:

- Lung sounds that are decreased or even absent on one side
- Hypotension
- Respiratory distress or arrest
- Cyanosis
- Jugular vein distention
- Pulsus paradoxus
- Tracheal deviation (a very late finding)

12-Lead ECG in Tension Pneumothorax

The 12-lead ECG is nonspecific, and tachycardia is the most common finding. Depending on whether a right or left pneumothorax has developed, clockwise or counterclockwise rotation of the electrical axis occurs as the heart is repositioned in the thorax.

Risk Stratification: Matching the Right Patient, the Right Therapy, at the Right Time: ECG and Troponin

Once a patient is thought to have an intermediate or high probability that chest discomfort is likely caused by CAD (Table 28), a second question is asked. This involves estimation of the probability that a MACE will occur. These events include death, nonfatal MI, and urgent need for coronary revascularization (Table 31).

Clinical indicators of high risk include an accelerating tempo of symptoms, such as occurrence with less exertion or at rest and prolonged episodes of pain or discomfort. Again, any evidence of LV dysfunction or worsening LV failure is serious. An elevated biomarker separates NSTEMI from UA and has incremental value in addition to the ECG.

ST-Segment Deviation and Risk Stratification

The ECG is not a perfect test for myocardial ischemia or infarction and has limitations. Cardiac ischemia is identified when horizontal ST-segment depression is present. In the past, consensus limits of ST-segment deviation were based on clinical data or trials with thresholds established to obtain adequate sensitivity (to detect patients with disease) and specificity (to identify patients who likely do not have the disease and will not benefit from therapy).

Measurement of ST-Segment Deviation

ST-segment depression often represents ischemia, and 1 mm of horizontal (flat) depression that persists for 0.08 second after the J point is used to define this abnormality in exercise stress testing. Some clinical ACS trials have used earlier measurements (0.02 second after the J point) to increase sensitivity. Compared with these ACS trials, others have used later measurements (0.06 second after the J point) to increase specificity. Clinical algorithms for acute chest discomfort in ACS have used ST-segment depression measured 0.04 second after the J point as representative and easy to measure (it is 1 horizontal small box on the ECG).

Clinical trials have found that 0.5 mm of ST depression is as predictive as 1 mm. Although this 0.5-mm ST-segment deviation threshold has not been subjected to the ECC

Table 31. Risk of Death or Nonfatal MI Over the Short Term in Patients With Chest Pain With High or Intermediate Likelihood of Ischemia*

	High Risk *Risk is high if patient has any of the following findings:*	**Intermediate Risk** *Risk is intermediate if patient has any of the following findings:*	**Low Risk** *Risk is low if patient has NO high- or intermediate-risk features; may have any of the following:*
History	• Accelerating tempo of ischemic symptoms over prior 48 hours	• Prior MI *or* • Peripheral artery disease *or* • Cerebrovascular disease *or* • CABG, prior aspirin use	
Character of Pain	• Prolonged, continuing (>20 min) rest pain	• Prolonged (>20 min) rest angina is now resolved (moderate to high likelihood of CAD) • Rest angina (<20 min) or relieved by rest or sublingual nitrates	• New-onset functional angina (Class III or IV) in past 2 weeks without prolonged rest pain (but with moderate or high likelihood of CAD)
Physical Exam	• Pulmonary edema secondary to ischemia • New or worse mitral regurgitation murmur • Hypotension, bradycardia, tachycardia • S_3 gallop or new or worsening rales • Age >75 years	• Age >70 years	
ECG	• Transient ST-segment deviation (≥0.5 mm) with rest angina • New or presumably new bundle branch block • Sustained VT	• T-wave inversion ≥2 mm • Pathologic Q waves or T waves that are not new	• Normal or unchanged ECG during an episode of chest discomfort
Cardiac Markers	• Elevated cardiac troponin I or T • Elevated CK-MB	*Any of the above findings PLUS* • Normal	• Normal

Abbreviations: CABG, coronary artery bypass grafting; CAD, coronary artery disease; CK-MB, MB fraction of creatine kinase; ECG, electrocardiogram; MI, myocardial infarction; VT, ventricular tachycardia.

*See columns A and B in Table 28 for definitions of high and intermediate likelihood of ischemia.

Modified from Braunwald et al.[110]

evidence evaluation process, it is the threshold recommended in the ACC/AHA guidelines[108] and the ACC/AHA guidelines update,[110] and the material in this text has been changed to reflect this threshold. Measurements of this small magnitude and ischemic characterization (horizontal flat depression) require careful review and interpretation by experienced ECG readers.

Dynamic T-Wave Changes

T waves may normally be inverted in lead III (and occasionally in lead II), and these T waves are often incorrectly interpreted as indicating ischemia. T-wave inversions that do reflect ischemia involve a widening of the normal QRS axis and T-wave vector for an individual ECG. This change occurs with ischemia and may also be associated with a prolonged corrected QT (QTc) interval. This diagnosis may be difficult for pattern ECG readers to make. But remember that T waves are normally upright in the leads that have dominant R waves (more of the QRS above baseline than below it). T-wave abnormalities may be difficult to identify unless a previous tracing is available for comparison. In outcome studies of ACS, T-wave abnormalities alone are not helpful in diagnosis or prognosis.

T-wave inversion is a nonspecific finding on the ECG. The mean QRS vector and the mean T-wave vector are related and called the QRS-T angle (normally approximately 45 to 60 degrees). In pattern recognition terms, this results in T waves that are upright in leads with predominantly upright or "dominant" R waves (2 mm or greater) and inverted in other leads.

- Ischemia causes a widening of the QRS-T angle. In pattern recognition terms, this causes T-wave inversion in leads with dominant R waves.
- This T-wave inversion is nonspecific with other causes.
- If dynamic T-wave inversion occurs and is associated with symptoms, it is strongly suggestive of ischemia.

Ischemic ST-segment depression more than 0.5 mm (0.05 mV) or dynamic T-wave inversion with pain or discomfort (Number 9 of the algorithm) is classified as UA/NSTEMI. Nonpersistent or transient ST-segment elevation of 0.5 mm or more for less than 20 minutes is also included in this category. Threshold values for ST-segment depression consistent with ischemia are J-point depression of 0.05 mV (–0.5 mm) in leads V_2 and V_3 and –0.1 mV (–1 mm) in all other leads (men and women).

Dynamic T-wave changes are important indicators of ischemia in patients with acute chest discomfort. In such patients the finding of widening of the angle between the QRS axis and the T-wave axis and resolution of this abnormality with rest or nitroglycerin are indicative of ischemia. To detect these dynamic changes, you must obtain an ECG *before* administration of nitroglycerin in patients with suspected ACS. Typical response to nitrates (in several minutes) is suggestive but not diagnostic of cardiac ischemia. If you fail to obtain an ECG tracing when the patient is in discomfort and a repeat ECG after resolution of the discomfort, you may miss a diagnostic abnormality and opportunity. T waves suggestive of ischemia are defined in the ACC/AHA guidelines.[108] Inverted T waves that are 2 mm or more in leads with dominant R waves are suggestive of ischemia and indicative of a widened QRS-T angle.

Nondiagnostic and Normal ECGs

Cardiologists vary in their criteria for diagnosis of nonspecific ST-segment and T-wave changes. Also, criteria may differ for some clinical situations. For example, ST-segment deviation in ACS is measured 0.04 second after the J point. A cardiologist performing a treadmill test measures ST-segment deviation at a point that is 0.08 second after the J point and does not count T waves at all.

A nonspecific or nondiagnostic ECG has the following characteristics:

- ST depression less than 0.5 mm, measured 0.04 second after the J point
- Upright T waves in leads with dominant R waves (normal) *or*
- T-wave inversion 2 mm or less in leads with dominant R waves

Prognostic Significance of ST-Segment Deviation and Prognosis

Although it can be nonspecific and has limitations, the ST segment can be a powerful prognostic tool and triage marker for patients with possible ACS. STEMI patients have a time-dependent critical factor inherent in the priority for rapid reperfusion. This does not and should not imply that patients with ST-segment depression have a better prognosis or can be the focus of casual evaluation and treatment. In fact, patients with NSTEMI may have a worse outcome and higher mortality than STEMI patients without reciprocal ST-segment depression (Figure 92).

Early Invasive vs Early Conservative Strategies

By 2002, treatment strategies had been developed with evidence-based trials and clinical bedside risk stratification of patients. An *early invasive strategy* recommends that patients with UA or NSTEMI *routinely* be taken to cardiac catheterization and that angiographically indicated

Prognostic Value of ECG Changes in ACS Patients: GUSTO IIb

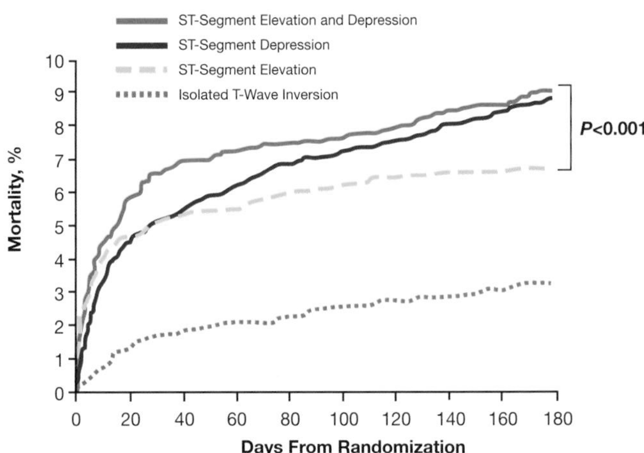

Figure 92. Percent mortality at 6 months based on initial ECG findings in the Global Utilization of Streptokinase and Tissue Plasminogen Activator for Occluded Coronary Arteries (GUSTO) IIb Trial. Patients with ST-segment depression have a higher mortality than "routine" patients with ST-segment elevation and rival STEMI patients with "reciprocal" ST-segment depression. These patients have reciprocal depression as a marker of large infarction or multivessel coronary disease. Isolated T-wave inversion has a lower prognostic value because it is nonspecific and includes patients without ACS. Reproduced from Savonitto et al.[128]

revascularization be performed. This could be PCI, CABG, or continued medical therapy, depending on the results of coronary angiography. The *early conservative strategy* recommends initial management of stable patients with antiplatelet, antithrombin, and antianginal therapy as indicated. The recurrence of symptoms despite adequate therapy or the finding of high-risk features (based on clinical criteria or stress testing) is then an indication for coronary angiography. Clinical trials comparing early conservative and early invasive strategies showed an improved outcome for patients at intermediate or high risk when assigned to the invasive strategy. For this reason, the 2012 Focused Update of the guidelines retains early invasive strategy as a Class I, LOE A recommendation for UA/NSTEMI patients who have an increased risk for clinical events.[129]

Indicators for Early Invasive Strategies

Risk stratification helps the clinician identify patients with NSTEMI and UA who should be managed with an invasive strategy. Coronary angiography then allows the clinician to determine whether patients are appropriate candidates for revascularization with PCI or CABG.

The following clinical indicators identify patients at increased risk:

- New ST-segment depression or positive troponins
- Persistent or recurrent ischemic symptoms
- Hemodynamic instability or VT
- Depressed LV function (ejection fraction less than 40%)
- ECG or functional study that suggests multivessel CAD

Recommendations

- An early invasive PCI strategy is indicated for patients with NSTEMI ACS who have no serious comorbidity and who have coronary lesions amenable to PCI and an elevated risk for clinical events.
- An early invasive strategy (ie, diagnostic angiography with intent to perform revascularization) is indicated in NSTEMI ACS patients who have refractory angina or hemodynamic or electric instability (without serious comorbidities or contraindications to such procedures).
- In initially stabilized patients, an initially conservative (ie, a selectively invasive) strategy may be considered as a treatment strategy for NSTEMI ACS patients (without serious comorbidities or contraindications to such procedures) who have an elevated risk for clinical events, including those with abnormal troponin elevations.
- The decision to implement an initial conservative (versus initial invasive) strategy in these patients may be made with consideration given to physician and patient preference.

TIMI Risk Score

The risk of MACE has been further studied and refined. Researchers who derived the important TIMI risk score used data from the TIMI-IIB and ESSENCE (Efficacy and Safety of Subcutaneous Enoxaparin in Non–Q-Wave Coronary Events) trials for NSTEMI and UA and from the In-TIME trial for STEMI. The TIMI risk score comprises 7 independent prognostic variables (Table 32).[130,131] These 7 variables were significantly associated with the occurrence within 14 days of at least 1 of the primary end points: death, new or recurrent MI, or need for urgent revascularization. The score is derived from complex multivariate logistic regression analysis and includes variables that seem historically counterintuitive. For example, it is useful to note that traditional cardiac risk factors are only weakly associated with MACE. Use of aspirin within the previous 7 days, for example, would not seem to be an indicator of a bad outcome, but aspirin use was found to be one of the most powerful predictors. It is possible that aspirin use identified a subgroup of patients at higher risk or who were undergoing active but failed therapy for CAD.

The creators of the TIMI risk score validated it with 3 groups of patients, and 4 clinical trials showed a significant interaction between the TIMI risk score and outcome. These findings confirm the value of the TIMI risk score as a guide to therapeutic decisions. A TIMI Risk Score Calculator is available at **www.TIMI.org.**

The Braunwald (Table 31) and TIMI (Table 32) risk scores serve as the dominant clinical guides for predicting the risk of MACE in patients with ACS. It is important to note that risk stratification is applicable to patients with an intermediate or high risk of symptoms caused by CAD, not the larger general population of patients presenting with chest discomfort or symptoms possibly caused by anginal equivalents. Risk stratification enables clinicians to direct therapy to those patients at intermediate or high risk of MACE and to avoid unnecessary therapy and the potential for adverse consequences in patients at lower risk.

The TIMI risk score has become the primary tool for evaluation of therapeutic recommendations. Some of the newer therapies may provide incrementally greater benefit for patients with higher risk scores.

One additional product of the TIMI trials is the TIMI grading system of coronary artery blood flow. TIMI investigators developed and validated a coronary artery perfusion scoring system that characterized the degree of reperfusion of a coronary artery on a scale of 0 (no flow) to 3 (complete, brisk flow). This grading system is now used as an outcome measure in many studies of ACS interventions.

Table 32. TIMI Risk Score for Patients With UA and NSTEMI: Predictor Variables

Predictor Variable	Point Value of Variable	Definition
Age ≥65 years	1	
≥3 Risk factors for CAD	1	Risk factors • Family history of CAD • Hypertension • Hypercholesterolemia • Diabetes • Current smoker
Aspirin use in last 7 days	1	
Recent, severe symptoms of angina	1	≥2 anginal events in past 24 hours
Elevated cardiac markers	1	CK-MB or cardiac-specific troponin level
ST deviation ≥0.5 mm	1	ST depression ≥0.5 mm is significant; transient ST elevation ≥0.5 mm for <20 minutes is treated as ST-segment depression and is high risk; ST elevation ≥1 mm for >20 minutes places these patients in the STEMI treatment category
Prior coronary artery stenosis ≥50%	1	Risk predictor remains valid even if this information is unknown
Calculated TIMI Risk Score	**Risk of ≥1 Primary End Point* in ≤14 Days**	**Risk Status**
0 or 1	5%	Low
2	8%	
3	13%	Intermediate
4	20%	
5	26%	High

Abbreviations: CAD, coronary artery disease; CK-MB, MB fraction of creatine kinase; NSTEMI, non–ST-segment elevation myocardial infarction; TIMI, Thrombolysis in Myocardial Infarction; UA, unstable angina.

*Primary end points: death, new or recurrent myocardial infarction, or need for urgent revascularization.

ECG: ST-Segment Depression or Dynamic T-Wave Inversion

When patients have ischemic ST depression or dynamic T-wave inversion, they are considered high risk (Figure 75, Numbers 9-12) and are candidates for intensive management with an early invasive strategy of cardiac catheterization and PCI (Figure 75, Number 12).

Integration of Cardiac Troponins With ECG Parameters

Serial cardiac biomarkers are diagnostic and prognostic, and they guide therapy.

- If troponin is positive on presentation, NSTEMI is present and the patient is already at high risk.
- If serial markers become positive, the patient has NSTEMI and an early invasive strategy is preferred.
- If serial markers remain negative in the patient with ST-segment depression, the patient has UA, unless ST-segment depression has another cause, such as secondary repolarization changes caused by LV hypertrophy.
- Some patients with positive serial markers will develop Q-wave MI.
- If patients with a normal or nondiagnostic ECG develop positive troponin, they have NSTEMI. These patients are now candidates for an invasive strategy rather than functional testing.

General Management: Start Adjunctive Treatments (Number 10)

Patients who are at high risk for complications of ACS receive intensive antiplatelet and antithrombotic therapy. Healthcare providers need to be aware that data are continually evolving, and individualization of therapy is necessary in the context of the risk-benefit assessment and a time-dependent strategy. If available, use an institutional protocol and consult with cardiology teams.

Treatment options include aspirin, ADP antagonists such as clopidogrel, heparin (UFH or LMWH), GP IIb/IIIa receptor inhibitors, parenteral nitroglycerin for recurrent or persistent discomfort, and β-adrenergic receptor blockers.

Antiplatelet and Antithrombin Therapy: Aspirin and Beyond

Aspirin

Although a time-dependent effect of aspirin in UA and NSTEMI is not supported by evidence, aspirin (160 to 325 mg PO) should be given as soon as possible to all patients with suspected ACS unless the patient has aspirin allergy or sensitivity, an active bleeding disorder, active peptic ulcer disease, or recent or acute gastrointestinal bleeding.

If patients are to be considered for an interventional strategy, after PCI, it is reasonable to use aspirin 81 mg per day in preference to higher maintenance doses.[132] This dose will be continued in conjunction with clopidogrel if a stent is placed.

Clopidogrel

Since 2000, several important studies of clopidogrel have been published that document its efficacy for both patients with UA/NSTEMI and those with STEMI. In these studies, patients with an ACS and a rise in serum levels of cardiac biomarkers or ECG changes consistent with ischemia had reduced stroke and MACE if clopidogrel was added to aspirin and heparin within 4 hours of hospital presentation.[133] One study confirmed that clopidogrel did not increase the risk of bleeding compared with aspirin.[134] Clopidogrel given 6 hours or more before elective PCI for patients with ACS without ST elevation has been shown to reduce adverse ischemic events at 28 days.[135]

The appropriate timing and dose of clopidogrel remain uncertain and are the subject of continuing investigation. The Clopidogrel for the Reduction of Events During Observation (CREDO) trial (post hoc analysis) found only a small clinical benefit unless the current loading dose of 300 mg was administered more than 15 hours before PCI. Clopidogrel resistance was present in approximately 25% of the patients.[136] Another trial used a 600 mg loading dose of clopidogrel given more than 12 hours before PCI and found an increased antiplatelet effect and fewer MACE at 1 month.[137]

Prasugrel

Prasugrel is an oral thienopyridine prodrug that irreversibly binds to the ADP receptor to inhibit platelet aggregation. Prasugrel may be associated with a reduction in combined event rate (cardiovascular mortality, nonfatal infarction, and nonfatal stroke) with no benefit in mortality compared with clopidogrel but with an overall resultant increase in major bleeding (compared with clopidogrel) when administered after angiography to patients with NSTEMI undergoing PCI. Risk factors associated with a higher rate of bleeding with prasugrel use are age 75 years or older, previous stroke or TIA, and body weight less than 60 kg. ACC/AHA 2011 NSTEMI guidelines recommend prasugrel as a reasonable alternative to clopidogrel for the initial treatment of the following groups of NSTEMI patients:

- Patients in whom an initial invasive strategy is planned (medium- or high-risk patients)
- Patients in whom PCI is planned

The recommended dose of prasugrel is a 60 mg loading dose followed by a 10 mg maintenance dose.[138]

In patients with UA/NSTEMI in whom PCI has been selected as a postangiography management strategy, healthcare providers should continue aspirin administration, administer a loading dose of an ADP antagonist if not started before diagnostic angiography, and discontinue anticoagulant therapy after PCI for uncomplicated cases.[138]

GP IIb/IIIa Inhibitors

After plaque rupture in the coronary artery, tissue factor in the lipid-rich core is exposed and forms complexes with or triggers other coagulation factors. Platelet adhesion, activation, and aggregation may result in formation of an arterial thrombus, and these processes are pivotal in the pathogenesis of ACS. The integrin GP IIb/IIIa receptor is the final common pathway to platelet aggregation, which leads to binding of circulating adhesive macromolecules. Administration of a GP IIb/IIIa receptor antagonist (inhibitor) is one way of reducing acute ischemic complications after plaque fissure or rupture.

Several large studies of GP IIb/IIIa inhibitors in UA/NSTEMI have shown a clear benefit of these agents when combined with standard aspirin and heparin and a strategy of mechanical reperfusion (PCI).[139] Severe bleeding complications in a minority of patients (but no increase in intracranial hemorrhage) in the GP IIb/IIIa group were offset by the large benefit of these agents. This benefit extends to high-risk patients with UA/NSTEMI treated with PCI.[140]

In UA/NSTEMI patients not treated with PCI, the effect of GP IIb/IIIa inhibitors has been mixed. One large meta-analysis[140] showed that GP IIb/IIIa inhibitors produced no mortality advantage and only a slight reduction in recurrent ischemic events, but a later, equally large meta-analysis showed a reduction in 30-day mortality.[141] Of note, the benefit of GP IIb/IIIa inhibitors was dependent on co-administration of UFH or LMWH. Interestingly, abciximab appears to behave differently from the other 2 GP IIb/IIIa inhibitors. In the Global Utilization of Streptokinase and Tissue Plasminogen Activator for Occluded Coronary Arteries (GUSTO) IV ACS trial and 1-year follow-up,[142,143] which involved 7800 patients, abciximab showed a lack of treatment effect compared with placebo in patients treated medically only; therefore, it should not be given unless PCI is planned.

The ACC/AHA NSTEMI guidelines[138] recommend

- The use of GP IIb/IIIa inhibitors as an alternative to clopidogrel or prasugrel in high-risk patients with NSTEMI who are being treated with an invasive strategy (these may be used at the time of PCI or upstream before PCI). Eptifibatide and tirofiban are preferred agents; abciximab should not be used.
- The addition of GP IIb/IIIa inhibitors to patients who are already taking aspirin and an ADP antagonist/prasugrel if they develop recurrent ischemia, hemodynamic instability, or arrhythmias
- Routine upstream use of GP IIb/IIIa inhibitors in high-risk UA/NSTEMI patients in addition to aspirin and an ADP antagonist/prasugrel
- Use of GP IIb/IIIa inhibitors in patients treated with an initial conservative strategy

These drugs should not be used in patients at low risk of ischemia (TIMI score less than 3) or at high risk of bleeding. For UA/NSTEMI patients in whom a conservative strategy is selected and who do not undergo angiography or stress testing, the patient should[138]

- Continue aspirin indefinitely
- Continue ADP antagonist for at least 1 month and ideally up to 1 year
- Discontinue IV GP IIb/IIIa inhibitor if started previously
- Continue UFH for 48 hours, or enoxaparin or fondaparinux should be administered for the duration of hospitalization, up to 8 days, and then the patient should discontinue anticoagulant therapy

Precautions and contraindications for the use of GP IIb/IIIa inhibitors include the following:

- Active internal bleeding or bleeding disorder in the past 30 days (thrombocytopenia, platelets less than 150 000)
- History of intracranial hemorrhage, neoplasm, arteriovenous malformation, or aneurysm, or stroke or major surgical procedure or trauma within the past 30 days
- Aortic dissection, pericarditis, and severe hypertension
- Hypersensitivity

Heparins

- Fondaparinux or enoxaparin is a reasonable alternative to UFH for in-hospital patients with NSTEMI managed with a planned initial conservative approach.
- Enoxaparin or UFH is a reasonable choice for in-hospital patients with NSTEMI managed with a planned invasive approach.
- Fondaparinux may be used in the setting of PCI but requires coadministration of UFH and does not appear to offer an advantage over UFH alone.
- Bivalirudin or UFH may be considered for in-hospital patients with NSTEMI and renal insufficiency.
- Fondaparinux or bivalirudin, as well as UFH, is reasonable and may be considered for in-hospital patients with NSTEMI and increased bleeding risk if anticoagulant therapy is not contraindicated.
- There is no specific evidence for or against anticoagulant use in NSTEMI in the prehospital setting.

Antianginal Therapy

Nitroglycerin IV Infusion

Nitroglycerin reduces myocardial oxygen demand while enhancing myocardial oxygen delivery. Nitroglycerin, an endothelium-independent vasodilator, has both peripheral and coronary vascular effects that contribute to increased oxygen delivery and reduced oxygen demand.

Treatment benefits of nitroglycerin are limited, and no conclusive evidence supports routine use of intravenous, oral, or topical nitrate therapy in patients with AMI. With this in mind, providers should carefully consider use of these agents, especially when low blood pressure precludes the use of other agents shown to be effective in reducing morbidity and mortality (eg, β-blockers and angiotensin-converting enzyme inhibitors).

Consider using IV nitroglycerin in the following circumstances:

- If discomfort is not controlled with up to 3 sublingual nitroglycerin tablets, 3 metered spray doses, or nitroglycerin paste
- If discomfort recurs after initial relief
- As an adjunct for blood pressure control after β-blockers have been given
- As an adjunct for treatment of CHF with ACS

Please consult the STEMI section of this chapter for the contraindications for nitrates.

β-Adrenoceptor Blocking Agents (β-Blockers)

β-Blockers block sympathetic nervous system stimulation of heart rate and contractility, which results in vasodilation and reduced ventricular afterload. They can reduce infarct size, decrease postinfarction ischemia, and reduce the incidence of ventricular ectopy and fibrillation. Oral β-blockers should be administered in the ED for ACS of all types unless contraindications are present (see above).

Analgesia

Analysis of retrospective registry data raised a question about the potentially adverse effects of morphine in patients with UA/NSTEMI; therefore, morphine is not highly recommended for this group of patients.

HMG-Coenzyme A Reductase Inhibitors (Statins)

A variety of studies documented consistent reduction in indicators of inflammation and complications such as reinfarction, recurrent angina, and arrhythmias when statin treatment was administered within a few days after onset of an ACS. Pretreatment with atorvastatin 80 mg 12 hours before and an additional 40 mg immediately before PCI for NSTEMI or documented ischemia has been shown to significantly decrease the 30-day composite of death, MI, and unplanned revascularization compared with placebo in a prospective randomized trial.[144]

Cardiac Catheterization (Number 12)

Coronary angiography identifies lesions at risk for occlusion or with a high level of ischemic potential. These are called "target lesions." When technically feasible, angioplasty is performed to dilate these target lesions. The majority of patients today also receive a stent to maintain vessel patency. This is possible in most patients with single-vessel disease and in some patients with more than 1 lesion. Coronary artery bypass surgery, if not contraindicated, is performed for patients with multiple target lesions, particularly diabetic patients.

Revascularization (Number 12)

When indicated, PCI or surgical revascularization may reduce the incidence of MACE and decrease the incidence of recurrent ischemia. CABG is indicated primarily for patients with stenosis of the left main coronary artery, for those with severe multivessel disease, or when PCI is not an option.

Additional Recommendations[138]

- Platelet function testing to determine platelet inhibitory response in patients with UA/NSTEMI (or after ACS and with PCI) who are undergoing thienopyridine therapy may be considered if results of testing may alter management.
- Genotyping for a CYP2C19 loss-of-function variant in patients with UA/NSTEMI (or after ACS and with PCI) who are undergoing clopidogrel therapy might be considered if results of testing may alter management.
- It is reasonable to use an insulin-based regimen to achieve and maintain glucose levels below 180 mg/dL while avoiding hypoglycemia for hospitalized patients with UA/NSTEMI with either a complicated or uncomplicated course.

Recommendations for Chronic Kidney Disease[138]

- Creatinine clearance should be estimated in UA/NSTEMI patients, and the doses of renally cleared medications should be adjusted according to the pharmacokinetic data for specific medications.
- Patients undergoing cardiac catheterization with receipt of contrast media should receive adequate preparatory hydration.
- Calculation of the ratio of contrast volume to creatinine clearance is useful to predict the maximum volume of contrast media that can be given without significantly increasing the risk of contrast-associated nephropathy.
- An invasive strategy is reasonable in patients with mild (stage II) and moderate (stage III) chronic kidney disease; there are insufficient data on benefit/risk of an invasive strategy in UA/NSTEMI patients with advanced (stages IV, V) chronic kidney disease.

Normal or Nondiagnostic ECG: Absence of Diagnostic Changes in ST Segment or T Waves (Intermediate/Low-Risk Unstable Angina) (Number 13)

Patients who present with possible or probable angina or with noncardiac chest discomfort who may have ischemia but have a normal or nondiagnostic ECG are rendered discomfort free and administered an aspirin if aspirin has not already been given. These patients are then further evaluated, and serial studies and functional testing are performed as indicated (Figure 75).

Patients who develop clinical indicators of instability or high risk, such as ECG changes with discomfort or positive troponin or CK-MB tests, are then managed similarly to patients initially presenting with ST-segment depression or dynamic T-wave inversion. Intensive medical therapy is indicated, as is an invasive strategy. Functional testing is contraindicated in these patients, who are unstable. If a conservative strategy is selected for indicated reasons or patient preference, functional testing is deferred until the patient has been discomfort free and stable for at least 24 hours on medical therapy.

Adjunctive treatments should continue or be started on the basis of specific indications (Number 14). Serial cardiac studies are obtained. If serial ECGs reveal development of persistent ST *elevation,* immediate reperfusion therapy is indicated. When patients in the ED/chest pain unit (CPU) are suspected of having ACS but have nonischemic ECGs and negative biomarkers, a noninvasive test for inducible myocardial ischemia or anatomic evaluation of the coronary arteries (eg, computed tomography [CT] angiography, cardiac magnetic resonance, myocardial perfusion imaging, stress echocardiography) can be useful in identifying patients suitable for discharge from the ED. This strategy may be considered to increase diagnostic accuracy for ACS, thereby decreasing costs, length of stay, and time to diagnosis, and can provide valuable short-term and long-term prognostic information of future major cardiac events.

Patients presenting with chest discomfort syndromes require continuous risk stratification during evaluation. In isolation, neither the history nor the ECG will identify patients at risk or free of disease, but once a noncardiac cause is identified during the evaluation, patients are treated for this diagnosis, and the chest discomfort evaluation protocol is no longer followed. A few clinical pearls assist in evaluation:

- Although the presence of ACS is low, a normal ECG does not rule out an ACS. For this reason, a second ECG is indicated if the chest discomfort persists or recurs to *any degree* during observation. A repeat ECG is obtained approximately 1 hour after admission or on anticipated discharge from the ED or transfer to another unit if ACS is suspected. If the discomfort recurs, obtain an ECG, preferably before administration of nitroglycerin, but do not significantly delay nitroglycerin administration solely for an "ECG during discomfort."
- Cardiac-specific markers of MI do not begin to become positive until several hours after damage to myocardial cells occurs. The ACC/AHA guidelines recommend that a *second* set of cardiac biomarkers (troponin I or T and CK-MB) be obtained when initial levels are not elevated. This testing is usually performed 6 to 8 hours after admission. Timing is important. The first ED sample may be equivalent to a 6-hour to 8-hour sample if the patient has had prolonged and continuous discomfort before presentation. It is important to note the time relationships, duration of discomfort, and episodic nature of the discomfort if present.
- Myocardial perfusion scintigraphy (MPS) can be used for risk stratification, especially when there is a low to intermediate likelihood of cardiac events according to traditional cardiac markers. Multidetector computed tomography (MDCT) can also be used in low-risk patients, which allows for safe early discharge.
- An institutional protocol is encouraged to define the type and time of testing in patients at low risk for ACS. Patients at low risk for symptoms caused by CAD and for MACE can be discharged and undergo functional testing within 48 to 72 hours if they are discomfort free, have normal ECGs, and have no elevation of cardiac markers (including "gray zone" troponin). Patients at high risk for MACE and those with positive markers do not usually undergo stress testing. Whether and when an individual patient at intermediate risk for ACS undergoes functional testing requires careful assessment and clinical judgment.

Discharge Acceptable (Number 17)

Patients to be discharged should have experienced complete relief of discomfort early after presenting unless a noncardiac cause of discomfort has been identified. If the discomfort was not quickly eliminated soon after presentation, or if possible ischemic discomfort recurs during evaluation, then the patient is considered to have at least intermediate risk.

If objective evidence (minimum of 2 normal ECGs with no ST-segment deviation or significant changes plus 2 sets of normal cardiac biomarkers obtained 6 or more hours apart) excludes myocardial necrosis and stratifies the patient as being at low risk for MACE, the patient can be discharged with specific instructions and follow-up. These actions not only constitute appropriate clinical care but also are a prudent risk management option.

- The responsible physician should arrange for timely follow-up of the patient, starting with outpatient testing 72 hours after discharge. Document these arrangements in writing in the medical record. If practical, communicate directly (voice to voice) with the physician who will take responsibility for the patient's continued evaluation.
- Ask the patient to sign a statement confirming the patient's understanding and acceptance of the follow-up plans, and place the statement in the medical record. In contemporary medicine practice, this statement most conveniently takes the form of a copy of the signed discharge instructions to the patient.
- Instruct patients to phone 911 and request EMS transport to return to the ED if any of their symptoms recur.
- It is reasonable for clinicians and hospitals that provide care to patients with UA/NSTEMI to participate in a standardized quality-of-care data registry designed to track and measure outcomes, complications, and adherence to evidence-based processes of care and quality improvement for UA/NSTEMI.[138]

Introduction to Heart Failure and Shock Complicating ACS

This section of the cardiovascular chapter describes complications of ACS: shock, pulmonary edema, and hypotension.

Critical Concept **"Rule Out" Is Now Ruled Out and ACS Is Now "Ruled In"**	Recently published consensus guidelines clearly establish that clinicians cannot rule out an ACS in patients with typical ischemic chest discomfort symptoms on the basis of history, physical examination, traditional risk factor evaluation, or clinical judgment alone. An institutional interdisciplinary protocol applied *routinely* to patients with chest discomfort suggestive of ischemia is recommended to guide the care of patients with possible ACS.

The first section discusses a general approach to the patient presenting in shock. The second section summarizes the pathophysiology and treatment of cardiogenic shock associated with STEMI and other ACS, with an emphasis on therapy unique to these patients. The last section reviews the Acute Pulmonary Edema, Hypotension, and Shock Algorithm and details initial evaluation and stabilization of any patient with pulmonary edema and shock or hypertensive urgency. This section contains more information about treatment decisions based on the initial response to therapy.

Key Points

- Cardiogenic shock is the leading cause of death in patients with AMI who survive to reach the hospital.
- The incidence of cardiogenic shock has largely remained unchanged, and mortality is high, approximately 50% in published trials.
- RV shock (usually found in association with inferior wall MI) has a high mortality rate similar to that of LV shock.
- Patients with cardiogenic shock and STEMI should be primarily transported or secondarily transferred (with a door-to-departure time of 30 minutes or less) to facilities capable of invasive strategies such as IABP, PCI, and CABG.
- An invasive strategy is recommended for patients 75 years of age or younger; carefully selected patients age 75 and older also can receive aggressive early revascularization.
- If heart failure and shock develop after hospital admission, the patient should undergo diagnostic angiography, and PCI or CABG if possible if shock develops within the first 36 hours of onset of MI.

Cardiogenic Shock, LV Failure, and CHF

Shock is a clinical condition characterized by a sustained and significant reduction in blood flow and oxygen delivery to organs and tissues. It is important to realize that shock and low blood pressure, although related, are not the same. In basic terms, shock is a condition in which tissue oxygenation (and cellular ventilation and nutrition) is inadequate for demand.

Patients frequently present with shock and no immediately obvious cause. Blood pressure alone can be misleading or "normal" for a variety of reasons. Hence, the diagnosis of shock is a clinical one characterized by several of the following findings:

- Clinically ill appearance or altered mental status
- Low blood pressure (defined as an SBP lower than 80 or 90 mm Hg)
- Tachycardia (heart rate higher than 100/min)
- Tachypnea (respiratory rate higher than 22 breaths/min or $Paco_2$ lower than 32 mm Hg)
- Systemic acidosis (serum lactate higher than 4 mmol/L)
- Decreased urine output (less than 0.5 mL/kg per hour)

Differential Diagnosis of Shock

Not all of these criteria may be present. For example, patients taking β-blockers may not have tachycardia. In early shock, blood pressure may be normal or only slightly low because of excess adrenergic drive, and it may not drop significantly until late in the process.

Blalock initially divided shock into 4 general categories,[145] and variations of these are still useful today during initial assessment of the patient in shock. Blalock's categories were hematologic, neurologic, vasogenic, and cardiogenic. Today we initially classify patients as those with volume problems, cardiac problems, or "distributive" problems. Consider the expanded systematic approach for perfusion assessment (volume, resistance, pump, rate):

- Volume—Inadequate intravascular volume relative to the vascular space (eg, hemorrhage, dehydration)
- Resistance—Inappropriate vascular resistance or maldistribution of blood flow (eg, septic shock)
- Pump—Inadequate cardiac output (contractility problem) caused by pump failure or obstruction (eg, cardiogenic shock, PE, tamponade)
- Rate—Bradycardia or tachycardia that reduces cardiac output (eg, complete atrioventricular block, VT)

The clinician can use these provisional etiologic mechanisms to characterize shock and to identify the appropriate initial focus of therapy:

- Hypovolemic shock → Volume therapy
- Cardiogenic shock → Support of pump function
- Distributive shock → Vasoactive drug therapy
- Obstructive shock → Correction of obstruction; cause-specific

An etiologic approach to shock often oversimplifies the problem. Any patient with severe or sustained shock will likely require some titration of fluid therapy to optimize intravascular volume, support of pump function, manipulation of vascular resistance and distribution of blood flow, or correction of specific obstruction. All patients with severe or sustained shock will have some myocardial failure or even necrosis. In fact, patients in ICUs with elevation of troponin in the absence of CAD have a worse prognosis.

Determinants of Cardiac Output

A more detailed diagnostic approach that defines the variable of cardiac output and allows for a more targeted approach to therapy is often required. Recall that blood pressure is only a surrogate for cardiac output.

Arterial Pressure = Cardiac Output × Total (Systemic) Vascular Resistance

Cardiac output is determined by stroke volume and heart rate.

Cardiac Output = Stroke Volume × Heart Rate

Stroke volume is determined by 3 variables:

- Intravascular volume (preload)
- Peripheral vascular resistance (afterload)
- Pump function (contractility)

Cardiac function and other variables that influence cardiac output are complex, but one major determinant relevant to the initial assessment is the volume-loading conditions of the heart. In normal volume-loading conditions, cardiac output is optimal at rest and in the absence of pathological conditions. As venous return decreases (low filling pressure), cardiac output falls. Compensatory mechanisms increase cardiac contractility and heart rate to maintain cardiac output. At the patient's bedside, a pulmonary arterial catheter can measure these filling pressures (central venous and pulmonary capillary wedge pressures) and cardiac output, with these measures used to calculate systemic vascular resistance when necessary and indicated. Cardiac echocardiography can also help differentiate underlying causes of low cardiac output or low blood pressure.

Interpretation can be complex, but 3 general divisions improve diagnostic accuracy (Table 33) and allow general classifications into hypovolemic, cardiogenic, and vasogenic shock. It should be remembered that insertion of a pulmonary artery catheter is a diagnostic, not a therapeutic, procedure with associated potential complications. In most patients, clinical assessment of filling pressure (central venous pressure, rales) and clinical circumstances are diagnostic.

Cardiogenic Shock Complicating AMI

Infarction of 40% or more of the LV myocardium in acute STEMI usually results in cardiogenic shock and death. Although the mortality rate of cardiogenic shock has decreased in selected recent trials, death rates still approximate 60%, and the overall incidence has decreased from 5.1% in 1999 to 3.6% in 2007.[146]

Cardiogenic Shock in NSTEMI ACS

It should also be appreciated that shock can occur in patients with NSTEMI, and even a small or modest infarct can cause hemodynamic instability if prior MI or LV dysfunction is present at the time of recurrent ACS. The mortality rate of these patients rivals that of those with large MIs because of delayed diagnosis and comorbidities, including renal dysfunction, bypass surgery, and peripheral vascular disease.[147,148] Moreover, patients with NSTEMI are significantly older and have more prior MI, heart failure, and 3-vessel disease than patients with STEMI. ECG findings for the circumflex distribution can be limited, and the circumflex artery is the cause of cardiogenic shock in approximately one third of patients.

Pathophysiology and Hemodynamics of Cardiogenic Shock

MI may result in hemodynamic instability and CHF. As described above, cardiogenic shock classically has been defined as a pump problem caused by "massive" heart attack. Cardiac output and ventricular ejection fraction fall, and heart rate increases to compensate for the fall in stroke volume in a reflex effort to maintain cardiac output. The damaged ventricle dilates, and the amount of blood ejected with each contraction decreases (ejection fraction).[149]

β-Blockade and Heart Failure

As noted, tachycardia may help maintain cardiac output despite the fall in ejection fraction and stroke volume. However, all compensatory changes are likely to increase myocardial oxygen consumption. They also can worsen ischemia in viable or distant myocardium and extend infarction. In some cases (eg, large anterior MI without CHF), a reduction in heart rate with β-blockade improves outcome. Blockade of excess sympathetic and neurohumoral

Table 33. **Hemodynamic Parameters in the 3 Major Categories of Shock***

Hypovolemic	Cardiogenic	Vasogenic
Low CVP/PCWP	High CVP/PCWP	Low CVP/PCWP
Low CO	Low CO	High CO
High SVR	High SVR	Low SVR

Abbreviations: CO, cardiac output; CVP, central venous pressure; PCWP, pulmonary capillary wedge pressure; SVR, systemic vascular resistance.

*In hypovolemic shock, filling pressure (CVP, PCWP) is low, which reduces CO. In an attempt to compensate and maintain arterial pressure, SVR increases. In cardiogenic shock, the pump is damaged and CO is low, which raises filling pressures (CVP, PCWP) and decreases CO. Because CO is low, SVR also increases to maintain arterial pressure. In vasogenic shock, seen in sepsis, for example, vasodilation occurs, which lowers SVR. This vasodilation causes a fall in vascular volume, and CO increases in an attempt to compensate and "fill the tank." CVP estimates right atrial pressure, and PCWP estimates left atrial pressure.

stimulation reduces myocardial oxygen consumption. In compensatory tachycardia, β-blockade can be life-threatening, such as in cardiogenic shock or severe heart failure, when the stroke volume is critically dependent on the tachycardia.

Hemodynamic Parameters of Cardiogenic Shock

When LV end-diastolic pressure increases substantially (more than 25 to 30 mm Hg), interstitial and then pulmonary edema develop. If RV end-diastolic pressure increases, peripheral edema will be observed. A fall in cardiac output also triggers an adrenergic response, which produces tachycardia and peripheral vasoregulatory changes that try to redistribute blood flow. Constriction of arteries to the skin, kidneys, and gut redistributes blood flow away from these tissues to maintain blood flow to the brain and heart. This systemic vasoconstriction may create increased LV *afterload,* which impedes LV ejection. As cardiac output continues to fall, hypotension and lactic acidosis develop. This combination of pulmonary edema with signs of inadequate systemic perfusion is the hallmark of cardiogenic shock.

The patient with LV dysfunction classically has been described as one with associated signs of hypoperfusion or a cardiac index (cardiac output corrected for body surface area) of 2.2 L/min per m^2 or less, pulmonary capillary wedge pressure more than 18 mm Hg, and SBP 90 mm Hg or less for 1 hour or more that is not responsive to fluid administration alone. When the cardiac index falls to 2.2 L/min per m^2 and SBP falls to 90 mm Hg, frank signs of poor peripheral perfusion are usually present.

Changing the Paradigm of Cardiogenic Shock

The changes described above for cardiogenic shock result from severe depression of myocardial contractility caused by MI. Cardiogenic shock remains the leading cause of in-hospital mortality from MI. In the SHOCK (Should We Emergently Revascularize Occluded Coronaries for Cardiogenic Shock) trial, the classic assumption that acute reduction in cardiac output leads to compensatory vasoconstriction in all patients was not confirmed, and a subgroup of patients was identified with low systemic vascular resistance.[150] New insights suggest that an inflammatory response and inappropriate vasodilation may play a role in these patients (Figure 93).[151]

Treatment of Cardiogenic Shock Associated With AMI

The mortality rate of AMI associated with cardiogenic shock is 50% or more in virtually every outcome report, and half of the deaths occur within the first 48 hours. Initial therapy for LV dysfunction without shock includes oxygen administration, IV administration of nitrates to reduce cardiac preload and afterload, and diuresis. Morphine is an adjunctive agent if the patient has continuing ischemia but should be used with caution. If SBP is less than 100 mm Hg, nitrates and morphine should be used with caution, if at all. When SBP is less than 90 mm Hg, they are contraindicated.

If the patient presents as or becomes markedly hypotensive, avoid or discontinue vasodilators and administer vasoactive drugs based on SBP to increase arterial tone (vasopressors), improve blood pressure, and redistribute cardiac output. If the patient does not respond to these initial therapies, be prepared to perform additional diagnostic studies, initiate advanced hemodynamic monitoring, and provide advanced therapies. In selected patients, mechanical circulatory assistance with intra-aortic balloon counterpulsation is an effective adjunct to reperfusion therapy. Results from the GUSTO-I and SHOCK trials[153] showed that an aggressive, early invasive approach increased survival for patients with cardiogenic shock and AMI (see below).

With increasing use of both fibrinolytic therapy and PCI, controversy arose over which technique was the better method of reperfusion. Retrospective and registry trial evidence has shown that for patients with AMI and cardiogenic shock, an aggressive early strategy of PCI is superior to medical therapy with fibrinolytics:

- The GUSTO-I investigators reported that mortality was lower in patients with cardiogenic shock treated with an aggressive PCI strategy than in similar patients given fibrinolytic therapy.[154]
- Investigators have reported higher survival rates for cardiogenic shock patients who undergo revascularization rather than fibrinolysis.[155]
- In the US Second National Registry of Myocardial Infarction, the mortality rate in patients with AMI and shock was lower in those treated with PCI as a primary strategy than in those treated with fibrinolytics.[155]
- In a large registry of patients with shock, mortality was lower in AMI patients who received early revascularization with either PCI or CABG.[156]
- Multiple investigators have reported reduced mortality in patients with cardiogenic shock and AMI who underwent IABP followed by cardiac catheterization and revascularization with PCI or CABG (when anatomy was suitable).[157]

Figure 94 gives recommendations for initial reperfusion therapy when cardiogenic shock complicates AMI.

The best method and timing of revascularization, as well as optimal therapy for shock, was a topic of controversy until evaluated and resolved by the randomized controlled SHOCK trial. This study compared early revascularization with IABP plus percutaneous transluminal coronary

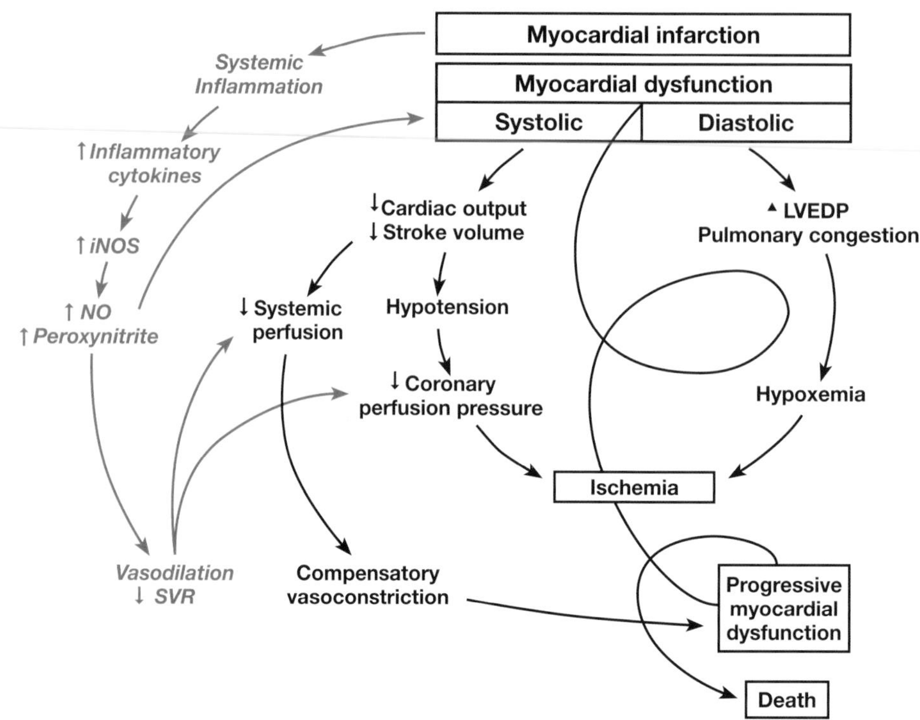

Figure 93. Classic shock paradigm, as illustrated by S. Hollenberg, is shown in black. The influence of the inflammatory response syndrome initiated by a large MI is illustrated in red. Abbreviations: iNOS, inducible nitric oxide synthase; LVEDP, left ventricular end-diastolic pressure; NO, nitric oxide; SVR, systemic vascular resistance. Adapted from Hollenberg et al.[152]

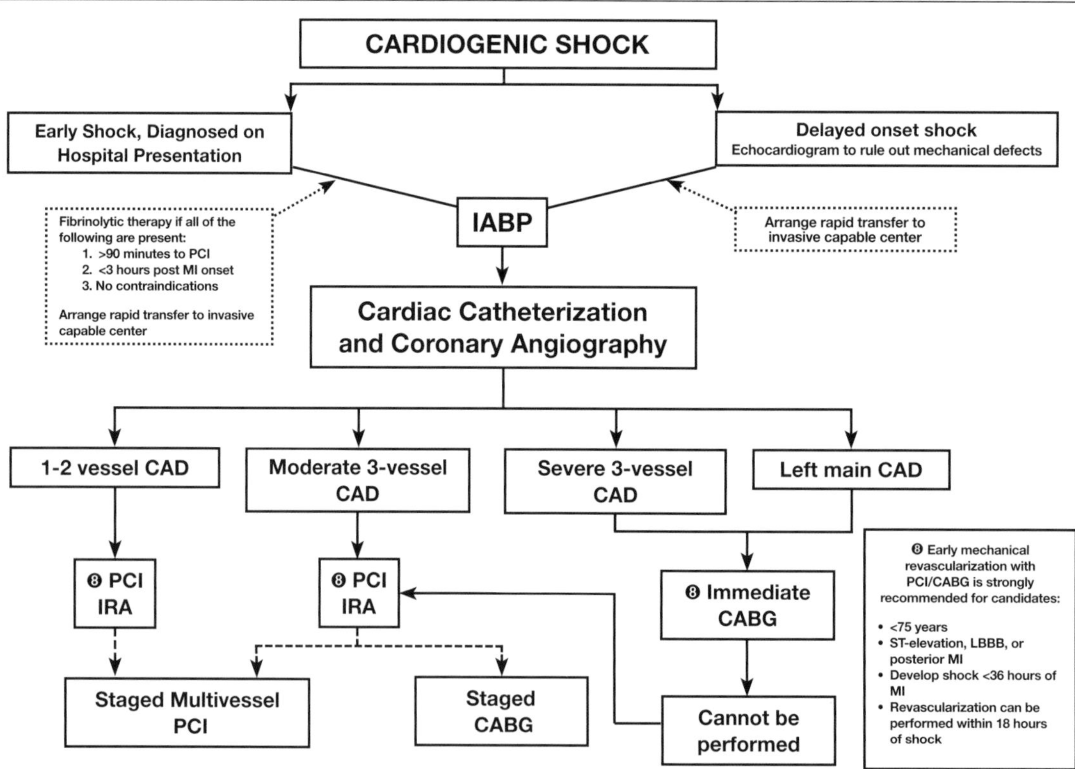

Figure 94. Recommendations for initial reperfusion therapy when cardiogenic shock complicates acute myocardial infarction (MI). Early mechanical revascularization with percutaneous coronary intervention (PCI) or coronary artery bypass grafting (CABG) is strongly recommended for suitable candidates less than 75 years of age and for selected elderly patients. Eighty-five percent of shock cases are diagnosed after initial therapy for acute MI, but most patients develop shock within 24 hours. Intra-aortic balloon pump (IABP) is recommended when shock is not quickly reversed with pharmacologic therapy, as a stabilizing measure for patients who are candidates for further invasive care. Dashed lines indicate that the procedure should be performed in patients with specific indications only. Abbreviations: CAD, coronary artery disease; IRA, infarct-related artery; LBBB, left bundle-branch block. Reproduced from Hochman.[151]

angioplasty or CABG with early medical stabilization by use of fibrinolytic therapy. Mortality at 6 months and at 1 year of follow-up was significantly lower in the early revascularization group than in the early medical therapy group (number needed to treat was approximately 8 at both time points). Follow-up data through 6 years are now available from this randomized trial. Almost two thirds of hospital survivors with cardiogenic shock who were treated with early revascularization were alive 6 years later. A strategy of early revascularization resulted in a 13.2% absolute and a 67% relative improvement in 6-year survival compared with initial medical stabilization.[158]

When possible, transfer patients at high risk for mortality or severe LV dysfunction with signs of shock, pulmonary congestion, heart rate more than 100/min, *and* SBP less than 100 mm Hg to a facility capable of performing PCI or CABG. Also consider triage or transfer for patients with a large anterior wall infarct, CHF, or pulmonary edema.

For a complete discussion of the diagnosis and management of cardiogenic shock complicating STEMI, see the ACC/AHA guidelines in *Circulation*.[15]

In 2004 the ACC/AHA Committee on Management of Acute Myocardial Infarction updated prior guidelines, and PCI remained a Class I recommendation for patients with ACS and shock who are younger than 75 years of age. Resuscitation experts reviewed and endorsed these recommendations at the 2010 International Consensus Conferences. The current recommendations from the updated ACC/AHA STEMI guidelines[15] are as follows:

- Provide early triage or transfer to cardiovascular facilities with cardiac catheterization suites and interventional capability.
- When possible, transfer patients at high risk for mortality or severe LV dysfunction with signs of shock, pulmonary congestion, heart rate more than 100/min, *and* SBP less than 100 mm Hg to a facility capable of performing PCI or CABG. This is highly recommended for patients younger than 75 years.
- PCI, including angioplasty with stent placement, is highly recommended for patients younger than 75 years of age with ACS and signs of shock.
- Use of IABP and diagnostic cardiac catheterization and coronary revascularization with PCI or CABG (if anatomy is suitable) may reduce mortality.
- The healthcare provider can use a checklist to identify patients who have contraindications to fibrinolytic therapy (Figure 85). If contraindications to fibrinolytic therapy exist, consider transfer to a cardiac intervention facility for reperfusion.

RV Shock

In the majority of persons, the right coronary artery supplies blood to the inferior wall and RV (Figure 95). When a thrombus occludes the proximal right coronary artery, ischemia and infarction of the RV occur. The RV marginal branch is

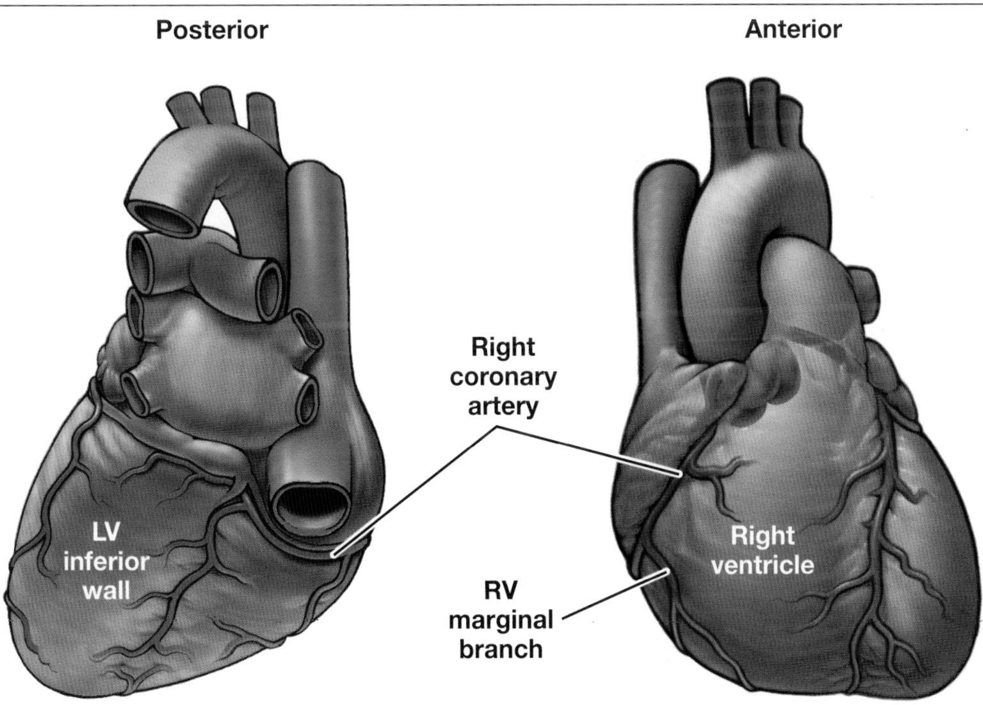

Figure 95. Anatomy of the heart showing the right coronary artery and RV marginal branch that supplies blood to the RV. A thrombus occluding the right coronary artery proximal to the RV marginal branch causes infarction of the inferior and posterior walls of the heart (if not supplied by the circumflex coronary artery) and the RV. In approximately 50% of patients, RV involvement leads to hemodynamic instability.

involved in approximately one third of patients with inferior infarction, and in one half of these patients occlusion is hemodynamically significant. Infarction of the RV has a favorable *long-term* prognosis, but hemodynamic infarction of the RV at the time of infarction more than doubles mortality. The RV is fairly resistant to infarction; most acute dysfunction is caused by ischemic but viable myocardium that can recover.

The SHOCK trial evaluated 933 patients in cardiogenic shock caused by predominant RV (n = 49) or LV (n = 884) failure. Patients with predominant RV shock were younger and had a lower prevalence of previous MI and multivessel disease. Despite the younger age, lower rate of anterior MI, and higher prevalence of single-vessel coronary disease of patients with RV shock and the similar benefit they receive from revascularization, mortality in these patients is unexpectedly high, similar to that in patients with LV shock.[159]

These patients have difficulty filling the lungs and returning blood to the left side of the heart. Only a small area of LV myocardium may be involved (inferior and posterior walls), and shock is caused by inadequate filling of the LV, which is caused by RV dysfunction. In patients with an inferior wall MI (Figure 96), RV involvement should be suspected and a right-sided 12-lead ECG performed (Figure 97). A 1-mm ST-segment elevation in lead V_4 is 88% sensitive and 78% specific for RV involvement.

Clinical findings are different in RV and LV shock. Lungs may be relatively clear because of the inability of the RV to pump blood to the pulmonary vasculature and the absence of LV dysfunction, which causes increased pulmonary capillary pressures. Paradoxically, neck veins may be distended because of high right atrial pressures. The triad of clear lungs, elevated jugular venous distention, and hypotension is present in only approximately 25% of patients.

Both RV and LV cardiogenic shock require emergent reperfusion; however, adjunctive medical management is different for each type. Vasodilation and low filling pressures are to be avoided in RV shock. The impaired RV requires

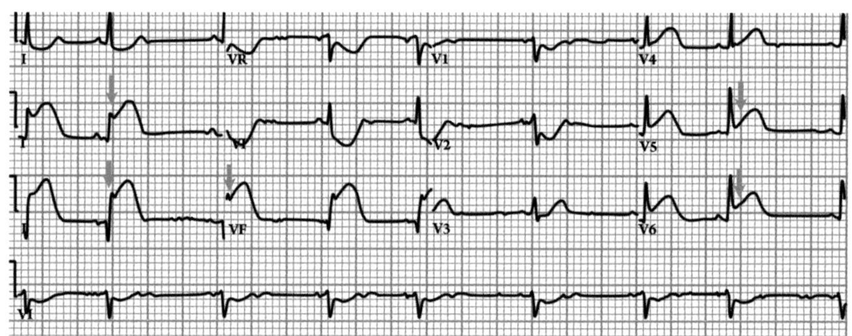

Figure 96. Twelve-lead ECG showing junctional ST-segment elevation in inferior leads II, III, and aVF. Note the ST-segment elevation in lateral leads V_5 and V_6, which indicates lateral wall involvement (inferolateral wall), and the ST-segment depression in precordial leads V_1 and V_2. These findings are not caused by anterior wall ischemia but by infarction of the posterior wall of the ventricle.

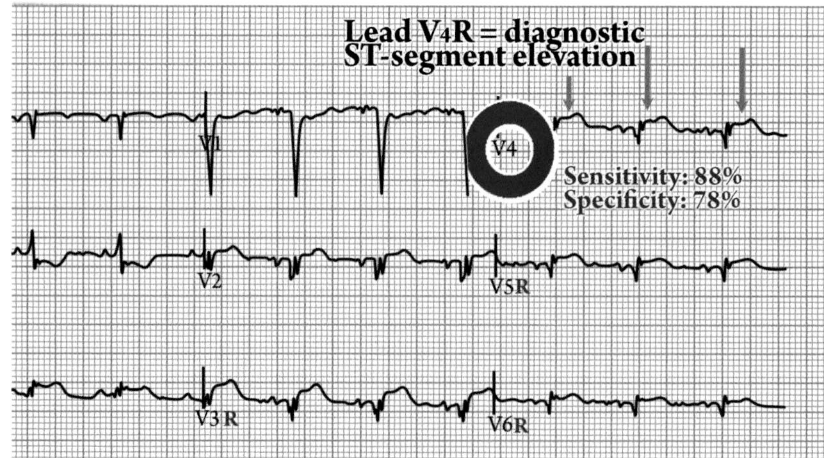

Figure 97. *Right-sided* 12-lead ECG showing junctional ST-segment elevation in leads over the right ventricle. Lead V_4R (blue circle) has 1 mm of ST-segment elevation. This elevation is 88% sensitive and 78% specific for right ventricular involvement.

optimal preload. Treatments that decrease preload, including nitrates, morphine, diuretics, and ACE inhibitors, may increase mortality and should be avoided. Optimal preload should be achieved with cautious and monitored volume replacement. Initially, 1 to 2 L of fluid may be required. This should be given in a 250 to 500 mL bolus, and vital signs and clinical assessment should be repeated. The rapid and injudicious administration of large amounts of fluid without clinical benefit should also be avoided, because high pressures and large amounts of volume will further impair RV function and recovery. In patients with multivessel involvement or prior MI, significant LV dysfunction may require additional measures such as IABP support. When initial measures do not improve hemodynamics, inotropic support of the RV with dobutamine may be beneficial. Dopamine can be added to augment arterial perfusion pressure if indicated.

Management of RV Infarction

In patients with inferior wall infarction, obtain an ECG with right-sided leads. ST-segment elevation (more than 1 mm) in lead V_4R is sensitive (sensitivity, 88%; specificity, 78%; diagnostic accuracy, 83%) for RV infarction and is a strong predictor of increased in-hospital complications and mortality.

The in-hospital mortality rate of patients with RV dysfunction is 25% to 30%; therefore, these patients should be routinely considered for reperfusion therapy. Fibrinolytic therapy reduces the incidence of RV dysfunction. Similarly, PCI is an alternative for patients with RV infarction and is preferred for patients in shock. Nitrates, diuretics, and other ACE inhibitors should be avoided because they may cause severe hypotension.

Acute Pulmonary Edema and Cardiogenic Shock

The Emergency Management of Complicated STEMI Algorithm (Figure 98) illustrates the management of patients who present with these complications of AMI. Based on clinical assessment and judgment, some of these recommendations will also be applicable to patients without

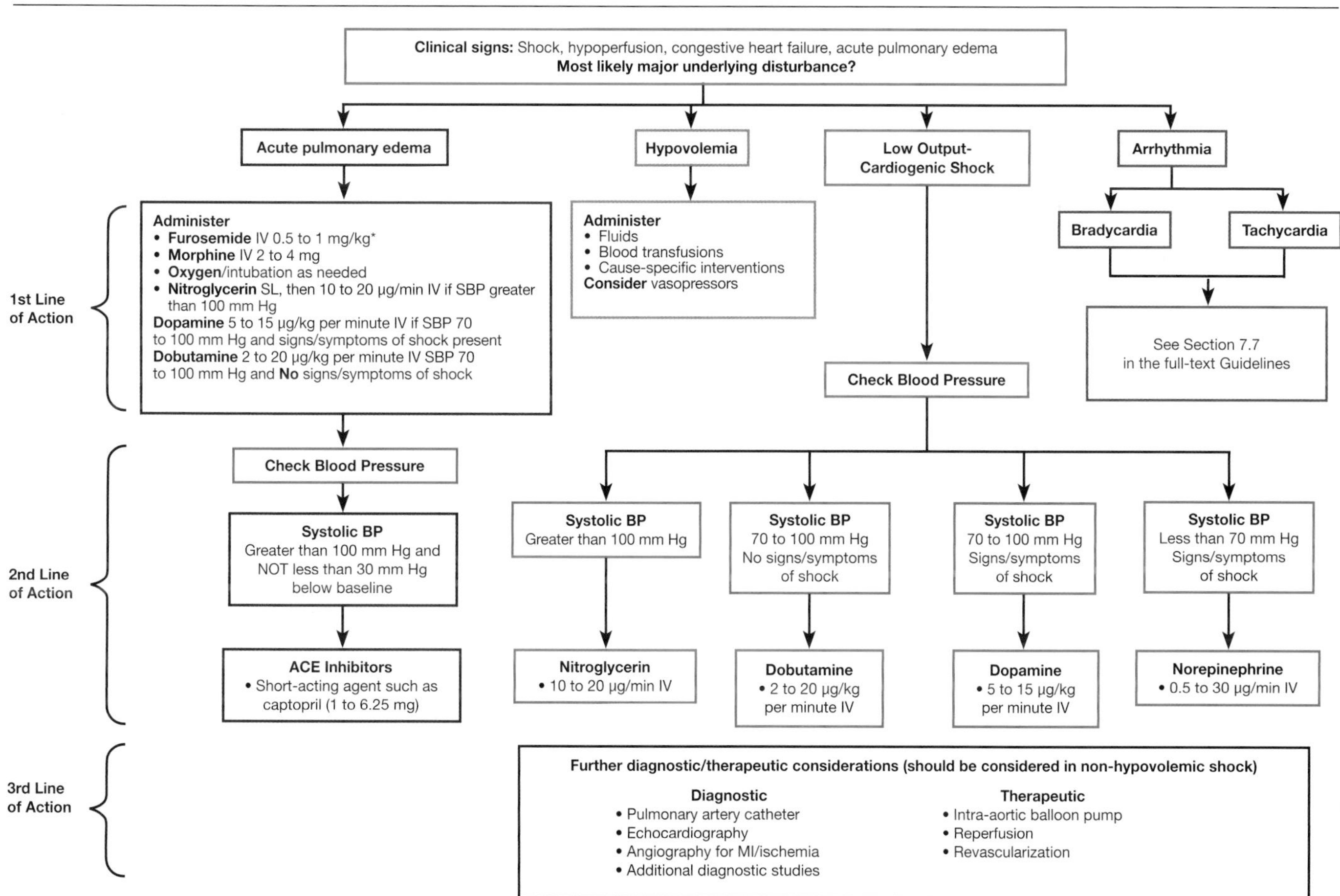

Figure 98. Emergency management of complicated STEMI. The emergency management of patients with cardiogenic shock or acute pulmonary edema, or both, is outlined.

*Give furosemide <0.5 mg/kg for new-onset acute pulmonary edema without hypovolemia; 1 mg/kg for acute or chronic volume overload or renal insufficiency. Nesiritide has not been studied adequately in patients with STEMI. Combinations of medications (eg, dobutamine and dopamine) may be used.

Modified from Guidelines 2000 for Cardiopulmonary Resuscitation and Emergency Cardiovascular Care.[160]

MI or applicable during the early evaluation for ACS. The following sections explain management of these patients in greater detail.

Clinical Signs

Shock and pulmonary edema are medical emergencies. Signs of shock include inadequate tissue perfusion (diminished peripheral pulses, cool extremities, delayed capillary refill, decreased urine output, and lactic acidosis). With CHF, signs of systemic and pulmonary venous congestion are present. Pulmonary edema produces tachypnea, labored respirations, rales, dyspnea, cyanosis, and hypoxemia. Frothy sputum may also be present. Providers should identify these conditions and begin treatment as soon as possible.

First-Line Actions

If signs of acute pulmonary edema are present, proceed with first-line actions if *low blood pressure and shock are absent*:

- Oxygen and positive pressure ventilation as needed
- Nitroglycerin SL or IV
- Furosemide IV 0.5 to 1 mg/kg
- Morphine IV 2 to 4 mg

If the patient's blood pressure is adequate, help the patient sit upright with the legs dependent. This position increases lung volume and vital capacity, diminishes the work of breathing, and decreases venous return to the heart. Administer morphine to dilate veins and arteries and to reduce cardiac preload and afterload.

Provide oxygen, establish IV access, and begin cardiac monitoring (ACLS providers treat "oxygen-IV-monitor" as a single word). Monitor oxyhemoglobin saturation with pulse oximetry, although results may be inaccurate and misleading if peripheral perfusion is poor. Oxyhemoglobin saturation does not provide information about hemoglobin concentration, oxygen content, ventilation, or acid-base status. Order additional laboratory studies to evaluate any significant comorbidity or complicating factors, such as anemia, renal dysfunction, or electrolyte imbalance.

Oxygen and Possible Intubation

Deliver oxygen at high flow rates, starting at 5 or 6 L/min by mask. Nonrebreathing masks with reservoir bags can provide oxygen concentrations of 90% to near 100%. A bag-mask may be used to provide assisted ventilation if the patient's ventilation is inadequate. If the patient is breathing spontaneously, consider continuous positive airway pressure by mask (noninvasive positive-pressure ventilation).

Be prepared to intubate the patient who has significant respiratory distress or respiratory failure. A need for intubation is particularly likely in situations that indicate progressive or imminent respiratory failure despite initial measures:

- PaO_2 cannot be maintained above 60 mm Hg despite 100% oxygen
- Signs of cerebral hypoxia (eg, lethargy or confusion) develop
- PCO_2 increases progressively
- Respiratory acidosis develops

Always verify successful intubation by use of both clinical confirmation and continuous waveform capnography. Pulmonary edema should not interfere with detection of exhaled CO_2.

Nitroglycerin

If SBP is adequate (usually more than 90 mm Hg) and the patient has no serious signs or symptoms of shock, then IV nitroglycerin is the drug of choice for acute pulmonary edema. Nitroglycerin reduces pulmonary congestion by dilating the venous capacitance vessels, which reduces preload. It also dilates systemic arteries, which decreases systemic vascular resistance. This effect can reduce afterload and increase cardiac output.

Nitroglycerin may initially be administered by sublingual tablets, oral spray, or the IV route as discussed above.

Furosemide

Loop diuretics, such as furosemide, have long been a mainstay in the treatment of acute pulmonary edema. Furosemide has a biphasic action. First, within approximately 5 minutes, it causes an immediate decrease in venous tone and an increase in venous capacitance. These changes lead to a fall in LV filling pressure (preload) that may improve clinical symptoms. Second, furosemide produces diuresis that begins within 5 to 10 minutes of IV administration. The diuresis need not be marked to be effective. If the patient is not already taking furosemide, a typical dose is 0.5 to 1 mg/kg given as a slow IV bolus over 1 to 2 minutes. If the response to this dose is inadequate after approximately 20 minutes, another bolus of 2 mg/kg is administered. If the patient is already taking oral furosemide, the clinical rule of thumb is to administer an initial dose that is twice the daily oral dose. If no effect occurs within approximately 20 minutes, double the initial dose. You may need to use higher doses if the patient has significant fluid retention, refractory heart failure, or renal insufficiency.

Nesiritide

Clinical trials have been conducted with nesiritide, a recombinant human brain natriuretic peptide, in patients hospitalized with decompensated CHF. Compared with placebo and "standard therapy," nesiritide was associated with improved hemodynamic function, decreased dyspnea and fatigue, and better global clinical status.

Morphine Sulfate

Morphine sulfate remains a part of the therapy for acute pulmonary edema, although recent research questions its effectiveness, especially outside the hospital. Morphine dilates the capacitance vessels of the peripheral venous bed. This dilatation reduces venous return to the central circulation and diminishes ventricular preload. Morphine also reduces afterload by causing mild arterial vasodilation. It also has a sedative effect. More effective vasodilators, such as ACE inhibitors, are now available, so morphine is considered an acceptable adjunct rather than a drug of choice for acute pulmonary edema.

Agents to Optimize Initial Blood Pressure

First-line actions include the administration of agents to optimize blood pressure. Patients with acute pulmonary edema have excess adrenergic drive, and many have preexisting hypertension. These patients can present with high blood pressures or accelerated hypertension. Often, treatment of the pulmonary edema itself will resolve high blood pressure, but initial therapy may include the use of IV nitroglycerin as an antihypertensive agent as well as a venodilator. Nitrates will reduce both preload and afterload to achieve this goal. In these patients the goal is to reduce blood pressure by no more than 30 mm Hg below the presentation blood pressure by titration of nitrates. IV nitroglycerin is initiated at 10 mcg/kg and titrated to this target goal. As mentioned, patients may respond to initial therapy with resolution of their elevated blood pressure, which would decrease or eliminate the need for IV nitrates. Use caution to avoid precipitating hypotension, because this may aggravate cardiac ischemia or precipitate organ ischemia in other vascular beds (eg, brain, kidneys, or gut).

Second-Line Actions

- Dopamine if SBP is 70 to 100 mm Hg with signs or symptoms of shock
- Dobutamine if SBP is 70 to 100 mm Hg with no signs or symptoms of shock
- ACE inhibitors if SBP is more than 100 mm Hg and not less than 30 mm Hg below baseline

Patients who respond to first-line actions for pulmonary edema may not require additional therapy unless otherwise indicated. If additional therapy is indicated, second-line actions are based on the patient's SBP and clinical response.

Patients Not in Shock With SBP More Than 100 mm Hg

- If SBP is more than 100 mm Hg and not less than 30 mm Hg below baseline, an ACE inhibitor is given to reduce afterload and attenuate LV remodeling in STEMI patients. Other agents can be used as indicated and tailored to the patient's clinical profile.
- Nitrates can be continued with the precautions noted under first-line actions. Tachyphylaxis (tolerance) to nitrates occurs in approximately 24 hours, so other agents are considered once the patient is stable. Contraindication and caution are as discussed above.
- IV nitroglycerin may be initiated at a rate of 10 mcg/min through continuous infusion with nonabsorbing tubing. Increase by 5 to 10 mcg/min every 3 to 5 minutes until a symptom or blood pressure response is noted. If no response is seen at 20 mcg/min, incremental increases of 10 mcg/min and later 20 mcg/min can be used. As the symptoms and signs of acute pulmonary edema or cardiac ischemia begin to resolve, there is no need to continue upward titration of nitroglycerin simply to obtain a fall in blood pressure.
  - When blood pressure reduction is a therapeutic goal, reduce the dosage when the blood pressure begins to fall. Frequently recommended limits for blood pressure reduction are 10% of baseline level in normotensive patients and 30% (or 30 mm Hg below baseline) in hypertensive patients.

Patients With SBP 70 to 100 mm Hg

If SBP is between 70 and 100 mm Hg and signs of shock *are* present, a dopamine infusion is recommended. If SBP is 70 to 100 mm Hg and the patient has *no signs of shock*, a dobutamine infusion is recommended as an inotropic agent to improve cardiac output or distribution of blood flow.

Third-Line Actions

Although called third-line actions, these diagnostic and therapeutic considerations or interventions may occur concurrent with first-line and second-line actions. For example, reperfusion in patients with pulmonary edema and STEMI is pursued without delay while treatment is initiated. An ECG is obtained within 10 minutes of presentation in patients with pulmonary edema to assess STEMI as a cause or complication. Any reversible or complicating conditions are identified and treated if possible. For example, mechanical complications of MI occur as the second-leading cause of in-hospital mortality. Patients with acute mitral regurgitation caused by rupture of a papillary muscle or chordae have conditions that are surgical emergencies. The use of echocardiography in the intensive care unit or ED on an emergent basis can identify these patients early. Patients on bed rest and those with heart failure are at increased risk for PE. An ED and hospital plan for rapid activation of cardiology and ancillary personnel and for IABP should be in place. Hospitals without LV assist devices, IABP, PCI, or cardiac surgery should also have an action plan to mobilize personnel and equipment for rapid transfer of STEMI patients to facilities with these capabilities.

References

1. Haryani A, Richmond T, Haw JM, Melgoza N, Purim-Shem-Tov Y, Calvin JE, Schaer GL. Patients developing STEMI in-hospital have delayed reperfusion and increased 1-year mortality compared to STEMI patients presenting to the emergency department. *Circulation*. 2009;120. Abstract 5102.
2. Nallamothu BK, Bates ER, Herrin J, Wang Y, Bradley EH, Krumholz HM. Times to treatment in transfer patients undergoing primary percutaneous coronary intervention in the United States: National Registry of Myocardial Infarction (NRMI)-3/4 analysis. *Circulation*. 2005;111:761-767.
3. Saczynski JS, Yarzebski J, Lessard D, Spencer FA, Gurwitz JH, Gore JM, Goldberg RJ. Trends in prehospital delay in patients with acute myocardial infarction (from the Worcester Heart Attack Study). *Am J Cardiol*. 2008;102:1589-1594.
4. Lefler LL, Bondy KN. Women's delay in seeking treatment with myocardial infarction: a meta-synthesis. *J Cardiovasc Nurs*. 2004;19:251-268.
5. McGinn AP, Rosamond WD, Goff DC Jr, Taylor HA, Miles JS, Chambless L. Trends in prehospital delay time and use of emergency medical services for acute myocardial infarction: experience in 4 US communities from 1987-2000. *Am Heart J*. 2005;150:392-400.
6. Jneid H, Fonarow GC, Cannon CP, Hernandez AF, Palacios IF, Maree AO, Wells Q, Bozkurt B, Labresh KA, Liang L, Hong Y, Newby LK, Fletcher G, Peterson E, Wexler L. Sex differences in medical care and early death after acute myocardial infarction. *Circulation*. 2008;118:2803-2810.
7. Foraker RE, Rose KM, McGinn AP, Suchindran CM, Goff DC Jr, Whitsel EA, Wood JL, Rosamond WD. Neighborhood income, health insurance, and prehospital delay for myocardial infarction: the atherosclerosis risk in communities study. *Arch Intern Med*. 2008;168:1874-1879.
8. Sari I, Acar Z, Ozer O, Erer B, Tekbas E, Ucer E, Genc A, Davutoglu V, Aksoy M. Factors associated with prolonged prehospital delay in patients with acute myocardial infarction. *Turk Kardiyol Dern Ars*. 2008;36:156-162.
9. Gibler WB, Armstrong PW, Ohman EM, Weaver WD, Stebbins AL, Gore JM, Newby LK, Califf RM, Topol EJ. Persistence of delays in presentation and treatment for patients with acute myocardial infarction: The GUSTO-I and GUSTO-III experience. *Ann Emerg Med*. 2002;39:123-130.
10. Mehta RH, Bufalino VJ, Pan W, Hernandez AF, Cannon CP, Fonarow GC, Peterson ED. Achieving rapid reperfusion with primary percutaneous coronary intervention remains a challenge: insights from American Heart Association's Get With the Guidelines program. *Am Heart J*. 2008;155:1059-1067.
11. Rathore SS, Curtis JP, Chen J, Wang Y, Nallamothu BK, Epstein AJ, Krumholz HM. Association of door-to–balloon time and mortality in patients admitted to hospital with ST elevation myocardial infarction: national cohort study. *BMJ*. 2009;338:b1807.
12. Song YB, Hahn JY, Gwon HC, Kim JH, Lee SH, Jeong MH. The impact of initial treatment delay using primary angioplasty on mortality among patients with acute myocardial infarction: from the Korea acute myocardial infarction registry. *J Korean Med Sci*. 2008;23:357-364.
13. Moser DK, Kimble LP, Alberts MJ, Alonzo A, Croft JB, Dracup K, Evenson KR, Go AS, Hand MM, Kothari RU, Mensah GA, Morris DL, Pancioli AM, Riegel B, Zerwic JJ. Reducing delay in seeking treatment by patients with acute coronary syndrome and stroke: a scientific statement from the American Heart Association Council on cardiovascular nursing and stroke council. *Circulation*. 2006;114:168-182.
14. Eisenberg MJ, Topal EJ. Prehospital administration of aspirin in patients with unstable angina and acute myocardial infarction. *Arch Intern Med*. 1996;156:1506-1510.
15. Antman EM, Anbe DT, Armstrong PW, Bates ER, Green LA, Hand M, Hochman JS, Krumholz HM, Kushner FG, Lamas GA, Mullany CJ, Ornato JP, Pearle DL, Sloan MA, Smith SC Jr, Alpert JS, Anderson JL, Faxon DP, Fuster V, Gibbons RJ, Gregoratos G, Halperin JL, Hiratzka LF, Hunt SA, Jacobs AK. ACC/AHA guidelines for the management of patients with ST-elevation myocardial infarction: a report of the American College of Cardiology/American Heart Association Task Force on Practice Guidelines (Committee to Revise the 1999 Guidelines for the Management of Patients with Acute Myocardial Infarction). *Circulation*. 2004;110:e82-e292.
16. Morrison LJ, Verbeek PR, McDonald AC, Sawadsky BV, Cook DJ. Mortality and prehospital thrombolysis for acute myocardial infarction: a meta-analysis. *JAMA*. 2000;283:2686-2692.
17. Dussoix P, Reuille O, Verin V, Gaspoz JM, Unger PF. Time savings with prehospital thrombolysis in an urban area. *Eur J Emerg Med*. 2003;10:2-5.
18. Feasibility, safety, and efficacy of domiciliary thrombolysis by general practitioners: Grampian region early anistreplase trial. GREAT Group. *BMJ*. 1992;305:548-553.
19. Libby P. Current concepts of the pathogenesis of the acute coronary syndromes. *Circulation*. 2001;104:365-372.
20. Wagner GS, Macfarlane P, Wellens H, Josephson M, Gorgels A, Mirvis DM, Pahlm O, Surawicz B, Kligfield P, Childers R, Gettes LS, Bailey JJ, Deal BJ, Hancock EW, Kors JA, Mason JW, Okin P, Rautaharju PM, van Herpen G. AHA/ACCF/HRS recommendations for the standardization and interpretation of the electrocardiogram: part VI: acute ischemia/infarction: a scientific statement from the American Heart Association Electrocardiography and Arrhythmias Committee, Council on Clinical Cardiology; the American College of Cardiology Foundation; and the Heart Rhythm Society. Endorsed by the International Society for Computerized Electrocardiology. *J Am Coll Cardiol*. 2009;53:1003-1011.
21. Wang K, Asinger RW, Marriott HJ. ST-segment elevation in conditions other than acute myocardial infarction. *N Engl J Med*. 2003;349:2128-2135.
22. Spodick DH. Differential characteristics of the electrocardiogram in early repolarization and acute pericarditis. *N Engl J Med*. 1976;295:523-526.
23. Libby P. Molecular bases of the acute coronary syndromes. *Circulation*. 1995;91:2844-2850.
24. Pantridge JF, Geddes JS. A mobile intensive-care unit in the management of myocardial infarction. *Lancet*. 1967;2:271-273.
25. Cohen MC, Rohtla KM, Lavery CE, Muller JE, Mittleman MA. Meta-analysis of the morning excess of acute myocardial infarction and sudden cardiac death. *Am J Cardiol*. 1997;79:1512-1516.
26. Colquhoun MC, Julien DG. Sudden death in the community—the arrhythmia causing cardiac arrest and results of immediate resuscitation. *Resuscitation*. 1992;24:177A.
27. Campbell RW, Murray A, Julian DG. Ventricular arrhythmias in first 12 hours of acute myocardial infarction. Natural history study. *Br Heart J*. 1981;46:351-357.

28. O'Doherty M, Tayler DI, Quinn E, Vincent R, Chamberlain DA. Five hundred patients with myocardial infarction monitored within one hour of symptoms. *Br Med J (Clin Res Ed)*. 1983;286:1405-1408.
29. Lie KI, Wellens HJ, Downar E, Durrer D. Observations on patients with primary ventricular fibrillation complicating acute myocardial infarction. *Circulation*. 1975;52:755-759.
30. Chiriboga D, Yarzebski J, Goldberg RJ, Gore JM, Alpert JS. Temporal trends (1975 through 1990) in the incidence and case-fatality rates of primary ventricular fibrillation complicating acute myocardial infarction. A communitywide perspective. *Circulation*. 1994;89:998-1003.
31. Kereiakes DJ, Weaver WD, Anderson JL, Feldman T, Gibler B, Aufderheide T, Williams DO, Martin LH, Anderson LC, Martin JS, et al. Time delays in the diagnosis and treatment of acute myocardial infarction: a tale of eight cities. Report from the Pre-hospital Study Group and the Cincinnati Heart Project. *Am Heart J*. 1990;120:773-780.
32. Goff DC Jr, Feldman HA, McGovern PG, Goldberg RJ, Simons-Morton DG, Cornell CE, Osganian SK, Cooper LS, Hedges JR. Prehospital delay in patients hospitalized with heart attack symptoms in the United States: the REACT trial. Rapid Early Action for Coronary Treatment (REACT) Study Group. *Am Heart J*. 1999;138:1046-1057.
33. Lee TH, Cook EF, Weisberg M, Sargent RK, Wilson C, Goldman L. Acute chest pain in the emergency room. Identification and examination of low-risk patients. *Arch Intern Med*. 1985;145:65-69.
34. Meine TJ, Roe MT, Chen AY, Patel MR, Washam JB, Ohman EM, Peacock WF, Pollack CV Jr, Gibler WB, Peterson ED. Association of intravenous morphine use and outcomes in acute coronary syndromes: results from the CRUSADE Quality Improvement Initiative. *Am Heart J*. 2005;149:1043-1049.
35. Hallstrom AP, Ornato JP, Weisfeldt M, Travers A, Christenson J, McBurnie MA, Zalenski R, Becker LB, Schron EB, Proschan M. Public-access defibrillation and survival after out-of-hospital cardiac arrest. *N Engl J Med*. 2004;351:637-646.
36. Karagounis L, Ipsen SK, Jessop MR, Gilmore KM, Valenti DA, Clawson JJ, Teichman S, Anderson JL. Impact of field-transmitted electrocardiography on time to in-hospital thrombolytic therapy in acute myocardial infarction. *Am J Cardiol*. 1990;66:786-791.
37. Kudenchuk PJ, Ho MT, Weaver WD, Litwin PE, Martin JS, Eisenberg MS, Hallstrom AP, Cobb LA, Kennedy JW. Accuracy of computer-interpreted electrocardiography in selecting patients for thrombolytic therapy. MITI Project Investigators. *J Am Coll Cardiol*. 1991;17:1486-1491.
38. Kereiakes DJ, Gibler WB, Martin LH, Pieper KS, Anderson LC. Relative importance of emergency medical system transport and the prehospital electrocardiogram on reducing hospital time delay to therapy for acute myocardial infarction: a preliminary report from the Cincinnati Heart Project. *Am Heart J*. 1992;123:835-840.
39. Aufderheide TP, Kereiakes DJ, Weaver WD, Gibler WB, Simoons ML. Planning, implementation, and process monitoring for prehospital 12-lead ECG diagnostic programs. *Prehosp Disaster Med*. 1996;11:162-171.
40. Aufderheide TP, Hendley GE, Thakur RK, Mateer JR, Stueven HA, Olson DW, Hargarten KM, Laitinen F, Robinson N, Preuss KC, et al. The diagnostic impact of prehospital 12-lead electrocardiography. *Ann Emerg Med*. 1990;19:1280-1287.
41. Grim PS, Feldman T, Childers RW. Evaluation of patients for the need of thrombolytic therapy in the prehospital setting. *Ann Emerg Med*. 1989;18:483-488.
42. Weaver WD, Cerqueira M, Hallstrom AP, Litwin PE, Martin JS, Kudenchuk PJ, Eisenberg M. Prehospital-initiated vs hospital-initiated thrombolytic therapy. The Myocardial Infarction Triage and Intervention Trial. *JAMA*. 1993;270:1211-1216.
43. Foster DB, Dufendach JH, Barkdoll CM, Mitchell BK. Prehospital recognition of AMI using independent nurse/paramedic 12-lead ECG evaluation: impact on in-hospital times to thrombolysis in a rural community hospital. *Am J Emerg Med*. 1994;12:25-31.
44. Aufderheide TP, Haselow WC, Hendley GE, Robinson NA, Armaganian L, Hargarten KM, Olson DW, Valley VT, Stueven HA. Feasibility of prehospital r-TPA therapy in chest pain patients. *Ann Emerg Med*. 1992;21:379-383.
45. Freimark D, Matetzky S, Leor J, Boyko V, Barbash IM, Behar S, Hod H. Timing of aspirin administration as a determinant of survival of patients with acute myocardial infarction treated with thrombolysis. *Am J Cardiol*. 2002;89:381-385.
46. Randomized trial of intravenous streptokinase, oral aspirin, both, or neither among 17,187 cases of suspected acute myocardial infarction: ISIS-2. ISIS-2 (Second International Study of Infarct Survival) Collaborative Group. *J Am Coll Cardiol*. 1988;12:3A-13A.
47. Gurfinkel EP, Manos EJ, Mejail RI, Cerda MA, Duronto EA, Garcia CN, Daroca AM, Mautner B. Low molecular weight heparin versus regular heparin or aspirin in the treatment of unstable angina and silent ischemia. *J Am Coll Cardiol*. 1995;26:313-318.
48. Collaborative meta-analysis of randomised trials of antiplatelet therapy for prevention of death, myocardial infarction, and stroke in high risk patients. *BMJ*. 2002;324:71-86.
49. Collaborative overview of randomised trials of antiplatelet therapy—I: Prevention of death, myocardial infarction, and stroke by prolonged antiplatelet therapy in various categories of patients. Antiplatelet Trialists' Collaboration. *BMJ*. 1994;308:81-106.
50. Kurth T, Glynn RJ, Walker AM, Chan KA, Buring JE, Hennekens CH, Gaziano JM. Inhibition of clinical benefits of aspirin on first myocardial infarction by nonsteroidal antiinflammatory drugs. *Circulation*. 2003;108:1191-1195.
51. MacDonald TM, Wei L. Effect of ibuprofen on cardioprotective effect of aspirin. *Lancet*. 2003;361:573-574.
52. Kimmel SE, Berlin JA, Reilly M, Jaskowiak J, Kishel L, Chittams J, Strom BL. The effects of nonselective non-aspirin non-steroidal anti-inflammatory medications on the risk of nonfatal myocardial infarction and their interaction with aspirin. *J Am Coll Cardiol*. 2004;43:985-990.
53. ISIS-4: a randomised factorial trial assessing early oral captopril, oral mononitrate, and intravenous magnesium sulphate in 58,050 patients with suspected acute myocardial infarction. ISIS-4 (Fourth International Study of Infarct Survival) Collaborative Group. *Lancet*. 1995;345:669-685.
54. Rawles JM. Quantification of the benefit of earlier thrombolytic therapy: five-year results of the Grampian Region Early Anistreplase Trial (GREAT). *J Am Coll Cardiol*. 1997;30:1181-1186.
55. Prehospital thrombolytic therapy in patients with suspected acute myocardial infarction. The European Myocardial Infarction Project Group. *N Engl J Med*. 1993;329:383-389.

56. Wallentin L, Goldstein P, Armstrong PW, Granger CB, Adgey AA, Arntz HR, Bogaerts K, Danays T, Lindahl B, Makijarvi M, Verheugt F, Van de Werf F. Efficacy and safety of tenecteplase in combination with the low-molecular-weight heparin enoxaparin or unfractionated heparin in the prehospital setting: the Assessment of the Safety and Efficacy of a New Thrombolytic Regimen (ASSENT)-3 PLUS randomized trial in acute myocardial infarction. *Circulation*. 2003;108:135-142.

57. Steg PG, Bonnefoy E, Chabaud S, Lapostolle F, Dubien PY, Cristofini P, Leizorovicz A, Touboul P. Impact of time to treatment on mortality after prehospital fibrinolysis or primary angioplasty: data from the CAPTIM randomized clinical trial. *Circulation*. 2003;108:2851-2856.

58. Morrow DA, Antman EM, Sayah A, Schuhwerk KC, Giugliano RP, deLemos JA, Waller M, Cohen SA, Rosenberg DG, Cutler SS, McCabe CH, Walls RM, Braunwald E. Evaluation of the time saved by prehospital initiation of reteplase for ST-elevation myocardial infarction: results of The Early Retavase-Thrombolysis in Myocardial Infarction (ER-TIMI) 19 trial. *J Am Coll Cardiol*. 2002;40:71-77.

59. Brouwer MA, Martin JS, Maynard C, Wirkus M, Litwin PE, Verheugt FW, Weaver WD. Influence of early prehospital thrombolysis on mortality and event-free survival (the Myocardial Infarction Triage and Intervention [MITI] Randomized Trial). MITI Project Investigators. *Am J Cardiol*. 1996;78:497-502.

60. An international randomized trial comparing four thrombolytic strategies for acute myocardial infarction. The GUSTO investigators. *N Engl J Med*. 1993;329:673-682.

61. O'Gara PT, Kushner FG, Ascheim DD, Casey DE Jr, Chung MK, de Lemos JA, Ettinger SM, Fang JC, Fesmire FM, Franklin BA, Granger CB, Krumholz HM, Linderbaum JA, Morrow DA, Newby LK, Ornato JP, Ou N, Radford MJ, Tamis-Holland JE, Tommaso CL, Tracy CM, Woo YJ, Zhao DX. 2013 ACCF/AHA guideline for the management of ST-elevation myocardial infarction: a report of the American College of Cardiology Foundation/American Heart Association Task Force on Practice Guidelines [published online ahead of print December 17, 2012]. *Circulation.* 2013. doi:10.1161/CIR.0b013e3182742cf6.

62. Emergency department: rapid identification and treatment of patients with acute myocardial infarction. National Heart Attack Alert Program Coordinating Committee, 60 Minutes to Treatment Working Group. *Ann Emerg Med*. 1994;23:311-329.

63. Pinto DS, Kirtane AJ, Nallamothu BK, Murphy SA, Cohen DJ, Laham RJ, Cutlip DE, Bates ER, Frederick PD, Miller DP, Carrozza JP Jr, Antman EM, Cannon CP, Gibson CM. Hospital delays in reperfusion for ST-elevation myocardial infarction: implications when selecting a reperfusion strategy. *Circulation*. 2006;114:2019-2025.

64. Kontos MC, McQueen RH, Jesse RL, Tatum JL, Ornato JP. Can myocardial infarction be rapidly identified in emergency department patients who have left bundle-branch block? *Ann Emerg Med*. 2001;37:431-438.

65. Gallagher EJ. Which patients with suspected myocardial ischemia and left bundle-branch block should receive thrombolytic agents? *Ann Emerg Med*. 2001;37:439-444.

66. Sgarbossa EB, Pinski SL, Wagner GS. Left bundle-branch block and the ECG in diagnosis of acute myocardial infarction. *JAMA*. 1999;282:1224-1225.

67. Sgarbossa EB. Recent advances in the electrocardiographic diagnosis of myocardial infarction: left bundle branch block and pacing. *Pacing Clin Electrophysiol*. 1996;19:1370-1379.

68. Sgarbossa EB. Value of the ECG in suspected acute myocardial infarction with left bundle branch block. *J Electrocardiol*. 2000;33:87-92.

69. Alpert JS, Thygesen K, Antman E, Bassand JP. Myocardial infarction redefined—a consensus document of The Joint European Society of Cardiology/American College of Cardiology Committee for the redefinition of myocardial infarction. *J Am Coll Cardiol*. 2000;36:959-969.

70. Wu AH, Apple FS, Gibler WB, Jesse RL, Warshaw MM, Valdes R Jr. National Academy of Clinical Biochemistry Standards of Laboratory Practice: recommendations for the use of cardiac markers in coronary artery diseases. *Clin Chem*. 1999;45:1104-1121.

71. Gibson CM, Murphy SA, Pride YB, Kirtane AJ, Aroesty JM, Stein EB, Ciaglo LN, Southard MC, Sabatine MS, Cannon CP, Braunwald E. Effects of pretreatment with clopidogrel on nonemergent percutaneous coronary intervention after fibrinolytic administration for ST-segment elevation myocardial infarction: a Clopidogrel as Adjunctive Reperfusion Therapy-Thrombolysis in Myocardial Infarction (CLARITY-TIMI) 28 study. *Am Heart J*. 2008;155:133-139.

72. Yusuf S, Zhao F, Mehta SR, Chrolavicius S, Tognoni G, Fox KK. Effects of clopidogrel in addition to aspirin in patients with acute coronary syndromes without ST-segment elevation. *N Engl J Med*. 2001;345:494-502.

73. Fox KA, Mehta SR, Peters R, Zhao F, Lakkis N, Gersh BJ, Yusuf S. Benefits and risks of the combination of clopidogrel and aspirin in patients undergoing surgical revascularization for non–ST-elevation acute coronary syndrome: the Clopidogrel in Unstable angina to prevent Recurrent ischemic Events (CURE) Trial. *Circulation*. 2004;110:1202-1208.

74. Sabatine MS, Cannon CP, Gibson CM, Lopez-Sendon JL, Montalescot G, Theroux P, Claeys MJ, Cools F, Hill KA, Skene AM, McCabe CH, Braunwald E. Addition of clopidogrel to aspirin and fibrinolytic therapy for myocardial infarction with ST-segment elevation. *N Engl J Med*. 2005;352:1179-1189.

75. O'Connor RE, Brady W, Brooks SC, Diercks D, Egan J, Ghaemmaghami C, Menon V, O'Neil BJ, Travers AH, Yannopoulos D. Part 10: acute coronary syndromes: 2010 American Heart Association Guidelines for Cardiopulmonary Resuscitation and Emergency Cardiovascular Care. *Circulation*. 2010;122:S787-S817.

76. Wiviott SD, Braunwald E, McCabe CH, Montalescot G, Ruzyllo W, Gottlieb S, Neumann FJ, Ardissino D, De Servi S, Murphy SA, Riesmeyer J, Weerakkody G, Gibson CM, Antman EM. Prasugrel versus clopidogrel in patients with acute coronary syndromes. *N Engl J Med*. 2007;357:2001-2015.

77. Antman EM, Wiviott SD, Murphy SA, Voitk J, Hasin Y, Widimsky P, Chandna H, Macias W, McCabe CH, Braunwald E. Early and late benefits of prasugrel in patients with acute coronary syndromes undergoing percutaneous coronary intervention: a TRITON-TIMI 38 (TRial to Assess Improvement in Therapeutic Outcomes by Optimizing Platelet InhibitioN with Prasugrel-Thrombolysis In Myocardial Infarction) analysis. *J Am Coll Cardiol*. 2008;51:2028-2033.

78. Murphy SA, Antman EM, Wiviott SD, Weerakkody G, Morocutti G, Huber K, Lopez-Sendon J, McCabe CH, Braunwald E. Reduction in recurrent cardiovascular events with prasugrel compared with clopidogrel in patients with acute coronary syndromes from the TRITON-TIMI 38 trial. *Eur Heart J*. 2008;29:2473-2479.

79. Wiviott SD, Braunwald E, Angiolillo DJ, Meisel S, Dalby AJ, Verheugt FW, Goodman SG, Corbalan R, Purdy DA, Murphy

SA, McCabe CH, Antman EM. Greater clinical benefit of more intensive oral antiplatelet therapy with prasugrel in patients with diabetes mellitus in the trial to assess improvement in therapeutic outcomes by optimizing platelet inhibition with prasugrel-Thrombolysis in Myocardial Infarction 38. *Circulation*. 2008;118:1626-1636.

80. Wiviott SD, Antman EM, Winters KJ, Weerakkody G, Murphy SA, Behounek BD, Carney RJ, Lazzam C, McKay RG, McCabe CH, Braunwald E. Randomized comparison of prasugrel (CS-747, LY640315), a novel thienopyridine P2Y12 antagonist, with clopidogrel in percutaneous coronary intervention: results of the Joint Utilization of Medications to Block Platelets Optimally (JUMBO)-TIMI 26 trial. *Circulation*. 2005;111:3366-3373.

81. Montalescot G, Wiviott SD, Braunwald E, Murphy SA, Gibson CM, McCabe CH, Antman EM. Prasugrel compared with clopidogrel in patients undergoing percutaneous coronary intervention for ST-elevation myocardial infarction (TRITON-TIMI 38): double-blind, randomised controlled trial. *Lancet*. 2009;373:723-731.

82. Wiviott SD, Braunwald E, McCabe CH, Horvath I, Keltai M, Herrman JP, Van de Werf F, Downey WE, Scirica BM, Murphy SA, Antman EM. Intensive oral antiplatelet therapy for reduction of ischaemic events including stent thrombosis in patients with acute coronary syndromes treated with percutaneous coronary intervention and stenting in the TRITON-TIMI 38 trial: a subanalysis of a randomised trial. *Lancet*. 2008;371:1353-1363.

83. Hjalmarson A, Herlitz J, Holmberg S, Ryden L, Swedberg K, Vedin A, Waagstein F, Waldenstrom A, Waldenstrom J, Wedel H, Wilhelmsen L, Wilhelmsson C. The Goteborg metoprolol trial. Effects on mortality and morbidity in acute myocardial infarction. *Circulation*. 1983;67:I26-32.

84. Hjalmarson A, Herlitz J. Limitation of infarct size by beta blockers and its potential role for prognosis. *Circulation*. 1983;67:I68-I71.

85. Metoprolol in acute myocardial infarction (MIAMI). A randomised placebo-controlled international trial. The MIAMI Trial Research Group. *Eur Heart J*. 1985;6:199-226.

86. Sleight P, Yusuf S, Peto R, Rossi P, Ramsdale D, Bennett D, Bray C, Furse L. Early intravenous atenolol treatment in suspected acute myocardial infarction. *Acta Med Scand Suppl*. 1981;651:185-192.

87. Randomised trial of intravenous atenolol among 16 027 cases of suspected acute myocardial infarction: ISIS-1. First International Study of Infarct Survival Collaborative Group. *Lancet*. 1986;2:57-66.

88. Rehnqvist N, Olsson G, Erhardt L, Ekman AM. Metoprolol in acute myocardial infarction reduces ventricular arrhythmias both in the early stage and after the acute event. *Int J Cardiol*. 1987;15:301-308.

89. Roberts R, Rogers WJ, Mueller HS, Lambrew CT, Diver DJ, Smith HC, Willerson JT, Knatterud GL, Forman S, Passamani E, et al. Immediate versus deferred beta-blockade following thrombolytic therapy in patients with acute myocardial infarction. Results of the Thrombolysis in Myocardial Infarction (TIMI) II-B Study. *Circulation*. 1991;83:422-437.

90. Al-Reesi A, Al-Zadjali N, Perry J, Fergusson D, Al-Shamsi M, Al-Thagafi M, Stiell I. Do beta-blockers reduce short-term mortality following acute myocardial infarction? A systematic review and meta-analysis. *CJEM*. 2008;10:215-223.

91. Chen ZM, Pan HC, Chen YP, Peto R, Collins R, Jiang LX, Xie JX, Liu LS. Early intravenous then oral metoprolol in 45 852 patients with acute myocardial infarction: randomised placebo-controlled trial. *Lancet*. 2005;366:1622-1632.

92. Wallentin L, Bergstrand L, Dellborg M, Fellenius C, Granger CB, Lindahl B, Lins LE, Nilsson T, Pehrsson K, Siegbahn A, Swahn E. Low molecular weight heparin (dalteparin) compared to unfractionated heparin as an adjunct to rt-PA (alteplase) for improvement of coronary artery patency in acute myocardial infarction-the ASSENT Plus study. *Eur Heart J*. 2003;24:897-908.

93. Ross AM, Molhoek P, Lundergan C, Knudtson M, Draoui Y, Regalado L, Le Louer V, Bigonzi F, Schwartz W, de Jong E, Coyne K. Randomized comparison of enoxaparin, a low-molecular-weight heparin, with unfractionated heparin adjunctive to recombinant tissue plasminogen activator thrombolysis and aspirin: second trial of Heparin and Aspirin Reperfusion Therapy (HART II). *Circulation*. 2001;104:648-652.

94. Van de Werf F, Armstrong PW, Granger C, Wallentin L. Efficacy and safety of tenecteplase in combination with enoxaparin, abciximab, or unfractionated heparin: the ASSENT-3 randomised trial in acute myocardial infarction. *Lancet*. 2001;358:605-613.

95. Theroux P, Welsh RC. Meta-analysis of randomized trials comparing enoxaparin versus unfractionated heparin as adjunctive therapy to fibrinolysis in ST-elevation acute myocardial infarction. *Am J Cardiol*. 2003;91:860-864.

96. Baird SH, Menown IB, McBride SJ, Trouton TG, Wilson C. Randomized comparison of enoxaparin with unfractionated heparin following fibrinolytic therapy for acute myocardial infarction. *Eur Heart J*. 2002;23:627-632.

97. Dickstein K, Kjekshus J. Effects of losartan and captopril on mortality and morbidity in high-risk patients after acute myocardial infarction: the OPTIMAAL randomised trial. Optimal Trial in Myocardial Infarction with Angiotensin II Antagonist Losartan. *Lancet*. 2002;360:752-760.

98. Correia LC, Sposito AC, Lima JC, Magalhaes LP, Passos LC, Rocha MS, D'Oliveira A, Esteves JP. Anti-inflammatory effect of atorvastatin (80 mg) in unstable angina pectoris and non-Q-wave acute myocardial infarction. *Am J Cardiol*. 2003;92:298-301.

99. Kayikcioglu M, Can L, Evrengul H, Payzin S, Kultursay H. The effect of statin therapy on ventricular late potentials in acute myocardial infarction. *Int J Cardiol*. 2003;90:63-72.

100. Kayikcioglu M, Can L, Kultursay H, Payzin S, Turkoglu C. Early use of pravastatin in patients with acute myocardial infarction undergoing coronary angioplasty. *Acta Cardiol*. 2002;57:295-302.

101. Kinlay S, Schwartz GG, Olsson AG, Rifai N, Leslie SJ, Sasiela WJ, Szarek M, Libby P, Ganz P. High-dose atorvastatin enhances the decline in inflammatory markers in patients with acute coronary syndromes in the MIRACL study. *Circulation*. 2003;108:1560-1566.

102. Mehta SR, Yusuf S, Diaz R, Zhu J, Pais P, Xavier D, Paolasso E, Ahmed R, Xie C, Kazmi K, Tai J, Orlandini A, Pogue J, Liu L. Effect of glucose-insulin-potassium infusion on mortality in patients with acute ST-segment elevation myocardial infarction: the CREATE-ECLA randomized controlled trial. *JAMA*. 2005;293:437-446.

103. Rationale and design of the magnesium in coronaries (MAGIC) study: A clinical trial to reevaluate the efficacy of early administration of magnesium in acute myocardial infarction. The MAGIC Steering Committee. *Am Heart J*. 2000;139:10-14.

104. Goodacre S, Locker T, Morris F, Campbell S. How useful are clinical features in the diagnosis of acute, undifferentiated chest pain? *Acad Emerg Med*. 2002;9:203-208.

105. Goodacre SW, Angelini K, Arnold J, Revill S, Morris F. Clinical predictors of acute coronary syndromes in patients with undifferentiated chest pain. *QJM*. 2003;96:893-898.

106. Everts B, Karlson BW, Wahrborg P, Hedner T, Herlitz J. Localization of pain in suspected acute myocardial infarction in relation to final diagnosis, age and sex, and site and type of infarction. *Heart Lung*. 1996;25:430-437.

107. McSweeney JC, Cody M, O'Sullivan P, Elberson K, Moser DK, Garvin BJ. Women's early warning symptoms of acute myocardial infarction. *Circulation*. 2003;108:2619-2623.

108. Braunwald E, Antman EM, Beasley JW, Califf RM, Cheitlin MD, Hochman JS, Jones RH, Kereiakes D, Kupersmith J, Levin TN, Pepine CJ, Schaeffer JW, Smith EE III, Steward DE, Theroux P, Gibbons RJ, Alpert JS, Eagle KA, Faxon DP, Fuster V, Gardner TJ, Gregoratos G, Russell RO, Smith SC Jr. ACC/AHA guidelines for the management of patients with unstable angina and non–ST-segment elevation myocardial infarction: executive summary and recommendations. A report of the American College of Cardiology/American Heart Association task force on practice guidelines (committee on the management of patients with unstable angina). *Circulation*. 2000;102:1193-1209.

109. Braunwald E. Unstable angina: an etiologic approach to management. *Circulation*. 1998;98:2219-2222.

110. Braunwald E, Antman EM, Beasley JW, Califf RM, Cheitlin MD, Hochman JS, Jones RH, Kereiakes D, Kupersmith J, Levin TN, Pepine CJ, Schaeffer JW, Smith EE III, Steward DE, Theroux P, Gibbons RJ, Alpert JS, Faxon DP, Fuster V, Gregoratos G, Hiratzka LF, Jacobs AK, Smith SC Jr. ACC/AHA guideline update for the management of patients with unstable angina and non–ST-segment elevation myocardial infarction—2002: summary article: a report of the American College of Cardiology/American Heart Association Task Force on Practice Guidelines (Committee on the Management of Patients With Unstable Angina). *Circulation*. 2002;106:1893-1900.

111. Peberdy MA, Ornato JP. Coronary artery disease in women. *Heart Dis Stroke*. 1992;1:315-319.

112. Douglas PS, Ginsburg GS. The evaluation of chest pain in women. *N Engl J Med*. 1996;334:1311-1315.

113. Sullivan AK, Holdright DR, Wright CA, Sparrow JL, Cunningham D, Fox KM. Chest pain in women: clinical, investigative, and prognostic features. *BMJ*. 1994;308:883-886.

114. Solomon CG, Lee TH, Cook EF, Weisberg MC, Brand DA, Rouan GW, Goldman L. Comparison of clinical presentation of acute myocardial infarction in patients older than 65 years of age to younger patients: the Multicenter Chest Pain Study experience. *Am J Cardiol*. 1989;63:772-776.

115. Khan IA, Nair CK. Clinical, diagnostic, and management perspectives of aortic dissection. *Chest*. 2002;122:311-328.

116. Hagan PG, Nienaber CA, Isselbacher EM, Bruckman D, Karavite DJ, Russman PL, Evangelista A, Fattori R, Suzuki T, Oh JK, Moore AG, Malouf JF, Pape LA, Gaca C, Sechtem U, Lenferink S, Deutsch HJ, Diedrichs H, Marcos y Robles J, Llovet A, Gilon D, Das SK, Armstrong WF, Deeb GM, Eagle KA. The International Registry of Acute Aortic Dissection (IRAD): new insights into an old disease. *JAMA*. 2000;283:897-903.

117. Podbregar M, Krivec B, Voga G. Impact of morphologic characteristics of central pulmonary thromboemboli in massive pulmonary embolism. *Chest*. 2002;122:973-979.

118. Goldhaber SZ, Visani L, De Rosa M. Acute pulmonary embolism: clinical outcomes in the International Cooperative Pulmonary Embolism Registry (ICOPER). *Lancet*. 1999;353:1386-1389.

119. Heit JA. The epidemiology of venous thromboembolism in the community: implications for prevention and management. *J Thromb Thrombolysis*. 2006;21:23-29.

120. Kucher N, Rossi E, De Rosa M, Goldhaber SZ. Massive pulmonary embolism. *Circulation*. 2006;113:577-582.

121. Thabut G, Thabut D, Myers RP, Bernard-Chabert B, Marrash-Chahla R, Mal H, Fournier M. Thrombolytic therapy of pulmonary embolism: a meta-analysis. *J Am Coll Cardiol*. 2002;40:1660-1667.

122. Piazza G, Goldhaber SZ. Acute pulmonary embolism: part I: epidemiology and diagnosis. *Circulation*. 2006;114:e28-e32.

123. Piazza G, Goldhaber SZ. Acute pulmonary embolism: part II: treatment and prophylaxis. *Circulation*. 2006;114:e42-e47.

124. Aikat S, Ghaffari S. A review of pericardial diseases: clinical, ECG and hemodynamic features and management. *Cleve Clin J Med*. 2000;67:903-914.

125. Bilchick KC, Wise RA. Paradoxical physical findings described by Kussmaul: pulsus paradoxus and Kussmaul's sign. *Lancet*. 2002;359:1940-1942.

126. Spittell JA Jr. Chest pain in patients with normal findings on angiography. *Mayo Clin Proc*. 2002;77:296.

127. King SB III, Smith SC Jr, Hirshfeld JW Jr, Jacobs AK, Morrison DA, Williams DO, Feldman TE, Kern MJ, O'Neill WW, Schaff HV, Whitlow PL, Adams CD, Anderson JL, Buller CE, Creager MA, Ettinger SM, Halperin JL, Hunt SA, Krumholz HM, Kushner FG, Lytle BW, Nishimura R, Page RL, Riegel B, Tarkington LG, Yancy CW. 2007 Focused Update of the ACC/AHA/SCAI 2005 Guideline Update for Percutaneous Coronary Intervention: a report of the American College of Cardiology/American Heart Association Task Force on Practice Guidelines: 2007 Writing Group to Review New Evidence and Update the ACC/AHA/SCAI 2005 Guideline Update for Percutaneous Coronary Intervention, Writing on Behalf of the 2005 Writing Committee. *Circulation*. 2008;117:261-295.

128. Savonitto S, Ardissino D, Granger CB, Morando G, Prando MD, Mafrici A, Cavallini C, Melandri G, Thompson TD, Vahanian A, Ohman EM, Califf RM, Van de Werf F, Topol EJ. Prognostic value of the admission electrocardiogram in acute coronary syndromes. *JAMA*. 1999;281:707-713.

129. Antman EM, Tanasijevic MJ, Thompson B, Schactman M, McCabe CH, Cannon CP, Fischer GA, Fung AY, Thompson C, Wybenga D, Braunwald E. Cardiac-specific troponin I levels to predict the risk of mortality in patients with acute coronary syndromes. *N Engl J Med*. 1996;335:1342-1349.

130. Antman EM, Cohen M, Bernink PJ, McCabe CH, Horacek T, Papuchis G, Mautner B, Corbalan R, Radley D, Braunwald E. The TIMI risk score for unstable angina/non–ST elevation MI: A method for prognostication and therapeutic decision making. *JAMA*. 2000;284:835-842.

131. A randomised, blinded, trial of clopidogrel versus aspirin in patients at risk of ischaemic events (CAPRIE). CAPRIE Steering Committee. *Lancet*. 1996;348:1329-1339.

132. Levine GN, Bates ER, Blankenship JC, Bailey SR, Bittl JA, Cercek B, Chambers CE, Ellis SG, Guyton RA, Hollenberg SM, Khot UN, Lange RA, Mauri L, Mehran R,

Moussa ID, Mukherjee D, Nallamothu BK, Ting HH. 2011 ACCF/AHA/SCAI Guideline for Percutaneous Coronary Intervention: executive summary: a report of the American College of Cardiology Foundation/American Heart Association Task Force on Practice Guidelines and the Society for Cardiovascular Angiography and Interventions. *Catheter Cardiovasc Interv*. 2012;79:453-495.

133. Steinhubl SR, Berger PB, Mann JT III, Fry ET, DeLago A, Wilmer C, Topol EJ. Early and sustained dual oral antiplatelet therapy following percutaneous coronary intervention: a randomized controlled trial. *JAMA*. 2002;288:2411-2420.

134. Steinhubl SR, Berger PB, Brennan DM, Topol EJ. Optimal timing for the initiation of pre-treatment with 300 mg clopidogrel before percutaneous coronary intervention. *J Am Coll Cardiol*. 2006;47:939-943.

135. Cuisset T, Frere C, Quilici J, Morange PE, Nait-Saidi L, Carvajal J, Lehmann A, Lambert M, Bonnet JL, Alessi MC. Benefit of a 600-mg loading dose of clopidogrel on platelet reactivity and clinical outcomes in patients with non–ST-segment elevation acute coronary syndrome undergoing coronary stenting. *J Am Coll Cardiol*. 2006;48:1339-1345.

136. Hochholzer W, Trenk D, Frundi D, Blanke P, Fischer B, Andris K, Bestehorn HP, Buttner HJ, Neumann FJ. Time dependence of platelet inhibition after a 600-mg loading dose of clopidogrel in a large, unselected cohort of candidates for percutaneous coronary intervention. *Circulation*. 2005;111:2560-2564.

137. Bosch X, Marrugat J. Platelet glycoprotein IIb/IIIa blockers for percutaneous coronary revascularization, and unstable angina and non–ST-segment elevation myocardial infarction. *Cochrane Database Syst Rev*. 2001:CD002130.

138. Jneid H, Anderson JL, Wright RS, Adams CD, Bridges CR, Casey DE, Ettinger SM, Fesmire FM, Ganiats TG, Lincoff AM, Peterson ED, Philippides GJ, Theroux P, Wenger NK, Zidar JP. 2012 ACCF/AHA Focused Update of the Guideline for the Management of Patients With Unstable Angina/Non–ST-Elevation Myocardial Infarction (Updating the 2007 Guideline and Replacing the 2011 Focused Update): a report of the American College of Cardiology Foundation/American Heart Association Task Force on Practice Guidelines. *Circulation.* 2012;126:875-910.

139. Boersma E, Harrington RA, Moliterno DJ, White H, Theroux P, Van de Werf F, de Torbal A, Armstrong PW, Wallentin LC, Wilcox RG, Simes J, Califf RM, Topol EJ, Simoons ML. Platelet glycoprotein IIb/IIIa inhibitors in acute coronary syndromes: a meta-analysis of all major randomised clinical trials. *Lancet*. 2002;359:189-198.

140. Simoons ML. Effect of glycoprotein IIb/IIIa receptor blocker abciximab on outcome in patients with acute coronary syndromes without early coronary revascularisation: the GUSTO IV-ACS randomised trial. *Lancet*. 2001;357:1915-1924.

141. Ottervanger JP, Armstrong P, Barnathan ES, Boersma E, Cooper JS, Ohman EM, James S, Topol E, Wallentin L, Simoons ML. Long-term results after the glycoprotein IIb/IIIa inhibitor abciximab in unstable angina: one-year survival in the GUSTO IV-ACS (Global Use of Strategies To Open Occluded Coronary Arteries IV—Acute Coronary Syndrome) Trial. *Circulation*. 2003;107:437-442.

142. Ferguson J. Low-molecular-weight heparins and glyco-protein IIb/IIIa antagonists in acute coronary syndromes. *J Invasive Cardiol*. 2004;16:136-144.

143. Ferguson JJ, Califf RM, Antman EM, Cohen M, Grines CL, Goodman S, Kereiakes DJ, Langer A, Mahaffey KW, Nessel CC, Armstrong PW, Avezum A, Aylward P, Becker RC, Biasucci L, Borzak S, Col J, Frey MJ, Fry E, Gulba DC, Guneri S, Gurfinkel E, Harrington R, Hochman JS, Kleiman NS, Leon MB, Lopez-Sendon JL, Pepine CJ, Ruzyllo W, Steinhubl SR, Teirstein PS, Toro-Figueroa L, White H. Enoxaparin vs unfractionated heparin in high-risk patients with non–ST-segment elevation acute coronary syndromes managed with an intended early invasive strategy: primary results of the SYNERGY randomized trial. *JAMA*. 2004;292:45-54.

144. Patti G, Pasceri V, Colonna G, Miglionico M, Fischetti D, Sardella G, Montinaro A, Di Sciascio G. Atorvastatin pretreatment improves outcomes in patients with acute coronary syndromes undergoing early percutaneous coronary intervention: results of the ARMYDA-ACS randomized trial. *J Am Coll Cardiol*. 2007;49:1272-1278.

145. Blalock A. *Principles of Surgical Care: Shock and Other Problems*. St Louis, MO: Mosby; 1940.

146. Awad HH, Anderson FA Jr, Gore JM, Goodman SG, Goldberg RJ. Cardiogenic shock complicating acute coronary syndromes: Insights from the Global Registry of Acute Coronary Events. *Am Heart J*. 2012;163:963-971.

147. Jacobs AK, French JK, Col J, Sleeper LA, Slater JN, Carnendran L, Boland J, Jiang X, LeJemtel T, Hochman JS. Cardiogenic shock with non–ST-segment elevation myocardial infarction: a report from the SHOCK Trial Registry. SHould we emergently revascularize Occluded coronaries for Cardiogenic shocK? *J Am Coll Cardiol*. 2000;36:1091-1096.

148. Holmes DR Jr, Berger PB, Hochman JS, Granger CB, Thompson TD, Califf RM, Vahanian A, Bates ER, Topol EJ. Cardiogenic shock in patients with acute ischemic syndromes with and without ST-segment elevation. *Circulation*. 1999;100:2067-2073.

149. Parrillo JE, Burch C, Shelhamer JH, Parker MM, Natanson C, Schuette W. A circulating myocardial depressant substance in humans with septic shock. Septic shock patients with a reduced ejection fraction have a circulating factor that depresses in vitro myocardial cell performance. *J Clin Invest*. 1985;76:1539-1553.

150. Menon V, Slater JN, White HD, Sleeper LA, Cocke T, Hochman JS. Acute myocardial infarction complicated by systemic hypoperfusion without hypotension: report of the SHOCK trial registry. *Am J Med*. 2000;108:374-380.

151. Hochman JS. Cardiogenic shock complicating acute myocardial infarction: expanding the paradigm. *Circulation*. 2003;107:2998-3002.

152. Hollenberg SM, Kavinsky CJ, Parrillo JE. Cardiogenic shock. *Ann Intern Med*. 1999;131:47-59.

153. Goldberg RJ, Samad NA, Yarzebski J, Gurwitz J, Bigelow C, Gore JM. Temporal trends in cardiogenic shock complicating acute myocardial infarction. *N Engl J Med*. 1999;340:1162-1168.

154. Berger PB, Holmes DR Jr, Stebbins AL, Bates ER, Califf RM, Topol EJ. Impact of an aggressive invasive catheterization and revascularization strategy on mortality in patients with cardiogenic shock in the Global Utilization of Streptokinase and Tissue Plasminogen Activator for Occluded Coronary Arteries (GUSTO-I) trial. An observational study. *Circulation*. 1997;96:122-127.

155. Tiefenbrunn AJ, Chandra NC, French WJ, Gore JM, Rogers WJ. Clinical experience with primary percutaneous transluminal coronary angioplasty compared with alteplase (recombinant tissue-type plasminogen activator) in patients with acute myocardial infarction: a report from the Second

National Registry of Myocardial Infarction (NRMI-2). *J Am Coll Cardiol*. 1998;31:1240-1245.

156. Lee L, Erbel R, Brown TM, Laufer N, Meyer J, O'Neill WW. Multicenter registry of angioplasty therapy of cardiogenic shock: initial and long-term survival. *J Am Coll Cardiol*. 1991;17:599-603.

157. Grines CL. Aggressive intervention for myocardial infarction: angioplasty, stents, and intra-aortic balloon pumping. *Am J Cardiol*. 1996;78:29-34.

158. Hochman JS, Sleeper LA, Webb JG, Dzavik V, Buller CE, Aylward P, Col J, White HD. Early revascularization and long-term survival in cardiogenic shock complicating acute myocardial infarction. *JAMA*. 2006;295:2511-2515.

159. Jacobs AK, Leopold JA, Bates E, Mendes LA, Sleeper LA, White H, Davidoff R, Boland J, Modur S, Forman R, Hochman JS. Cardiogenic shock caused by right ventricular infarction: a report from the SHOCK registry. *J Am Coll Cardiol*. 2003;41:1273-1279.

160. Guidelines 2000 for Cardiopulmonary Resuscitation and Emergency Cardiovascular Care. Part 7: the era of reperfusion: section 1: acute coronary syndromes (acute myocardial infarction). The American Heart Association in collaboration with the International Liaison Committee on Resuscitation. *Circulation*. 2000;102:I172-I203.

Chapter 12

Stroke

This Chapter

- **How to Identify Patients With Ischemic Stroke**
- **Whom to Transport to an Appropriate Facility for Stroke Care**
- **How to Minimize Disability From Stroke**

Key Points

- Emergency medical services (EMS) activation and transport results in faster hospital arrival and decreased emergency department (ED) evaluation time.
- EMS dispatchers can identify 50% of patients with stroke.
- With standard training in stroke recognition, paramedics demonstrated a sensitivity of 61% to 66% for identifying patients with stroke, and the sensitivity increased to 86% to 97% after receipt of training in use of a stroke assessment tool.
- Public education programs result in sustained identification and treatment of stroke patients.
- Designation of *primary stroke centers* for emergency stroke care is strongly recommended.

Introduction

Each year in the United States, approximately 795 000 people have a new or repeat stroke.[1] Mortality data from 2009 indicate that stroke accounted for approximately 1 of every 19 deaths in the United States. On average, someone has a stroke every 40 seconds.[1] Many advances have been made in stroke prevention, treatment, and rehabilitation.[2,3] For example, fibrinolytic therapy can limit the extent of neurologic damage from stroke and improve outcome, but the time available for treatment is limited.[3,4]

Stroke Facts[1]

- On average, every 40 seconds someone in the United States has a stroke.
- Each year approximately 795 000 people experience a new or recurrent stroke. Approximately 610 000 of these are first attacks, and 185 000 are recurrent attacks.
- Each year, approximately 55 000 more women than men have a stroke. Blacks and Hispanics have almost twice the risk of first-ever stroke as whites.

Activation of the 911 system and brief EMS assessment and transport of potential stroke patients to the closest stroke centers are recommended. Healthcare providers, hospitals, and communities must develop systems to increase the efficiency and effectiveness of stroke care. The 8 D's of Stroke Care—detection, dispatch, delivery, door, data, decision, drug, and disposition (Table 34)—highlight the major steps in diagnosis and treatment and the key points at which delays can occur.[5] Additionally, educational programs to increase public awareness are encouraged because they increase the number of patients evaluated and treated for stroke. This chapter describes the management of acute stroke in the adult patient. It summarizes out-of-hospital care through the first hours of therapy and focuses treatment on rapid identification of acute ischemic stroke while allowing evaluation for reperfusion therapy. Highlights and updates from the *2010 American Heart Association (AHA) Guidelines for Cardiopulmonary Resuscitation (CPR) and Emergency Cardiovascular Care (ECC)* and the *AHA/American Stroke Association (ASA) Guidelines for the Early Management of Adults With Ischemic Stroke* are included. For additional information about the management of acute ischemic stroke, consult these guidelines.[6]

The Stroke Chain of Survival

The goal of stroke care is to minimize brain injury and maximize the patient's recovery. The time-sensitive nature of stroke care is central to the establishment of successful stroke systems, hence the commonly used refrain, "Time is Brain." Therefore, the AHA and ASA have developed a community-oriented Stroke Chain of Survival (Figure 99) that links specific actions to be taken by patients and family members with recommended actions by out-of-hospital healthcare responders, ED personnel, and in-hospital specialty services:

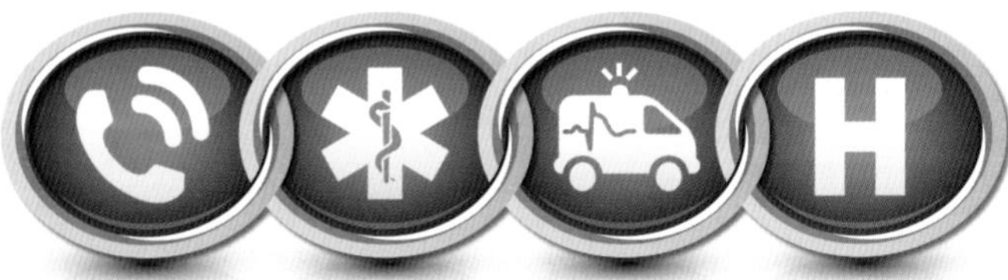

Figure 99. The Stroke Chain of Survival.

- Rapid recognition and reaction to stroke warning signs
- Rapid EMS dispatch
- Rapid EMS system transport and prearrival notification to the receiving hospital
- Rapid diagnosis and treatment in hospital

The first 3 points constitute out-of-hospital acute stroke care. The in-hospital acute stroke care (point 4) includes the

- Ability to rapidly determine patient eligibility for fibrinolytic therapy
- Administration of fibrinolytic therapy to appropriate candidates within target times
- Initiation of the stroke pathway and patient admission to a stroke unit if available

The AHA ECC stroke guidelines focus on the initial out-of-hospital and ED assessment and management of the patient with acute stroke as depicted in the Suspected Stroke Algorithm (Figure 100). The target times and goals are recommended by the National Institute of Neurological Disorders and Stroke (NINDS) and are illustrated on the left side of the algorithm as clocks. The NINDS has recommended measurable goals for the evaluation of stroke patients. These targets or goals should be achieved for at least 80% of patients with acute stroke.

The 8 D's of Stroke Care

In ST-segment elevation myocardial infarction (STEMI), time is muscle. When acute ischemic stroke occurs, time is brain, so the reperfusion concept was expanded to include not only patients with acute coronary syndromes (STEMI) but also highly selected stroke patients.[5] Hazinski was the first to describe an analogous series of linked actions to guide ACLS stroke care. Borrowing from the "door-to-drug" theme of the National Heart Attack Alert Program for fibrinolytic treatment of STEMI,[7] the 8 D's of Stroke Care were created. At each step, care must be organized and efficient to avoid needless delays.

Table 34. The 8 D's of Stroke Care

The 8 D's of Stroke Care highlight the major steps in diagnosis and treatment of stroke and key points at which delays can occur:

- **Detection:** Rapid recognition of stroke symptoms
- **Dispatch:** Early activation and dispatch of EMS by calling 911
- **Delivery:** Rapid EMS identification, management, and transport
- **Door:** Appropriate triage to stroke center
- **Data:** Rapid triage, evaluation, and management within the ED
- **Decision:** Stroke expertise and therapy selection
- **Drug:** Fibrinolytic therapy, intra-arterial strategies
- **Disposition:** Rapid admission to the stroke unit or critical care unit

Abbreviations: ED, emergency department; EMS, emergency medical services.

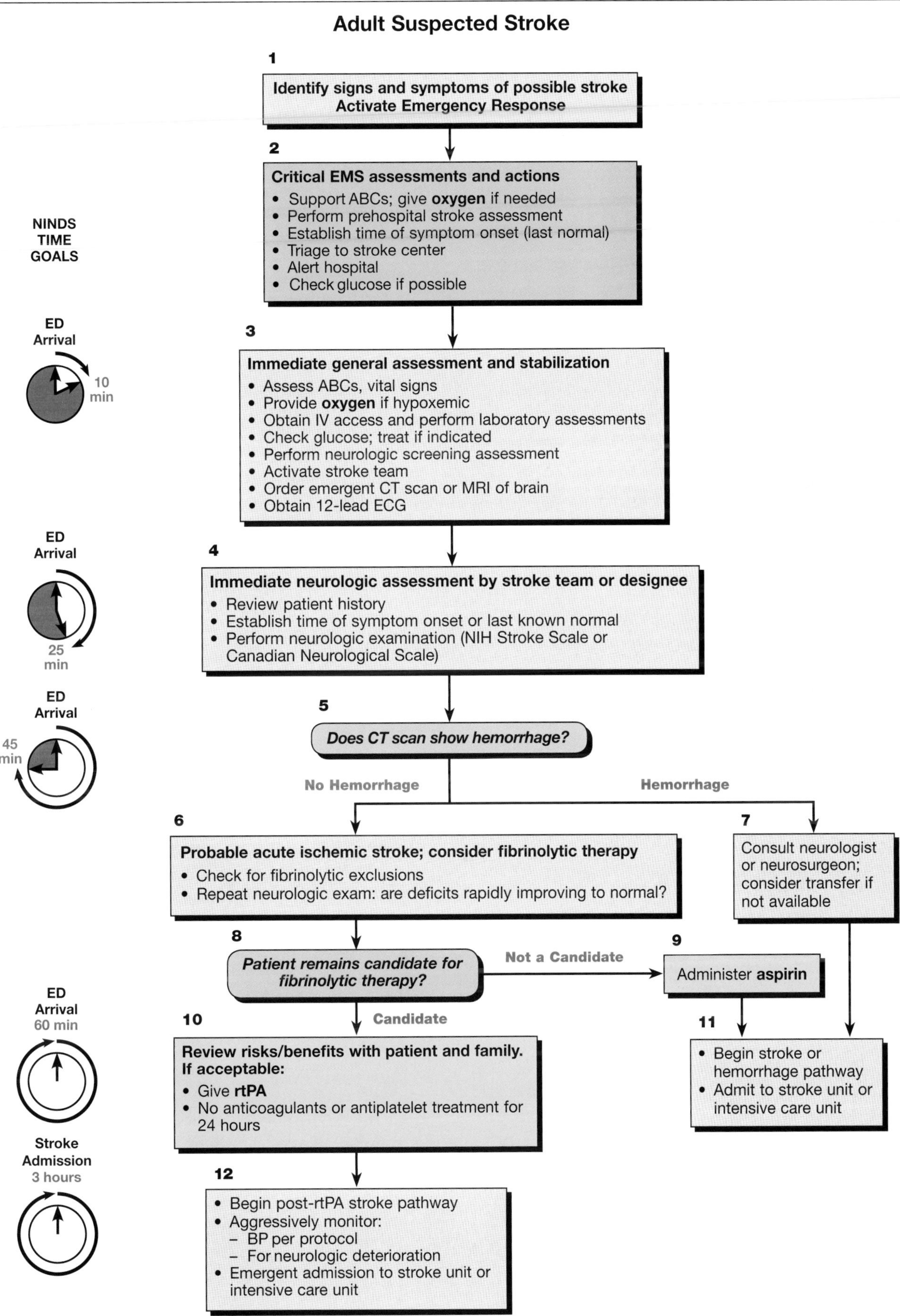

Adult Suspected Stroke
1
Identify signs and symptoms of possible stroke
Activate Emergency Response
2
Critical EMS assessments and actions
• Support ABCs; give oxygen if needed
• Perform prehospital stroke assessment
• Establish time of symptom onset (last normal)
• Triage to stroke center
• Alert hospital
• Check glucose if possible
NINDS TIME GOALS
ED Arrival
10 min
3
Immediate general assessment and stabilization
• Assess ABCs, vital signs
• Provide oxygen if hypoxemic
• Obtain IV access and perform laboratory assessments
• Check glucose; treat if indicated
• Perform neurologic screening assessment
• Activate stroke team
• Order emergent CT scan or MRI of brain
• Obtain 12-lead ECG
ED Arrival
25 min
4
Immediate neurologic assessment by stroke team or designee
• Review patient history
• Establish time of symptom onset or last known normal
• Perform neurologic examination (NIH Stroke Scale or Canadian Neurological Scale)
ED Arrival
45 min
5
Does CT scan show hemorrhage?
No Hemorrhage
Hemorrhage
6
Probable acute ischemic stroke; consider fibrinolytic therapy
• Check for fibrinolytic exclusions
• Repeat neurologic exam: are deficits rapidly improving to normal?
7
Consult neurologist or neurosurgeon; consider transfer if not available
8
Patient remains candidate for fibrinolytic therapy?
Not a Candidate
9
Administer aspirin
ED Arrival
60 min
10
Candidate
Review risks/benefits with patient and family. If acceptable:
• Give rtPA
• No anticoagulants or antiplatelet treatment for 24 hours
11
• Begin stroke or hemorrhage pathway
• Admit to stroke unit or intensive care unit
Stroke Admission
3 hours
12
• Begin post-rtPA stroke pathway
• Aggressively monitor:
– BP per protocol
– For neurologic deterioration
• Emergent admission to stroke unit or intensive care unit

Figure 100. The Suspected Stroke Algorithm.

Definitions

A *cerebrovascular accident or stroke* refers to the acute neurologic impairment that follows an interruption in blood supply or a rupture of a blood vessel to a specific region of the brain. Experts and clinicians most often classify strokes as either *ischemic* or *hemorrhagic* (Figure 101). The causes of stroke are numerous, but the initial therapy is based on the presence or absence of bleeding and a presumed ischemic stroke regardless of cause.

The distinction between ischemic and hemorrhagic stroke is important for these reasons:

- Reperfusion therapy with recombinant tissue plasminogen activator (rtPA) is appropriate for ischemic stroke only.
- Hemorrhagic stroke is an absolute contraindication to rtPA therapy.
- rtPA can be fatal if given mistakenly to a patient having a hemorrhagic stroke.

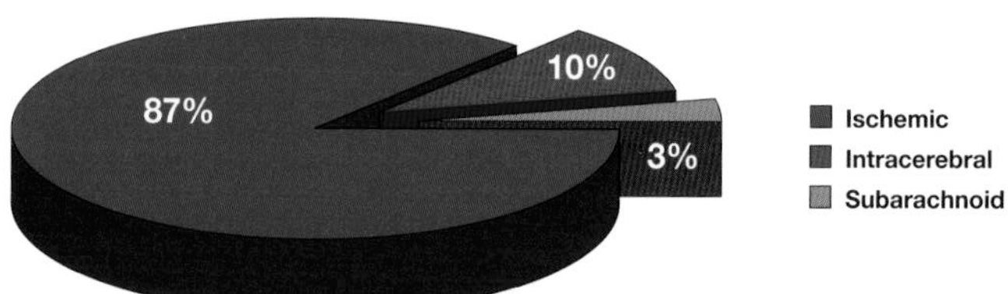

Figure 101. Type of stroke. Eighty-seven percent of strokes are ischemic and potentially eligible for fibrinolytic therapy if patients otherwise qualify. Thirteen percent of strokes are hemorrhagic (10% intracerebral and 3% subarachnoid). The male/female incidence ratio was 1.25 in those 55 to 64 years of age, 1.50 in those 65 to 74, 1.07 in those 75 to 84, and 0.76 in those 85 years of age and older, and blacks and Hispanics had a much higher risk of first-ever stroke than whites.

Ischemic Stroke

Definition and Categories of Ischemic Stroke

In an ischemic stroke (87% of all strokes), interruption in blood supply is caused by occlusion of an artery to a region of the brain. Ischemic stroke rarely leads to death within the first hour.

Ischemic strokes can be defined on the basis of cause and duration of symptoms. They are generally subdivided into the following categories (Figure 102):

- **Thrombotic stroke:** An acute clot that occludes an artery is superimposed on chronic arterial narrowing, acutely altered endothelial lining, or both. This pathophysiology parallels that for acute coronary syndromes (ACS), in which a ruptured or eroded plaque is the proximate cause of most episodes of ACS.
- **Embolic stroke:** Intravascular material, most often a blood clot, separates from a proximal source and flows through an artery until it occludes an artery in the brain. Many of these are cardioembolic—originating from the heart—in patients with atrial fibrillation, valvular heart disease, acute myocardial infarction (AMI), or rarely, endocarditis.
- **Transient ischemic attack (TIA) (sometimes called "mini-stroke"):** A transient episode of neurologic dysfunction caused by focal brain, spinal cord, or retinal ischemia, without acute infarction. Clinically, most TIAs resolve completely and spontaneously within 1 hour.
- **Reversible ischemic neurologic deficit (RIND): Any focal neurologic deficit** that resolves completely and spontaneously within 24 hours. (RINDS were **previously called TIAs.**) **Any patient with a persistent neurologic deficit** beyond 24 hours is said to have had a stroke. New diagnostic techniques have shown that 60% of patients with a TIA or RIND have definite evidence of brain infarction.
- **Hypoperfusion stroke:** A more global pattern of brain infarction that results from low blood flow or intermittent periods of no flow. Hypoperfusion stroke often occurs in patients who recover cardiac function after sudden cardiac arrest.

Classification by Vascular Supply

Strokes are also classified by vascular supply and anatomic location:

- **Anterior circulation (carotid artery territory) stroke:** Stroke that follows occlusion of branches of the *carotid artery*. This accounts for about 80% of strokes and usually involves the cerebral hemispheres.
- **Posterior circulation (vertebrobasilar artery territory) stroke:** Stroke that follows occlusion of branches of the *vertebrobasilar artery*. These strokes usually involve the brainstem or cerebellum. Approximately 20% of strokes belong to this group.

Hemorrhagic Stroke

Hemorrhagic strokes (13% of all strokes) occur when a blood vessel in the brain suddenly ruptures with hemorrhage into the surrounding tissue. Damage results from direct trauma to brain cells; expanding mass effects, which lead to elevated intracranial pressure; release of damaging mediators; local vascular spasm; and loss of blood supply to brain tissue downstream from the ruptured vessel.

There are 2 types of hemorrhagic stroke, based on the location of the arterial rupture:

- **Intracerebral hemorrhagic stroke (10%):** Occurs when blood leaks directly into the brain parenchyma, usually from small intracerebral arterioles damaged by chronic hypertension.
  - Hypertension is the most common cause of intracerebral hemorrhage.

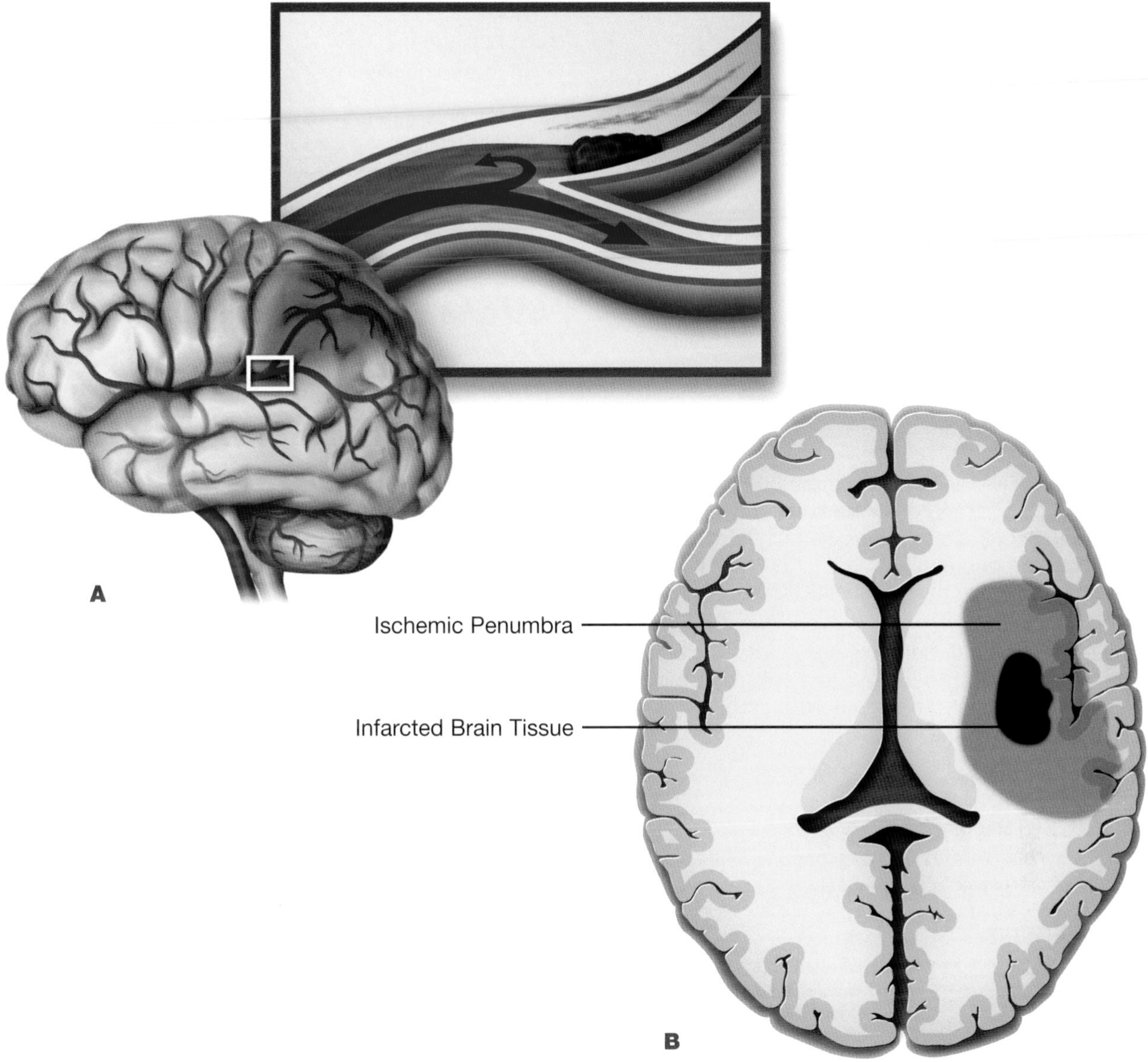

Figure 102. Occlusion in the middle cerebral artery by a thrombus: **A,** Area of ischemic penumbra (ischemic, but not yet infarcted [dead] brain tissue) surrounding areas of infarction. **B,** Area of infarction surrounding immediate site and distal portion of brain tissue after occlusion. This ischemic penumbra is alive but dysfunctional because of altered membrane potentials. The dysfunction is potentially reversible. Current stroke treatment tries to keep the area of permanent brain infarction as small as possible by preventing the areas of reversible brain ischemia in the penumbra from transforming into larger areas of irreversible brain infarction.

  - Among the elderly, amyloid angiopathy appears to play a major role in intracerebral hemorrhage.
- **Subarachnoid hemorrhagic stroke (3%):** Occurs when blood leaks from a cerebral vessel into the subarachnoid space. If the rupture occurs in a cerebral artery, the blood is released at systemic arterial pressure, which causes sudden, painful, and dramatic symptoms.
  - Aneurysms cause most subarachnoid hemorrhages.
  - Arteriovenous malformations cause approximately 5% of subarachnoid hemorrhages.

Pathophysiology

The Evolving "Ruptured Plaque" Concept

An ulcerated, ruptured plaque is the key mechanism of most thrombotic and embolic strokes in patients without valvular heart disease or atrial fibrillation. In thrombotic stroke, complete occlusion develops at an atherosclerotic plaque. In embolic stroke the developing thrombus breaks off and heads downstream. Ruptured plaques occur not only in the intracranial branches of the carotid and vertebrobasilar arteries but also in the extracranial portions of the carotid arteries and in the ascending and transverse aorta.

The "ruptured plaque" concept, the pathophysiologic foundation of ACS, explains many features of ischemic stroke[8-10] (see Chapter 11, Figure 76). The effects of stroke result from interaction between blood vessels, the coagulation components of blood, inflammatory cells, and chemical mediators of inflammation.

- The most common cause of acute ischemic stroke is atherosclerosis of the carotid or vertebrobasilar artery. Varying degrees of inflammation in vulnerable atherosclerotic plaques predispose these arteries to endothelial erosion, plaque rupture, and platelet activation and aggregation.
- The ensuing development of a thrombus, composed of platelets, fibrin, and other elements, can completely occlude an artery already narrowed by atherosclerosis. This occlusion of blood flow leads to rapid infarction of downstream brain tissue cells, producing a thrombotic stroke.
- The thrombus, either before or immediately after it becomes completely occlusive, may dislodge and travel to more distal cerebral arteries, producing an embolic stroke (Figure 102).

Postocclusion Dynamics

Downstream from the thrombotic or embolic obstruction, brain cells begin to die and necrosis occurs. With persistent occlusion, a central area of irreversible brain damage (infarction or necrosis) develops.

- Surrounding the central area of necrosis or infarction is an area of ischemia called the *ischemic penumbra* or *shadow*.
- This area of "threatened" brain tissue is an area of *potentially reversible* brain damage.
- Until the arrival of rtPA therapy, practitioners had few effective methods to reduce the area of threatened brain tissue and to abort the progression from reversible brain damage to irreversible, permanent brain necrosis.

Other Pathophysiologic Processes

Atrial Fibrillation

Atrial fibrillation remains the most frequent cause of cardioembolic stroke.

- The noncontracting walls of the fibrillating left atrium and left atrial appendage serve as both a stimulus and a reservoir for small emboli.
- The risk of stroke in patients with nonvalvular atrial fibrillation averages 5% per year, 2 to 7 times that of people without atrial fibrillation.

Hypertension

Hypertension causes a thickening of the walls of small cerebral arteries, leading to reduced flow and a predisposition to thrombosis.

- Lacunar infarcts are one example of the type of thrombotic stroke caused by chronic hypertension. They are thought to result from occlusion of a small perforating artery to the subcortical areas of the brain.
- A major cerebrovascular burden imposed by chronic hypertension is hemorrhagic stroke.

Stroke Risk Factors

Risk factors can be identified in most stroke patients.[15] Stroke prevention requires identification of a patient's risk factors, followed by elimination, control, or treatment of as many factors as possible:

- Elimination (eg, smoking)
- Control (eg, hypertension, diabetes mellitus)
- Treatment (eg, antiplatelet therapy, carotid endarterectomy when indicated)

Physical activities may protect against stroke as demonstrated by a meta-analysis of 31 observational studies conducted mainly in the United States and Europe. The meta-analysis found that moderate and high levels of leisure-time and occupational physical activity protected against total stroke, hemorrhagic stroke, and ischemic stroke.[14] Additionally, results from the Physicians' Health Study showed a lower stroke risk associated with vigorous exercise among men.[15] The Harvard Alumni Study also showed a decrease in total stroke risk in men who were highly physically active.[16]

Table 35 lists the major stroke risk factors that are amenable to modification.

Stroke Management

Stroke intervention begins with the recognition of the symptoms of stroke. An important component in this initial step is education—of the patient, family, community, and healthcare provider (out-of-hospital care). Once recognition of potential stroke symptoms occurs, management involves expeditious transfer of the patient to an appropriate facility (out-of-hospital care) and rapid assessment of the patient for reperfusion therapy (in-hospital care). Figure 100 is the Suspected Stroke Algorithm, which identifies treatment goals for these patients.

Patients with acute ischemic stroke have a time-dependent benefit for fibrinolytic therapy similar to that of patients with STEMI, but this time-dependent benefit is much shorter. The NINDS has established critical in-hospital time periods for assessment and management of patients with suspected stroke:

1. Immediate general assessment by the stroke team, emergency physician, or another expert within *10 minutes* of arrival; order urgent noncontrast computed tomography (CT) scan.
2. Neurologic assessment by the stroke team or their designee and CT scan performed within *25 minutes* of hospital arrival.
3. Interpretation of the CT scan within *45 minutes* of ED arrival.
4. Initiation of fibrinolytic therapy in appropriate patients (those without contraindications) within 1 hour of hospital arrival and within 3 hours from symptom onset.
5. Door-to-admission time of 3 hours.

Table 35. **Stroke Risk Factors That Can Be Modified**

Risk Factor	Comments
Hypertension	• One of the most important modifiable risk factors for ischemic and spontaneous hemorrhagic stroke • Risk of hemorrhagic stroke increases markedly with elevations in systolic pressure • Control of hypertension significantly decreases the risk of stroke
Cigarette smoking	• All of the following smoking effects have been linked to stroke: – Accelerated atherosclerosis – Transient elevations in blood pressure – Release of toxic enzymes (linked to formation of aneurysms) – Altered platelet function and reduced platelet survival • Cessation of cigarette smoking reduces the risk of stroke
Transient ischemic attack	• Highly significant indicator of a person at increased risk for stroke • 25% of stroke patients have had a previous TIA • 10% of patients presenting to an ED with TIA will have a completed stroke within 90 days; half of these within the first 2 days • Antiplatelet agents (eg, aspirin, clopidogrel) can reduce the risk of stroke in patients with TIA
Heart disease	• Coronary artery disease and heart failure double the risk of stroke • Atrial fibrillation increases the risk of embolic stroke • Oral anticoagulants, given to patients with atrial fibrillation, reduce the risk of embolic stroke
Diabetes mellitus	• Highly associated with accelerated atherosclerosis • Careful monitoring and control of hyperglycemia reduce the risk of microvascular complications due to diabetes, and reduction of microvascular complications reduces stroke risk
Hypercoagulopathy	• Any hypercoagulative state (eg, protein S or C deficiency, cancer, pregnancy) increases the risk of stroke
High RBC count and sickle cell anemia	• A moderate increase in RBC count increases the risk of stroke • Increases in RBC count can be treated by removing blood and replacing it with intravenous fluid or by administering an anticoagulant • Sickle cell anemia increases the risk of stroke because "sickled" red blood cells can clump, causing arterial occlusion. Stroke risk from sickle cell anemia may be reduced by maintaining adequate oxygenation and hydration and by providing exchange transfusions.
Carotid bruit	• Carotid bruits often indicate partial obstruction (atherosclerosis) of an artery • Carotid bruits are associated with an increased risk of stroke • This risk is reduced by surgical endarterectomy but only in symptomatic patients with >70% stenosis • Some evidence suggests that carotid endarterectomy is beneficial in selected asymptomatic patients with high-grade stenosis

Abbreviations: ED, emergency department; RBC, red blood cell; TIA, transient ischemic attack.

Critical Concept "Time Is Brain"	• The recently coined term *brain attack* and the phrase *time is brain* convey the sense of urgency in stroke therapy. • Once occlusion occurs, an inexorable countdown begins; there is only a limited time available to recognize, evaluate, and treat reversible brain damage.[11-13]

Identification of Signs of Possible Stroke (Number 1)

The warning signs of an ischemic stroke or TIA may be varied, subtle, and transient, but they foretell a potentially life-threatening neurologic illness. Similar to symptoms of ACS, symptoms of ischemic stroke can be misinterpreted and denied. Emergency healthcare providers should recognize the importance of these symptoms and respond quickly with medical or surgical measures that have proven efficacy in stroke management. The signs and symptoms of a stroke may be subtle:

- Sudden weakness or numbness of the face, arm, or leg, especially on one side of the body
- Sudden confusion
- Trouble speaking or understanding
- Sudden trouble seeing in one or both eyes
- Sudden trouble walking
- Dizziness or loss of balance or coordination
- Sudden severe headache with no known cause

✓ Detection: Rapid Recognition of Stroke Symptoms

Early treatment of stroke depends on the patient, family members, or other bystanders recognizing the event. Patients will often ignore the initial signs and symptoms of a stroke, and most delay access to care for several hours after the onset of symptoms. Because of these time delays, many patients with ischemic stroke cannot benefit from fibrinolytic treatment, which must be started within 3 hours of symptom onset.

In one study of 100 stroke patients, only 8% had received information about the signs of stroke, yet nearly half had previously had a TIA or stroke. Unlike a heart attack, in which chest pain can be a dramatic and unrelenting symptom, a stroke may have a subtle presentation with only mild facial paralysis or speech difficulty. Mild signs or symptoms may go unnoticed or be denied by the patient or bystander. Strokes that occur while the patient is asleep or when the patient is alone further hamper prompt recognition and action.[17,18]

Public education, an essential part of any strategy to ensure timely access to care for stroke patients, has been successful in reducing the time to arrival in the ED. In the Temple Foundation Stroke Project (TLL), rtPA use increased from 15% to 52% after patient and physician educational initiatives, and this increase was sustained at 6 months.[17,18]

Critical EMS Assessments and Actions (Number 2)

The Important Role of the Community EMS System in Stroke Care

Three of the 4 links in the Stroke Chain of Survival and the first 3 D's of the 8 D's of Stroke Care (**D**etection, **D**ispatch, and **D**elivery) require effective operation of the EMS system. For this reason, the *2010 AHA Guidelines for CPR and ECC* and the AHA/ASA Guidelines for the Early Management of Adults With Ischemic Stroke strongly emphasize the important role of these personnel and services. Recent data show that 29% to 65% of patients with signs and symptoms of stroke contact local EMS, but only 14% to 32% of them arrive within 2 hours of symptom onset.[19,20] Use of EMS is strongly associated with decreased time to initial physician assessment, computed tomography (CT) imaging for stroke, and neurologic evaluation.[21,22]

EMS Assessments and Actions

EMS assessments and actions for patients with suspected stroke include the following steps:

- Rapid identification of patients with signs and symptoms of acute stroke (✓ *Detection*)
- Support of vital functions
- Prearrival notification of the receiving facility
- Rapid transport of the patient to the receiving facility

✓ Dispatch: Early Activation and Dispatch of EMS by Calling 911

Stroke patients and their families must understand the need to activate the EMS system as soon as they suspect stroke signs or symptoms. The EMS system provides the safest and most efficient method for transporting the patient to the hospital.[23]

Emergency medical dispatchers play a critical role in the timely treatment of potential stroke patients. Data show that dispatchers correctly identify stroke symptoms on the basis of just the initial phone description in more than half the cases of stroke.[19,24] Current literature suggests that 911 telecommunicators may benefit from the use of scripted stroke-specific screens during a 911 call.[25] Studies are ongoing to investigate the effectiveness of such a stroke assessment tool for 911 telecommunicators. Dispatchers can triage emergencies over the telephone and prioritize calls to ensure a rapid response by the EMS system. Specific educational efforts about stroke are encouraged, and stroke dispatch should be given a priority similar to that for AMI and trauma.

✔ Delivery: Rapid EMS Identification, Management, and Transport

Leaders in EMS and emergency medicine must develop training programs and patient care protocols to guide the actions of prehospital care providers. After the ACLS EP Survey and appropriate actions have been performed for airway, breathing, and circulation, EMS providers should immediately obtain a focused history and patient assessment (Table 36). A key component of the patient's history is the *time of symptom onset.* The history *must* include this information. The provider may need to obtain this and other details of the patient's history from family or the appropriate bystander. Preferably, this person should be transported with the patient. Prehospital providers can help establish the precise time of stroke onset or the last time the patient was noted to be neurologically normal. This time point is viewed as "time zero," a starting point that is critical for time-dependent treatment with fibrinolytic agents.

Table 36. **Key Components of a Focused Stroke Patient History**

- Time of symptom onset
- Recent past medical history
- Stroke
- Transient ischemic attack
- Atrial fibrillation
- Acute coronary syndromes (myocardial infarction)
- Trauma or surgery
- Bleeding disorder
- Complicating disease
- Hypertension
- Diabetes mellitus
- Medication use
- Anticoagulants (warfarin) or newer anticoagulant agents (direct thrombin inhibitors or factor Xa inhibitors)
- Antiplatelet agents (aspirin, clopidogrel, ticagrelor)
- Antihypertensives

Out-of-Hospital Stroke Scales for Early Detection and Delivery

The assessment includes a brief and focused examination for stroke. Providers can conduct a rapid neurologic assessment by using validated tools such as the Cincinnati Prehospital Stroke Scale (CPSS)[26,27] or the Los Angeles Prehospital Stroke Screen (LAPSS).[28,29] Studies have confirmed the sensitivity and specificity of these 2 scales for prehospital identification of patients with ischemic stroke.

The CPSS (Table 37) is based on physical examination only, and it can be completed in 30 to 60 seconds.[26] The EMS responder checks for 3 physical findings:

- Facial droop (Figure 103)
- Arm drift (Figure 104)
- Abnormal speech

If any 1 of these 3 signs is abnormal, the probability of a stroke is 72%. The presence of all 3 findings indicates that the probability of stroke is higher than 85%.

Table 37. **Cincinnati Prehospital Stroke Scale**

Test	Findings
Facial droop: Have the patient show teeth or smile (Figure 103)	❑ **Normal**—both sides of face move equally ❑ **Abnormal**—one side of face does not move as well as the other side
Arm drift: Patient closes eyes and extends both arms straight out, with palms up, for 10 seconds (Figure 104)	❑ **Normal**—both arms move the same or both arms do not move at all (other findings, such as pronator drift, may be helpful) ❑ **Abnormal**—one arm does not move or one arm drifts down compared with the other
Abnormal speech: Have the patient say "you can't teach an old dog new tricks"	❑ **Normal**—patient uses correct words with no slurring ❑ **Abnormal**—patient slurs words, uses the wrong words, or is unable to speak

From Kothari et al,[14] with permission from Elsevier.

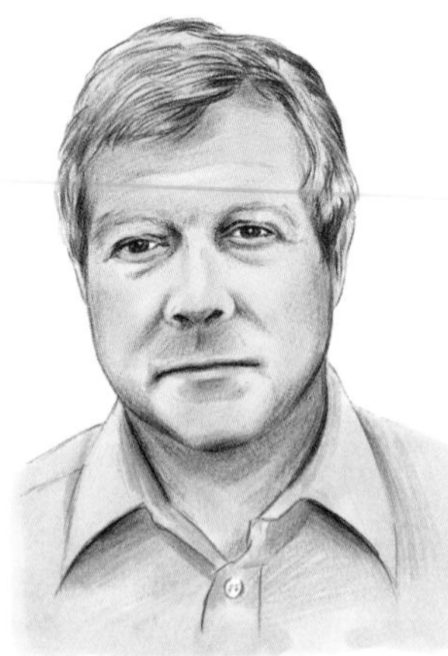
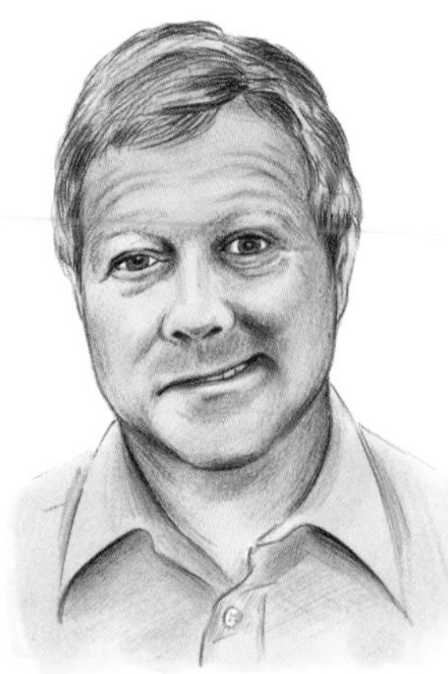

Figure 103. Facial droop.

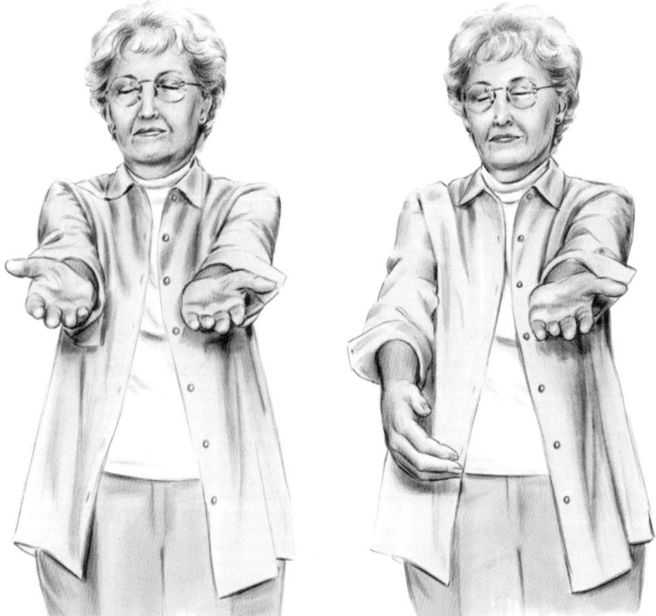

Figure 104. One-sided motor weakness (right arm).

Destination Hospital Protocols

Once a patient with probable stroke is identified, transport the patient to the nearest *most appropriate* facility. Prearrival notification to the facility is key to speeding patient evaluation, CT imaging, and reperfusion therapy. An ambulance may bypass a hospital that does not have the resources or the institutional commitment to treat patients with a stroke if a more appropriate hospital is available within a reasonable transport interval. Multiple randomized clinical trials and meta-analyses in adults have shown consistent improvement in 1-year survival rate, functional outcome, and quality of life when patients hospitalized with acute stroke are cared for in a dedicated stroke unit by a multidisciplinary team that is experienced in managing stroke care. Therefore, an ambulance may bypass a hospital if

- The facility does not have the resources for acute stroke care.
- The facility lacks an institutional commitment to treat patients with a stroke.
- A more appropriate hospital is available within a reasonable transport interval.

Air medical transport appears to be beneficial, but studies are limited. Helicopters may extend the range of reperfusion therapy to rural areas, delivering teams to administer rtPA or rapidly transferring patients to appropriate facilities.[30-33] Helicopter transfer of patients has been shown to be cost-effective.[33]

Prehospital Initial Studies

Prehospital care and assessment beyond initial management should be completed during patient transport and should not delay departure for the hospital. Establish intravenous (IV) access and administer normal saline. Avoid glucose-containing fluids unless hypoglycemia is strongly suspected or present (excess glucose may be harmful to stroke patients). Checking blood glucose in suspected stroke patients is prudent. Also initiate cardiac monitoring. Obtain a 12-lead electrocardiogram (ECG) if the patient has ongoing ischemic-type chest discomfort.

Patients with acute stroke are at risk for respiratory compromise from aspiration, upper airway obstruction, hypoventilation, and (rarely) neurogenic pulmonary edema. The combination of poor perfusion and hypoxemia will exacerbate and extend ischemic brain injury and has been associated with worse outcome from stroke. Therefore, both out-of-hospital and in-hospital medical personnel should administer supplemental oxygen to hypoxemic (ie, oxygen saturation is less than 94%) stroke patients or those with unknown oxygen saturation.

In-Hospital Management

✓ *Door: Appropriate Triage to Stroke Center*

Immediate General Assessment and Stabilization *(Number 3)*

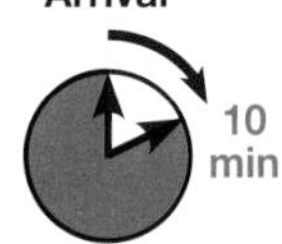

As a goal, ED personnel should assess the patient with suspected stroke within 10 minutes of arrival in the ED. The ED physician should perform a neurologic screening assessment, order an emergent CT scan of the brain, and activate the stroke team or arrange consultation with a stroke expert. General care includes assessment and support of airway, breathing, and circulation and evaluation of baseline vital signs. Oxygen is administered to hypoxemic patients in the ED but is not recommended for patients without hypoxemia. Oxygen saturation should be monitored and maintained at 94% or higher. A Cheyne-Stokes pattern of respirations can be reversed with oxygen supplementation. Establish (or confirm) IV access, and obtain blood samples for baseline studies (blood count, coagulation studies, blood glucose, etc). Treat hypoglycemia immediately if present.

A 12-lead ECG and other ancillary studies do not take priority over the CT scan and are performed as indicated and concomitant with expedited stroke care. The ECG may identify a recent AMI or arrhythmias (eg, atrial fibrillation) as the cause of a cardioembolic stroke. If the patient is hemodynamically stable, treatment of other arrhythmias, including bradycardia, premature atrial or ventricular contractions, or defects or blocks in atrioventricular conduction, may be unnecessary.[35] There is general agreement that cardiac monitoring should be done during the initial 24 hours of evaluation of patients with acute ischemic stroke to detect atrial fibrillation and potentially life-threatening arrhythmias.[36]

Data: Rapid Triage, Evaluation, and Management Within the ED

Immediately initiate diagnostic studies in all patients to assess conditions that may mimic stroke and comorbid problems that can complicate management. Consider the need for additional studies and perform them in selected patients as indicated. These tests may include the following:

All Patients
• Noncontrast brain CT or MRI • Blood glucose • Serum electrolytes • Renal function • CBC and platelet count • Coagulation studies (PTT, PT, INR) • Oxygen saturation • ECG
Selected Patients
• Chest x-ray • Hepatic function • Blood alcohol and toxicology screen • Arterial blood gas • Lumbar puncture • EEG • Pregnancy test

Abbreviations: CBC, complete blood count; CT, computed tomography; ECG, electrocardiogram; EEG, electroencephalogram; INR, international normalized ratio; MRI, magnetic resonance imaging; PPT, partial thromboplastin time; PT, prothrombin time.

Establish Time of Onset (Less Than 3 Hours Required for Fibrinolytics, Less Than 4.5 Hours in Selected Patients)

Protocols for EMS personnel should direct them to ask the patient and family about when they first noted any stroke symptoms. Neither the patient nor family members may recall the exact hour and minute. But they may be able to relate the onset of symptoms to other events, such as a television or radio program that was playing, a telephone

Critical Concept **ED Assessment Priorities**	Use protocols in the ED to minimize delay to definitive diagnosis and therapy.[34] Diagnostic studies ordered in the ED are aimed at **1.** Establishing stroke as the cause of the patient's symptoms **2.** Determining the exact time of onset **3.** Differentiating ischemic from hemorrhagic stroke **4.** Rapidly administering rtPA to patients with ischemic stroke if no contraindications are present

Critical Concept **Diagnostic Studies—Do Not Delay CT Imaging or Fibrinolytic Therapy**	Other routine and selected diagnostic studies are important, but they should not delay CT imaging or fibrinolytic therapy unless **1.** There is clinical suspicion of a bleeding disorder **2.** The patient has received heparin or warfarin **3.** Anticoagulant status is uncertain

call, or someone's arrival or departure. Be aware that time of onset is difficult to establish for patients who are discovered unconscious or unable to communicate or for patients who awaken from sleep with neurologic abnormalities. For these patients, the time of onset of symptoms is defined as the last time the patient was observed as normal.

Immediate Neurologic Screening Assessment

The immediate neurologic stroke assessment should focus on 5 key assessments:

1. Onset of symptoms or when the patient was last seen functioning normally
2. Level of consciousness
3. Level of stroke severity
4. Type of stroke: ischemic versus hemorrhagic
5. Location of stroke: anterior (carotid) versus posterior (vertebrobasilar)

The clinical status of stroke patients often fluctuates. Clinicians should perform several focused neurologic examinations to detect any deterioration or improvement.

Determine Level of Consciousness (Glasgow Coma Scale)

Altered consciousness or the appearance of confusion can complicate and delay evaluation. The Glasgow Coma Scale (GCS) (Table 38) provides a way to establish the severity of neurologic compromise in patients with altered consciousness and is a reliable tool to assess serial changes

Table 38. Glasgow Coma Scale[37]

Eye opening	Score
Spontaneous	4
In response to speech	3
In response to pain	2
None	1
Best verbal response	
Oriented conversation	5
Confused conversation	4
Inappropriate words	3
Incomprehensible sounds	2
None	1
Best motor response	
Obeys	6
Localizes	5
Withdraws	4
Abnormal flexion	3
Abnormal extension	2
None	1

in function over time. The total score ranges from 3 to 15. It is the sum of the best response the patient displays for 3 functions: eye opening (1 through 4), verbal responses (1 through 5), and motor function (1 through 6).[37] The patient who has no verbal response, has no eye opening, and is flaccid has a GCS score of 3. In general, a GCS score of 8 or less is associated with an ominous prognosis.

Immediate Neurologic Assessment by Stroke Team or Designee (Number 4)

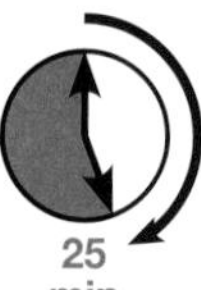

The goal for neurologic assessment is within 25 minutes of the patient's arrival in the ED. *"Time is Brain."* The stroke team, another expert, or an emergency physician with access to remote stroke expert support will review the patient's history and verify time of onset of symptoms (Number 4). This may require interviewing out-of-hospital providers, witnesses, and family members to establish the time that the patient was last known to be normal. Neurologic assessment is performed incorporating either the National Institutes of Health (NIH) Stroke Scale or Canadian Neurological Scale.

Determine Severity of Stroke (NIH Stroke Scale)

The NIH Stroke Scale (Table 39) involves 15 items used to assess the responsive stroke patient. This is a validated measure of stroke severity based on a detailed neurologic examination (cranial nerve and gait testing are omitted).[11] The NIH Stroke Scale allows either nurse stroke specialists or physicians to perform standardized neurologic evaluations of a patient.[11,38] The score correlates with long-term outcome in patients with ischemic stroke[38-40] and is designed to provide a reliable,[41] valid, and easy-to-perform alternative to the standard neurologic examination. The NIH Stroke Scale can be performed in less than 7 minutes. The NIH Stroke Scale received further validation during the landmark NINDS trial of rtPA for acute ischemic stroke.[4]

The total score ranges from 0 (normal) to 42 points. The scale covers the following major areas:

- **Level of consciousness:** Alert, drowsy; knows month, age; performs tasks correctly
- **Visual assessment:** Follows finger with or without gaze palsy, forced deviation; hemianopsia (none, partial, complete, bilateral)
- **Motor function:** Face, arm, leg strength and movement
- **Sensation:** Pin prick to face, arm, trunk, leg; compare side to side
- **Cerebellar function:** Finger-nose; heel down shin
- **Language:** Aphasia (name items, describe a picture, read sentences); dysarthria (evaluate speech clarity by having patient repeat listed words)

Table 39. National Institutes of Health Stroke Scale

Instructions	Scale Definition	Score
1a. Level of Consciousness: The investigator must choose a response if a full evaluation is prevented by such obstacles as an endotracheal tube, language barrier, orotracheal trauma/bandages. A 3 is scored only if the patient makes no movement (other than reflexive posturing) in response to noxious stimulation.	0 = **Alert;** keenly responsive. 1 = **Not alert;** but arousable by minor stimulation to obey, answer, or respond. 2 = **Not alert;** requires repeated stimulation to attend, or is obtunded and requires strong or painful stimulation to make movements (not stereotyped). 3 = Responds only with reflex motor or autonomic effects or totally unresponsive, flaccid, and areflexic.	____
1b. LOC Questions: The patient is asked the month and his/her age. The answer must be correct—there is no partial credit for being close. Aphasic and stuporous patients who do not comprehend the questions will score 2. Patients unable to speak because of endotracheal intubation, orotracheal trauma, severe dysarthria from any cause, language barrier, or any other problem not secondary to aphasia are given a 1. It is important that only the initial answer be graded and that the examiner not "help" the patient with verbal or non-verbal cues.	0 = **Answers** both questions correctly. 1 = **Answers** one question correctly. 2 = **Answers** neither question correctly.	____
1c. LOC Commands: The patient is asked to open and close the eyes and then to grip and release the non-paretic hand. Substitute another one step command if the hands cannot be used. Credit is given if an unequivocal attempt is made but not completed due to weakness. If the patient does not respond to command, the task should be demonstrated to him or her (pantomime), and the result scored (i.e., follows none, one or two commands). Patients with trauma, amputation, or other physical impediments should be given suitable one-step commands. Only the first attempt is scored.	0 = **Performs** both tasks correctly. 1 = **Performs** one task correctly. 2 = **Performs** neither task correctly.	____
2. Best Gaze: Only horizontal eye movements will be tested. Voluntary or reflexive (oculocephalic) eye movements will be scored, but caloric testing is not done. If the patient has a conjugate deviation of the eyes that can be overcome by voluntary or reflexive activity, the score will be 1. If a patient has an isolated peripheral nerve paresis (CN III, IV or VI), score a 1. Gaze is testable in all aphasic patients. Patients with ocular trauma, bandages, pre-existing blindness, or other disorder of visual acuity or fields should be tested with reflexive movements, and a choice made by the investigator. Establishing eye contact and then moving about the patient from side to side will occasionally clarify the presence of a partial gaze palsy.	0 = **Normal.** 1 = **Partial gaze palsy;** gaze is abnormal in one or both eyes, but forced deviation or total gaze paresis is not present. 2 = **Forced deviation,** or total gaze paresis not overcome by the oculocephalic maneuver.	____
3. Visual: Visual fields (upper and lower quadrants) are tested by confrontation, using finger counting or visual threat, as appropriate. Patients may be encouraged, but if they look at the side of the moving fingers appropriately, this can be scored as normal. If there is unilateral blindness or enucleation, visual fields in the remaining eye are scored. Score 1 only if a clear-cut asymmetry, including quadrantanopia, is found. If patient is blind from any cause, score 3. Double simultaneous stimulation is performed at this point. If there is extinction, patient receives a 1, and the results are used to respond to item 11.	0 = **No visual loss.** 1 = **Partial hemianopia.** 2 = **Complete hemianopia.** 3 = **Bilateral hemianopia** (blind including cortical blindness).	____

(continued)

(continued)

Instructions	Scale Definition	Score
4. **Facial Palsy:** Ask—or use pantomime to encourage—the patient to show teeth or raise eyebrows and close eyes. Score symmetry of grimace in response to noxious stimuli in the poorly responsive or non-comprehending patient. If facial trauma/bandages, orotracheal tube, tape or other physical barriers obscure the face, these should be removed to the extent possible.	0 = **Normal** symmetrical movements. 1 = **Minor paralysis** (flattened nasolabial fold, asymmetry on smiling). 2 = **Partial paralysis** (total or near-total paralysis of lower face). 3 = **Complete paralysis** of one or both sides (absence of facial movement in the upper and lower face).	____
5. **Motor Arm:** The limb is placed in the appropriate position: extend the arms (palms down) 90 degrees (if sitting) or 45 degrees (if supine). Drift is scored if the arm falls before 10 seconds. The aphasic patient is encouraged using urgency in the voice and pantomime, but not noxious stimulation. Each limb is tested in turn, beginning with the non-paretic arm. Only in the case of amputation or joint fusion at the shoulder, the examiner should record the score as untestable (UN), and clearly write the explanation for this choice.	0 = **No drift;** limb holds 90 (or 45) degrees for full 10 seconds. 1 = **Drift;** limb holds 90 (or 45) degrees, but drifts down before full 10 seconds; does not hit bed or other support. 2 = **Some effort against gravity;** limb cannot get to or maintain (if cued) 90 (or 45) degrees, drifts down to bed, but has some effort against gravity. 3 = **No effort against gravity;** limb falls. 4 = **No movement.** UN = **Amputation** or joint fusion, explain: ________________ **5a. Left Arm** **5b. Right Arm**	____
6. **Motor Leg:** The limb is placed in the appropriate position: hold the leg at 30 degrees (always tested supine). Drift is scored if the leg falls before 5 seconds. The aphasic patient is encouraged using urgency in the voice and pantomime, but not noxious stimulation. Each limb is tested in turn, beginning with the non-paretic leg. Only in the case of amputation or joint fusion at the hip, the examiner should record the score as untestable (UN), and clearly write the explanation for this choice.	0 = **No drift;** leg holds 30-degree position for full 5 seconds. 1 = **Drift;** leg falls by the end of the 5-second period but does not hit bed. 2 = **Some effort against gravity;** leg falls to bed by 5 seconds, but has some effort against gravity. 3 = **No effort against gravity;** leg falls to bed immediately. 4 = **No movement.** UN = **Amputation** or joint fusion, explain: ________________ **6a. Left Leg** **6b. Right Leg**	____
7. **Limb Ataxia:** This item is aimed at finding evidence of a unilateral cerebellar lesion. Test with eyes open. In case of visual defect, ensure testing is done in intact visual field. The finger-nose-finger and heel-shin tests are performed on both sides, and ataxia is scored only if present out of proportion to weakness. Ataxia is absent in the patient who cannot understand or is paralyzed. Only in the case of amputation or joint fusion, the examiner should record the score as untestable (UN), and clearly write the explanation for this choice. In case of blindness, test by having the patient touch nose from extended arm position.	0 = **Absent.** 1 = **Present in one limb.** 2 = **Present in two limbs.** UN = **Amputation** or joint fusion, explain: ________________	____

(continued)

(continued)

Instructions	Scale Definition	Score
8. Sensory: Sensation or grimace to pinprick when tested, or withdrawal from noxious stimulus in the obtunded or aphasic patient. Only sensory loss attributed to stroke is scored as abnormal and the examiner should test as many body areas (arms [not hands], legs, trunk, face) as needed to accurately check for hemisensory loss. A score of 2, "severe or total sensory loss," should only be given when a severe or total loss of sensation can be clearly demonstrated. Stuporous and aphasic patients will, therefore, probably score 1 or 0. The patient with brainstem stroke who has bilateral loss of sensation is scored 2. If the patient does not respond and is quadriplegic, score 2. Patients in a coma (item 1a = 3) are automatically given a 2 on this item.	0 = **Normal;** no sensory loss. 1 = **Mild-to-moderate sensory loss;** patient feels pinprick is less sharp or is dull on the affected side; or there is a loss of superficial pain with pinprick, but patient is aware of being touched. 2 = **Severe to total sensory loss;** patient is not aware of being touched in the face, arm, and leg.	____
9. Best Language: A great deal of information about comprehension will be obtained during the preceding sections of the examination. For this scale item, the patient is asked to describe what is happening in the attached picture, to name the items on the attached naming sheet and to read from the attached list of sentences. Comprehension is judged from responses here, as well as to all of the commands in the preceding general neurological exam. If visual loss interferes with the tests, ask the patient to identify objects placed in the hand, repeat, and produce speech. The intubated patient should be asked to write. The patient in a coma (item 1a = 3) will automatically score 3 on this item. The examiner must choose a score for the patient with stupor or limited cooperation, but a score of 3 should be used only if the patient is mute and follows no one-step commands.	0 = **No aphasia;** normal. 1 = **Mild-to-moderate aphasia;** some obvious loss of fluency or facility of comprehension, without significant limitation on ideas expressed or form of expression. Reduction of speech and/or comprehension, however, makes conversation about provided materials difficult or impossible. For example, in conversation about provided materials, examiner can identify picture or naming card content from patient's response. 2 = **Severe aphasia;** all communication is through fragmentary expression; great need for inference, questioning, and guessing by the listener. Range of information that can be exchanged is limited; listener carries burden of communication. Examiner cannot identify materials provided from patient response. 3 = **Mute, global aphasia;** no usable speech or auditory comprehension.	____
10. Dysarthria: If patient is thought to be normal, an adequate sample of speech must be obtained by asking patient to read or repeat words from the attached list. If the patient has severe aphasia, the clarity of articulation of spontaneous speech can be rated. Only if the patient is intubated or has other physical barriers to producing speech, the examiner should record the score as untestable (UN), and clearly write an explanation for this choice. Do not tell the patient why he or she is being tested.	0 = **Normal.** 1 = **Mild-to-moderate dysarthria;** patient slurs at least some words and, at worst, can be understood with some difficulty. 2 = **Severe dysarthria;** patient's speech is so slurred as to be unintelligible in the absence of or out of proportion to any dysphasia, or is mute/anarthric. UN = **Intubated** or other physical barrier, explain: ____________	____
11. Extinction and Inattention (formerly Neglect): Sufficient information to identify neglect may be obtained during the prior testing. If the patient has a severe visual loss preventing visual double simultaneous stimulation, and the cutaneous stimuli are normal, the score is normal. If the patient has aphasia but does appear to attend to both sides, the score is normal. The presence of visual spatial neglect or anosagnosia may also be taken as evidence of abnormality. Since the abnormality is scored only if present, the item is never untestable.	0 = **No abnormality.** 1 = **Visual, tactile, auditory, spatial, or personal inattention** or extinction to bilateral simultaneous stimulation in one of the sensory modalities. 2 = **Profound hemi-inattention or extinction to more than one modality;** does not recognize own hand or orients to only one side of space.	____

Full scale with attachments can be found at National Institute of Neurological Disorders and Stroke website. NIH Stroke Scale. http://www.ninds.nih.gov/doctors/NIH_Stroke_Scale.pdf. Revised October 1, 2003. Accessed November 13, 2012.

Critical Concept **Time of Symptom Onset Is Crucial**	• Inability to establish the time of symptom onset with accuracy is a contraindication to rtPA therapy! • If prehospital care personnel cannot reliably determine a specific time, ED personnel should continue the inquiries. Call or speak directly with a family member, coworker, or bystander.

An NIH Stroke Scale score of less than 4 usually indicates minor neurologic deficits, such as sensory losses, dysarthria, or some manual clumsiness. Fibrinolytic agents are not recommended for these patients because treatment offers minimal benefits relative to the risks. Some disabling neurologic deficits, such as isolated severe aphasia (score of 3) or the visual field losses of hemianopsia (score of 2 or 3), can be associated with a low score on the NIH Stroke Scale. Patients with these deficits may be exceptions to the recommendation against fibrinolytic agents for patients with an NIH Stroke Scale score of less than 4.

Severe deficits (score greater than 22) indicate large areas of ischemic damage. Patients with such deficits face an increased risk of brain hemorrhage. In general, the use of fibrinolytic treatment in these patients should follow careful discussion with the patient, the patient's spouse and family, and the admitting physicians to ensure that everyone understands the risk and benefits. For some patients with severe deficits, the probability of harm outweighs the potential for significant benefit. A favorable risk-benefit ratio varies from patient to patient. The responsible clinician should always evaluate therapeutic decisions on an individual basis in close collaboration with the patient and family.

Management of Hypertension

Management of hypertension in the stroke patient is controversial. For patients eligible for fibrinolytic therapy, however, control of blood pressure is required to reduce the risk of bleeding. If a patient who is otherwise eligible for treatment with rtPA has elevated blood pressure, providers can try to lower it to a systolic pressure of 185 mm Hg or less and a diastolic blood pressure of 110 mm Hg or less (Table 40). Because the maximum interval from onset of stroke until effective treatment with rtPA is limited, most patients with sustained hypertension above these levels (ie, systolic blood pressure higher than 185 mm Hg or diastolic blood pressure higher than 110 mm Hg) cannot be treated with IV rtPA (Table 41).[42-44] Consider lowering blood pressure in acute ischemic stroke patients who are not candidates for acute perfusion therapy when systolic blood pressure is higher than 220 mm Hg or diastolic blood pressure is higher than 120 mm Hg. Consider blood pressure reduction as indicated for other concomitant organ system injury (eg, AMI, congestive heart failure, acute aortic dissection). A reasonable target is to lower blood pressure by only 15% to 25% within the first day.

Imaging *(Number 5)*

The most commonly obtained brain imaging test is a non–contrast-enhanced CT scan, but some centers can now obtain a magnetic resonance imaging (MRI) scan with efficiency equal to CT scanning. The noncontrast CT scan accurately identifies most cases of intracranial hemorrhage and discriminates nonvascular causes of neurologic symptoms mimicking stroke (eg, brain tumor). Ongoing research is evaluating MRI, magnetic resonance angiography, and multimodal CT, which includes noncontrast CT, perfusion CT, and CT angiographic studies. Centers may perform more advanced neurologic imaging (multimodal MRI, CT perfusion, and CT angiography), but obtaining these studies should not delay initiation of IV rtPA in eligible patients.

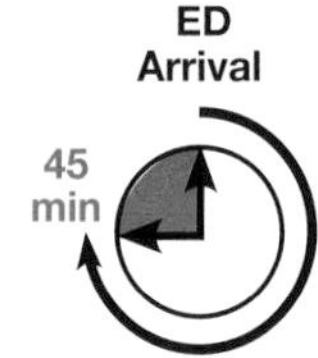

Ideally the CT scan should be completed within 25 minutes of the patient's arrival in the ED and should be read within 45 minutes of ED arrival (Number 5). Emergent CT or MRI scans of patients with suspected stroke should be promptly evaluated by a physician with expertise in interpretation of these studies.[45,46] During the first few hours of an ischemic stroke, the noncontrast CT scan may not show signs of brain ischemia.

The CT scan is central to the triage and therapy of the stroke patient (hemorrhage or no hemorrhage):

- If the CT scan shows no evidence of hemorrhage, the patient may be a candidate for fibrinolytic therapy (Numbers 6 and 8).
- If hemorrhage (intracerebral or subarachnoid hemorrhage) is noted on the CT scan, the patient is not a candidate for fibrinolytic therapy. Consult a neurologist or neurosurgeon and consider transfer as needed for appropriate care (Number 7).
- If hemorrhage is not present on the initial CT scan and the patient is not a candidate for fibrinolytic therapy for other reasons, consider administration of aspirin (Number 9) either rectally or orally after the patient is screened for dysphagia. Admit the patient to a stroke unit (if available) for careful monitoring (Number 11).

The Initial Noncontrast CT Scan

On CT images, blood from a hemorrhagic stroke has a density that is only about 3% greater than the density of brain tissue. On modern CT scanners, this 3% difference in density can be manipulated so that the hemorrhage and

Table 40. Potential Approaches to Arterial Hypertension in Acute Ischemic Stroke Patients Who Are Potential Candidates for Acute Reperfusion Therapy[6]

1. Patient otherwise eligible for acute reperfusion therapy except that blood pressure is >185/110 mm Hg:
   - Labetalol 10 to 20 mg IV over 1 to 2 min, may repeat once, or
   - Nicardipine IV 5 mg/h, titrate up by 2.5 mg/h every 5 to 15 minutes, maximum 15 mg/h; when desired blood pressure is reached, lower to 3 mg/h, or
   - Other agents (hydralazine, enalapril, etc) may be considered when appropriate.
2. If blood pressure is not maintained at or below 185/110 mm Hg, do not administer rtPA.
3. Management of blood pressure during and after rtPA or other acute reperfusion therapy:

   Monitor blood pressure every 15 minutes for 2 hours from the start of rtPA therapy, then every 30 minutes for 6 hours, and then every hour for 16 hours.
4. If systolic blood pressure is 180 to 230 mm Hg or diastolic blood pressure is 105 to 120 mm Hg, give
   - Labetalol 10 mg IV followed by continuous IV infusion 2 to 8 mg/min, or
   - Nicardipine IV 5 mg/h, titrate up to desired effect by 2.5 mg/h every 5 to 15 min, maximum 15 mg/h.
5. If blood pressure is not controlled or diastolic blood pressure is >140 mm Hg, consider sodium nitroprusside.

Abbreviation: rtPA, recombinant tissue plasminogen activator.

free blood will appear distinctly white in comparison with surrounding tissues. Contrast agents also "light up" on CT scans. Because these agents would obscure the high-contrast areas of free blood, the initial CT scan is made without contrast enhancement. Acute intracranial complications of stroke, such as hydrocephalus, edema, mass effect, or shift of normal brain structures, can also be seen with CT.

During the first few hours of a thrombotic or embolic stroke, the noncontrast CT scan will generally appear *normal*. Brain structures without normal blood flow appear initially the same as structures with good blood flow on the CT scan. For this reason the CT scan will continue to appear normal for a few hours after blood flow is blocked or reduced to an area of the brain. A well-defined area of hypodensity, purported to be caused by lack of blood flow past an occlusion, will rarely develop within the first 3 hours of a stroke. The brain tissue downstream from an occlusion is indeed ischemic and damaged. It soon begins to swell with edema and inflammation.

A hypodense area on the CT scan generally excludes a patient from fibrinolytic therapy as it typically takes 6 to 12 hours for the edema and swelling to produce the hypodensity. Larger infarctions can cause early CT changes. But these changes are often subtle, such as obscuration of the gray-white matter junction, sulcal effacement, or early hypodensity.

Table 41. Approach to Arterial Hypertension in Acute Ischemic Stroke Patients Who Are *Not* Potential Candidates for Acute Reperfusion Therapy[6]

Consider lowering blood pressure in patients with acute ischemic stroke if systolic blood pressure is >220 mm Hg or diastolic blood pressure is >120 mm Hg.

Consider blood pressure reduction as indicated for other concomitant organ system injury:

- AMI
- Congestive heart failure
- Acute aortic dissection

A reasonable target is to lower blood pressure by 15% to 25% within the first day.

Abbreviation: AMI, acute myocardial infarction.

Decision: Stroke Expertise and Therapy Selection

Risk Assessment and Administration of IV rtPA (Number 10)

When the CT scan shows no hemorrhage, the probability of acute ischemic stroke is high. The physician or stroke team should review the inclusion and exclusion criteria for IV fibrinolytic therapy (Tables 42 and 43) and perform a repeat neurologic examination (incorporating the NIH Stroke Scale or Canadian Neurological Scale). If the patient's neurologic signs are spontaneously clearing (ie, function is rapidly improving toward normal) and are near baseline, fibrinolytic administration is not recommended (Number 6).

Major Benefit: Improved Neurologic Outcome Without Mortality

Several studies have documented a higher likelihood of good to excellent functional outcome when rtPA is administered to adults with acute ischemic stroke within 3 hours of symptom onset. Such results are obtained when rtPA is administered by physicians in hospitals with a stroke protocol that rigorously adheres to the eligibility criteria and therapeutic regimen of the NINDS protocol. These results have been supported by a subsequent 1-year follow-up study, reanalysis of the NINDS data, and a meta-analysis. Evidence from prospective, randomized studies in adults also documents a greater likelihood of benefit the earlier treatment is begun. Many physicians have emphasized the flaws in the NINDS trials, but additional analyses of the original NINDS data by an independent group of investigators confirmed the validity of the results, verifying that improved outcomes in the rtPA treatment arm persist even when imbalances in baseline stroke severity among treatment groups are corrected.

Major Risk: Intracranial Hemorrhage and Death

Like all medications, fibrinolytics have potential adverse effects. The physician must verify that there are no exclusion criteria, consider the risks and benefits to the patient, and be prepared to monitor and treat any potential complications. The major complication of IV rtPA for stroke is symptomatic intracranial hemorrhage. This complication occurred in 6.4% of the 312 patients treated in the NINDS trial[4] and 4.6% of the 1135 patients treated in 60 Canadian centers.[47] A meta-analysis of 15 published case series on the open-label use of rtPA for acute ischemic stroke in general clinical practice shows a symptomatic hemorrhage rate of 5.2% of 2639 patients treated.[48] Other complications include orolingual angioedema (occurs in about 1.5% of patients), acute hypotension, and systemic bleeding. In one large prospective registry, major systemic bleeding was uncommon (0.4%) and usually occurred at the site of femoral groin puncture for acute angiography.[47,49]

How to Minimize Risks and Maximize Benefits of rtPA for Acute Stroke

In the NINDS trial, fatal intracranial hemorrhage occurred in approximately 3 of every 100 patients treated with rtPA (3%) but only 3 of every 1000 (0.3%) receiving placebo. This means that the risk of fatal bleeding into the brain was 10 times greater in the rtPA-treated patients. But it is important to note that overall mortality was not increased in the rtPA-treated group. For a perspective on this risk, consider that the rate of fatal hemorrhagic stroke in patients given rtPA within 12 hours of acute coronary artery occlusion averages less than 1%. To minimize the risks and maximize the benefits, responsible clinicians must adhere strictly to the inclusion and exclusion criteria (Tables 42 and 43). rtPA therapy is acceptable only with strict adherence to these criteria.

Strategies for Success

Administration of IV rtPA to patients with acute ischemic stroke who meet the NINDS eligibility criteria is recommended if rtPA is administered by physicians in the setting of a clearly defined protocol, a knowledgeable team, and institutional commitment. It is important to note that the superior outcomes reported in both community and tertiary care hospitals in the NINDS trials have been difficult to replicate in hospitals with less experience in, and institutional commitment to, acute stroke care.[50,51] Failure to adhere to protocol is associated with an increased rate of complications, particularly the risk of symptomatic intracranial hemorrhage.[52,53] There is also strong evidence to avoid all delays and treat patients as soon as possible.

Community hospitals have reported outcomes comparable to the results of the NINDS trials after implementing a stroke program with a focus on quality improvement.[47,54,55] The experience of the Cleveland Clinic system is instructive.[51,55] A quality improvement program increased compliance with the rtPA treatment protocol in 9 community hospitals, and the rate of symptomatic intracerebral hemorrhage fell from 13.4% to 6.4%.[55]

There is a relationship between violations of the NINDS treatment protocol and increased risk of symptomatic intracerebral hemorrhage and death.[48] In Germany, there was an increased risk of death after administration of rtPA for acute ischemic stroke in hospitals that treated 5 or fewer patients per year, which suggests that clinical experience is an important factor in ensuring adherence to protocol.[49] Adding a dedicated stroke team to a community hospital can increase the number of patients with acute stroke treated with fibrinolytic therapy and produce excellent clinical outcomes.[56] These findings show that it is important to have an institutional commitment to ensure optimal patient outcomes.

To provide standardized and comprehensive stroke care, the Brain Attack Coalition published criteria for primary stroke centers and comprehensive stroke centers—PSCs and CSCs. A PSC has resources to care for many patients with uncomplicated stroke.[57] A CSC provides comprehensive and specialized care for patients with a complicated stroke and those requiring specialized care, such as surgery or stroke intensive care.

Recommendations for stroke care include

- Transport to the closest facility with resources to care for stroke patients (ie, hospital bypass)
- Development of PSCs—strongly recommended
- Certification of stroke centers by external agency—strongly encouraged

Critical Concept **Normal CT = Candidate for Fibrinolytic Therapy**	An important, if somewhat counterintuitive, point to remember is that a completely normal CT scan—no sign of hemorrhage, no large areas of no flow, and no hypodense areas—is supportive of rtPA administration in a stroke patient who otherwise meets the criteria for fibrinolytic therapy.

Table 42. **Fibrinolytic Checklist Inclusion and Exclusion Characteristics of Patients With Ischemic Stroke Who Could Be Treated With rtPA Within *3 Hours* From Symptom Onset**[6]

Inclusion Criteria
• Diagnosis of ischemic stroke causing measurable neurologic deficit • Onset of symptoms less than 3 hours before beginning treatment • Age 18 years or older
Exclusion Criteria
• Major surgery in the previous 14 days • Head trauma or prior stroke in previous 3 months • Symptoms suggest subarachnoid hemorrhage • Arterial puncture at noncompressible site in previous 7 days • History of previous intracranial hemorrhage • Elevated blood pressure (systolic above 185 mm Hg or diastolic above 110 mm Hg) • Evidence of active bleeding on examination • Acute bleeding diathesis, including but not limited to – Platelet count <100 000/mm^3 – Heparin received within 48 hours, resulting in an aPTT above the upper limit of normal – Current use of anticoagulant with INR more than 1.7 or PT more than 15 seconds • Blood glucose concentration below 50 mg/dL (2.7 mmol/L) • CT demonstrates multilobar infarction (hypodensity more than ⅓ cerebral hemisphere)
Relative Exclusion Criteria
Recent experience suggests that under some circumstances—with careful consideration and weighing of risk to benefit—patients may receive fibrinolytic therapy despite 1 or more relative contraindications. Consider risk to benefit of rtPA administration carefully if any of these relative contraindications is present: • Only minor or rapidly improving stroke symptoms (clearing spontaneously) • Seizure at onset with postictal residual neurologic impairments • Major surgery or serious trauma within previous 14 days • Recent gastrointestinal or urinary tract hemorrhage (within previous 21 days) • Recent AMI (within previous 3 months)

Abbreviations: AMI, acute myocardial infarction; aPTT, activated partial thromboplastin time; CT, computed tomography; INR, international normalized ratio; PT, prothrombin time; rtPA, recombinant tissue plasminogen activator.

✓ Drug: Fibrinolytic Therapy and Intra-arterial Strategies

Additional Actions Before Fibrinolytic Therapy

Review for CT Exclusions: Are Any Observed?

- Hemorrhage, either intracerebral or subarachnoid, must be excluded. Failure to identify a small area of hemorrhage could be a **fatal error.**

- Areas of well-defined hypodensity are generally CT exclusions because they indicate either that more than 3 hours has passed since the infarction or that a large area of the brain is threatened.

- CT indications of a large infarction (early hypodensity, obscured junction between gray and white matter, or sulcal effacement) are relative contraindications to rtPA. Larger brain infarctions are prone to undergo hemorrhagic transformation, exposing a patient receiving a fibrinolytic agent to the risk of fatal intracerebral hemorrhage. These patients, however, have a poor outcome without intervention, so some authors have concluded that patients with severe deficit or CT findings of hypodensity or mass effect can be candidates for rtPA therapy, with both greater possibility of benefit and greater risk of harm.

Repeat Neurologic Exam: Are Deficits Variable or Rapidly Improving?

- The risk of harm from rtPA is not justified for patients with a TIA or rapidly improving deficits. These patients usually have lesions or partial occlusions that are not resolved by rtPA. However, some stroke experts consider administration of rtPA if there is a low NIH Stroke Scale score or if the patient is aphasic.

Review Fibrinolytic Exclusions: Are Any Observed?

- Tables 42 and 43 list the major exclusions for the use of rtPA. These should be available wherever stroke patients might be treated with fibrinolytics.

- One of the clinicians responsible for final decisions about rtPA should personally complete this or a similar checklist, sign it, and make it a part of the formal medical record.

Review Patient Data: Is Time Since Symptom Onset Now More Than 3 Hours?

- This step reminds the clinician to make one last review of all the information gathered during the patient assessments. In particular, document the estimated length of time that has passed since the onset of the stroke.

- IV infusion of the rtPA must begin within 180 minutes of the beginning of stroke symptoms.

Drug: Administration and Monitoring of rtPA Infusion

Fibrinolytic therapy is recommended for a highly selected, well-defined subset of ischemic stroke patients. Treatment with IV rtPA within 3 hours of the onset of ischemic stroke improved clinical outcome at 3 months. ED-based or hospital-based stroke specialists should aim to start the initial bolus within 60 minutes of arrival in the ED. Ten percent of a total dose of 0.9 mg/kg (maximum 90 mg) is given by bolus administration and the remainder over 60 minutes.

During rtPA infusion

- Monitor neurologic status; if any signs of deterioration develop, obtain an emergent CT scan.
- Monitor blood pressure, which may increase during fibrinolytic treatment. Initiate antihypertensive treatment for blood pressure of 180 to 230 mm Hg systolic or 105 to 120 mm Hg diastolic (see Table 42).
- Admit patient to the critical care unit, stroke unit, or other skilled facility capable of careful observation, frequent neurologic assessments, and cardiovascular monitoring.

Avoid anticoagulant or antiplatelet treatment for the next 24 hours. Treatment of carefully selected acute ischemic stroke patients with IV rtPA between 3 and 4.5 hours after onset of symptoms has also been shown to improve clinical outcome, although the degree of clinical benefit is smaller than that achieved with treatment within 3 hours. Data supporting treatment in this time window come from a large, randomized trial—the third European Cooperative Acute Stroke Study (ECASS-3)—that specifically enrolled patients between 3 and 4.5 hours after symptom onset, as well as a meta-analysis of previous trials.

At present, use of IV rtPA within the 3- to 4.5-hour window has not yet been FDA approved, although it is recommended by a current AHA/ASA science advisory.[58] Administration of IV rtPA to patients with acute ischemic stroke who meet the NINDS or ECASS-3 eligibility criteria (Table 43) is recommended if rtPA is administered by physicians in the setting of a clearly defined protocol, a knowledgeable team, and institutional commitment.

Intra-arterial rtPA

For patients with acute ischemic stroke who are not candidates for standard IV fibrinolysis, administration of intra-arterial fibrinolysis in centers that have the resources and expertise available is reasonable (Class I, LOE B). A recent trial has shown improved outcomes even when this is done within the first 8 hours after the onset of symptoms.[59] To date, intra-arterial administration of rtPA has not yet been approved by the FDA.

Transition to Critical Care and Rehabilitation (Numbers 11 and 12)

Disposition: Rapid Admission to Stroke Unit or Critical Care Unit

General Stroke Care

Given the requirements for frequent neurologic assessment and vital sign measurements, especially after administration of IV rtPA, patients should be admitted as quickly as possible, ideally within 3 hours from arrival. If the patient's neurologic status deteriorates, an emergent CT scan is required to determine if cerebral edema or hemorrhage is responsible for the deterioration. Treatment of hemorrhage or edema should be started immediately as indicated.

Additional stroke care includes support of the airway, oxygenation and ventilation, and nutritional support. Normal saline is administered at approximately 75 to 100 mL/h to maintain euvolemia if needed. The reported frequency of seizures during the first days of stroke ranges from 2% to 23%. Most seizures occur during the first day and can recur. Seizure prophylaxis is not recommended. Treatment of acute seizures followed by administration of anticonvulsants to prevent further seizures is recommended, consistent with the established management of seizures. Monitor the patient for signs of increased intracranial pressure. Continued control of blood pressure is required to reduce the risk of bleeding.

Critical Concept

Anticoagulants and Antiplatelet Therapy

Neither anticoagulants nor antiplatelet treatment is administered for 24 hours after administration of rtPA, typically until a follow-up CT scan at 24 hours shows no hemorrhage (Number 10).

- If the patient has brain hemorrhage, DO NOT GIVE ASPIRIN (Number 7).
- If the patient has ischemic stroke but is not a candidate for rtPA, consider aspirin or another antiplatelet agent.
- DO NOT administer heparin (unfractionated or low molecular weight). Heparin is associated with an increased risk of bleeding within the first 24 hours.

Table 43. Inclusion and Exclusion Characteristics of Patients With Ischemic Stroke Who Could Be Treated With rtPA From *3 to 4.5 Hours* From Symptom Onset[58]

Inclusion Criteria
• Diagnosis of ischemic stroke causing measurable neurologic deficit • Onset of symptoms 3 to 4.5 hours before beginning treatment
Exclusion Criteria
• Age older than 80 years • Severe stroke (NIH Stroke Scale score less than 25) • Taking an oral anticoagulant regardless of INR • History of both diabetes and prior ischemic stroke
Notes • The checklist includes some FDA-approved indications and contraindications for administration of rtPA for acute ischemic stroke. Recent guideline revisions have modified the original FDA criteria. A physician with expertise in acute stroke care may modify this list. • Onset time is either witnessed or last known normal. • In patients without recent use of oral anticoagulants or heparin, treatment with rtPA can be initiated before availability of coagulation study results but should be discontinued if INR is more than 1.7 or PT is elevated by local laboratory standards. • In patients without a history of thrombocytopenia, treatment with rtPA can be initiated before availability of platelet count but should be discontinued if platelet count is less than 100 000/mm^3.

Abbreviations: FDA, Food and Drug Administration; INR, international normalized ratio; NIH, National Institutes of Health; PT, prothrombin time; rtPA, recombinant tissue plasminogen activator.

Hyperglycemia

Hyperglycemia is present in about one third of patients admitted with stroke. Hyperglycemia is associated with worse clinical outcome in patients with acute ischemic stroke than is normoglycemia, but there is no direct evidence that active glucose control improves clinical outcome.[60,61] There is evidence that insulin treatment of hyperglycemia in other critically ill patients improves survival rates. For this reason the AHA/ASA recommend the use of insulin when the serum glucose level is greater than 185 mg/dL in patients with acute stroke; however, the utility of administration of IV or subcutaneous insulin to lower blood glucose in patients with acute ischemic stroke when serum glucose is 185 mg/dL or higher remains uncertain.[62,63]

Temperature Control

Increased temperature in stroke is associated with poor neurologic outcome. No data have demonstrated that lowering temperature improves outcome, but an elevated temperature of 37.5°C (99.5°F) or higher should be treated and the source of fever identified and treated if possible.

Induced hypothermia can exert neuroprotective effects after a stroke. Hypothermia has been shown to improve survival and functional outcome in patients following resuscitation from sudden cardiac arrest caused by ventricular fibrillation, but it has not been shown in controlled human trials to be effective for acute ischemic stroke. In some small human pilot studies and in animal models, hypothermia (33°C to 36°C [91.4°F to 96.8°F]) for acute ischemic stroke has been shown to be relatively safe and feasible (level of evidence 3 to 5). Although the effects of hypothermia on both global and focal cerebral ischemia in animals have been promising, cooling to 33°C (91.4°F) and lower appears to be associated with increased complications, including hypotension, cardiac arrhythmias, cardiac failure, pneumonia, thrombocytopenia, and a rebound increase in intracranial pressure during rewarming. At present there is insufficient scientific evidence to recommend for or against the use of hypothermia in the treatment of acute ischemic stroke.

Dysphagia Screening

All patients with stroke should be screened for dysphagia before anything is given by mouth. A simple bedside screening evaluation involves asking the patient to sip water from a cup. If the patient can sip and swallow without difficulty, the patient is asked to take a large gulp of water and swallow. If there are no signs of coughing or aspiration after 30 seconds, then it is safe for the patient to have a thickened diet until formally assessed by a speech pathologist. Medications may be given in applesauce or jam. Any patient who fails a swallow test may be given medications such as aspirin rectally or if appropriate via the IV, intramuscular, or subcutaneous route.

Stroke System of Care

Substantial progress has been made toward regionalization of stroke care. Several states have passed legislation requiring prehospital providers to triage patients with suspected stroke to designated stroke centers. This is contingent on the accuracy of dispatch, an area where further improvement is needed. Please see Chapter 4 of this text for a detailed description of the stroke system of care.

References

1. Go AS, Mozaffarian D, Roger VL, Benjamin EJ, Berry JD, Borden WB, Bravata DM, Dai S, Ford ES, Fox CS, Franco S, Fullerton HJ, Gillespie C, Hailpern SM, Heit JA, Howard VJ, Huffman MD, Kissela BM, Kittner SJ, Lackland DT, Lichtman JH, Lisabeth LD, Magid D, Marcus GM, Marelli A, Matchar DB, McGuire D, Mohler E, Moy CS, Mussolino ME, Nichol G, Paynter NP, Schreiner PJ, Sorlie PD, Stein J, Turan TN, Virani SS, Wong ND, Woo D, Turner MB; on behalf of the American Heart Association Statistics Committee and Stroke Statistics Subcommittee. Heart disease and stroke statistics—2013 update: a report from the American Heart Association [published online ahead of print December 12, 2012]. *Circulation*. 2013. doi:10.1161/CIR.0b013e31828124ad.
2. Schwamm LH, Pancioli A, Acker JE III, Goldstein LB, Zorowitz RD, Shephard TJ, Moyer P, Gorman M, Johnston SC, Duncan PW, Gorelick P, Frank J, Stranne SK, Smith R, Federspiel W, Horton KB, Magnis E, Adams RJ. Recommendations for the establishment of stroke systems of care: recommendations from the American Stroke Association's Task Force on the Development of Stroke Systems. *Circulation.* 2005;111:1078-1091.
3. Dobkin BH. Clinical practice. Rehabilitation after stroke. *N Engl J Med.* 2005;352:1677-1684.
4. Tissue plasminogen activator for acute ischemic stroke. The National Institute of Neurological Disorders and Stroke rt-PA Stroke Study Group. *N Engl J Med.* 1995;333:1581-1587.
5. Hazinski M. D-mystifying recognition and management of stroke. *Curr Emerg Cardiac Care.* 1996;7:8.
6. Adams HP Jr, del Zoppo G, Alberts MJ, Bhatt DL, Brass L, Furlan A, Grubb RL, Higashida RT, Jauch EC, Kidwell C, Lyden PD, Morgenstern LB, Qureshi AI, Rosenwasser RH, Scott PA, Wijdicks EF. Guidelines for the early management of adults with ischemic stroke: a guideline from the American Heart Association/American Stroke Association Stroke Council, Clinical Cardiology Council, Cardiovascular Radiology and Intervention Council, and the Atherosclerotic Peripheral Vascular Disease and Quality of Care Outcomes in Research Interdisciplinary Working Groups. *Stroke.* 2007;38:1655-1711.
7. Emergency department: rapid identification and treatment of patients with acute myocardial infarction. National Heart Attack Alert Program Coordinating Committee, 60 Minutes to Treatment Working Group. *Ann Emerg Med.* 1994;23:311-329.
8. Carr S, Farb A, Pearce WH, Virmani R, Yao JS. Atherosclerotic plaque rupture in symptomatic carotid artery stenosis. *J Vasc Surg.* 1996;23:755-765.
9. Spagnoli LG, Mauriello A, Sangiorgi G, Fratoni S, Bonanno E, Schwartz RS, Piepgras DG, Pistolese R, Ippoliti A, Holmes DR Jr. Extracranial thrombotically active carotid plaque as a risk factor for ischemic stroke. *JAMA.* 2004;292:1845-1852.
10. Redgrave JN, Lovett JK, Gallagher PJ, Rothwell PM. Histological assessment of 526 symptomatic carotid plaques in relation to the nature and timing of ischemic symptoms: the Oxford plaque study. *Circulation.* 2006;113:2320-2328.
11. Brott T, Adams HP Jr, Olinger CP, Marler JR, Barsan WG, Biller J, Spilker J, Holleran R, Eberle R, Hertzberg V, et al. Measurements of acute cerebral infarction: a clinical examination scale. *Stroke.* 1989;20:864-870.
12. Brott TG, Haley EC Jr, Levy DE, Barsan W, Broderick J, Sheppard GL, Spilker J, Kongable GL, Massey S, Reed R, et al. Urgent therapy for stroke. Part I. Pilot study of tissue plasminogen activator administered within 90 minutes. *Stroke.* 1992;23:632-640.
13. Zachariah BS, Pepe PE. The development of emergency medical dispatch in the USA: a historical perspective. *Eur J Emerg Med.* 1995;2:109-112.
14. Wendel-Vos GC, Schuit AJ, Feskens EJ, Boshuizen HC, Verschuren WM, Saris WH, Kromhout D. Physical activity and stroke. A meta-analysis of observational data. *Int J Epidemiol.* 2004;33:787-798.
15. Lee IM, Hennekens CH, Berger K, Buring JE, Manson JE. Exercise and risk of stroke in male physicians. *Stroke.* 1999;30:1-6.
16. Lee IM, Paffenbarger RS Jr. Physical activity and stroke incidence: the Harvard Alumni Health Study. *Stroke.* 1998;29:2049-2054.
17. Morgenstern LB, Bartholomew LK, Grotta JC, Staub L, King M, Chan W. Sustained benefit of a community and professional intervention to increase acute stroke therapy. *Arch Intern Med.* 2003;163:2198-2202.
18. Morgenstern LB, Staub L, Chan W, Wein TH, Bartholomew LK, King M, Felberg RA, Burgin WS, Groff J, Hickenbottom SL, Saldin K, Demchuk AM, Kalra A, Dhingra A, Grotta JC. Improving delivery of acute stroke therapy: the TLL Temple Foundation Stroke Project. *Stroke.* 2002;33:160-166.
19. Handschu R, Poppe R, Rauss J, Neundorfer B, Erbguth F. Emergency calls in acute stroke. *Stroke.* 2003;34:1005-1009.
20. Williams JE, Rosamond WD, Morris DL. Stroke symptom attribution and time to emergency department arrival: the delay in accessing stroke healthcare study. *Acad Emerg Med.* 2000;7:93-96.
21. Morris DL, Rosamond W, Madden K, Schultz C, Hamilton S. Prehospital and emergency department delays after acute stroke: the Genentech Stroke Presentation Survey. *Stroke.* 2000;31:2585-2590.
22. Schroeder EB, Rosamond WD, Morris DL, Evenson KR, Hinn AR. Determinants of use of emergency medical services in a population with stroke symptoms: the Second Delay in Accessing Stroke Healthcare (DASH II) Study. *Stroke.* 2000;31:2591-2596.
23. Barsan WG, Brott TG, Broderick JP, Haley EC, Levy DE, Marler JR. Time of hospital presentation in patients with acute stroke. *Arch Intern Med.* 1993;153:2558-2561.
24. Kothari R, Barsan W, Brott T, Broderick J, Ashbrock S. Frequency and accuracy of prehospital diagnosis of acute stroke. *Stroke.* 1995;26:937-941.
25. Buck BH, Starkman S, Eckstein M, Kidwell CS, Haines J, Huang R, Colby D, Saver JL. Dispatcher recognition of stroke using the National Academy Medical Priority Dispatch System. *Stroke.* 2009;40:2027-2030.
26. Kothari RU, Pancioli A, Liu T, Brott T, Broderick J. Cincinnati Prehospital Stroke Scale: reproducibility and validity. *Ann Emerg Med.* 1999;33:373-378.
27. Kothari R, Hall K, Brott T, Broderick J. Early stroke recognition: developing an out-of-hospital NIH Stroke Scale. *Acad Emerg Med.* 1997;4:986-990.
28. Kidwell CS, Saver JL, Schubert GB, Eckstein M, Starkman S. Design and retrospective analysis of the Los Angeles Prehospital Stroke Screen (LAPSS). *Prehosp Emerg Care.* 1998;2:267-273.
29. Kidwell CS, Starkman S, Eckstein M, Weems K, Saver JL. Identifying stroke in the field. Prospective validation of the

Los Angeles prehospital stroke screen (LAPSS). *Stroke.* 2000;31:71-76.

30. Chalela JA, Kasner SE, Jauch EC, Pancioli AM. Safety of air medical transportation after tissue plasminogen activator administration in acute ischemic stroke. *Stroke.* 1999;30:2366-2368.
31. Conroy MB, Rodriguez SU, Kimmel SE, Kasner SE. Helicopter transfer offers a potential benefit to patients with acute stroke. *Stroke.* 1999;30:2580-2584.
32. Silbergleit R, Scott PA. Thrombolysis for acute stroke: the incontrovertible, the controvertible, and the uncertain. *Acad Emerg Med.* 2005;12:348-351.
33. Silbergleit R, Scott PA, Lowell MJ, Silbergleit R. Cost-effectiveness of helicopter transport of stroke patients for thrombolysis. *Acad Emerg Med.* 2003;10:966-972.
34. A systems approach to immediate evaluation and management of hyperacute stroke. Experience at eight centers and implications for community practice and patient care. The National Institute of Neurological Disorders and Stroke (NINDS) rt-PA Stroke Study Group. *Stroke.* 1997;28:1530-1540.
35. Oppenheimer SM, Cechetto DF, Hachinski VC. Cerebrogenic cardiac arrhythmias. Cerebral electrocardiographic influences and their role in sudden death. *Arch Neurol.* 1990;47:513-519.
36. Adams HP Jr, Brott TG, Crowell RM, Furlan AJ, Gomez CR, Grotta J, Helgason CM, Marler JR, Woolson RF, Zivin JA, et al. Guidelines for the management of patients with acute ischemic stroke. A statement for healthcare professionals from a special writing group of the Stroke Council, American Heart Association. *Stroke.* 1994;25:1901-1914.
37. Teasdale G, Jennett B. Assessment of coma and impaired consciousness: a practical scale. *Lancet.* 1974;2(7872):81-84.
38. Lyden P, Rapp K, Babcock T, Rothrock J. Ultra-rapid identification, triage, and enrollment of stroke patients into clinical trials. *J Stroke Cerebrovasc Dis.* 1974;2:106-113.
39. Brott T. Utility of the NIH stroke scale. *Cerebrovasc Dis.* 1992;2:241-242.
40. Lyden P, Lu M, Jackson C, Marler J, Kothari R, Brott T, Zivin J. Underlying structure of the National Institutes of Health Stroke Scale: results of a factor analysis. NINDS tPA Stroke Trial Investigators. *Stroke.* 1999;30:2347-2354.
41. Goldstein LB, Bertels C, Davis JN. Interrater reliability of the NIH stroke scale. *Arch Neurol.* 1989;46:660-662.
42. Adams H, Adams R, Del Zoppo G, Goldstein LB. Guidelines for the early management of patients with ischemic stroke: 2005 guidelines update: a scientific statement from the Stroke Council of the American Heart Association/American Stroke Association. *Stroke.* 2005;36:916-923.
43. Adams HP Jr, Adams RJ, Brott T, del Zoppo GJ, Furlan A, Goldstein LB, Grubb RL, Higashida R, Kidwell C, Kwiatkowski TG, Marler JR, Hademenos GJ. Guidelines for the early management of patients with ischemic stroke: a scientific statement from the Stroke Council of the American Stroke Association. *Stroke.* 2003;34:1056-1083.
44. Part 6: advanced cardiovascular life support. Section 1: Introduction to ACLS 2000: overview of recommended changes in ACLS from the guidelines 2000 conference. European Resuscitation Council. *Resuscitation.* 2000;46:103-107.
45. Connors JJ III, Sacks D, Furlan AJ, Selman WR, Russell EJ, Stieg PE, Hadley MN. Training, competency, and credentialing standards for diagnostic cervicocerebral angiography, carotid stenting, and cerebrovascular intervention: a joint statement from the American Academy of Neurology, American Association of Neurological Surgeons, American Society of Interventional and Therapeutic Radiology, American Society of Neuroradiology, Congress of Neurological Surgeons, AANS/CNS Cerebrovascular Section, and Society of Interventional Radiology. *Radiology.* 2005;234:26-34.
46. Schriger DL, Kalafut M, Starkman S, Krueger M, Saver JL. Cranial computed tomography interpretation in acute stroke: physician accuracy in determining eligibility for thrombolytic therapy. *JAMA.* 1998;279:1293-1297.
47. Hill MD, Buchan AM. Thrombolysis for acute ischemic stroke: results of the Canadian Alteplase for Stroke Effectiveness Study. *CMAJ.* 2005;172:1307-1312.
48. Graham GD. Tissue plasminogen activator for acute ischemic stroke in clinical practice: a meta-analysis of safety data. *Stroke.* 2003;34:2847-2850.
49. Heuschmann PU, Berger K, Misselwitz B, Hermanek P, Leffmann C, Adelmann M, Buecker-Nott HJ, Rother J, Neundoerfer B, Kolominsky-Rabas PL. Frequency of thrombolytic therapy in patients with acute ischemic stroke and the risk of in-hospital mortality: the German Stroke Registers Study Group. *Stroke.* 2003;34:1106-1113.
50. Bravata DM, Kim N, Concato J, Krumholz HM, Brass LM. Thrombolysis for acute stroke in routine clinical practice. *Arch Intern Med.* 2002;162:1994-2001.
51. Katzan IL, Furlan AJ, Lloyd LE, Frank JI, Harper DL, Hinchey JA, Hammel JP, Qu A, Sila CA. Use of tissue-type plasminogen activator for acute ischemic stroke: the Cleveland area experience. *JAMA.* 2000;283:1151-1158.
52. Katzan IL, Hammer MD, Hixson ED, Furlan AJ, Abou-Chebl A, Nadzam DM. Utilization of intravenous tissue plasminogen activator for acute ischemic stroke. *Arch Neurol.* 2004;61:346-350.
53. Lopez-Yunez AM, Bruno A, Williams LS, Yilmaz E, Zurru C, Biller J. Protocol violations in community-based rtPA stroke treatment are associated with symptomatic intracerebral hemorrhage. *Stroke.* 2001;32:12-16.
54. Asimos AW, Norton HJ, Price MF, Cheek WM. Therapeutic yield and outcomes of a community teaching hospital code stroke protocol. *Acad Emerg Med.* 2004;11:361-370.
55. Katzan IL, Hammer MD, Furlan AJ, Hixson ED, Nadzam DM. Quality improvement and tissue-type plasminogen activator for acute ischemic stroke: a Cleveland update. *Stroke.* 2003;34:799-800.
56. Lattimore SU, Chalela J, Davis L, DeGraba T, Ezzeddine M, Haymore J, Nyquist P, Baird AE, Hallenbeck J, Warach S. Impact of establishing a primary stroke center at a community hospital on the use of thrombolytic therapy: the NINDS Suburban Hospital Stroke Center experience. *Stroke.* 2003;34:e55-e57.
57. Alberts MJ, Hademenos G, Latchaw RE, Jagoda A, Marler JR, Mayberg MR, Starke RD, Todd HW, Viste KM, Girgus M, Shephard T, Emr M, Shwayder P, Walker MD. Recommendations for the establishment of primary stroke centers. Brain Attack Coalition. *JAMA.* 2000;283:3102-3109.
58. del Zoppo GJ, Saver JL, Jauch EC, Adams HP Jr. Expansion of the time window for treatment of acute ischemic stroke with intravenous tissue plasminogen activator: a science advisory from the American Heart Association/American Stroke Association. *Stroke.* 2009;40:2945-2948.
59. Saver JL, Jahan R, Levy EI, Jovin TG, Baxter B, Nogueira RG, Clark W, Budzik R, Zaidat OO; for the SWIFT Trialists. Solitaire flow restoration device versus the Merci Retriever in patients

with acute ischaemic stroke (SWIFT): a randomised, parallel-group, non-inferiority trial. *Lancet.* 2012;380(9849):1241-1249.

60. Scott JF, Robinson GM, French JM, O'Connell JE, Alberti KG, Gray CS. Glucose potassium insulin infusions in the treatment of acute stroke patients with mild to moderate hyperglycemia: the Glucose Insulin in Stroke Trial (GIST). *Stroke.* 1999;30:793-799.
61. Gray CS, Hildreth AJ, Alberti GK, O'Connell JE. Poststroke hyperglycemia: natural history and immediate management. *Stroke.* 2004;35:122-126.
62. Van den Berghe G, Wouters PJ, Bouillon R, Weekers F, Verwaest C, Schetz M, Vlasselaers D, Ferdinande P, Lauwers P. Outcome benefit of intensive insulin therapy in the critically ill: insulin dose versus glycemic control. *Crit Care Med.* 2003;31:359-366.
63. van den Berghe G, Wouters P, Weekers F, Verwaest C, Bruyninckx F, Schetz M, Vlasselaers D, Ferdinande P, Lauwers P, Bouillon R. Intensive insulin therapy in critically ill patients. *N Engl J Med.* 2001;345:1359-1367.

Chapter 13

Post–Cardiac Arrest Care

This Chapter

- The Immediate Post–Cardiac Arrest Care Algorithm
- Therapeutic Hypothermia
- Percutaneous Coronary Intervention (PCI)
- Post-ROSC Integrated System of Care

Introduction

There is increasing recognition that systematic post–cardiac arrest care after return of spontaneous circulation (ROSC) can improve the likelihood of patient survival with good quality of life. Positive correlations have been observed between the likelihood of survival and the number of cardiac arrest cases treated at any individual hospital.[1,2] Studies show most deaths occur during the first 24 hours after resuscitation from cardiac arrest.[3,4] Post–cardiac arrest care has a significant potential to reduce early mortality caused by hemodynamic instability and later morbidity and mortality caused by multiorgan failure and brain injury.[5,6] This chapter summarizes the hemodynamic, neurologic, and metabolic abnormalities initially encountered in patients who are resuscitated from cardiac arrest.

There is a growing body of research focused on the identification and optimization of practices that improve outcomes of patients who achieve ROSC after cardiac arrest (Table 44).[7] Mere restoration of blood pressure and gas exchange does not ensure survival and functional recovery. Significant cardiovascular dysfunction can develop after ROSC that requires active support of blood flow and ventilation, including intravascular volume expansion, vasoactive and inotropic drugs, and invasive devices. Therapeutic hypothermia and treatment of the underlying cause of cardiac arrest impact survival and neurologic outcome. Protocolized hemodynamic optimization and multifaceted early goal-directed therapy protocols have been introduced as part of a bundle of care to improve survival.[8-10] The data suggest that proactive management of post–cardiac arrest physiology can improve outcomes by ensuring organ oxygenation and perfusion and by avoiding and managing complications.

Overview of Post–Cardiac Arrest Care

Providers should ensure an adequate airway and support breathing immediately after ROSC. Unconscious patients usually require an advanced airway for mechanical support of breathing. Methods for securing an advanced airway are discussed in Chapter 6, "Airway Management." Providers should also elevate the head of the bed 30° if tolerated to reduce the incidence of cerebral edema, aspiration, and ventilatory-associated pneumonia. Proper placement of an advanced airway, particularly during patient transport, should be monitored by waveform capnography as described in the *2010 AHA Guidelines for CPR and ECC*. Oxygenation of the patient should be monitored continuously with pulse oximetry.

Although 100% oxygen may have been used during initial resuscitation, providers should titrate inspired oxygen to the lowest level required to achieve an arterial oxygen saturation of 94% or higher to avoid potential oxygen toxicity. Hyperventilation is common after cardiac arrest and should be avoided because of the potential for adverse hemodynamic effects. Hyperventilation increases intrathoracic

Table 44. **Multiple System Approach to Post–Cardiac Arrest Care**

Ventilation	Hemodynamics	Cardiovascular	Neurological	Metabolic
• Capnography	• Frequent Blood Pressure Monitoring/Arterial-line	• Continuous Cardiac Monitoring	• Serial Neurological Exam	• Serial Lactate
• Rationale: Confirm secure airway and titrate ventilation	• Rationale: Maintain perfusion and prevent recurrent hypotension	• Rationale: Detect recurrent arrhythmia	• Rationale: Serial examinations define coma, brain injury, and prognosis	• Rationale: Confirm adequate perfusion
• Endotracheal tube when possible for comatose patients	• Mean arterial pressure ≥65 mm Hg or systolic blood pressure ≥90 mm Hg	• No prophylactic antiarrhythmics	• Response to verbal commands or physical stimulation	
• P_{ETCO_2}~35–40 mm Hg		• Treat arrhythmias as required	• Pupillary light and corneal reflex, spontaneous eye movement	
• Pa_{CO_2}~40–45 mm Hg		• Remove reversible causes	• Gag, cough, spontaneous breaths	
• Chest X-ray	• Treat Hypotension	• 12-lead ECG/Troponin	• EEG Monitoring If Comatose	• Serum Potassium
• Rationale: Confirm secure airway and detect causes or complications of arrest: pneumonitis, pneumonia, pulmonary edema	• Rationale: Maintain perfusion	• Rationale: Detect Acute Coronary Syndrome/ST-Elevation Myocardial Infarction; Assess QT interval	• Rationale: Exclude seizures	• Rationale: Avoid hypokalemia which promotes arrhythmias
	• Fluid bolus if tolerated		• Anticonvulsants if seizing	• Replace to maintain K >3.5 mEq/L
	• Dopamine 5–10 mcg/kg per min			
	• Norepinephrine 0.1–0.5 mcg/kg per min			
	• Epinephrine 0.1–0.5 mcg/kg per min			
• Pulse Oximetry/ABG	...	• Treat Acute Coronary Syndrome	• Core Temperature Measurement If Comatose	• Urine Output, Serum Creatinine
• Rationale: Maintain adequate oxygenation and minimize F_{IO_2}	...	• Aspirin/heparin	• Rationale: Minimize brain injury and improve outcome	• Rationale: Detect acute kidney injury
• Sp_{O_2} ≥94%	...	• Transfer to acute coronary treatment center	• Prevent hyperpyrexia >37.7°C	• Maintain euvolemia
• Pa_{O_2}~100 mm Hg	...	• Consider emergent PCI or fibrinolysis	• Induce therapeutic hypothermia if no contraindications	• Renal replacement therapy if indicated
• Reduce F_{IO_2} as tolerated	...		• Cold IV fluid bolus 30 mL/kg if no contraindication	
• Pa_{O_2}/F_{IO_2} ratio to follow acute lung injury	...		• Surface or endovascular cooling for 32°C–34°C×24 hours	
	...		• After 24 hours, slow rewarming 0.25°C/hr	
• Mechanical Ventilation	...	• Echocardiogram	• Consider Non-enhanced CT Scan	• Serum Glucose
• Rationale: Minimize acute lung injury, potential oxygen toxicity	...	• Rationale: Detect global stunning, wall-motion abnormalities, structural problems or cardiomyopathy	• Rationale: Exclude primary intracranial process	• Rationale: Detect hyperglycemia and hypoglycemia
• Tidal Volume 6–8 mL/kg	...			• Treat hypoglycemia (<80 mg/dL) with dextrose
• Titrate minute ventilation to P_{ETCO_2}~35–40 mm Hg Pa_{CO_2}~40–45 mm Hg	...			• Treat hyperglycemia to target glucose 144–180 mg/dL
• Reduce F_{IO_2} as tolerated to keep Sp_{O_2} or Sa_{O_2} ≥94%	...			• Local insulin protocols
	...	• Treat Myocardial Stunning	• Sedation/Muscle Relaxation	• Avoid Hypotonic Fluids
	...	• Fluids to optimize volume status (requires clinical judgment)	• Rationale: To control shivering, agitation, or ventilator desynchrony as needed	• Rationale: May increase edema, including cerebral edema
	...	• Dobutamine 5–10 mcg/kg per min		
	...	• Mechanical augmentation (IABP)		

A comprehensive, structured, multidisciplinary system of care should be implemented in a consistent manner for the treatment of post–cardiac arrest patients (Class I, LOE B). Programs should include therapeutic hypothermia, optimization of hemodynamics and gas exchange, immediate coronary reperfusion when indicated for restoration of coronary blood flow with percutaneous coronary intervention (PCI), glycemic control, neurologic diagnosis, critical care management, and prognostication.

Abbreviations: CT, computed tomography; ECG, electrocardiogram; EEG, electroencephalographic; IABP, intra-aortic balloon pump; IV, intravenous.

pressure, which decreases preload and lowers cardiac output. The decrease in Pa_{CO_2} seen with hyperventilation can also decrease cerebral blood flow directly. Ventilation should be started at 10 to 12 breaths per minute and titrated to achieve a P_{ETCO_2} of 35 to 40 mm Hg or a Pa_{CO_2} of 40 to 45 mm Hg.

Healthcare providers should frequently reassess vital signs and monitor for recurrent cardiac arrhythmias using continuous electrocardiographic (ECG) monitoring. If the patient is hypotensive (systolic blood pressure [SBP] less than 90 mm Hg), fluid boluses can be administered. If therapeutic hypothermia is indicated, cold fluids may be helpful for initial induction of hypothermia. If the patient's volume status is adequate, infusions of vasoactive agents may be initiated and titrated to achieve a minimum SBP of 90 mm Hg or greater or a mean arterial pressure of 65 mm Hg or more. Some advocate higher mean arterial pressures to promote cerebral blood flow.

Brain injury and cardiovascular instability are the major factors that determine survival after cardiac arrest.[11] Because therapeutic hypothermia is currently the only intervention demonstrated to improve neurologic recovery, it should be considered for any patient who is unable to follow verbal commands after ROSC. The patient should be transported to a location that reliably provides this therapy in addition to coronary reperfusion (eg, PCI) and other goal-directed postarrest care therapies.

Clinicians should treat the precipitating cause of cardiac arrest after ROSC and initiate or request studies that will further aid in evaluation of the patient. It is essential to identify and treat any cardiac, electrolyte, toxicologic, pulmonary, and neurologic precipitants of arrest. Overall, the most common cause of cardiac arrest is cardiovascular disease and associated coronary ischemia.[12,13] Therefore, a 12-lead ECG should be obtained as soon as possible to detect ST elevation or left bundle branch block. When there is high suspicion of acute myocardial infarction (AMI), local protocols for treatment of AMI and coronary reperfusion should be activated. Even in the absence of ST elevation, medical or interventional treatments should be considered for treatment of ACS[13-15] and should not be deferred in the presence of coma. Concurrent PCI and hypothermia are safe, with good outcomes reported for some comatose patients who have undergone PCI.

Critical care facilities that treat patients after cardiac arrest should use a comprehensive care plan that includes acute cardiovascular interventions, use of therapeutic hypothermia, standardized medical goal-directed therapies, and advanced neurologic monitoring and care. Neurologic prognosis may be difficult to determine during the first 72 hours following resuscitation. This time frame for prognostication is likely to be extended in patients undergoing therapeutic hypothermia.[16] Many initially comatose survivors of cardiac arrest have the potential for full recovery.[8,17,18] Therefore, it is important to place patients in a hospital critical care unit where expert care and neurologic evaluation can be performed and where appropriate testing to aid prognosis is performed in a timely manner.

Managing Post–Cardiac Arrest Care: The Immediate Post–Cardiac Arrest Care Algorithm

The Immediate Post–Cardiac Arrest Care Algorithm (Figure 105) outlines the recommended steps for the immediate assessment and management of post–cardiac arrest patients with ROSC.

Introduction

The algorithm begins with a patient who has achieved ROSC after being resuscitated from cardiac arrest (Number 1).

Ventilation and Oxygenation

Ensure an adequate airway and support breathing immediately after ROSC (Number 2).

If an advanced airway is needed, use continuous waveform capnography to confirm and monitor correct placement. Although capnography to confirm and monitor correct placement of supraglottic airways has not been studied, effective ventilation through a supraglottic airway device should result in a capnography waveform during cardiopulmonary resuscitation (CPR) and after ROSC. Continuous waveform capnography is recommended in the *2010 AHA Guidelines for CPR and ECC,* in addition to clinical assessment, as the most reliable method to confirm and monitor correct placement of an endotracheal tube or other advanced airway. Healthcare providers should observe a persistent capnographic waveform with ventilation to confirm and monitor endotracheal tube placement in the field, in the transport vehicle, on arrival at the hospital, and after any patient transfer to reduce the risk of unrecognized tube displacement.

Avoid excessive ventilation of the patient (do not ventilate too fast; avoid large tidal volumes). Excessive ventilation can potentially lead to decreases in cerebral blood flow when Pa_{CO_2} decreases. Adverse hemodynamic effects may be seen when intrathoracic pressures are increased, which causes reduced preload. Providers may begin ventilations at 10 to 12 breaths/min (not to exceed 20/min) and titrate to achieve a P_{ETCO_2} of 35 to 40 mm Hg or a Pa_{CO_2} of 40 to 45 mm Hg. Slightly higher Pa_{CO_2} allows for temperature correction when hypothermia is used (real Pa_{CO_2} at the

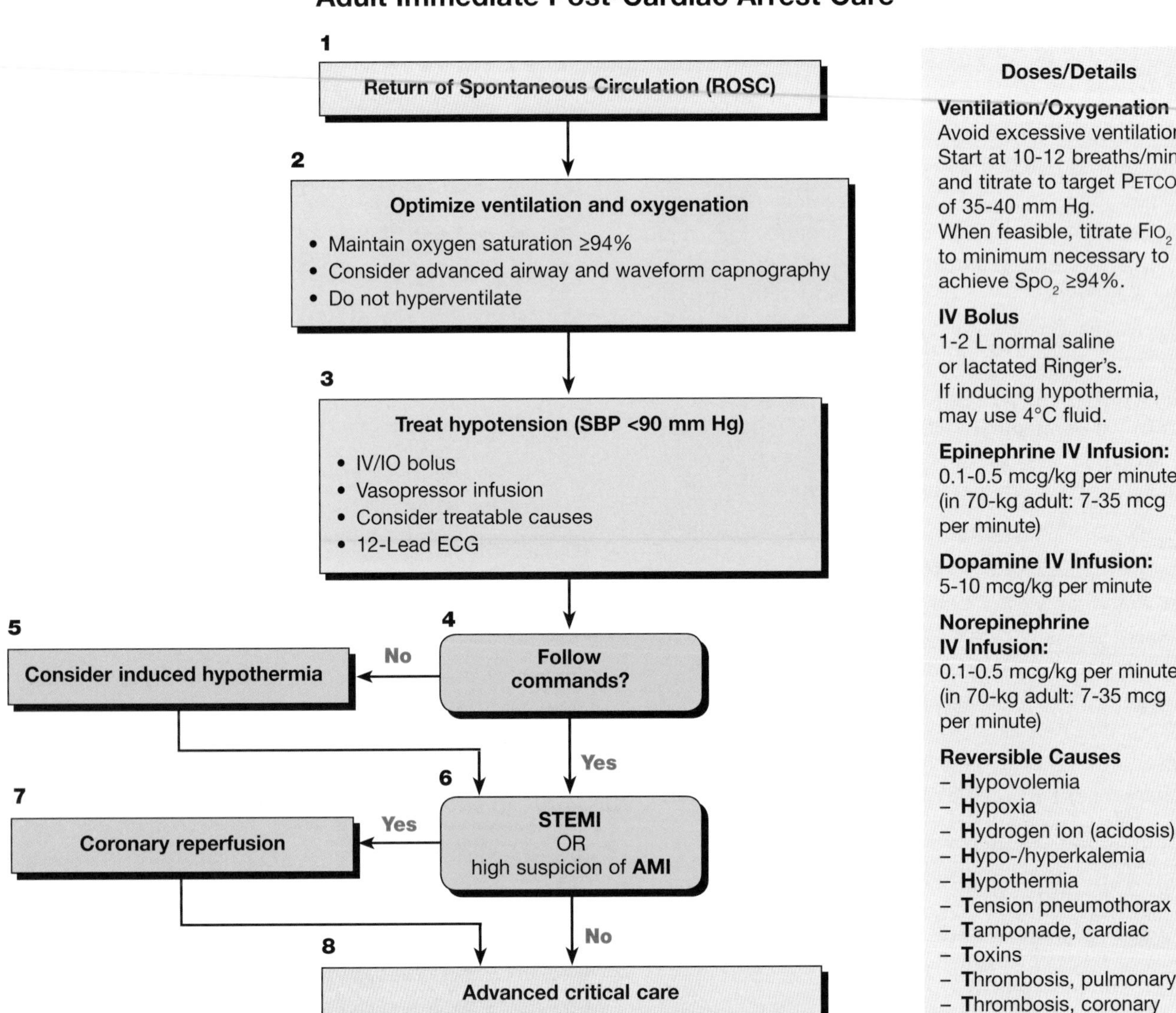

Adult Immediate Post-Cardiac Arrest Care
1
Return of Spontaneous Circulation (ROSC)
2
Optimize ventilation and oxygenation
• Maintain oxygen saturation ≥94%
• Consider advanced airway and waveform capnography
• Do not hyperventilate
3
Treat hypotension (SBP <90 mm Hg)
• IV/IO bolus
• Vasopressor infusion
• Consider treatable causes
• 12-Lead ECG
4
Follow commands?
No
5
Consider induced hypothermia
Yes
6
STEMI OR high suspicion of AMI
Yes
7
Coronary reperfusion
No
8
Advanced critical care
Doses/Details
Ventilation/Oxygenation
Avoid excessive ventilation. Start at 10-12 breaths/min and titrate to target PETCO2 of 35-40 mm Hg.
When feasible, titrate FIO2 to minimum necessary to achieve SpO2 ≥94%.
IV Bolus
1-2 L normal saline or lactated Ringer's.
If inducing hypothermia, may use 4°C fluid.
Epinephrine IV Infusion:
0.1-0.5 mcg/kg per minute (in 70-kg adult: 7-35 mcg per minute)
Dopamine IV Infusion:
5-10 mcg/kg per minute
Norepinephrine IV Infusion:
0.1-0.5 mcg/kg per minute (in 70-kg adult: 7-35 mcg per minute)
Reversible Causes
– Hypovolemia
– Hypoxia
– Hydrogen ion (acidosis)
– Hypo-/hyperkalemia
– Hypothermia
– Tension pneumothorax
– Tamponade, cardiac
– Toxins
– Thrombosis, pulmonary
– Thrombosis, coronary

Figure 105. The Adult Immediate Post–Cardiac Arrest Care Algorithm.

patient temperature will be lower than the value reported by the machine). When securing an advanced airway, avoid using ties that risk obstructing venous return from the brain.

If the appropriate equipment is available, adjust the FIO_2 after ROSC has been achieved to the minimum concentration needed to achieve an arterial oxyhemoglobin saturation of 94% or more. Because an oxygen saturation of 100% may correspond to a PaO_2 from 80 to 500 mm Hg, in general it is appropriate to wean FIO_2 to the lowest level needed to consistently keep the oxyhemoglobin saturation at 94% or greater according to a pulse oximeter. The goal is to avoid hyperoxia while ensuring adequate oxygen delivery. When titration of inspired oxygen is not feasible, it is reasonable to empirically use 100% oxygen until the patient is placed on a ventilator.

Hypotension

The patient's blood pressure should be reassessed regularly and frequently. Since blood pressure can be quite labile in post-cardiac arrest patients, an arterial line may be indicated for continuous blood pressure monitoring. Treat hypotension when SBP is less than 90 mm Hg (Number 3).

ECG monitoring should continue after ROSC. At this stage, continue to look for and treat any reversible causes that might have precipitated the cardiac arrest but persist after ROSC, such as dysrhythmias or ST changes consistent with ischemia. Providers should obtain IV/IO access if not already established or verify the patency of any IV/IO lines already in place.

Critical Concept Waveform Capnography	• Continuous waveform capnography can provide immediate recognition if the advanced airway has been displaced or if an acute change in cardiac output has occurred. • Over time, the capnography trend can indicate whether a patient is being hyperventilated or hypoventilated.

Management of hypotension:

- **IV bolus** 1 to 2 L of normal saline or lactated Ringer's. If therapeutic hypothermia is indicated, cold (4°C) fluids are useful as an initial treatment to induce cooling. Use caution and/or avoid fluid bolus treatment in patients with renal failure or known volume overload.

Options for vasopressor infusion:

- **Epinephrine** 0.1 to 0.5 mcg/kg per minute (in 70-kg adult: 7 to 35 mcg/min) IV.

Titrate the infusion to achieve a minimum SBP of more than 90 mm Hg or a mean arterial pressure of more than 65 mm Hg.

- **Dopamine** 5 to 10 mcg/kg per minute IV. Titrate the infusion to achieve a minimum SBP of more than 90 mm Hg or a mean arterial pressure of more than 65 mm Hg.
- **Norepinephrine** 0.1 to 0.5 mcg/kg per minute (in 70-kg adult: 7 to 35 mcg/min) IV.

Titrate the infusion to achieve a minimum SBP of more than 90 mm Hg or a mean arterial pressure of more than 65 mm Hg.

Therapeutic Hypothermia

After ROSC, if the patient fails to follow verbal commands (Number 4), initiate therapeutic hypothermia (Number 5) after out-of-hospital cardiac arrest precipitated by ventricular fibrillation (VF) and consider therapeutic hypothermia after out-of-hospital cardiac arrest with an initial rhythm of pulseless electrical activity or asystole. When ROSC occurs in the out-of-hospital setting, emergency medical services (EMS) personnel may initiate the cooling process and should transport the patient to a facility that can reliably continue this therapy. Therapeutic hypothermia may be considered for patients with ROSC after in-hospital cardiac arrest as well. The optimal timing to initiate therapeutic hypothermia is not currently known.

Identify and Treat STEMI or AMI

A 12-lead ECG should be obtained as soon as possible after ROSC to identify those patients with ST-segment elevation myocardial infarction (STEMI) or with symptoms strongly suggestive of AMI (Number 6). Once such patients have been identified, hospital personnel should attempt coronary reperfusion (Number 7). EMS personnel should transport these patients to a facility that can reliably provide this type of therapy. If STEMI or AMI is detected after ROSC, aggressive treatment of STEMI or AMI, including coronary reperfusion with PCI, should be initiated regardless of coma or induced hypothermia. In the case of out-of-hospital STEMI, provide advance notification to receiving facilities for patients diagnosed with STEMI to reduce reperfusion delay.

The healthcare team should transfer the patient to an intensive care unit after coronary reperfusion interventions or directly in cases in which the post–cardiac arrest patient has no evidence of acute ischemia (Number 8). There is currently no evidence to support the continued prophylactic administration of antiarrhythmic medications once a patient achieves ROSC; therefore, infusions of amiodarone or lidocaine should not be started simply because these were given during the resuscitation. Antiarrhythmic therapy should be administered only as needed to treat ongoing arrhythmias.

The remaining sections will provide additional material on different aspects of post–cardiac arrest care.

Targeted Temperature Management

Induced Hypothermia

Therapeutic hypothermia is recommended for the protection of the brain and other organs in patients who remain comatose after ROSC. The strongest evidence for improved neurologic outcome after therapeutic hypothermia exists for comatose survivors of VF cardiac arrest.[19,20] Therapeutic hypothermia has also been shown to provide a beneficial effect on outcome in comatose survivors of out-of-hospital cardiac arrest associated with any arrest rhythm.[9,21-25] A potential benefit of hypothermia has been observed after in- and out-of-hospital cardiac arrest associated with non-VF initial rhythms.[26,27]

The optimal duration of induced hypothermia is at least 12 hours and may be longer than 24 hours. Hypothermia was maintained for 12 or 24 hours in studies of out-of-hospital patients who presented in VF.[18,28] Most therapeutic hypothermia protocols in current practice recommend a cooling duration of 24 hours from the time that target temperature is established. The effect of a longer duration of cooling on outcome has not been studied in adults, but hypothermia for up to 72 hours was used safely in newborns.[29,30] Healthcare providers should cool patients to a target temperature of 32°C to 34°C (89.6°F to 93.2°F).

Although the optimal method of achieving the target temperature is unknown, any combination of rapid infusion of chilled, isotonic, non–glucose-containing fluid (30 mL/kg),[31-33] endovascular catheters, feedback-controlled surface cooling devices,[34-36] or simple surface interventions (eg, ice bags, cooling blankets) appears to be safe and effective. Avoid active rewarming in comatose patients who spontaneously develop a mild degree of hypothermia (above 32°C [89.6°F]) after resuscitation from cardiac arrest during the first 48 hours after ROSC. If nonthermostatically controlled methods such as ice bags are employed, care should be taken to avoid hypothermia "overshoot" or a temperature below 32°C.

Healthcare providers should monitor the patient's core temperature during induced hypothermia with an esophageal thermometer, a temperature-sensing urinary catheter in nonanuric patients, or a central venous catheter if present.[18,28] Axillary, tympanic, and oral temperatures are inadequate for measurement of core temperature changes during the use of therapeutic hypothermia.[37,38]

Therapeutic hypothermia is feasible after cardiogenic shock with ROSC[23,39,40] and in combination with emergent PCI.[9,41-44] Fibrinolytic therapy has been used successfully for AMI after ROSC.[45,46]

A number of potential complications are associated with therapeutic hypothermia, including coagulopathy, arrhythmias, and hyperglycemia, particularly with an unintended drop below target temperature.[44] The likelihood of pneumonia and sepsis may increase in patients who have undergone therapeutic hypothermia.[18,28] Infections are common in this population, and prolonged hypothermia is known to decrease immune function. Because hypothermia impairs coagulation, ongoing bleeding should be controlled before a cooling protocol is initiated.

In summary, therapeutic hypothermia is the only intervention demonstrated to improve neurologic recovery after cardiac arrest. It is recommended that comatose adult patients with ROSC after out-of-hospital VF-associated cardiac arrest be cooled to 32°C to 34°C (89.6°F to 93.2°F) for 12 to 24 hours (Class I, LOE B). Therapeutic hypothermia also may be considered for comatose adult patients with ROSC after in-hospital cardiac arrest of any initial rhythm or after out-of-hospital cardiac arrest with an initial rhythm of pulseless electrical activity or asystole (Class IIb, LOE B). After resuscitation from cardiac arrest and during the first 48 hours after ROSC, active rewarming should be avoided in comatose patients who spontaneously develop a mild degree of hypothermia (more than 32°C [89.6°F]) (Class III, LOE C).

Sample Post-ROSC Care Protocol

- Patient is eligible for post-ROSC therapeutic hypothermia if
  - **a.** Patient has experienced cardiac arrest, defined as a period of absent pulses that requires chest compressions, regardless of location or presenting rhythm, followed by return of spontaneous circulation (ROSC)
  - **b.** Status before cardiac arrest is not DNAR (do not attempt resuscitation)
  - **c.** Prearrest cognitive status is not severely impaired
  - **d.** Signs of neurologic impairment with a Glasgow Coma Motor Score <6 before sedation (ie, does not follow commands: two thumbs up, squeeze and release); no other obvious reasons for coma
  - **e.** No uncontrolled bleeding
  - **f.** Goals of care do not include long-term support because of other disease processes or advanced directives
  - **g.** Less than 4 hours since ROSC; cool patients as soon as possible after arrest
- Personnel caring for patient (emergency department, floor, or catheterization laboratory) should initiate and continue to implement the therapeutic hypothermia protocol until an intensive care unit (ICU) bed is available and all equipment is ready for patient.
- Place arterial line while initiating cooling (may be very difficult to place once the patient is at target temperature).
- Measures should be taken to avoid shivering in the patient. Many places use paralytics (muscle relaxants) as cooling is initiated in addition to sedation. Maintain sedation and/or paralysis until after rewarming is complete (36°C).
- Cooling is best managed with a thermostatically controlled feedback loop device that cools and maintains target temperature automatically. Initial cooling can be done rapidly. (Goal is target temperature of 32°C to 34°C within 4 hours after ROSC.)
- Out-of-hospital cardiac arrest patients have a high incidence of acute coronary syndrome, and early coronary revascularization may improve survival.[47]
- Patient should be managed in the appropriate critical care setting.

1. *Early Goal-Directed Therapy*

Postresuscitation syndrome has many pathophysiologic features in common with acute sepsis.[48] Early goal-directed therapy has been demonstrated to decrease in-hospital mortality of patients with severe sepsis with an elevated lactate level or septic shock.[49] A similar approach to optimize oxygen delivery may have the same beneficial effects in postresuscitation syndrome.

2. *Glycemic Control*

Avoidance of hyperglycemia and hypoglycemia is a reasonable goal during postarrest resuscitation and therapeutic hypothermia. This should be accomplished with hyperglycemia management protocols commonly employed in critical care settings.[50,51]

3. *Management of Adrenal Insufficiency*

Acute adrenal insufficiency may occur as part of postresuscitation syndrome. In patients with fluid and vasopressor refractory septic shock, treatment with "stress dose" corticosteroids significantly reduces mortality.[52] Thus, in post–cardiac arrest patients with hemodynamic instability associated with vasodilation, diagnosis and treatment of acute adrenal insufficiency should be considered.

- Continuous electroencephalographic (EEG) monitoring should be considered because of an enhanced risk of seizures that may be undetected in a patient who has been given paralytics. The EEG is monitored for 24 hours after the patient has reached normothermia. The EEG should not be discontinued until the patient has been rewarmed and paralytics have been discontinued or until malignant patterns have been controlled.
- Rewarming is begun 24 hours after target temperature is reached. Warming should not proceed too quickly (1°C every 3 hours), and rebound pyrexia (fever) should be avoided. (Goal is **target temperature of 36°C to 37°C.**) Maintain sedation and paralysis until temperature reaches 36°C to avoid shivering and rapid rewarming.
- Pregnancy is not an absolute contraindication for post-ROSC therapeutic hypothermia. Two published case reports suggest that therapeutic hypothermia can be performed safely on a pregnant female.[14,53] If a β-HCG test is positive, consult with appropriate obstetric services if therapeutic hypothermia is instituted.
- The neurologic prognosis of the comatose cardiac arrest survivor cannot be predicted reliably until at least 72 hours after resuscitation.[54] In addition, the reliability of the routinely used neurologic prognostic parameters has not been evaluated as thoroughly in patients treated with therapeutic hypothermia; therefore, DNAR status should not be established and care should not be withdrawn ***on the basis of neurologic prognosis*** until at least 72 hours after rewarming.

—Contributed by Benjamin S. Abella, MD, MPhil, University of Pennsylvania

Hyperthermia

After ROSC, a temperature elevation above normal can impair brain recovery. The cause of fever after cardiac arrest may be related to activation of inflammatory cytokines in a pattern similar to that reported in sepsis.[55,56] There is an association between poor survival outcomes and pyrexia of 37.6°C or more.[57-67] Patients with elevated temperatures and a cerebrovascular event that leads to brain ischemia experience worsened short-term outcome and increased long-term mortality.[62-67] These patients can also develop hyperthermia after being rewarmed after hypothermia treatment. Providers should closely monitor patient core temperature after ROSC and actively intervene to avoid hyperthermia (Class I, LOE C).

Organ-Specific Evaluation and Support

Pulmonary System

Pulmonary complications after cardiac arrest are common. Causes include hydrostatic pulmonary edema, noncardiogenic edema, severe pulmonary atelectasis, or aspiration that occurs during cardiac arrest or resuscitation. Patients can develop regional mismatch of ventilation and perfusion, which contributes to decreased arterial oxygen content. The severity of pulmonary dysfunction is often measured in terms of the PaO_2/FIO_2 ratio (300 mm Hg or less usually defines acute lung injury). The acute onset of bilateral infiltrates on chest x-ray and a pulmonary artery pressure of 18 mm Hg or less or no evidence of left atrial hypertension are common to both acute lung injury and acute respiratory distress syndrome (ARDS). A PaO_2/FIO_2 ratio less than 300 or less than 200 mm Hg separates acute lung injury from ARDS, respectively.[68] Positive end-expiratory pressure (PEEP) and titrated FIO_2 are strategies that can be used to improve pulmonary function and PaO_2 while the practitioner is determining the pathophysiology of the pulmonary dysfunction.

Recommended diagnostic tests for intubated patients include chest radiographs and arterial blood gas measurements. Other diagnostic tests may be added at the discretion of the clinician based on history, physical examination, and clinical circumstances. Providers should adjust the level of mechanical ventilatory support on the basis of the measured oxyhemoglobin saturation, blood gas values (FIO_2, SpO_2, $PETCO_2$), minute ventilation (respiratory rate and tidal volume), and patient-ventilator synchrony.

The optimal FIO_2 during the immediate period after cardiac arrest is still unknown. The beneficial effect of high FIO_2 on systemic oxygen delivery should be weighed against the deleterious effect of the generation of oxygen-derived free radicals during the reperfusion phase. Ventilation with 100% oxygen (which generates PaO_2 more than 350 mm Hg at 15 to 60 minutes after ROSC) increases brain lipid peroxidation, metabolic dysfunction, and neurologic degeneration and worsens short-term functional outcome compared with ventilation with room air or an inspired oxygen fraction titrated to a pulse oximeter reading between 94% and 96%.[69-74]

Once the circulation is restored, systemic arterial oxyhemoglobin saturation should be monitored. Because an arterial oxyhemoglobin saturation of 100% may correspond to a PaO_2 anywhere between approximately 80 and 500 mm Hg, it is usually appropriate to wean FIO_2 to the lowest concentration that maintains SpO_2 at 94% or more.

Because patients may have significant metabolic acidosis after cardiac arrest, clinicians may be tempted to institute hyperventilation to normalize blood pH. However, metabolic acidosis is likely to be reversed once adequate perfusion is restored, and there are several physiologic reasons why hyperventilation may be detrimental. Minute ventilation alters the partial pressure of carbon dioxide ($PaCO_2$), which in turn can affect cerebral blood flow. After ROSC there is an initial hyperemic blood flow response (10 to 30 minutes), followed by a more prolonged period of low blood flow.[75,76] During this latter period of late hypoperfusion, a mismatch between blood flow (as a component of oxygen delivery) and oxygen requirement can occur. Hyperventilation can cause additional cerebral ischemia in the post–cardiac arrest patient because sustained hypocapnia (low PCO_2) may reduce cerebral blood flow.[77,78]

Hyperventilation can compromise systemic blood flow because of occult or auto-PEEP and is deleterious in all low-flow states, including CPR[79,80] and hypovolemia.[81,82] Auto-PEEP occurs more often in patients with obstructive lung disease and is aggravated by hyperventilation, which may not allow sufficient time for complete exhalation. Hyperventilation should be avoided, especially in hypotensive patients.

Other ventilatory parameters may affect the outcome of patients on mechanical ventilation after cardiac arrest, particularly when acute lung injury or ARDS develops. Over the last decade attention has focused on low-volume/high-rate ventilation. Patient ventilation can be targeted to maintain tidal volume (V_T) of 6 to 8 mL/kg predicted body weight and inspiratory plateau pressure of 30 cm H_2O or less to reduce ventilator-associated lung injury.[83,84] Because low V_T ventilation (6 mL/kg) is associated with an increased incidence of atelectasis, PEEP and other lung "recruitment maneuver" procedures may be warranted.[85]

Post–cardiac arrest patients are at risk of acute lung injury and ARDS; however, refractory hypoxemia is not a frequent mode of death after cardiac arrest. There is no reason to recommend hyperventilation or "permissive hypercapnia" (hypoventilation) for these patients, and normocapnia should be considered the standard.

Routine hyperventilation with hypocapnia should be avoided after ROSC because it may worsen global brain ischemia by causing excessive cerebral vasoconstriction (Class III, LOE C). Hyperventilation or excessive tidal volumes that result in increased intrathoracic pressure may also contribute to hemodynamic instability in some patients. Ventilation rate and volume may be titrated to maintain high-normal $Paco_2$ (40 to 45 mm Hg) or $PETCO_2$ (35 to 40 mm Hg) while avoiding hemodynamic compromise (Class IIb, LOE C).

Treatment of Pulmonary Embolism After CPR

The use of fibrinolytics may benefit patients with massive pulmonary emboli who have not had CPR.[86] Fibrinolytics have also been used to treat pulmonary embolism after CPR.[87] CPR itself does not appear to pose an unacceptable risk of bleeding when fibrinolytics are used during CPR.[88-96] Alternatively, surgical embolectomy has also been used successfully in some patients after pulmonary embolism–induced cardiac arrest.[95,97-100] In post–cardiac arrest patients with arrest caused by pulmonary embolism, fibrinolytics may be considered (Class IIb, LOE C).

Sedation After Cardiac Arrest

Patients intubated and maintained on mechanical ventilation for a period of time can experience discomfort, pain, and anxiety. Intermittent or continuous sedation and/or analgesia can be beneficial. Opioids, anxiolytics, and sedative-hypnotic agents can be used to improve patient-ventilator interaction and blunt the stress-related surge of endogenous catecholamines. Other agents with sedative and antipsychotic-tranquilizer properties, such as α_2-adrenergic agonists[101] and butyrophenones,[102] can also be used based on individual clinical circumstances.

If patient agitation is life-threatening, neuromuscular blocking agents can be used for short intervals with adequate sedation. Post-ROSC patients have a high risk of seizures, and neuromuscular blocking agents should be used with caution unless continuous EEG monitoring is available. The duration of use of neuromuscular blocking agents should be kept to a minimum.

Consider the titrated use of sedation and analgesia in critically ill patients who require mechanical ventilation or shivering suppression during induced hypothermia after cardiac arrest (Class IIb, LOE C). Sedation scales[103-108] and motor activity scales[109] have been developed to titrate these pharmacological interventions to a clinical goal.

Cardiovascular System

ACS is a common cause of cardiac arrest.[13,15,43,44,109-122] Obtain a 12-lead ECG as soon as possible after ROSC to determine whether acute ST elevation is present (Class I, LOE B). Because it is impossible to determine the final neurologic status of comatose patients after ROSC, treatment of STEMI should begin as with non–cardiac arrest patients, regardless of coma or induced hypothermia. Because of the high incidence of coronary ischemia, consideration of acute coronary angiography may be reasonable even in the absence of STEMI.[13,15] Notably, PCI, alone or as part of a bundle of care, is associated with improved myocardial function[13] and neurologic outcomes.[9,15] Therapeutic hypothermia can be safely combined with primary PCI after cardiac arrest caused by AMI.[9,39,42-44]

Antiarrhythmic drugs such as amiodarone can be administered to patients with cardiac arrest during initial resuscitation. There is no evidence to support continued or prophylactic administration of these medications after ROSC.[7,123-127]

Vasoactive Drugs for Post–Cardiac Arrest Patients

Vasopressors

Vasoactive drugs may be administered after ROSC to support cardiac output and provide blood flow to the heart and brain. Drugs may be selected to improve heart rate, myocardial contractility, or arterial pressure or to reduce afterload.

Some commonly used initial dose ranges are listed in Table 45. Vasoactive drugs must be titrated to secure the desired response while limiting side effects. In general, adrenergic drugs should not be mixed with sodium bicarbonate or other alkaline solutions in the IV line because they may become inactivated.[128,129] Administration through a central line is preferred whenever possible for norepinephrine (levarterenol) and other catecholamines that activate α-adrenergic receptors because these agents may cause necrosis if extravasation occurs.

Table 45. Medications Commonly Used for Post-ROSC Cardiovascular Support

Drug	Typical Starting Dose (then titrate to response)
Epinephrine	0.1-0.5 mcg/kg per minute • Acts at alpha and beta receptors to provide vasoconstriction and increased cardiac output • Used to treat severe hypotension (eg, systolic blood pressure <70 mm Hg) • Useful for anaphylaxis associated with hemodynamic instability or respiratory distress
Norepinephrine	0.1-0.5 mcg/kg per minute • Has a potent alpha effect that causes vasoconstriction with a lesser beta effect so that cardiac output tends to be maintained • Used to treat severe hypotension (eg, systolic blood pressure <70 mm Hg) and a low total peripheral resistance • Usually induces renal and mesenteric vasoconstriction; in sepsis, however, norepinephrine improves renal blood flow and urine output[130,131]
Dopamine	5-10 mcg/kg per minute • Acts at alpha, beta, and dopaminergic receptors • Increases heart rate and contractility • Vasoconstrictor
Phenylephrine	0.5-2.0 mcg/kg per minute • Acts at alpha receptors only, less potent than norepinephrine • Vasoconstrictor • Used to treat mild hypotension
Dobutamine	5-10 mcg/kg per minute • Acts at beta receptors only • Increases cardiac contractility and heart rate • Mild vasodilator
Milrinone	Load 50 mcg/kg over 10 minutes, and then infuse at 0.375 mcg/kg per minute • Phosphodiesterase inhibitor • Increases cardiac contractility • Vasodilator
Vasopressin	0.01-0.04 units/min • Acts at V_1 receptors • Potent vasoconstrictor • Relatively long half-life (about 20 minutes); do not titrate quickly • Useful in sepsis

Use of Vasoactive Drugs After Cardiac Arrest

Hemodynamic instability often occurs after cardiac arrest.[3] The ischemia/reperfusion of cardiac arrest and electrical defibrillation both can cause transient myocardial stunning and dysfunction[132] that can last many hours but may improve with the use of vasoactive drugs.[133] Early echocardiographic evaluation within the first 24 hours after arrest is a useful way to assess myocardial function in order to guide ongoing management.[12,13] Fluid administration and vasoactive (eg, norepinephrine), inotropic (eg, dobutamine), and inodilator (eg, milrinone) agents should be titrated as needed to optimize blood pressure, cardiac output, and systemic perfusion (Class I, LOE B). Although ideal targets for blood pressure or blood oxygenation have not been established in human studies,[8,9] a mean arterial pressure of 65 mm Hg or more and an $ScvO_2$ of 70% or more are generally considered reasonable goals.

Modifying Outcomes From Critical Illness

Cardiac arrest is thought to involve multiorgan ischemic injury and microcirculatory dysfunction.[55,56,134] Implementation of a protocol for goal-directed therapy with fluid and vasoactive drug administration along with monitoring of central venous oxygen saturation may improve survival from sepsis.[135] A similar approach may benefit post–cardiac arrest patients.

Glucose Control

Higher than normal blood glucose levels have been associated with increased mortality or worse neurologic outcomes.[7,60,136-138] Intensive therapy leads to more frequent episodes of severe hypoglycemia (usually defined as a blood glucose level of 40 mg/dL [2.2 mmol/L] or less).[139-147] Hypoglycemia may be associated with worse outcomes in critically ill patients.[148,149]

Strategies to target moderate glycemic control (144 to 180 mg/dL [8 to 10 mmol/L]) may be considered in adult patients with ROSC after cardiac arrest (Class IIb, LOE B). Attempts to control the glucose concentration within a lower range (80 to 110 mg/dL [4.4 to 6.1 mmol/L]) should not be implemented after cardiac arrest because of the increased risk of hypoglycemia (Class III, LOE B).

Steroids

Corticosteroids have an important role in the physiological response to severe stress, including maintenance of vascular tone and capillary permeability. The post–cardiac arrest syndrome has similarities to septic shock,[150,151] but the efficacy of corticosteroids remains controversial in patients with sepsis.[56,152-154] It is unknown whether the provision of corticosteroids in the post–cardiac arrest phase improves outcomes. Therefore, the routine use of corticosteroids for patients with ROSC and without adrenal insufficiency after cardiac arrest is uncertain.

Hemofiltration

Hemofiltration has been proposed as a method to modify the humoral response to the ischemic-reperfusion injury that occurs after cardiac arrest. In a single randomized controlled trial, there was no difference in 6-month survival among the groups (LOE 1).[155] Another study suggested improved survival and neurologic outcome in patients treated with high-volume hemofiltration after resuscitation from cardiac arrest (LOE 2).[156] Future investigations are required to determine whether hemofiltration will improve outcome for post–cardiac arrest patients.

Central Nervous System

Brain injury is a common cause of morbidity and mortality in post–cardiac arrest patients.[11] Clinical manifestations of post–cardiac arrest brain injury include coma, seizures, myoclonus, various degrees of neurocognitive dysfunction, and brain death.[6]

Seizure Management

Seizures are common after ROSC, occurring in 5% to 20% of comatose cardiac arrest survivors with or without therapeutic hypothermia.[9,157,158] The true incidence of post–cardiac arrest electrographic seizures may be higher, because the clinical diagnosis of seizures may not be readily apparent. Several studies have suggested that post–cardiac arrest seizures may be refractory to traditional anticonvulsant agents.[159-161] An EEG for the diagnosis of seizure should be performed with prompt interpretation as soon as possible and should be monitored frequently or continuously in comatose patients after ROSC (Class I, LOE C). The same anticonvulsant regimens for the treatment of seizures used for status epilepticus from other causes may be considered after cardiac arrest (Class IIb, LOE C).

Prognostication of Neurologic Outcome in Comatose Cardiac Arrest Survivors

The primary goal of post–cardiac arrest management is to return patients to their prearrest functional level. Poor outcome is generally defined as death, persistent unresponsiveness, or the inability to undertake independent activities after 6 months.[162] No prearrest or intra-arrest parameters (including arrest duration, bystander CPR, or presenting rhythm) alone or in combination can accurately predict outcome in individual patients who achieve ROSC.

A thorough neurologic evaluation is needed to obtain an accurate prognostic assessment. After 24 hours, somatosensory evoked potentials and select physical examination findings at specific time points after ROSC in the absence of confounders (such as hypotension, sedatives, seizures, or neuromuscular blockers) are the most reliable predictors of poor outcome for patients not undergoing therapeutic hypothermia. However, the decision to limit care should never be made on the basis of a single prognostic parameter, and expert consultation may be needed.

Neurologic Assessment

The neurologic examination is the most widely studied parameter to predict outcome in comatose post–cardiac arrest patients. Currently, no clinical neurologic signs reliably predict poor outcome less than 24 hours after cardiac arrest.[163,164] The absence of both pupillary light and corneal reflexes at 72 hours or more after cardiac arrest predicted poor outcome with high reliability for adult patients who were comatose and had not been treated with hypothermia.[163] The absence of vestibulo-ocular reflexes at 24 hours or more[164,165] or a Glasgow Coma Scale score less than 5 at 72 hours or more[163,166,167] is less reliable for prediction of poor outcome or was studied only in limited numbers of patients. Other clinical signs, including myoclonus,[168-172] are not recommended for prediction of poor outcome (Class III, LOE C). Current recommendations from the American Academy of Neurology stress that neuroprognostication based on clinical examination should be avoided in the first 72 hours following resuscitation because clinical findings (eg, papillary or gag reflexes) are poorly predictive of recovery.

EEG

In normothermic patients without significant confounders, an EEG pattern that shows generalized suppression to less than 20 μV, a burst-suppression pattern associated with generalized epileptic activity, or diffuse periodic complexes on a flat background is associated with a poor outcome.[162] One week after the initial arrest event, specific EEG findings may be useful for prediction of poor outcomes in comatose cardiac arrest survivors.[162,163,165,173-181] The metabolism of sedatives may be prolonged in patients with therapeutic hypothermia. Therefore, care should be taken to allow additional time for the effect of these drugs to subside before neurologic function is assessed for the purposes of prognostication. In the absence of confounding factors such as sedatives, hypotension, neuromuscular blockade, seizures, or hypoxemia, it may be helpful to use an unprocessed EEG interpretation observed 24 hours or more after ROSC to assist with the prediction of a poor outcome in comatose survivors of cardiac arrest not treated with hypothermia (Class IIb, LOE B).

Evoked Potentials

Abnormalities in cortical evoked potentials measured more than 24 hours after ROSC are associated with poor outcomes in comatose cardiac arrest survivors. Specifically, bilateral absence of an N20 cortical response after median nerve stimulation is very predictive of poor outcome in patients not treated with hypothermia.[163] Fewer data are available for patients treated with hypothermia.

Neuroimaging

Extensive cortical and subcortical lesions on magnetic resonance imaging are associated with poor neurologic outcome.[182-212] These studies varied widely in the magnetic resonance imaging parameters used, sample size, and interval after arrest when testing occurred.

The use of computed tomography imaging for detection of brain injury and prediction of functional outcome has been reported in several studies.[202,204,210-226] Computed tomography parameters associated with poor outcome were varied and included quantitative measure of gray matter:white matter ratio (in Hounsfield units) and qualitative description of brain structures. Other less common neuroimaging modalities include single-photon emission computed tomography,[209,225,227] cerebral angiography,[211] and transcranial Doppler.[198]

Despite its tremendous potential, neuroimaging has yet to be proved as an independently accurate modality for prediction of outcome in individual comatose survivors of cardiac arrest, and specific neuroimaging modalities cannot be recommended at this time for prediction of poor outcome after cardiac arrest.

Blood and Cerebrospinal Fluid Biomarkers

Biomarkers in the blood (plasma or serum) and cerebrospinal fluid have been studied for their utility as early predictors of poor outcome in comatose cardiac arrest survivors. These compounds are typically released from dying neurons or glial cells in the brain (eg, neuron-specific enolase [NSE], S100B, glial fibrillary acidic protein, the BB isoenzyme of creatine kinase) and can be measured in the blood or cerebrospinal fluid. The primary advantage of biomarkers is that levels are unlikely to be confounded by sedation or neuromuscular blockade, both of which are commonly used in the first few days after cardiac arrest.

The most promising and extensively studied biomarker is serum NSE, which had a 0% false-positive rate (95% confidence interval, 0% to 3%) for prediction of poor outcome in one study when measured between 24 and 72 hours after cardiac arrest.[162,163] However, the primary limitation of serum NSE is the variability among studies in both the assays used and the cutoff value that resulted in a false-positive rate of 0% for prediction of poor outcome.[228-239] Therefore, the routine use of any serum or cerebrospinal

Critical Concept **Duration of Observation After ROSC**	Durations of observation greater than 72 hours after ROSC should be considered before predicting poor outcome in patients treated with hypothermia (Class I, Level C).

fluid biomarker as a sole predictor of poor outcome in comatose patients after cardiac arrest is not recommended (Class III, LOE B).

Changes in Prognostication With Hypothermia

There is a paucity of data regarding the utility of physical examination, EEG, and evoked potentials for patients who have undergone induced hypothermia. Durations of observation greater than 72 hours after ROSC should be considered before poor outcome is predicted in patients treated with hypothermia (Class I, Level C).

Organ Donation After Cardiac Arrest

There is no difference in functional outcomes of organs transplanted from patients who are brain-dead as a consequence of cardiac arrest compared with donors who are brain-dead of other causes.[240-243] Therefore, adult patients who progress to brain death after resuscitation from cardiac arrest should be considered for organ donation (Class I, LOE B).

Summary

The goals of immediate post–cardiac arrest care are to optimize systemic perfusion, restore metabolic homeostasis, and support organ system function to increase the likelihood of intact neurologic survival. Support and treatment of acute myocardial dysfunction and acute myocardial ischemia can increase the probability of survival. Interventions to reduce post–cardiac arrest brain injury, such as therapeutic hypothermia, can improve survival and neurologic recovery. The treatment of diverse problems after cardiac arrest involves multidisciplinary aspects of emergency medicine, critical care, cardiology, and neurology with a comprehensive plan of care. It is more challenging to determine the prognosis of patients after cardiac arrest than before because of the success of new therapies; therefore, expert evaluation of neurologic status is required.

References

1. Callaway CW, Schmicker R, Kampmeyer M, Powell J, Rea TD, Daya MR, Aufderheide TP, Davis DP, Rittenberger JC, Idris AH, Nichol G. Receiving hospital characteristics associated with survival after out-of-hospital cardiac arrest. *Resuscitation*. 2010;81:524-529.
2. Carr BG, Kahn JM, Merchant RM, Kramer AA, Neumar RW. Inter-hospital variability in post–cardiac arrest mortality. *Resuscitation*. 2009;80:30-34.
3. Laurent I, Monchi M, Chiche JD, Joly LM, Spaulding C, Bourgeois B, Cariou A, Rozenberg A, Carli P, Weber S, Dhainaut JF. Reversible myocardial dysfunction in survivors of out-of-hospital cardiac arrest. *J Am Coll Cardiol*. 2002;40:2110-2116.
4. Negovsky VA. The second step in resuscitation—the treatment of the 'post-resuscitation disease.' *Resuscitation*. 1972;1:1-7.
5. Safar P. Resuscitation from clinical death: pathophysiologic limits and therapeutic potentials. *Crit Care Med*. 1988;16:923-941.
6. Neumar RW, Nolan JP, Adrie C, Aibiki M, Berg RA, Bottiger BW, Callaway C, Clark RS, Geocadin RG, Jauch EC, Kern KB, Laurent I, Longstreth WT Jr, Merchant RM, Morley P, Morrison LJ, Nadkarni V, Peberdy MA, Rivers EP, Rodriguez-Nunez A, Sellke FW, Spaulding C, Sunde K, Vanden Hoek T. Post–cardiac arrest syndrome: epidemiology, pathophysiology, treatment, and prognostication. A consensus statement from the International Liaison Committee on Resuscitation (American Heart Association, Australian and New Zealand Council on Resuscitation, European Resuscitation Council, Heart and Stroke Foundation of Canada, InterAmerican Heart Foundation, Resuscitation Council of Asia, and the Resuscitation Council of Southern Africa); the American Heart Association Emergency Cardiovascular Care Committee; the Council on Cardiovascular Surgery and Anesthesia; the Council on Cardiopulmonary, Perioperative, and Critical Care; the Council on Clinical Cardiology; and the Stroke Council. *Circulation*. 2008;118:2452-2483.
7. Skrifvars MB, Pettila V, Rosenberg PH, Castren M. A multiple logistic regression analysis of in-hospital factors related to survival at six months in patients resuscitated from out-of-hospital ventricular fibrillation. *Resuscitation*. 2003;59:319-328.
8. Gaieski DF, Band RA, Abella BS, Neumar RW, Fuchs BD, Kolansky DM, Merchant RM, Carr BG, Becker LB, Maguire C, Klair A, Hylton J, Goyal M. Early goal-directed hemodynamic optimization combined with therapeutic hypothermia in comatose survivors of out-of-hospital cardiac arrest. *Resuscitation*. 2009;80:418-424.
9. Sunde K, Pytte M, Jacobsen D, Mangschau A, Jensen LP, Smedsrud C, Draegni T, Steen PA. Implementation of a standardised treatment protocol for post resuscitation care after out-of-hospital cardiac arrest. *Resuscitation*. 2007;73:29-39.
10. Kirves H, Skrifvars MB, Vahakuopus M, Ekstrom K, Martikainen M, Castren M. Adherence to resuscitation guidelines during prehospital care of cardiac arrest patients. *Eur J Emerg Med*. 2007;14:75-81.
11. Laver S, Farrow C, Turner D, Nolan J. Mode of death after admission to an intensive care unit following cardiac arrest. *Intensive Care Med*. 2004;30:2126-2128.
12. Anyfantakis ZA, Baron G, Aubry P, Himbert D, Feldman LJ, Juliard JM, Ricard-Hibon A, Burnod A, Cokkinos DV, Steg PG. Acute coronary angiographic findings in survivors of out-of-hospital cardiac arrest. *Am Heart J*. 2009;157:312-318.
13. Spaulding CM, Joly LM, Rosenberg A, Monchi M, Weber SN, Dhainaut JF, Carli P. Immediate coronary angiography in survivors of out-of-hospital cardiac arrest. *N Engl J Med*. 1997;336:1629-1633.
14. Dumas F, Cariou A, Manzo-Silberman S, Grimaldi D, Vivien B, Rosencher J, Empana JP, Carli P, Mira JP, Jouven X, Spaulding C. Immediate percutaneous coronary intervention is associated with better survival after out-of-hospital cardiac arrest: insights from the PROCAT (Parisian Region Out of hospital Cardiac ArresT) registry. *Circ Cardiovasc Interv*. 2010;3:200-207.
15. Reynolds JC, Callaway CW, El Khoudary SR, Moore CG, Alvarez RJ, Rittenberger JC. Coronary angiography predicts

improved outcome following cardiac arrest: propensity-adjusted analysis. *J Intensive Care Med*. 2009;24:179-186.

16. Booth CM, Boone RH, Tomlinson G, Detsky AS. Is this patient dead, vegetative, or severely neurologically impaired? Assessing outcome for comatose survivors of cardiac arrest. *JAMA*. 2004;291:870-879.
17. Bunch TJ, White RD, Gersh BJ, Meverden RA, Hodge DO, Ballman KV, Hammill SC, Shen WK, Packer DL. Long-term outcomes of out-of-hospital cardiac arrest after successful early defibrillation. *N Engl J Med*. 2003;348:2626-2633.
18. Hypothermia After Cardiac Arrest Study Group. Mild therapeutic hypothermia to improve the neurologic outcome after cardiac arrest. *N Engl J Med*. 2002;346:549-556.
19. Belliard G, Catez E, Charron C, Caille V, Aegerter P, Dubourg O, Jardin F, Vieillard-Baron A. Efficacy of therapeutic hypothermia after out-of-hospital cardiac arrest due to ventricular fibrillation. *Resuscitation*. 2007;75:252-259.
20. Castrejon S, Cortes M, Salto ML, Benittez LC, Rubio R, Juarez M, Lopez de Sa E, Bueno H, Sanchez PL, Fernandez Aviles F. Improved prognosis after using mild hypothermia to treat cardiorespiratory arrest due to a cardiac cause: comparison with a control group. *Rev Esp Cardiol*. 2009;62:733-741.
21. Don CW, Longstreth WT Jr, Maynard C, Olsufka M, Nichol G, Ray T, Kupchik N, Deem S, Copass MK, Cobb LA, Kim F. Active surface cooling protocol to induce mild therapeutic hypothermia after out-of-hospital cardiac arrest: a retrospective before-and-after comparison in a single hospital. *Crit Care Med*. 2009;37:3062-3069.
22. Bernard SA, Jones BM, Horne MK. Clinical trial of induced hypothermia in comatose survivors of out-of-hospital cardiac arrest. *Ann Emerg Med*. 1997;30:146-153.
23. Oddo M, Schaller MD, Feihl F, Ribordy V, Liaudet L. From evidence to clinical practice: effective implementation of therapeutic hypothermia to improve patient outcome after cardiac arrest. *Crit Care Med*. 2006;34:1865-1873.
24. Busch M, Soreide E, Lossius HM, Lexow K, Dickstein K. Rapid implementation of therapeutic hypothermia in comatose out-of-hospital cardiac arrest survivors. *Acta Anaesthesiol Scand*. 2006;50:1277-1283.
25. Storm C, Steffen I, Schefold JC, Krueger A, Oppert M, Jorres A, Hasper D. Mild therapeutic hypothermia shortens intensive care unit stay of survivors after out-of-hospital cardiac arrest compared to historical controls. *Crit Care*. 2008;12:R78.
26. Arrich J. Clinical application of mild therapeutic hypothermia after cardiac arrest. *Crit Care Med*. 2007;35:1041-1047.
27. Holzer M, Mullner M, Sterz F, Robak O, Kliegel A, Losert H, Sodeck G, Uray T, Zeiner A, Laggner AN. Efficacy and safety of endovascular cooling after cardiac arrest: cohort study and Bayesian approach. *Stroke*. 2006;37:1792-1797.
28. Bernard SA, Gray TW, Buist MD, Jones BM, Silvester W, Gutteridge G, Smith K. Treatment of comatose survivors of out-of-hospital cardiac arrest with induced hypothermia. *N Engl J Med*. 2002;346:557-563.
29. Gluckman PD, Wyatt JS, Azzopardi D, Ballard R, Edwards AD, Ferriero DM, Polin RA, Robertson CM, Thoresen M, Whitelaw A, Gunn AJ. Selective head cooling with mild systemic hypothermia after neonatal encephalopathy: multicentre randomised trial. *Lancet*. 2005;365:663-670.
30. Shankaran S, Laptook AR, Ehrenkranz RA, Tyson JE, McDonald SA, Donovan EF, Fanaroff AA, Poole WK, Wright LL, Higgins RD, Finer NN, Carlo WA, Duara S, Oh W, Cotten CM, Stevenson DK, Stoll BJ, Lemons JA, Guillet R, Jobe AH. Whole-body hypothermia for neonates with hypoxic-ischemic encephalopathy. *N Engl J Med*. 2005;353:1574-1584.
31. Kliegel A, Losert H, Sterz F, Kliegel M, Holzer M, Uray T, Domanovits H. Cold simple intravenous infusions preceding special endovascular cooling for faster induction of mild hypothermia after cardiac arrest—a feasibility study. *Resuscitation*. 2005;64:347-351.
32. Kliegel A, Janata A, Wandaller C, Uray T, Spiel A, Losert H, Kliegel M, Holzer M, Haugk M, Sterz F, Laggner AN. Cold infusions alone are effective for induction of therapeutic hypothermia but do not keep patients cool after cardiac arrest. *Resuscitation*. 2007;73:46-53.
33. Kim F, Olsufka M, Carlbom D, Deem S, Longstreth WT Jr, Hanrahan M, Maynard C, Copass MK, Cobb LA. Pilot study of rapid infusion of 2 L of 4 degrees C normal saline for induction of mild hypothermia in hospitalized, comatose survivors of out-of-hospital cardiac arrest. *Circulation*. 2005;112:715-719.
34. Heard KJ, Peberdy MA, Sayre MR, Sanders A, Geocadin RG, Dixon SR, Larabee TM, Hiller K, Fiorello A, Paradis NA, O'Neil BJ. A randomized controlled trial comparing the Arctic Sun to standard cooling for induction of hypothermia after cardiac arrest. *Resuscitation*. 2010;81:9-14.
35. Pichon N, Amiel JB, Francois B, Dugard A, Etchecopar C, Vignon P. Efficacy of and tolerance to mild induced hypothermia after out-of-hospital cardiac arrest using an endovascular cooling system. *Crit Care*. 2007;11:R71.
36. Flint AC, Hemphill JC, Bonovich DC. Therapeutic hypothermia after cardiac arrest: performance characteristics and safety of surface cooling with or without endovascular cooling. *Neurocrit Care*. 2007;7:109-118.
37. Imamura M, Matsukawa T, Ozaki M, Sessler DI, Nishiyama T, Kumazawa T. The accuracy and precision of four infrared aural canal thermometers during cardiac surgery. *Acta Anaesthesiol Scand*. 1998;42:1222-1226.
38. Pujol A, Fusciardi J, Ingrand P, Baudouin D, Le Guen AF, Menu P. Afterdrop after hypothermic cardiopulmonary bypass: the value of tympanic membrane temperature monitoring. *J Cardiothorac Vasc Anesth*. 1996;10:336-341.
39. Hovdenes J, Laake JH, Aaberge L, Haugaa H, Bugge JF. Therapeutic hypothermia after out-of-hospital cardiac arrest: experiences with patients treated with percutaneous coronary intervention and cardiogenic shock. *Acta Anaesthesiol Scand*. 2007;51:137-142.
40. Skulec R, Kovarnik T, Dostalova G, Kolar J, Linhart A. Induction of mild hypothermia in cardiac arrest survivors presenting with cardiogenic shock syndrome. *Acta Anaesthesiol Scand*. 2008;52:188-194.
41. Batista LM, Lima FO, Januzzi JL Jr, Donahue V, Snydeman C, Greer DM. Feasibility and safety of combined percutaneous coronary intervention and therapeutic hypothermia following cardiac arrest. *Resuscitation*. 2010;81:398-403.
42. Wolfrum S, Pierau C, Radke PW, Schunkert H, Kurowski V. Mild therapeutic hypothermia in patients after out-of-hospital cardiac arrest due to acute ST-segment elevation myocardial infarction undergoing immediate percutaneous coronary intervention. *Crit Care Med*. 2008;36:1780-1786.
43. Knafelj R, Radsel P, Ploj T, Noc M. Primary percutaneous coronary intervention and mild induced hypothermia in comatose survivors of ventricular fibrillation with ST-elevation acute myocardial infarction. *Resuscitation*. 2007;74:227-234.
44. Nielsen N, Hovdenes J, Nilsson F, Rubertsson S, Stammet P, Sunde K, Valsson F, Wanscher M, Friberg H. Outcome, timing and adverse events in therapeutic hypothermia after

out-of-hospital cardiac arrest. *Acta Anaesthesiol Scand*. 2009;53:926-934.

45. Voipio V, Kuisma M, Alaspaa A, Manttari M, Rosenberg P. Thrombolytic treatment of acute myocardial infarction after out-of-hospital cardiac arrest. *Resuscitation*. 2001;49:251-258.

46. Weston CF, Avery P. Thrombolysis following pre-hospital cardiopulmonary resuscitation. *Int J Cardiol*. 1992;37:195-198.

47. Spaulding CM, Joly LM, Rosenberg A, Monchi M, Weber SN, Dhainaut JF, Carli P. Immediate coronary angiography in survivors of out-of-hospital cardiac arrest. *New England Journal of Medicine*. 1997;336:1629-1633.

48. Adrie C, Laurent I, Monchi M, Cariou A, Dhainaou J-F, Spaulding C. Postresuscitation disease after cardiac arrest: a sepsis-like syndrome? *Current Opinion in Critical Care*. 2004;10:208-212.

49. Rivers E, Nguyen B, Havstad S, Ressler J, Muzzin A, Knoblich B, Peterson E, Tomlanovich M, Early Goal-Directed Therapy Collaborative Group. Early goal-directed therapy in the treatment of severe sepsis and septic shock. *New England Journal of Medicine*. 2001;345:1368-1377.

50. van den Berghe G, Wouters P, Weekers F, Verwaest C, Bruyninckx F, Schetz M, Vlasselaers D, Ferdinande P, Lauwers P, Bouillon R. Intensive insulin therapy in the critically ill patients. *New England Journal of Medicine*. 2001;345:1359-1367.

51. Van den Berghe G, Wouters PJ, Bouillon R, Weekers F, Verwaest C, Schetz M, Vlasselaers D, Ferdinande P, Lauwers P. Outcome benefit of intensive insulin therapy in the critically ill: Insulin dose versus glycemic control. *Critical Care Medicine*. 2003;31:359-366.

52. Annane D, Sebille V, Charpentier C, Bollaert PE, Francois B, Korach JM, Capellier G, Cohen Y, Azoulay E, Troche G, Chaumet-Riffaut P, Bellissant E. Effect of treatment with low doses of hydrocortisone and fludrocortisone on mortality in patients with septic shock. *JAMA*. 2002;288:862-871.

53. Sogut O, Kamaz A, Erdogan MO, Sezen Y. Successful cardiopulmonary resuscitation in pregnancy: a case report. *J Clin Med Res*. 2010;2:50-52.

54. Zandbergen EG, de Haan RJ, Stoutenbeek CP, Koelman JH, Hijdra A. Systematic review of early prediction of poor outcome in anoxic-ischaemic coma. *Lancet*. 1998;352:1808-1812.

55. Adrie C, Laurent I, Monchi M, Cariou A, Dhainaou JF, Spaulding C. Postresuscitation disease after cardiac arrest: a sepsis-like syndrome? *Curr Opin Crit Care*. 2004;10:208-212.

56. Adrie C, Adib-Conquy M, Laurent I, Monchi M, Vinsonneau C, Fitting C, Fraisse F, Dinh-Xuan AT, Carli P, Spaulding C, Dhainaut JF, Cavaillon JM. Successful cardiopulmonary resuscitation after cardiac arrest as a "sepsis-like" syndrome. *Circulation*. 2002;106:562-568.

57. Takino M, Okada Y. Hyperthermia following cardiopulmonary resuscitation. *Intensive Care Med*. 1991;17:419-420.

58. Zeiner A, Holzer M, Sterz F, Schorkhuber W, Eisenburger P, Havel C, Kliegel A, Laggner AN. Hyperthermia after cardiac arrest is associated with an unfavorable neurologic outcome. *Arch Intern Med*. 2001;161:2007-2012.

59. Hickey RW, Kochanek PM, Ferimer H, Graham SH, Safar P. Hypothermia and hyperthermia in children after resuscitation from cardiac arrest. *Pediatrics*. 2000;106:118-122.

60. Langhelle A, Tyvold SS, Lexow K, Hapnes SA, Sunde K, Steen PA. In-hospital factors associated with improved outcome after out-of-hospital cardiac arrest. A comparison between four regions in Norway. *Resuscitation*. 2003;56:247-263.

61. Takasu A, Saitoh D, Kaneko N, Sakamoto T, Okada Y. Hyperthermia: is it an ominous sign after cardiac arrest? *Resuscitation*. 2001;49:273-277.

62. Wang Y, Lim LL, Levi C, Heller RF, Fisher J. Influence of admission body temperature on stroke mortality. *Stroke*. 2000;31:404-409.

63. Diringer MN. Treatment of fever in the neurologic intensive care unit with a catheter-based heat exchange system. *Crit Care Med*. 2004;32:559-564.

64. Diringer MN, Reaven NL, Funk SE, Uman GC. Elevated body temperature independently contributes to increased length of stay in neurologic intensive care unit patients. *Crit Care Med*. 2004;32:1489-1495.

65. Reith J, Jorgensen HS, Pedersen PM, Nakayama H, Raaschou HO, Jeppesen LL, Olsen TS. Body temperature in acute stroke: relation to stroke severity, infarct size, mortality, and outcome. *Lancet*. 1996;347:422-425.

66. Hanchaiphiboolkul S. Body temperature and mortality in acute cerebral infarction. *J Med Assoc Thai*. 2005;88:26-31.

67. Kammersgaard LP, Jorgensen HS, Rungby JA, Reith J, Nakayama H, Weber UJ, Houth J, Olsen TS. Admission body temperature predicts long-term mortality after acute stroke: the Copenhagen Stroke Study. *Stroke*. 2002;33:1759-1762.

68. Bernard GR, Artigas A, Brigham KL, Carlet J, Falke K, Hudson L, Lamy M, Legall JR, Morris A, Spragg R. The American-European Consensus Conference on ARDS. Definitions, mechanisms, relevant outcomes, and clinical trial coordination. *Am J Respir Crit Care Med*. 1994;149:818-824.

69. Liu Y, Rosenthal RE, Haywood Y, Miljkovic-Lolic M, Vanderhoek JY, Fiskum G. Normoxic ventilation after cardiac arrest reduces oxidation of brain lipids and improves neurological outcome. *Stroke*. 1998;29:1679-1686.

70. Marsala J, Marsala M, Vanicky I, Galik J, Orendacova J. Post cardiac arrest hyperoxic resuscitation enhances neuronal vulnerability of the respiratory rhythm generator and some brainstem and spinal cord neuronal pools in the dog. *Neurosci Lett*. 1992;146:121-124.

71. Zwemer CF, Whitesall SE, D'Alecy LG. Cardiopulmonary-cerebral resuscitation with 100% oxygen exacerbates neurological dysfunction following nine minutes of normothermic cardiac arrest in dogs. *Resuscitation*. 1994;27:159-170.

72. Vereczki V, Martin E, Rosenthal RE, Hof PR, Hoffman GE, Fiskum G. Normoxic resuscitation after cardiac arrest protects against hippocampal oxidative stress, metabolic dysfunction, and neuronal death. *J Cereb Blood Flow Metab*. 2006;26:821-835.

73. Richards EM, Fiskum G, Rosenthal RE, Hopkins I, McKenna MC. Hyperoxic reperfusion after global ischemia decreases hippocampal energy metabolism. *Stroke*. 2007;38:1578-1584.

74. Richards EM, Rosenthal RE, Kristian T, Fiskum G. Postischemic hyperoxia reduces hippocampal pyruvate dehydrogenase activity. *Free Radic Biol Med*. 2006;40:1960-1970.

75. Fischer M, Hossmann KA. No-reflow after cardiac arrest. *Intensive Care Med*. 1995;21:132-141.

76. Wolfson SK Jr, Safar P, Reich H, Clark JM, Gur D, Stezoski W, Cook EE, Krupper MA. Dynamic heterogeneity of cerebral hypoperfusion after prolonged cardiac arrest in dogs measured by the stable xenon/CT technique: a preliminary study. *Resuscitation*. 1992;23:1-20.

77. Yundt KD, Diringer MN. The use of hyperventilation and its impact on cerebral ischemia in the treatment of traumatic brain injury. *Crit Care Clin*. 1997;13:163-184.

78. Ausina A, Baguena M, Nadal M, Manrique S, Ferrer A, Sahuquillo J, Garnacho A. Cerebral hemodynamic changes during sustained hypocapnia in severe head injury: can hyperventilation cause cerebral ischemia? *Acta Neurochir Suppl*. 1998;71:1-4.

79. Yannopoulos D, Tang W, Roussos C, Aufderheide TP, Idris AH, Lurie KG. Reducing ventilation frequency during cardiopulmonary resuscitation in a porcine model of cardiac arrest. *Respir Care*. 2005;50:628-635.

80. Yannopoulos D, Aufderheide TP, Gabrielli A, Beiser DG, McKnite SH, Pirrallo RG, Wigginton J, Becker L, Vanden Hoek T, Tang W, Nadkarni VM, Klein JP, Idris AH, Lurie KG. Clinical and hemodynamic comparison of 15:2 and 30:2 compression-to-ventilation ratios for cardiopulmonary resuscitation. *Crit Care Med*. 2006;34:1444-1449.

81. Pepe PE, Raedler C, Lurie KG, Wigginton JG. Emergency ventilatory management in hemorrhagic states: elemental or detrimental? *J Trauma*. 2003;54:1048-1055; discussion 1055-1047.

82. Herff H, Paal P, von Goedecke A, Lindner KH, Severing AC, Wenzel V. Influence of ventilation strategies on survival in severe controlled hemorrhagic shock. *Crit Care Med*. 2008;36:2613-2620.

83. Ventilation with lower tidal volumes as compared with traditional tidal volumes for acute lung injury and the acute respiratory distress syndrome. The Acute Respiratory Distress Syndrome Network. *N Engl J Med*. 2000;342:1301-1308.

84. Tremblay LN, Slutsky AS. Ventilator-induced lung injury: from the bench to the bedside. *Intensive Care Med*. 2006;32:24-33.

85. Borges JB, Okamoto VN, Matos GF, Caramez MP, Arantes PR, Barros F, Souza CE, Victorino JA, Kacmarek RM, Barbas CS, Carvalho CR, Amato MB. Reversibility of lung collapse and hypoxemia in early acute respiratory distress syndrome. *Am J Respir Crit Care Med*. 2006;174:268-278.

86. Wan S, Quinlan DJ, Agnelli G, Eikelboom JW. Thrombolysis compared with heparin for the initial treatment of pulmonary embolism: a meta-analysis of the randomized controlled trials. *Circulation*. 2004;110:744-749.

87. Scholz KH, Hilmer T, Schuster S, Wojcik J, Kreuzer H, Tebbe U. Thrombolysis in resuscitated patients with pulmonary embolism [in German]. *Dtsch Med Wochenschr*. 1990;115:930-935.

88. Bottiger BW, Bode C, Kern S, Gries A, Gust R, Glatzer R, Bauer H, Motsch J, Martin E. Efficacy and safety of thrombolytic therapy after initially unsuccessful cardiopulmonary resuscitation: a prospective clinical trial. *Lancet*. 2001;357:1583-1585.

89. Fatovich DM, Dobb GJ, Clugston RA. A pilot randomised trial of thrombolysis in cardiac arrest (The TICA trial). *Resuscitation*. 2004;61:309-313.

90. Fava M, Loyola S, Bertoni H, Dougnac A. Massive pulmonary embolism: percutaneous mechanical thrombectomy during cardiopulmonary resuscitation. *J Vasc Interv Radiol*. 2005;16:119-123.

91. Janata K, Holzer M, Kurkciyan I, Losert H, Riedmuller E, Pikula B, Laggner AN, Laczika K. Major bleeding complications in cardiopulmonary resuscitation: the place of thrombolytic therapy in cardiac arrest due to massive pulmonary embolism. *Resuscitation*. 2003;57:49-55.

92. Lederer W, Lichtenberger C, Pechlaner C, Kinzl J, Kroesen G, Baubin M. Long-term survival and neurological outcome of patients who received recombinant tissue plasminogen activator during out-of-hospital cardiac arrest. *Resuscitation*. 2004;61:123-129.

93. Zahorec R. Rescue systemic thrombolysis during cardiopulmonary resuscitation. *Bratisl Lek Listy*. 2002;103:266-269.

94. Spohr F, Bottiger BW. Thrombolytic therapy during or after cardiopulmonary resuscitation. Efficacy and safety of a new therapeutic approach. *Minerva Anestesiol*. 2003;69:357-364.

95. Konstantinov IE, Saxena P, Koniuszko MD, Alvarez J, Newman MA. Acute massive pulmonary embolism with cardiopulmonary resuscitation: management and results. *Tex Heart Inst J*. 2007;34:41-45; discussion 45-46.

96. Lederer W, Lichtenberger C, Pechlaner C, Kroesen G, Baubin M. Recombinant tissue plasminogen activator during cardiopulmonary resuscitation in 108 patients with out-of-hospital cardiac arrest. *Resuscitation*. 2001;50:71-76.

97. Schmid C, Zietlow S, Wagner TO, Laas J, Borst HG. Fulminant pulmonary embolism: symptoms, diagnostics, operative technique, and results. *Ann Thorac Surg*. 1991;52:1102-1105; discussion 1105-1107.

98. Doerge HC, Schoendube FA, Loeser H, Walter M, Messmer BJ. Pulmonary embolectomy: review of a 15-year experience and role in the age of thrombolytic therapy. *Eur J Cardiothorac Surg*. 1996;10:952-957.

99. Ullmann M, Hemmer W, Hannekum A. The urgent pulmonary embolectomy: mechanical resuscitation in the operating theatre determines the outcome. *Thorac Cardiovasc Surg*. 1999;47:5-8.

100. Dauphine C, Omari B. Pulmonary embolectomy for acute massive pulmonary embolism. *Ann Thorac Surg*. 2005;79:1240-1244.

101. Hall JE, Uhrich TD, Barney JA, Arain SR, Ebert TJ. Sedative, amnestic, and analgesic properties of small-dose dexmedetomidine infusions. *Anesth Analg*. 2000;90:699-705.

102. Milbrandt EB, Kersten A, Kong L, Weissfeld LA, Clermont G, Fink MP, Angus DC. Haloperidol use is associated with lower hospital mortality in mechanically ventilated patients. *Crit Care Med*. 2005;33:226-229; discussion 263-265.

103. De Jonghe B, Cook D, Griffith L, Appere-de-Vecchi C, Guyatt G, Theron V, Vagnerre A, Outin H. Adaptation to the Intensive Care Environment (ATICE): development and validation of a new sedation assessment instrument. *Crit Care Med*. 2003;31:2344-2354.

104. Weinert C, McFarland L. The state of intubated ICU patients: development of a two-dimensional sedation rating scale for critically ill adults. *Chest*. 2004;126:1883-1890.

105. Ramsay MA, Savege TM, Simpson BR, Goodwin R. Controlled sedation with alphaxalone-alphadolone. *Br Med J*. 1974;2:656-659.

106. Sessler CN, Gosnell MS, Grap MJ, Brophy GM, O'Neal PV, Keane KA, Tesoro EP, Elswick RK. The Richmond Agitation-Sedation Scale: validity and reliability in adult intensive care unit patients. *Am J Respir Crit Care Med*. 2002;166:1338-1344.

107. Riker RR, Fraser GL, Cox PM. Continuous infusion of haloperidol controls agitation in critically ill patients. *Crit Care Med*. 1994;22:433-440.

108. de Lemos J, Tweeddale M, Chittock D. Measuring quality of sedation in adult mechanically ventilated critically ill patients.

the Vancouver Interaction and Calmness Scale. Sedation Focus Group. *J Clin Epidemiol*. 2000;53:908-919.

109. Devlin JW, Boleski G, Mlynarek M, Nerenz DR, Peterson E, Jankowski M, Horst HM, Zarowitz BJ. Motor Activity Assessment Scale: a valid and reliable sedation scale for use with mechanically ventilated patients in an adult surgical intensive care unit. *Crit Care Med*. 1999;27:1271-1275.

110. Rello J, Diaz E, Roque M, Valles J. Risk factors for developing pneumonia within 48 hours of intubation. *Am J Respir Crit Care Med*. 1999;159:1742-1746.

111. Gorjup V, Radsel P, Kocjancic ST, Erzen D, Noc M. Acute ST-elevation myocardial infarction after successful cardiopulmonary resuscitation. *Resuscitation*. 2007;72:379-385.

112. Lettieri C, Savonitto S, De Servi S, Guagliumi G, Belli G, Repetto A, Piccaluga E, Politi A, Ettori F, Castiglioni B, Fabbiocchi F, De Cesare N, Sangiorgi G, Musumeci G, Onofri M, D'Urbano M, Pirelli S, Zanini R, Klugmann S. Emergency percutaneous coronary intervention in patients with ST-elevation myocardial infarction complicated by out-of-hospital cardiac arrest: early and medium-term outcome. *Am Heart J*. 2009;157:569-575 e561.

113. Kahn JK, Glazier S, Swor R, Savas V, O'Neill WW. Primary coronary angioplasty for acute myocardial infarction complicated by out-of-hospital cardiac arrest. *Am J Cardiol*. 1995;75:1069-1070.

114. Marcusohn E, Roguin A, Sebbag A, Aronson D, Dragu R, Amikam S, Boulus M, Grenadier E, Kerner A, Nikolsky E, Markiewicz W, Hammerman H, Kapeliovich M. Primary percutaneous coronary intervention after out-of-hospital cardiac arrest: patients and outcomes. *Isr Med Assoc J*. 2007;9:257-259.

115. McCullough PA, Prakash R, Tobin KJ, O'Neill WW, Thompson RJ. Application of a cardiac arrest score in patients with sudden death and ST segment elevation for triage to angiography and intervention. *J Interv Cardiol*. 2002;15:257-261.

116. Nagao K, Hayashi N, Kanmatsuse K, Arima K, Ohtsuki J, Kikushima K, Watanabe I. Cardiopulmonary cerebral resuscitation using emergency cardiopulmonary bypass, coronary reperfusion therapy and mild hypothermia in patients with cardiac arrest outside the hospital. *J Am Coll Cardiol*. 2000;36:776-783.

117. Peels HO, Jessurun GA, van der Horst IC, Arnold AE, Piers LH, Zijlstra F. Outcome in transferred and nontransferred patients after primary percutaneous coronary intervention for ischaemic out-of-hospital cardiac arrest. *Catheter Cardiovasc Interv*. 2008;71:147-151.

118. Pleskot M, Babu A, Hazukova R, Stritecky J, Bis J, Matejka J, Cermakova E. Out-of-hospital cardiac arrests in patients with acute ST elevation myocardial infarctions in the East Bohemian region over the period 2002-2004. *Cardiology*. 2008;109:41-51.

119. Quintero-Moran B, Moreno R, Villarreal S, Perez-Vizcayno MJ, Hernandez R, Conde C, Vazquez P, Alfonso F, Banuelos C, Escaned J, Fernandez-Ortiz A, Azcona L, Macaya C. Percutaneous coronary intervention for cardiac arrest secondary to ST-elevation acute myocardial infarction. Influence of immediate paramedical/medical assistance on clinical outcome. *J Invasive Cardiol*. 2006;18:269-272.

120. Bendz B, Eritsland J, Nakstad AR, Brekke M, Klow NE, Steen PA, Mangschau A. Long-term prognosis after out-of-hospital cardiac arrest and primary percutaneous coronary intervention. *Resuscitation*. 2004;63:49-53.

121. Engdahl J, Abrahamsson P, Bang A, Lindqvist J, Karlsson T, Herlitz J. Is hospital care of major importance for outcome after out-of-hospital cardiac arrest? Experience acquired from patients with out-of-hospital cardiac arrest resuscitated by the same Emergency Medical Service and admitted to one of two hospitals over a 16-year period in the municipality of Göteborg. *Resuscitation*. 2000;43:201-211.

122. Garot P, Lefevre T, Eltchaninoff H, Morice MC, Tamion F, Abry B, Lesault PF, Le Tarnec JY, Pouges C, Margenet A, Monchi M, Laurent I, Dumas P, Garot J, Louvard Y. Six-month outcome of emergency percutaneous coronary intervention in resuscitated patients after cardiac arrest complicating ST-elevation myocardial infarction. *Circulation*. 2007;115:1354-1362.

123. Connolly SJ, Gent M, Roberts RS, Dorian P, Roy D, Sheldon RS, Mitchell LB, Green MS, Klein GJ, O'Brien B. Canadian implantable defibrillator study (CIDS): a randomized trial of the implantable cardioverter defibrillator against amiodarone. *Circulation*. 2000;101:1297-1302.

124. Kuck KH, Cappato R, Siebels J, Ruppel R. Randomized comparison of antiarrhythmic drug therapy with implantable defibrillators in patients resuscitated from cardiac arrest: the Cardiac Arrest Study Hamburg (CASH). *Circulation*. 2000;102:748-754.

125. Wever EF, Hauer RN, van Capelle FL, Tijssen JG, Crijns HJ, Algra A, Wiesfeld AC, Bakker PF, Robles de Medina EO. Randomized study of implantable defibrillator as first-choice therapy versus conventional strategy in postinfarct sudden death survivors. *Circulation*. 1995;91:2195-2203.

126. A comparison of antiarrhythmic-drug therapy with implantable defibrillators in patients resuscitated from near-fatal ventricular arrhythmias. The Antiarrhythmics versus Implantable Defibrillators (AVID) Investigators. *N Engl J Med*. 1997;337:1576-1583.

127. Buxton AE, Lee KL, Fisher JD, Josephson ME, Prystowsky EN, Hafley G. A randomized study of the prevention of sudden death in patients with coronary artery disease. Multicenter Unsustained Tachycardia Trial Investigators. *N Engl J Med*. 1999;341:1882-1890.

128. Bonhomme L, Benhamou D, Comoy E, Preaux N. Stability of epinephrine in alkalinized solutions. *Ann Emerg Med*. 1990;19:1242-1244.

129. Grillo JA, Gonzalez ER, Ramaiya A, Karnes HT, Wells B. Chemical compatibility of inotropic and vasoactive agents delivered via a multiple line infusion system. *Crit Care Med*. 1995;23:1061-1066.

130. Gisvold SE, Sterz F, Abramson NS, Bar-Joseph G, Ebmeyer U, Gervais H, Ginsberg M, Katz LM, Kochanek PM, Kuboyama K, Miller B, Obrist W, Roine RO, Safar P, Sim KM, Vandevelde K, White RJ, Xiao F. Cerebral resuscitation from cardiac arrest: treatment potentials. *Crit Care Med*. 1996;24:S69-S80.

131. del Zoppo GJ, Mabuchi T. Cerebral microvessel responses to focal ischemia. *J Cereb Blood Flow Metab*. 2003;23:879-894.

132. Weaver WD, Cobb LA, Copass MK, Hallstrom AP. Ventricular defibrillation—a comparative trial using 175-J and 320-J shocks. *N Engl J Med*. 1982;307:1101-1106.

133. Vasquez A, Kern KB, Hilwig RW, Heidenreich J, Berg RA, Ewy GA. Optimal dosing of dobutamine for treating post-resuscitation left ventricular dysfunction. *Resuscitation*. 2004;61:199-207.

134. Dellinger RP, Carlet JM, Masur H, Gerlach H, Calandra T, Cohen J, Gea-Banacloche J, Keh D, Marshall JC, Parker MM, Ramsay G, Zimmerman JL, Vincent JL, Levy MM. Surviving

Sepsis Campaign guidelines for management of severe sepsis and septic shock. *Crit Care Med*. 2004;32:858-873.

135. Rivers E, Nguyen B, Havstad S, Ressler J, Muzzin A, Knoblich B, Peterson E, Tomlanovich M. Early goal-directed therapy in the treatment of severe sepsis and septic shock. *N Engl J Med*. 2001;345:1368-1377.

136. Nolan JP, Laver SR, Welch CA, Harrison DA, Gupta V, Rowan K. Outcome following admission to UK intensive care units after cardiac arrest: a secondary analysis of the ICNARC Case Mix Programme Database. *Anaesthesia*. 2007;62:1207-1216.

137. Mullner M, Sterz F, Binder M, Schreiber W, Deimel A, Laggner AN. Blood glucose concentration after cardiopulmonary resuscitation influences functional neurological recovery in human cardiac arrest survivors. *J Cereb Blood Flow Metab*. 1997;17:430-436.

138. Losert H, Sterz F, Roine RO, Holzer M, Martens P, Cerchiari E, Tiainen M, Mullner M, Laggner AN, Herkner H, Bischof MG. Strict normoglycaemic blood glucose levels in the therapeutic management of patients within 12h after cardiac arrest might not be necessary. *Resuscitation*. 2008;76:214-220.

139. Griesdale DE, de Souza RJ, van Dam RM, Heyland DK, Cook DJ, Malhotra A, Dhaliwal R, Henderson WR, Chittock DR, Finfer S, Talmor D. Intensive insulin therapy and mortality among critically ill patients: a meta-analysis including NICE-SUGAR study data. *CMAJ*. 2009;180:821-827.

140. Wiener RS, Wiener DC, Larson RJ. Benefits and risks of tight glucose control in critically ill adults: a meta-analysis. *JAMA*. 2008;300:933-944.

141. Oksanen T, Skrifvars MB, Varpula T, Kuitunen A, Pettila V, Nurmi J, Castren M. Strict versus moderate glucose control after resuscitation from ventricular fibrillation. *Intensive Care Med*. 2007;33:2093-2100.

142. van den Berghe G, Wouters P, Weekers F, Verwaest C, Bruyninckx F, Schetz M, Vlasselaers D, Ferdinande P, Lauwers P, Bouillon R. Intensive insulin therapy in critically ill patients. *N Engl J Med*. 2001;345:1359-1367.

143. Van den Berghe G, Wilmer A, Hermans G, Meersseman W, Wouters PJ, Milants I, Van Wijngaerden E, Bobbaers H, Bouillon R. Intensive insulin therapy in the medical ICU. *N Engl J Med*. 2006;354:449-461.

144. Arabi YM, Dabbagh OC, Tamim HM, Al-Shimemeri AA, Memish ZA, Haddad SH, Syed SJ, Giridhar HR, Rishu AH, Al-Daker MO, Kahoul SH, Britts RJ, Sakkijha MH. Intensive versus conventional insulin therapy: a randomized controlled trial in medical and surgical critically ill patients. *Crit Care Med*. 2008;36:3190-3197.

145. Brunkhorst FM, Engel C, Bloos F, Meier-Hellmann A, Ragaller M, Weiler N, Moerer O, Gruendling M, Oppert M, Grond S, Olthoff D, Jaschinski U, John S, Rossaint R, Welte T, Schaefer M, Kern P, Kuhnt E, Kiehntopf M, Hartog C, Natanson C, Loeffler M, Reinhart K. Intensive insulin therapy and pentastarch resuscitation in severe sepsis. *N Engl J Med*. 2008;358:125-139.

146. Preiser JC, Devos P, Ruiz-Santana S, Melot C, Annane D, Groeneveld J, Iapichino G, Leverve X, Nitenberg G, Singer P, Wernerman J, Joannidis M, Stecher A, Chiolero R. A prospective randomised multi-centre controlled trial on tight glucose control by intensive insulin therapy in adult intensive care units: the Glucontrol study. *Intensive Care Med*. 2009;35:1738-1748.

147. Finfer S, Chittock DR, Su SY, Blair D, Foster D, Dhingra V, Bellomo R, Cook D, Dodek P, Henderson WR, Hebert PC, Heritier S, Heyland DK, McArthur C, McDonald E, Mitchell I, Myburgh JA, Norton R, Potter J, Robinson BG, Ronco JJ. Intensive versus conventional glucose control in critically ill patients. *N Engl J Med*. 2009;360:1283-1297.

148. Krinsley JS, Grover A. Severe hypoglycemia in critically ill patients: risk factors and outcomes. *Crit Care Med*. 2007;35:2262-2267.

149. Arabi YM, Tamim HM, Rishu AH. Hypoglycemia with intensive insulin therapy in critically ill patients: predisposing factors and association with mortality. *Crit Care Med*. 2009;37:2536-2544.

150. Schultz CH, Rivers EP, Feldkamp CS, Goad EG, Smithline HA, Martin GB, Fath JJ, Wortsman J, Nowak RM. A characterization of hypothalamic-pituitary-adrenal axis function during and after human cardiac arrest. *Crit Care Med*. 1993;21:1339-1347.

151. Kim JJ, Lim YS, Shin JH, Yang HJ, Kim JK, Hyun SY, Rhoo I, Hwang SY, Lee G. Relative adrenal insufficiency after cardiac arrest: impact on postresuscitation disease outcome. *Am J Emerg Med*. 2006;24:684-688.

152. Sprung CL, Annane D, Keh D, Moreno R, Singer M, Freivogel K, Weiss YG, Benbenishty J, Kalenka A, Forst H, Laterre PF, Reinhart K, Cuthbertson BH, Payen D, Briegel J. Hydrocortisone therapy for patients with septic shock. *N Engl J Med*. 2008;358:111-124.

153. Minneci PC, Deans KJ, Banks SM, Eichacker PQ, Natanson C. Corticosteroids for septic shock. *Ann Intern Med*. 2004;141:742-743.

154. Annane D, Sebille V, Charpentier C, Bollaert PE, Francois B, Korach JM, Capellier G, Cohen Y, Azoulay E, Troche G, Chaumet-Riffaud P, Bellissant E. Effect of treatment with low doses of hydrocortisone and fludrocortisone on mortality in patients with septic shock. *JAMA*. 2002;288:862-871.

155. Laurent I, Adrie C, Vinsonneau C, Cariou A, Chiche JD, Ohanessian A, Spaulding C, Carli P, Dhainaut JF, Monchi M. High-volume hemofiltration after out-of-hospital cardiac arrest: a randomized study. *J Am Coll Cardiol*. 2005;46:432-437.

156. Huang D, Xu R. et al. Effect of high-volume hemofiltration on outcome of cerebral edema following cerebral reperfusion injury [in Chinese]. *Chin J Clin Rehabil*. 2004;4:3796 –3797.

157. Randomized clinical study of thiopental loading in comatose survivors of cardiac arrest. Brain Resuscitation Clinical Trial I Study Group. *N Engl J Med*. 1986;314:397-403.

158. Holzer M, Sterz F, Behringer W, Oschatz E, Kofler J, Eisenburger P, Kittler H, Konschitzky R, Laggner AN. Endothelin-1 elevates regional cerebral perfusion during prolonged ventricular fibrillation cardiac arrest in pigs. *Resuscitation*. 2002;55:317-327.

159. Krumholz A, Stern BJ, Weiss HD. Outcome from coma after cardiopulmonary resuscitation: relation to seizures and myoclonus. *Neurology*. 1988;38:401-405.

160. Wijdicks EF, Parisi JE, Sharbrough FW. Prognostic value of myoclonus status in comatose survivors of cardiac arrest. *Ann Neurol*. 1994;35:239-243.

161. Hui AC, Cheng C, Lam A, Mok V, Joynt GM. Prognosis following Postanoxic Myoclonus Status epilepticus. *Eur Neurol*. 2005;54:10-13.

162. Wijdicks EF, Hijdra A, Young GB, Bassetti CL, Wiebe S. Practice parameter: prediction of outcome in comatose survivors after cardiopulmonary resuscitation (an evidence-based review): report of the Quality Standards Subcommittee of the American Academy of Neurology. *Neurology*. 2006;67:203-210.

163. Zandbergen EG, Hijdra A, Koelman JH, Hart AA, Vos PE, Verbeek MM, de Haan RJ. Prediction of poor outcome within the first 3 days of postanoxic coma. *Neurology*. 2006;66:62-68.

164. Edgren E, Hedstrand U, Nordin M, Rydin E, Ronquist G. Prediction of outcome after cardiac arrest. *Crit Care Med*. 1987;15:820-825.

165. Young GB, Doig G, Ragazzoni A. Anoxic-ischemic encephalopathy: clinical and electrophysiological associations with outcome. *Neurocrit Care*. 2005;2:159-164.

166. Bassetti C, Bomio F, Mathis J, Hess CW. Early prognosis in coma after cardiac arrest: a prospective clinical, electrophysiological, and biochemical study of 60 patients. *J Neurol Neurosurg Psychiatry*. 1996;61:610-615.

167. Edgren E, Hedstrand U, Kelsey S, Sutton-Tyrrell K, Safar P. Assessment of neurological prognosis in comatose survivors of cardiac arrest. BRCT I Study Group. *Lancet*. 1994;343:1055-1059.

168. English WA, Giffin NJ, Nolan JP. Myoclonus after cardiac arrest: pitfalls in diagnosis and prognosis. *Anaesthesia*. 2009;64:908-911.

169. Arnoldus EP, Lammers GJ. Postanoxic coma: good recovery despite myoclonus status. *Ann Neurol*. 1995;38:697-698.

170. Celesia GG, Grigg MM, Ross E. Generalized status myoclonicus in acute anoxic and toxic-metabolic encephalopathies. *Arch Neurol*. 1988;45:781-784.

171. Datta S, Hart GK, Opdam H, Gutteridge G, Archer J. Post-hypoxic myoclonic status: the prognosis is not always hopeless. *Crit Care Resusc*. 2009;11:39-41.

172. Morris HR, Howard RS, Brown P. Early myoclonic status and outcome after cardiorespiratory arrest. *J Neurol Neurosurg Psychiatry*. 1998;64:267-268.

173. Zandbergen EG, de Haan RJ, Stoutenbeek CP, Koelman JH, Hijdra A. Systematic review of early prediction of poor outcome in anoxic-ischaemic coma. *Lancet*. 1998;352:1808-1812.

174. Rundgren M, Rosen I, Friberg H. Amplitude-integrated EEG (aEEG) predicts outcome after cardiac arrest and induced hypothermia. *Intensive Care Med*. 2006;32:836-842.

175. Shibata S, Imota T, Shigeomi S, Sato W, Enzan K. Use of the bispectral index during the early postresuscitative phase after out-of-hospital cardiac arrest. *J Anesth*. 2005;19:243-246.

176. Stammet P, Werer C, Mertens L, Lorang C, Hemmer M. Bispectral index (BIS) helps predicting bad neurological outcome in comatose survivors after cardiac arrest and induced therapeutic hypothermia. *Resuscitation*. 2009;80:437-442.

177. Ajisaka H. Early electroencephalographic findings in patients with anoxic encephalopathy after cardiopulmonary arrest and successful resusitation. *J Clin Neurosci*. 2004;11:616-618.

178. Rossetti AO, Logroscino G, Liaudet L, Ruffieux C, Ribordy V, Schaller MD, Despland PA, Oddo M. Status epilepticus: an independent outcome predictor after cerebral anoxia. *Neurology*. 2007;69:255-260.

179. Thomke F, Brand A, Weilemann SL. The temporal dynamics of postanoxic burst-suppression EEG. *J Clin Neurophysiol*. 2002;19:24-31.

180. Fatovich DM, Jacobs IG, Celenza A, Paech MJ. An observational study of bispectral index monitoring for out of hospital cardiac arrest. *Resuscitation*. 2006;69:207-212.

181. Berkhoff M, Donati F, Bassetti C. Postanoxic alpha (theta) coma: a reappraisal of its prognostic significance. *Clin Neurophysiol*. 2000;111:297-304.

182. Allen JS, Tranel D, Bruss J, Damasio H. Correlations between regional brain volumes and memory performance in anoxia. *J Clin Exp Neuropsychol*. 2006;28:457-476.

183. De Volder AG, Michel C, Guerit JM, Bol A, Georges B, de Barsy T, Laterre C. Brain glucose metabolism in postanoxic syndrome due to cardiac arrest. *Acta Neurol Belg*. 1994;94:183-189.

184. Fujioka M, Nishio K, Miyamoto S, Hiramatsu KI, Sakaki T, Okuchi K, Taoka T, Fujioka S. Hippocampal damage in the human brain after cardiac arrest. *Cerebrovasc Dis*. 2000;10:2-7.

185. Tommasino C, Grana C, Lucignani G, Torri G, Fazio F. Regional cerebral metabolism of glucose in comatose and vegetative state patients. *J Neurosurg Anesthesiol*. 1995;7:109-116.

186. Lovblad K, Senn P, Walpoth BH, Walpotth BN, Mattle HP, Radanov BP, Ozdoba C, Schroth G. Increased brain tolerance for ischemia in accidental deep hypothermia and circulatory arrest. *Riv Neuroradiol*. 1998;11:224-226.

187. Edgren E, Enblad P, Grenvik A, Lilja A, Valind S, Wiklund L, Hedstrand U, Stjernstrom H, Persson L, Ponten U, Langstrom B. Cerebral blood flow and metabolism after cardiopulmonary resuscitation. A pathophysiologic and prognostic positron emission tomography pilot study. *Resuscitation*. 2003;57:161-170.

188. Grubb NR, Fox KA, Smith K, Best J, Blane A, Ebmeier KP, Glabus MF, O'Carroll RE. Memory impairment in out-of-hospital cardiac arrest survivors is associated with global reduction in brain volume, not focal hippocampal injury. *Stroke*. 2000;31:1509-1514.

189. Gut E, Fritz R, Leyhe T, Manzl G, Schönle PW. MRT after cerebral hypoxia. Correlation of imaging findings with clinical outcome and functional rehabilitation. *Klin Neuroradiol*. 1999;9:147-152.

190. Els T, Kassubek J, Kubalek R, Klisch J. Diffusion-weighted MRI during early global cerebral hypoxia: a predictor for clinical outcome? *Acta Neurol Scand*. 2004;110:361-367.

191. Kano H, Houkin K, Harada K, Koyanagi I, Nara S, Itou Y, Imaizumi H, Asai Y, Saitou M. Neuronal cell injury in patients after cardiopulmonary resuscitation: evaluation by diffusion-weighted imaging and magnetic resonance spectroscopy. *Neurosurg Rev*. 2006;29:88-92.

192. Wijdicks EF, Campeau NG, Miller GM. MR imaging in comatose survivors of cardiac resuscitation. *AJNR Am J Neuroradiol*. 2001;22:1561-1565.

193. Wijman CA, Mlynash M, Caulfield AF, Hsia AW, Eyngorn I, Bammer R, Fischbein N, Albers GW, Moseley M. Prognostic value of brain diffusion-weighted imaging after cardiac arrest. *Ann Neurol*. 2009;65:394-402.

194. Wu O, Sorensen AG, Benner T, Singhal AB, Furie KL, Greer DM. Comatose patients with cardiac arrest: predicting clinical outcome with diffusion-weighted MR imaging. *Radiology*. 2009;252:173-181.

195. Arbelaez A, Castillo M, Mukherji SK. Diffusion-weighted MR imaging of global cerebral anoxia. *AJNR Am J Neuroradiol*. 1999;20:999-1007.

196. Barrett KM, Freeman WD, Weindling SM, Brott TG, Broderick DF, Heckman MG, Crook JE, Divertie GD, Meschia JF. Brain injury after cardiopulmonary arrest and its assessment

with diffusion-weighted magnetic resonance imaging. *Mayo Clin Proc*. 2007;82:828-835.

197. Berek K, Lechleitner P, Luef G, Felber S, Saltuari L, Schinnerl A, Traweger C, Dienstl F, Aichner F. Early determination of neurological outcome after prehospital cardiopulmonary resuscitation. *Stroke*. 1995;26:543-549.
198. Iida K, Satoh H, Arita K, Nakahara T, Kurisu K, Ohtani M. Delayed hyperemia causing intracranial hypertension after cardiopulmonary resuscitation. *Crit Care Med*. 1997;25:971-976.
199. Ettl A, Fischer-Klein C, Chemelli A, Daxer A, Felber S. Proton relaxation times of the vitreous body in hereditary vitreoretinal dystrophy. *Ophthalmologica*. 1994;208:195-197.
200. Greer DM. MRI in anoxic brain injury. *Neurocrit Care*. 2004;1:213-215.
201. Kuoppamaki M, Bhatia KP, Quinn N. Progressive delayed-onset dystonia after cerebral anoxic insult in adults. *Mov Disord*. 2002;17:1345-1349.
202. Verslegers W, Crols R, van den Kerchove M, de Potter W, Appel B, Lowenthal A. Parkinsonian syndrome after cardiac arrest: radiological and neurochemical changes. *Clin Neurol Neurosurg*. 1988;90:177-179.
203. Bolouri MR, Small GA. Neuroimaging of hypoxia and cocaine-induced hippocampal stroke. *J Neuroimaging*. 2004;14:290-291.
204. Fujioka M, Okuchi K, Sakaki T, Hiramatsu K, Miyamoto S, Iwasaki S. Specific changes in human brain following reperfusion after cardiac arrest. *Stroke*. 1994;25:2091-2095.
205. Johkura K, Naito M. Wernicke's encephalopathy-like lesions in global cerebral hypoxia. *J Clin Neurosci*. 2008;15:318-319.
206. Konaka K, Miyashita K, Naritomi H. Changes in diffusion-weighted magnetic resonance imaging findings in the acute and subacute phases of anoxic encephalopathy. *J Stroke Cerebrovasc Dis*. 2007;16:82-83.
207. Singhal AB, Topcuoglu MA, Koroshetz WJ. Diffusion MRI in three types of anoxic encephalopathy. *J Neurol Sci*. 2002;196:37-40.
208. Wartenberg KE, Patsalides A, Yepes MS. Is magnetic resonance spectroscopy superior to conventional diagnostic tools in hypoxic-ischemic encephalopathy? *J Neuroimaging*. 2004;14:180-186.
209. Zhang YX, Liu JR, Jiang B, Liu HQ, Ding MP, Song SJ, Zhang BR, Zhang H, Xu B, Chen HH, Wang ZJ, Huang JZ. Lance-Adams syndrome: a report of two cases. *J Zhejiang Univ Sci B*. 2007;8:715-720.
210. Nogami K, Fujii M, Kato S, Nishizaki T, Suzuki M, Yamashita S, Oda Y, Sadamitsu D, Maekawa T. Analysis of magnetic resonance imaging (MRI) morphometry and cerebral blood flow in patients with hypoxic-ischemic encephalopathy. *J Clin Neurosci*. 2004;11:376-380.
211. Arishima H, Ishii H, Kubota T, Maeda H, Shigemori K. Angiographic features of anoxic encephalopathy in the acute phase: a case report [in Japanese]. *No To Shinkei*. 2003;55:977-982.
212. Hung GU, Lee JD, Lee JK. Bilateral cranial Tc-99m MDP uptake due to hypoxic-ischemic encephalopathy. *Clin Nucl Med*. 2007;32:328-329.
213. Choi SP, Park HK, Park KN, Kim YM, Ahn KJ, Choi KH, Lee WJ, Jeong SK. The density ratio of grey to white matter on computed tomography as an early predictor of vegetative state or death after cardiac arrest. *Emerg Med J*. 2008;25:666-669.
214. De Reuck J, Decoo D, Vienne J, Strijckmans K, Lemahieu I. Significance of white matter lucencies in posthypoxic-ischemic encephalopathy: comparison of clinical status and of computed and positron emission tomographic findings. *Eur Neurol*. 1992;32:334-339.
215. Inoue Y, Shiozaki T, Irisawa T, Mohri T, Yoshiya K, Ikegawa H, Tasaki O, Tanaka H, Shimazu T, Sugimoto H. Acute cerebral blood flow variations after human cardiac arrest assessed by stable xenon enhanced computed tomography. *Curr Neurovasc Res*. 2007;4:49-54.
216. Nunes B, Pais J, Garcia R, Magalhaes Z, Granja C, Silva MC. Cardiac arrest: long-term cognitive and imaging analysis. *Resuscitation*. 2003;57:287-297.
217. Yanagawa Y, Un-no Y, Sakamoto T, Okada Y. Cerebral density on CT immediately after a successful resuscitation of cardiopulmonary arrest correlates with outcome. *Resuscitation*. 2005;64:97-101.
218. Della Corte F, Barelli A, Giordano A, Iacobucci T, Valente MR, Pennisi MA. CBF determination in post-ischemic-anoxic comatose patients. *Minerva Anestesiol*. 1993;59:637-641.
219. Kjos BO, Brant-Zawadzki M, Young RG. Early CT findings of global central nervous system hypoperfusion. *AJR Am J Roentgenol*. 1983;141:1227-1232.
220. Morimoto Y, Kemmotsu O, Kitami K, Matsubara I, Tedo I. Acute brain swelling after out-of-hospital cardiac arrest: pathogenesis and outcome. *Crit Care Med*. 1993;21:104-110.
221. Torbey MT, Geocadin R, Bhardwaj A. Brain arrest neurological outcome scale (BrANOS): predicting mortality and severe disability following cardiac arrest. *Resuscitation*. 2004;63:55-63.
222. Imaizumi H, Tsuruoka K, Ujike Y, Kaneko M, Namiki A. Hypoxic brain damage after prolonged cardiac arrest during anesthesia—changes in CT and serum NSE concentration [in Japanese]. *Masui*. 1994;43:1256-1260.
223. Kelsen J, Obel A. Images in clinical medicine. Fatal cerebral hypoxemia after cardiac arrest. *N Engl J Med*. 2003;348:817.
224. Schwab SA, Richter G, Bautz WA, Uder M, Alibek S. Hypoxic injury of all deep nuclei of the brain—a case report from computed tomography [in German]. *Rontgenpraxis*. 2008;56:245-248.
225. Tanaka H, Masugata H, Fukunaga R, Mandai K, Sueyoshi K, Abe H. Sequential change of heterogeneous cerebral blood blow patterns after diffuse brain ischemia. *Resuscitation*. 1992;24:273-281.
226. Torbey MT, Selim M, Knorr J, Bigelow C, Recht L. Quantitative analysis of the loss of distinction between gray and white matter in comatose patients after cardiac arrest. *Stroke*. 2000;31:2163-2167.
227. Heckmann JG, Lang CJ, Pfau M, Neundorfer B. Electrocerebral silence with preserved but reduced cortical brain perfusion. *Eur J Emerg Med*. 2003;10:241-243.
228. Grubb NR, Simpson C, Sherwood RA, Abraha HD, Cobbe SM, O'Carroll RE, Deary I, Fox KA. Prediction of cognitive dysfunction after resuscitation from out-of-hospital cardiac arrest using serum neuron-specific enolase and protein S-100. *Heart*. 2007;93:1268-1273.
229. Reisinger J, Hollinger K, Lang W, Steiner C, Winter T, Zeindlhofer E, Mori M, Schiller A, Lindorfer A, Wiesinger K, Siostrzonek P. Prediction of neurological outcome after cardiopulmonary resuscitation by serial determination of serum neuron-specific enolase. *Eur Heart J*. 2007;28:52-58.
230. Prohl J, Rother J, Kluge S, de Heer G, Liepert J, Bodenburg S, Pawlik K, Kreymann G. Prediction of short-term and

long-term outcomes after cardiac arrest: a prospective multivariate approach combining biochemical, clinical, electrophysiological, and neuropsychological investigations. *Crit Care Med*. 2007;35:1230-1237.

231. Rech TH, Vieira SR, Nagel F, Brauner JS, Scalco R. Serum neuron-specific enolase as early predictor of outcome after in-hospital cardiac arrest: a cohort study. *Crit Care*. 2006;10:R133.
232. Pfeifer R, Borner A, Krack A, Sigusch HH, Surber R, Figulla HR. Outcome after cardiac arrest: predictive values and limitations of the neuroproteins neuron-specific enolase and protein S-100 and the Glasgow Coma Scale. *Resuscitation*. 2005;65:49-55.
233. Meynaar IA, Oudemans-van Straaten HM, van der Wetering J, Verlooy P, Slaats EH, Bosman RJ, van der Spoel JI, Zandstra DF. Serum neuron-specific enolase predicts outcome in post-anoxic coma: a prospective cohort study. *Intensive Care Med*. 2003;29:189-195.
234. Zingler VC, Krumm B, Bertsch T, Fassbender K, Pohlmann-Eden B. Early prediction of neurological outcome after cardiopulmonary resuscitation: a multimodal approach combining neurobiochemical and electrophysiological investigations may provide high prognostic certainty in patients after cardiac arrest. *Eur Neurol*. 2003;49:79-84.
235. Rosen H, Sunnerhagen KS, Herlitz J, Blomstrand C, Rosengren L. Serum levels of the brain-derived proteins S-100 and NSE predict long-term outcome after cardiac arrest. *Resuscitation*. 2001;49:183-191.
236. Schoerkhuber W, Kittler H, Sterz F, Behringer W, Holzer M, Frossard M, Spitzauer S, Laggner AN. Time course of serum neuron-specific enolase. A predictor of neurological outcome in patients resuscitated from cardiac arrest. *Stroke*. 1999;30:1598-1603.
237. Fogel W, Krieger D, Veith M, Adams HP, Hund E, Storch-Hagenlocher B, Buggle F, Mathias D, Hacke W. Serum neuron-specific enolase as early predictor of outcome after cardiac arrest. *Crit Care Med*. 1997;25:1133-1138.
238. Martens P, Raabe A, Johnsson P. Serum S-100 and neuron-specific enolase for prediction of regaining consciousness after global cerebral ischemia. *Stroke*. 1998;29:2363-2366.
239. Dauberschmidt R, Zinsmeyer J, Mrochen H, Meyer M. Changes of neuron-specific enolase concentration in plasma after cardiac arrest and resuscitation. *Mol Chem Neuropathol*. 1991;14:237-245.
240. Ali AA, Lim E, Thanikachalam M, Sudarshan C, White P, Parameshwar J, Dhital K, Large SR. Cardiac arrest in the organ donor does not negatively influence recipient survival after heart transplantation. *Eur J Cardiothorac Surg*. 2007;31:929-933.
241. Matsumoto CS, Kaufman SS, Girlanda R, Little CM, Rekhtman Y, Raofi V, Laurin JM, Shetty K, Fennelly EM, Johnson LB, Fishbein TM. Utilization of donors who have suffered cardiopulmonary arrest and resuscitation in intestinal transplantation. *Transplantation*. 2008;86:941-946.
242. Adrie C, Haouache H, Saleh M, Memain N, Laurent I, Thuong M, Darques L, Guerrini P, Monchi M. An underrecognized source of organ donors: patients with brain death after successfully resuscitated cardiac arrest. *Intensive Care Med*. 2008;34:132-137.
243. Mercatello A, Roy P, Ng-Sing K, Choux C, Baude C, Garnier JL, Colpart JJ, Finaz J, Petit P, Moskovtchenko JF, et al. Organ transplants from out-of-hospital cardiac arrest patients. *Transplant Proc*. 1988;20:749-750.

Chapter 14

Toxicologic Emergencies

This Chapter

- **Common Poisonings Affecting the Cardiovascular System**
- **Intentional and Unintentional Toxins, Chemical Exposures, or Medications Causing Patient Harm**
- **The Toxidrome Concept in Poisoning and Overdose**
- **Emergency Cardiovascular Care for the Poisoned Patient—General Principles and Treatment**

General Considerations

ACLS providers frequently encounter cardiopulmonary problems and imminent cardiac or pulmonary emergencies caused by intentional, unintentional, or iatrogenic poisoning. For the purposes of this chapter, the term "poisoning" includes intentional or unintentional exposure to any toxin, chemical, or medication that causes harm to a patient. This could be related to an overdose, an adverse drug reaction, or a medication error. It might also include exposure to chemical toxins.

Toxidrome Identification

Although immediate identification of the specific toxin is not always possible, patients still require immediate treatment. In these situations it may be helpful to identify a *toxidrome*.[1] A toxidrome is a set of signs and symptoms commonly caused by a specific toxin (eg, cocaine) or group of toxins (eg, β-blockers). Identification of a toxidrome allows provision of sign- or symptom-based therapy until the specific toxin is identified.

- The clinician must have a high index of suspicion for poisonings in appropriate clinical situations. A toxidrome is often suggested by the history and presentation or by the circumstances before the event.
- Examine the patient for a constellation of signs and symptoms usually observed after exposure to a potentially toxic substance.
- Physiologically group abnormalities according to the following physical findings:
  - Vital signs
  - Skin and mucous membranes
  - Pupils
  - Cardiovascular system
  - Gastrointestinal and genitourinary systems
  - Neurologic findings/mental status

Use of standard ACLS protocols for all patients who are critically poisoned may not result in an optimal outcome. Care of patients with severe poisoning can be enhanced by consultation with a medical toxicologist or regional poison center. Alternative approaches that may be effective in severely poisoned patients include

- Higher doses of medication than what is recommended in standard ACLS guidelines
- Therapies with drugs such as calcium chloride, glucagon, insulin, labetalol, phenylephrine, physostigmine, lipid emulsion, or sodium bicarbonate that are not routinely part of ACLS
- Use of specific antagonists or antidotes
- Extraordinary measures, such as prolonged CPR and possibly use of circulatory assist devices (eg, extracorporeal membrane oxygenation)

Critical Concept **Be Suspicious of Poisoning**	• Suspect poisoning in appropriate or suspicious clinical settings. • Look for groups of signs and symptoms that may be markers of a specific toxin or toxidrome. • Begin appropriate supportive therapy immediately while attempting to identify the specific toxin. • Keep in mind that a mass exposure with multiple patients may occur with some toxins. • Exposure to multiple agents may render the toxidrome concept less useful.

Major Toxidromes

Table 46 shows examples of major toxidromes.

Table 46. Examples of Major Toxidromes

Toxidrome	Findings	Examples	Possible Therapy
Sympathomimetic	Tachycardia Arrhythmias Agitation Diaphoresis Mydriasis Hypertension Hyperthermia	Amphetamine Cocaine Ephedrine	Benzodiazepines Cooling
Cholinergic	**"SLUDGE"** syndrome **S**alivation **L**acrimation **U**rination **D**efecation **G**astrointestinal symptoms **E**mesis	Organophosphates Insecticides	Atropine Pralidoxime
Anticholinergic	*"Mad as a hatter, blind as a bat, red as a beet, hot as a hare, dry as a bone"* Mental status changes Mydriasis Dry/flushed skin Hyperthermia Decreased bowel sounds	Diphenhydramine Scopolamine Atropine Jimson weed	Physostigmine Benzodiazepine Cooling
Opioid	CNS depression Respiratory depression Miosis	Heroin Morphine Fentanyl derivatives	Naloxone
Sedative/hypnotic	CNS depression (sedation, coma) Respiratory depression (apnea) Confusion Delirium Hallucinations	Ethanol Benzodiazepines Barbiturates Anticonvulsants	Supportive therapy Flumazenil (with caution)

Abbreviation: CNS, central nervous system.

This section reviews some major toxidromes. If you suspect a toxidrome, initiate the following general treatment measures:

- Identify need for decontamination and personal protective measures.
- Initiate the systematic approach, which includes BLS and ACLS EP Surveys and support.
- Attempt to identify a specific antidote or therapy while continuing to provide necessary supportive care.

The BLS and ACLS EP Surveys provide an excellent initial approach to any life-threatening problem. Be prepared to support oxygenation, ventilation, and circulation as needed. Establish vascular access and provide vasopressor and rhythm support when clinically indicated. Attempt to determine the presence of a common toxidrome or history of drug ingestion, medication administration, or toxic exposure that would explain the clinical findings or failure to respond to initial therapy. If a toxidrome is identified or suspected during consideration of the differential diagnosis, therapy can be modified to include a specific treatment or antidote.

Ingested Toxins

Gastrointestinal decontamination, previously one of the most common treatments for ingested toxins, now has a smaller role in the management of poisoning. Except in rare cases, gastric lavage and syrup of ipecac administration are no longer recommended.[2-4] In life-threatening poisons for which no adequate antidote is available, single-dose activated charcoal may be used if it can be administered within 1 hour of the toxin ingestion.[5] Multiple-dose activated charcoal should be considered for patients who have ingested a life-threatening amount of specific toxins (eg, carbamazepine, dapsone, phenobarbital, quinine, or theophylline) for which a benefit of this strategy has been established.[6,7] Charcoal should only be administered to patients with a protected or intact airway and is not recommended for caustic substances, hydrocarbons, lithium, or metals.[5] Follow local protocols and consult the poison control center for recommendations.

Symptom-Based Therapy for Toxicologic Emergencies

Practically every sign and symptom observed in poisoning can be produced by natural disease, and many clinical presentations associated with natural disease can be mimicked by some poison.[8] It is important to maintain a broad differential diagnosis, particularly when the history of toxic chemical exposure is unclear. Table 47 lists common signs and symptoms associated with toxicologic emergencies. By recognizing these presentations, the clinician can establish a working diagnosis that guides initial management.

Drug-Induced Cardiac Arrest

Cardiac arrest associated with drugs or poisonings may be associated with any of the arrest rhythms: asystole, pulseless electrical activity, or VF/pulseless ventricular tachycardia (VT). This is discussed in greater detail later.

Cardioversion/Defibrillation

Electrical defibrillation is appropriate for pulseless patients with drug-induced VT or VF and for unstable patients with polymorphic VT. In cases of sympathomimetic poisoning with refractory VF, increase the interval between doses of epinephrine and use only standard dosing. Propranolol is contraindicated in cocaine overdose; however, some case reports suggest that this agent may be useful in the treatment of ephedrine and pseudoephedrine overdose.[9]

Prolonged CPR and Resuscitation

Patients with cardiac arrest that results from poisoning or overdose, especially those with calcium channel blocker poisoning,[10] may warrant more prolonged cardiopulmonary resuscitation (CPR) and resuscitation efforts. Recovery with good neurologic outcomes has been reported in severely poisoned patients who received prolonged CPR (eg, 3 to 5 hours).[11,12]

Critical Concept Poison Control Number	***A certified poison control center can be contacted by calling*** **1-800-222-1222 in the United States**

Critical Concept ACLS Toxicologic Emergency Management Principles	• Initiate the Expanded Systematic Approach with the BLS and ACLS-EP Surveys and provide support. • During the differential diagnosis, attempt to identify a possible toxidrome and a specific antidote or therapy. • Outpatients may be exposed intentionally or unintentionally to toxins or experience toxic effects from medications. • Hospital inpatients may experience adverse drug effects as a result of clinician-caused medication errors or overdose, as well as subversive self-administration.

Intra-Aortic Balloon Pumps and Cardiopulmonary Bypass

Intra-aortic balloon pump (IABP) circulatory assist devices have been used successfully in critical poisonings refractory to maximal medical care. These techniques, however, are expensive and manpower intensive and have significant associated morbidity. To be effective, these devices must be used early in the resuscitative effort, before the irreversible effects of severe shock or cardiac arrest develop. If IABP support is planned, the patient must have an intrinsic cardiac rhythm, because balloon inflation is synchronized with the electrocardiogram (ECG) to provide diastolic augmentation. Cardiopulmonary bypass has been used successfully in the resuscitation of patients with severe poisoning.[13]

Brain Death and Organ Donation Criteria

Brain death criteria based only on an electroencephalogram and neurologic examination are invalid during acute toxic encephalopathy. These brain death criteria apply only when drug levels are no longer toxic. In the presence of toxic drug levels, the only valid confirmatory test for brain death is absent cerebral blood flow.

Organ transplantation after a fatal poisoning from agents capable of causing severe end-organ damage, such as carbon monoxide, cocaine, and iron, is controversial. In a case like this, consultation with transplantation and toxicology experts may be warranted. When organ function is evaluated carefully, successful transplantation of some organs from patients with fatal poisoning with *acetaminophen, cyanide, methanol,* and *carbon monoxide* is possible.[14] However, transplantation of known *target* organs after a fatal poisoning is unlikely to succeed. These target organs include the heart in carbon monoxide poisoning, the heart and liver in cocaine and iron poisonings, and the liver and kidneys in acetaminophen poisonings.

Ventricular Tachycardia/Fibrillation

It is not possible to distinguish drug-induced VT and ventricular fibrillation (VF) from drug-induced wide-complex conduction impairments from the electrocardiogram alone. The patient's history and circumstances may provide clues to the cause of the arrhythmia.

Table 47. **Common Signs and Symptoms Associated With Toxidromes**[1]

Cardiovascular Signs		
Tachycardia and/or Hypertension	**Bradycardia and/or Hypotension**	**Cardiac Conduction Delays (Wide QRS)**
Amphetamines Anticholinergic drugs Antihistamines Cocaine Theophylline/caffeine Withdrawal states	β-Blockers Calcium channel blockers Clonidine Digoxin and related glycosides Organophosphates and carbamates	Cocaine Cyclic antidepressants Local anesthetics Propoxyphene Antiarrhythmics (eg quinidine, flecainide)
CNS/Metabolic Signs		
Seizures	**CNS and/or Respiratory Depression**	**Metabolic Acidosis**
Cyclic antidepressants Isoniazid Local anesthetics Selective and nonselective norepinephrine reuptake inhibitors (eg, bupropion) Withdrawal states	Antidepressants (several classes) Benzodiazepines Carbon monoxide Ethanol Methanol Opioids Oral hypoglycemics	Cyanide Ethylene glycol Metformin Methanol Salicylates

Abbreviation: CNS, central nervous system.

*Differential diagnosis lists are partial.

Reproduced from Vanden Hoek et al.[1]

Treatment

Cardioversion or Defibrillation

The presence or absence of hemodynamic stability determines the treatment of patients with drug-induced VT. Perform immediate shock for VF or VT without pulses. Perform electrical cardioversion for hemodynamically unstable VT with pulses according to ACLS algorithms. Keep in mind that the arrhythmia may be refractory in the continuing presence of a toxin.

Antiarrhythmics

Antiarrhythmics are indicated for most cases of hemodynamically stable drug-induced VT. Vaughan Williams class I_A and I_C and other antiarrhythmics that block the fast sodium channel (eg, sotalol) are contraindicated in cases of poisoning with TCAs or other fast sodium channel blockers (eg, sympathomimetics such as cocaine) because of the risk of synergistic toxicity.[15] Phenytoin is no longer recommended for TCA poisoning.[16,17] Magnesium has beneficial effects in certain cases of drug-induced VT, but it may also aggravate drug-induced hypotension.[18,19]

Lidocaine

To prevent arrhythmias that are secondary to cocaine-induced myocardial infarction, consider a lidocaine bolus followed by a lidocaine infusion. Current evidence neither supports nor refutes a role for lidocaine in the management of wide-complex tachycardia caused by cocaine.

Propranolol

In sympathomimetic poisonings (especially with cocaine), propranolol is contraindicated.[20-24]

Procainamide

Procainamide is contraindicated in poisonings from TCAs and other drugs with similar antiarrhythmic (Vaughan Williams type Ia_{vw}) properties because it can cause a prolongation in the QRS interval.

Magnesium

Magnesium has demonstrated beneficial effects for drug-induced VT, but it may aggravate drug-induced hypotension.[18,19]

Amiodarone

A handful of cases of refractory drug-induced VT or VF have been reported to respond to amiodarone. Amiodarone should be used with caution because it may worsen drug-induced hypotension and may have proarrhythmic effects.

Epinephrine

In sympathomimetic poisonings with refractory VF, the risk-benefit ratio of epinephrine in management is unknown. If epinephrine is used, increase the interval between doses and use only standard dose amounts (1 mg IV). Avoid high-dose epinephrine.

Sodium bicarbonate

Extrapolation from evidence for the treatment of wide-complex tachycardia caused by other agents suggests that hypertonic sodium bicarbonate may be beneficial for wide-complex tachycardia.[25]

Torsades de Pointes

Torsades de pointes can occur with either therapeutic or toxic exposure to many drugs (Table 48). Contributing factors for torsades de pointes include hypoxemia, hypokalemia, and hypomagnesemia. High-quality research has not yet established the safety and efficacy of many of these recommended therapies for drug-induced polymorphic VT, and most therapies are Class IIb, LOE C. However, administration of magnesium is recommended for patients with torsades de pointes even when the serum magnesium concentration is normal. A reasonable strategy for the management of torsades de pointes caused by drug exposure is

- Correct hypoxia, hypokalemia, and hypomagnesemia if present.
- Administer magnesium 1 to 2 g diluted in 10 mL D_5W IV push, even when the serum magnesium concentration is normal.
- Consider lidocaine.
- Consider electrical overdrive pacing at rates of 100 to 120/min.
- Consider pharmacologic overdrive pacing with isoproterenol at 2 to 10 mcg/kg per minute; titrate to increase heart rate until VT is suppressed.[26]
- Some toxicologists recommend supplemental potassium administration even when the serum potassium concentration is normal.

Critical Concept **Drug-Induced VT**	Suspect drug-induced VT whenever a poisoned patient demonstrates a sudden conversion to a wide-complex rhythm with hypotension. If the patient is unstable and polymorphic VT is present, use high-energy unsynchronized shocks (defibrillation doses).

Table 48. Most Common Medications Associated With Torsades de Pointes[27]

Sotalol	Digoxin
Cisapride	Procainamide
Amiodarone	Terodiline
Erythromycin	Fluconazole
Ibutilide	Disopyramide
Terfenadine	Bepridil
Quinidine	Furosemide
Clarithromycin	Thioridazine
Haloperidol	Flecanide
Fluoxetine	Loratidine

Reproduced from Yap and Camm,[27] with permission from BMJ Publishing Group Ltd.

Shock

Drug-induced shock results from 1 of 3 mechanisms or from a combination of factors. The drug induces

- A *decrease in intravascular volume*
- A *fall in systemic vascular resistance*
- *Diminished myocardial contractility*

These combined aspects of cardiovascular dysfunction render drug-induced shock refractory to many standard therapies.

Drug-Induced Hypovolemic Shock (With Normal Systemic Vascular Resistance)

Ingestion and overdose of some drugs or poisoning with chemicals (eg, zinc salts) can cause excessive fluid loss through the gastrointestinal tract, which results in pure hypovolemia. However, drug-induced shock typically includes cardiovascular dysfunction with decreased myocardial contractility and low systemic vascular resistance (SVR), which necessitates the use of a combination of volume therapy and myocardial support.

Fluid Challenge

Initial treatment must include a fluid challenge (250 to 500 mL of normal saline) to correct hypovolemia and optimize cardiac preload. If the offending agent is cardiotoxic, it will reduce the patient's ability to tolerate excess intravascular volume. Volume therapy may lead to iatrogenic congestive heart failure with pulmonary edema.

Vasopressors and Inotropes

If shock persists after an adequate fluid challenge, start an infusion to maintain blood pressure and cardiac output. Most patients with drug-induced shock have decreased myocardial contractility and decreased SVR. Dopamine is an effective vasopressor and inotrope in mild to moderate poisonings.[28,29] The usual infusion rate is 2 to 20 mcg/kg per minute titrated to response. When drug-induced shock is unresponsive to volume loading and conventional doses of dopamine, a potent vasoconstrictor such as norepinephrine may be needed if the primary toxic effect is vasodilation. If both vasoconstriction and inotropic support are needed, a mixed adrenergic drug such as epinephrine may be the best choice. Central hemodynamic monitoring with a pulmonary artery or central venous catheter may be helpful, but do not delay treatment of hypotension. Optimize cardiac preload quickly, making sure that hypovolemia is treated, then use calculated cardiac output and SVR to guide selection and titration of a vasopressor and inotropic agent.

Drug-Induced Distributive Shock (Normal Volume With Decreased SVR)

Distributive shock is associated with normal or even high cardiac output and low SVR and requires treatment with α-adrenergic drugs such as norepinephrine. Vasopressin may also be useful.[30] More powerful vasoconstrictors such as endothelin have not been well studied. Monitor for the development of ventricular arrhythmias with the use of these agents.

Norepinephrine or Phenylephrine

In distributive shock, use more potent vasoconstrictive agents with greater α-adrenergic effect (norepinephrine or phenylephrine). Increase the dose of the α-adrenergic vasopressor until the shock is adequately treated or adverse effects (eg, ventricular arrhythmias) begin to appear. Some poisoned patients require doses of vasopressors far above conventional doses, so-called high-dose vasopressor therapy. Consider use of powerful vasoconstrictors, such as *vasopressin*, in severely poisoned patients if other adrenergic agents produce ventricular arrhythmias before the shock is adequately treated.

Drug-Induced Cardiogenic Shock (Low Cardiac Output, Low SVR)

Drug-induced cardiogenic shock can be associated with low cardiac output and low SVR. Cardiac ischemia may also be present in these patients. In addition to volume titration and use of sympathomimetic drugs such as dobutamine, agents such as milrinone, calcium, glucagon, insulin, or even isoproterenol may provide inotropic support.[11,12] Concurrent vasopressor therapy is often required.[31]

Inotropic and Vasopressor Agents

Agents used successfully in some studies include *inamrinone* and *dobutamine*, as well as *calcium, glucose,* and *insulin.*[32-34] In some patients more than 1 agent is necessary. Often a concomitant vasopressor is required.[31]

Critical Concept Drug-Induced Distributive Shock	Distributive shock is associated with normal or even high cardiac output and low SVR. • Treatment with α-adrenergic drugs such as norepinephrine or phenylephrine may be needed. • Avoid dobutamine and isoproterenol, which may worsen hypotension by further decreasing SVR.

Acute Coronary Syndromes

Chest discomfort is a common complaint of cocaine users. The vast majority of patients have only transient chest pain with no evidence of acute ischemia on ECG. In some patients, an acute coronary syndrome (ACS) may be due to sympathomimetic-induced coronary artery vasospasm. Although rare, an acute myocardial infarction (AMI) may occur in cocaine users. (See "Cocaine Toxicity" for more information.)

ACS can result from ischemia caused by the combined effects of cocaine: stimulation of β-adrenergic myocardial receptors results in increased myocardial oxygen demand, and α-adrenergic and serotonin-agonist actions cause coronary artery constriction.

Treatment

Treatment should be provided for both the direct and indirect effects of drug toxicity. Indirect effects may include coronary artery vasospasm, ischemia, and cardiac arrhythmias.

Benzodiazepines and Nitroglycerin

These agents are the first-line agents for treatment of drug-induced ACS.[35,36] Nitroglycerin has been shown to reverse cocaine-induced vasoconstriction when studied in the cardiac catheterization suite.[37] Intra-arterially administered nifedipine for coronary artery vasospasm has been documented.

Phentolamine

Phentolamine, a potent pure α-blocker, has a nitroglycerin-like ability to reverse cocaine-induced vasoconstriction.[38] Consider phentolamine as a second-line therapy.

Precautions

Several studies suggest that administration of β-blockers may worsen cardiac perfusion or produce paradoxical hypertension when cocaine is present.[39,40] Although contradictory evidence exists,[22,23] current recommendations are that pure β-blocker medications in the setting of cocaine are not indicated (Class IIb, LOE C).[24]

Fibrinolytics

The management of ST-elevation myocardial infarction (STEMI) that occurs as a result of cocaine use can be challenging. Although the initial mechanism that reduces coronary flow involves spasm, thrombus evolves in the infarct-related coronary artery because of stasis. Although fibrinolytic therapy has been used in small numbers of reported patients, fibrinolytics are contraindicated if uncontrolled, severe drug-induced hypertension is present. When percutaneous coronary intervention (PCI) is not available, fibrinolytic therapy may be appropriate if no contraindications are present and the risk-benefit ratio is favorable.

Aortic dissection has been reported with cocaine use. Fibrinolytics should be avoided in patients at risk for, or suspected to have, aortic dissection or cerebral hemorrhage. Careful physical examination and chest x-ray should be obtained before intiation of fibrinolytic therapy. Emergent ultrasound imaging of the chest and aorta should be obtained when aortic dissection is suspected, if possible. Focal neurologic signs or symptoms should prompt appropriate emergent imaging to rule out carotid artery dissection or intracerebral bleeding.

Most experts prefer PCI for drug-induced ACS, especially when coronary atherosclerosis is known to be present or may be present (older age, risk factors). If emergency cardiac catheterization reveals a thrombus without atherosclerotic disease, PCI with intracoronary antithrombin may be used. If a heavy thrombus load is present, antiplatelet therapy (eg, abciximab) may be needed.

Hemodynamically Significant Tachycardia

Tachycardia secondary to drug ingestion or poisoning is common. Hemodynamically significant tachycardia is much less common. It rarely may cause myocardial ischemia, myocardial infarction, or ventricular arrhythmias and may lead to high-output heart failure and shock. Adenosine and synchronized cardioversion are unlikely to be of benefit in this context given the ongoing presence of a toxin, although some drug-induced tachyarrhythmias may be treated successfully with adenosine.[41] In patients with borderline hypotension, diltiazem and verapamil are contraindicated because they may further lower blood pressure. Mild tachycardia by itself, in the absence of other symptoms, may not require direct therapy.

Treatment

Benzodiazepines

Benzodiazepines such as diazepam or lorazepam are generally safe and effective for the treatment of symptomatic drug-induced tachycardia that results from excess cathecholamine release due to sympathomimetic agents. Benzodiazepines are particularly helpful in the treatment of cocaine toxicity because they appear to attenuate the toxic myocardial and CNS effects of cocaine.[36,42,43] When large quantities of benzodiazepines are used to treat poisoning or overdose, providers must closely monitor the patient's level of consciousness, ventilatory effort, and respiratory function because of the sedative effects of benzodiazepines.

Physostigmine

Physostigmine is a specific antidote that may be preferable for drug-induced hemodynamically significant tachycardia and central anticholinergic syndrome caused by pure anticholinergic poisoning, such as with diphenhydramine or Jimson weed.[44] Use with caution because it may produce symptoms of cholinergic crisis, such as copious tracheobronchial secretions, seizures, bradycardia, and even asystole if given in excessive doses or too rapidly. Do not administer physostigmine for anticholinergic symptoms associated with TCA overdose. Consultation with a medical toxicologist or regional poison center is strongly recommended.

Propranolol

Nonselective β-blockers such as propranolol may be effective in drug-induced tachycardia caused by some poisonings, but they should not be administered for cocaine intoxication[20] or amphetamine or ephedrine poisoning. β-Blockers may worsen cardiac perfusion or produce paradoxical hypertension in patients with cocaine intoxication.[20,21]

Hypertensive Emergencies

Drug-induced hypertensive emergencies are frequently short-lived. When treatment is indicated, administer a benzodiazepine, because this class of medication decreases the effects of endogenous catecholamine release. Hypertensive emergencies frequently develop in patients with cocaine toxicity.

Treatment

Initiate antihypertensive therapy when hypertension is severe or coexisting conditions require lowering of blood pressure. If the high blood pressure is refractory to adequate treatment with benzodiazepines, begin treatment with antihypertensive agents. Use short-acting antihypertensive agents because of the short-lived nature of many hypertensive episodes and the possible occurrence of hypotension after resolution.

Benzodiazepines

Most toxicology experts consider benzodiazepines the first-line therapy for hypertension in cases of sympathomimetic overdose (eg, cocaine or amphetamine intoxication).

Nitroprusside

In drug-induced hypertensive emergencies refractory to benzodiazepines, use a short-acting antihypertensive such as nitroprusside as the second line of therapy.

Combined α/β-Blockade

Administration of phentolamine and a nonselective α-antagonist, such as labetalol, can provide both α- and β-blockade. However, most experts now recommend against the use of *any* β-blocker if a sympathomimetic such as cocaine is the suspected cause of the hypertensive emergency.[45]

Cocaine Toxicity

Although arrhythmias and cardiac arrest caused by cocaine are relatively uncommon, cocaine use of any type by any route can cause disastrous complications.[46,47]

Cocaine first stimulates the release and then blocks the reuptake of norepinephrine, epinephrine, dopamine, and serotonin[46,48] (Figure 106). Cocaine abusers experience an elevation in blood pressure, tachycardia, and feelings of euphoria coupled with decreased fatigue. Seizures, myocardial infarctions, and deaths have occurred in users who have taken only small quantities of the drug.[46,49,50]

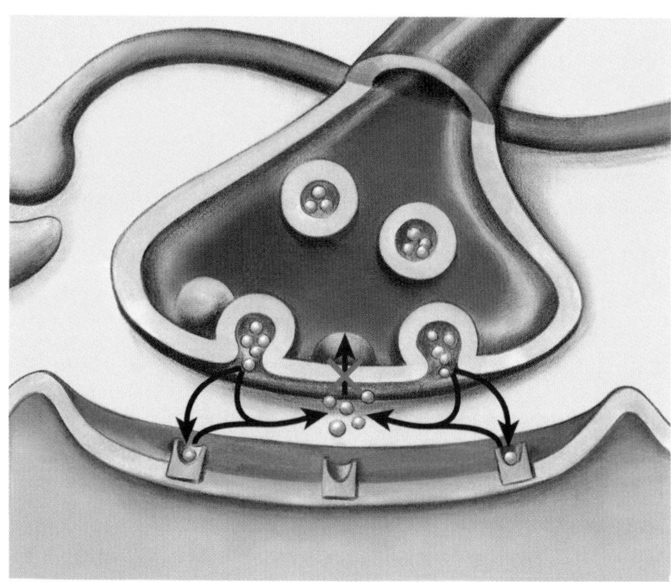

Figure 106. Mechanism of cocaine toxicity. Reproduced from Lange and Hillis,[42] copyright © 2001 Massachusetts Medical Society. With permission from Massachusetts Medical Society.

Cardiac Toxicity

Serious cocaine-induced cardiac toxicity stems from the direct effect of cocaine on the heart. Cocaine causes myocardial ischemia through complex pathophysiologic mechanisms[42] and provokes the CNS to stimulate the cardiovascular system. The β-adrenergic effects of cocaine increase heart rate and myocardial contractility. The α-adrenergic effects of cocaine decrease coronary blood flow and may induce coronary artery spasm. Cocaine increases platelet adhesiveness, which leads to increased risk of coronary thrombosis. These mechanisms lead to decreased coronary artery perfusion at a time of increased myocardial oxygen demand. Hypoxia from pulmonary edema and acidosis from cocaine-induced seizures may exacerbate the cardiotoxicity of cocaine. In long-term cocaine users, atherosclerosis and left ventricular hypertrophy develop at an accelerated pace.

Cocaine toxicity may cause thermoregulatory problems, including hyperpyrexia. A rise in the patient's body temperature can worsen existing tachycardia and neurologic symptoms. High ambient temperatures have also been associated with a significant increase in mortality in patients with cocaine toxicity.[42,49]

Cocaine-Induced Arrhythmias

All patients with cocaine-induced CNS symptoms or cardiovascular complications require close observation. Treat fever and cool patients who present with agitation, delirium, seizures, and elevated body temperature. If an arrhythmia or ACS is present, administer oxygen and provide continuous ECG monitoring.

Supraventricular Arrhythmias

Cocaine-induced supraventricular arrhythmias include paroxysmal supraventricular tachycardia, rapid atrial fibrillation, and atrial flutter.[51] These arrhythmias are often short-lived and seldom require therapy unless hemodynamic compromise is also present.[52-54]

Benzodiazepine

Treat persistent supraventricular arrhythmias in hemodynamically stable patients with a benzodiazepine, such as *diazepam* in a dose of 5 to 20 mg IV over 5 to 20 minutes.

Stable Ventricular Tachycardia

Nonarrest ventricular arrhythmias caused by cocaine include ventricular ectopy, episodes of nonsustained VT, and stable monomorphic and polymorphic VT.[55,56]

Benzodiazepine

Like supraventricular arrhythmias, ventricular ectopy and tachycardia are often transient and may require only careful observation. Most experienced clinicians will administer a benzodiazepine in a titrated fashion.

Antiarrhythmic Therapy

In severe overdose, cocaine acts as a Vaughan Williams class Ic antiarrhythmic, producing wide-complex tachycardia through several mechanisms, including blockade of cardiac sodium channels.[57] Although there is no human evidence of its benefit in cocaine poisoning, extrapolation from evidence in the treatment of wide-complex tachycardia caused by other class Ic agents (flecainide) and TCAs suggests that administration of hypertonic sodium bicarbonate may be beneficial.[57] A typical treatment strategy used for these other sodium channel blockers involves administration of 1 mL/kg sodium bicarbonate solution (8.4%, 1 mEq/mL) IV as a bolus, repeated as needed until hemodynamic stability is restored and QRS duration is 120 ms.[58-65]

Many experts recommend lidocaine at the standard dose of 1 to 1.5 mg/kg for treatment of ventricular arrhythmias unresponsive to a titrated benzodiazepine. Cocaine, an anesthetic agent, has properties of a sodium channel blocker (class I_{VW} antiarrhythmic). Lidocaine, which acts as a similar sodium channel blocker (class I_{VW} antiarrhythmic), competes with cocaine at the sodium channel, thus decreasing the effects of cocaine. Current evidence neither supports nor refutes a role for lidocaine in the management of wide-complex tachycardia caused by cocaine.

Sodium Bicarbonate

Some experimental animal studies and human case reports[66,67] support the use of sodium bicarbonate (1 to 2 mEq/kg) in the treatment of cocaine-induced VF and VT.[68] Most toxicologists agree with early use of sodium bicarbonate in the management of ventricular tachycardias that result from the use of cocaine.[42,68,69]

Defibrillation

As a precaution, have a defibrillator available at the bedside. Healthcare providers can preattach adhesive defibrillator pads and perform cardiac monitoring by conventional defibrillator/monitors.

Critical Concept Nonselective β-Blocking Agents (Propranolol)	*Propranolol* (a nonselective β-blocker) is contraindicated for drug-induced hypertension. It may block only β-receptors, leaving unopposed α-adrenergic stimulation and worsening cardiac output and perfusion.[20,21]

VF

There are no data to support the use of cocaine-specific interventions in the setting of cardiac arrest due to cocaine overdose. Resuscitation from cardiac arrest should follow standard BLS and ACLS algorithms, with specific antidotes used in the postresuscitation phase if severe cardiotoxicity or neurotoxicity is encountered. A single case series demonstrated excellent overall and neurologically intact survival (55%) in patients with cardiac arrest associated with cocaine overdose who were treated with standard therapy.[70]

Cocaine-Induced Hypertension and Pulmonary Edema

Cocaine-Induced Hypertension

Cocaine toxicity can produce hypertensive emergencies through effects on the CNS and peripheral α-agonist stimulation. Hypertensive patients should initially be treated with a benzodiazepine in an attempt to minimize the stimulatory effects of cocaine on the CNS and cardiovascular system.[71,72]

Patients who require additional therapy should be treated with a vasodilator such as nitroglycerin or nitroprusside in a titrated dose. Nitroglycerin is preferable in patients with superimposed chest pain.

Although contradictory evidence exists,[22,23] current recommendations are that pure β-blocker medications in the setting of cocaine are not indicated (Class IIb, LOE C).[24] They have the potential to raise blood pressure by antagonizing cocaine-induced β-receptor stimulation and allowing unopposed cocaine-induced α-receptor stimulation. Labetalol, with both α- and β-blocker effects, has shown inferior results compared with *nitroglycerin* or *nitroprusside* and should be avoided.[73,74] A pure α-blocker such as phentolamine (1 mg every 2 to 3 minutes; up to 10 mg) may be used.[75]

Cocaine-Induced Pulmonary Edema

Pulmonary edema can occur from the effects of cocaine on pulmonary dynamics, from a cocaine-induced myocardial infarction, as a result of associated subarachnoid hemorrhage, or as a consequence of additional drugs of abuse.[48,76-78] *Positive-pressure ventilation* with a continuous positive airway pressure mask or intubation supplemented by positive end-expiratory pressure will usually rapidly correct hypoxemia.

Cocaine-Induced ACS

Although rare, AMIs do occur in cocaine users. Most cocaine-related infarctions occur in patients who smoke cigarettes or who have other cardiac risk factors.[50,79,80] The risk of myocardial infarction can increase as much as 24-fold in the first hour after cocaine use,[81] and most cocaine-associated myocardial infarctions occur within 24 hours of use.[80] Nonetheless, spontaneous episodes of ST-segment elevation have been documented on ambulatory monitoring up to 6 weeks after last use of cocaine.[82]

Cocaine-related myocardial ischemia should be treated with *oxygen, aspirin, nitrates,* and a titrated dose of a *benzodiazepine*.[37,72] β-Blockers should *not* be used because of the possibility of α-mediated vasospasm.[20] Because of its antispasmodic effects and its beneficial role in myocardial infarction, *magnesium* can also be used for cocaine-related ischemia and infarction.[83,84] *Morphine* should be administered for continued pain.

STEMI and Reperfusion Therapy in Cocaine Toxicity

Perhaps half of all cocaine-related myocardial infarctions appear to be caused by spasm, not plaque rupture. Indications for fibrinolytic therapy must be reviewed in light of the fact that "false-positive" ST-segment changes are common in cocaine users.[85] Before starting fibrinolytic therapy, some clinicians require a diagnostic echocardiogram or evidence of infarction by a rapid assay technique of cardiac markers. These dilemmas have led many experts to prefer cardiac catheterization with coronary angiography.

Treatment Considerations of the Cardiovascular Complications of Cocaine Use

Evidence-Based Treatment?

High-quality, prospective, multicenter cohort evaluations have provided valuable information regarding the treatment of cocaine-associated ACS.[86,87] Most consensus recommendations, however, are supported by evidence from case series, reasonable extrapolations from existing data, and rational conjecture (common sense) or common practices accepted before evidence-based guidelines.

Treatment Comparisons: Cocaine-Related vs Cocaine-Unrelated ACS

Benzodiazepines. Benzodiazepines are recommended for patients with cocaine-associated ACS even though these agents are not routinely used in patients with ACS unrelated to cocaine.[42,53,88,89]

β-Blockers. Despite the success of β-blockers in AMI unrelated to cocaine, they are contraindicated for cocaine-associated ACS. See "The Evidence Against Use of β-Adrenergic Antagonists (β-Blockers) in Cocaine-Related AMI."[20,21,90]

Reperfusion Therapy. Reperfusion therapy for patients with STEMI in the setting of cocaine use or toxicity has the same priority as reperfusion therapy in general. Coronary flow to the ischemic region should be established as soon as possible. In patients using cocaine, the proximate cause of STEMI may be coronary spasm, which when combined with decreased coronary blood flow eventually causes intracoronary thrombus. Many experts prefer PCI to assess the status of the coronary artery involved.

Emergency Treatment of Cocaine-Induced ACS

Attempts to reduce is reverse the coronary vasoconstriction, hypertension, tachycardia, and predisposition to thrombus formation are the mainstays of cocaine-associated myocardial ischemia treatment. The objective is to improve coronary artery perfusion and oxygen delivery while reducing myocardial oxygen demand.

Benzodiazepines. Diazepam is the initial agent for treating all cocaine-intoxicated patients.[36,53] Benzodiazepines protect the CNS while decreasing sympathetic outflow, which calms the patient and returns vital signs to the normal range.

Nitroglycerin. Specific anti-ischemic therapy begins with *nitroglycerin*. The recommendation for nitrates is based on experimental reversal of coronary vasoconstriction in humans and clinical relief of chest pain.[35-37]

Antiplatelet and Antithrombotic Agents. Attempts to decrease the acute coagulability of blood with *aspirin* or *heparin* are recommended with some support from clinical reports specific to cocaine users.[91] The current understanding of the pharmacology of these agents suggests some value.

Management of Refractory ACS

Patients with ischemia refractory to the above measures can be treated with either *phentolamine*, *calcium antagonists*, or *reperfusion therapy*.[88]

Phentolamine. Phentolamine blocks the α-adrenergic effects of cocaine and reverses the coronary vasoconstrictive effects of cocaine.[38] Because phentolamine may result in hypotension, use of small incremental doses (1 mg every 2 to 3 minutes) is recommended.

Calcium Antagonists. Data on the efficacy of *calcium channel blockers* for the treatment of cocaine toxicity are contradictory.

- In a human cardiac catheterization model of cocaine toxicity, verapamil successfully reversed cocaine-induced coronary artery vasoconstriction.[92]
- In multicenter clinical trials in patients with ACS *not* associated with cocaine toxicity, researchers found no benefit from calcium channel blockers on important outcomes such as survival.
- In studies of cocaine-poisoned animals pretreated with calcium channel blockers, investigators have observed favorable results for a variety of end points, such as better survival, fewer seizures, and fewer cardiac arrhythmias, but in other studies investigators have found adverse effects.

The Evidence Against Use of β-Adrenergic Antagonists (β-Blockers) in Cocaine-Related AMI

Despite the success of β-blockers in patients with AMI unrelated to cocaine, β-blockers are contraindicated in recent cocaine users.[88] Clinicians should not administer β-blockers or mixed α/β-blockers to patients who have recently used cocaine.

- β-Blockers increase CNS toxicity and exacerbate coronary artery vasospasm in animal models of cocaine toxicity.
- β-blockers do not reverse the hypertensive and tachycardic effects of cocaine.[21]
- Studies in human volunteers show that β-blockers exacerbate cocaine-induced coronary artery vasoconstriction.[20]
- Scientific agreement has not been established on the role, if any, of either pure β- or mixed α/β-blockers in the treatment of cocaine intoxication. Labetalol does not appear to offer any advantages over pure β-antagonists even though it produced no adverse outcomes in some cases.[73,93,94] The evidence does not support the use of labetalol.

Hemodynamically Significant Bradycardia

Hemodynamically significant bradycardia from poisoning or drug overdose may be refractory to standard ACLS protocols because some toxins bind receptors or produce direct cellular toxicity. In these cases, specific antidote therapy may be needed. For example, therapeutic options for refractory hemodynamic instability caused by β-blocker overdose include glucagon, high-dose insulin, or IV calcium salts. Calcium channel blocker overdose has been treated with calcium and high-dose insulin when routine measures have been ineffective. Digoxin-specific antibody (Fab) can neutralize digoxin and other plant- and animal-derived cardiac glycosides.

Treatments

Atropine

The administration of atropine may be lifesaving in poisoning from cholinesterase inhibitors such as organophosphate, carbamate, or nerve agents. The recommended starting adult dose for insecticide poisoning from cholinesterase inhibitors is 2 to 4 mg or higher. In these cases, doses well in excess of accepted maximums may be required.

Pacing

Transcutaneous cardiac pacing may be effective in cases of mild to moderate drug-induced bradycardia. Prophylactic transvenous pacing is not recommended because the tip of the transvenous catheter may trigger ventricular arrhythmias when the myocardium is irritable (eg, as in digoxin toxicity). However, transvenous pacing is needed if transcutaneous pacing fails or is poorly tolerated or if electrical capture is difficult to maintain.

β-Agonists

In drug-induced bradycardia resistant to atropine and pacing, chronotropic drugs with β-adrenergic agonist activity are indicated. The most commonly used infusions are dopamine and epinephrine titrated to response. Doses much larger than usual may be needed in cases of β-blocker or calcium channel blocker overdose. Norepinephrine has also been used.

Isoproterenol is contraindicated in most drug-induced bradycardias, including acetylcholinesterase-induced bradycardias, because it causes vasodilation that may induce or aggravate hypotension and ventricular arrhythmias. However, it may be useful at high doses in refractory bradycardia induced by β-antagonist receptor blockade.

Digoxin-Specific Antibody (Fab) Fragments

This therapy is extremely effective for life-threatening ventricular arrhythmias and atrioventricular (AV) nodal blockade caused by digoxin and cardiac glycoside poisoning. AV block and ventricular arrhythmias associated with certain Chinese herbal medications, digoxin, or other plant- or animal-derived cardiac glycoside poisoning may be treated effectively with digoxin-specific antibody fragment therapy (Fab).[95-99] These plant and animal sources include oleander, squill, lily-of-the-valley, and toad skin.

Calcium Channel Blocker and β-Blocker Toxicity

Both calcium channel blockers and β-blockers have negative inotropic (contractility) and negative chronotropic (heart rate) effects. Whereas calcium channel blockers possess varying degrees of direct vasodilatory properties,[100] β-blockers do not.[101]

Toxicity from calcium channel blockers and β-blockers can produce the following signs and symptoms:

- Hypotension
- Depression of myocardial contractility
- Bradycardias from depression of sinoatrial nodal, AV nodal, and intraventricular conduction; heart block
- Decreased level of consciousness, lethargy, or even coma
- Seizures (which may be the initial sign of serious toxicity), usually caused by hypoperfusion of the CNS
- Hypoglycemia, hyperkalemia with β-blocker overdose
- Hyperglycemia associated with calcium channel blocker overdose
- Sudden decompensation to profound shock within minutes
- Cardiac arrest caused by refractory AV block or pulseless electrical activity

β-Blocker overdose may also cause a variety of arrhythmias, including torsades de pointes, VF, AV block, and in rare cases asystole.

Time Course

Signs and symptoms of overdose from either calcium channel blockers or β-blockers typically develop within 2 to 4 hours of ingestion of *regular-release* preparations. Failure to develop symptoms within 4 to 6 hours of regular-release ingestion indicates that moderate to severe toxicity is unlikely to occur. Toxic effects of controlled-release and long-acting preparations, however, may not be seen for up to 6 to 18 hours after ingestion.

Common Therapy for Calcium Channel and β-Blocker Overdoses

There are no data to support the use of specific antidotes in the setting of cardiac arrest caused by calcium channel blocker overdose. Resuscitation from cardiac arrest should follow standard BLS and ACLS algorithms.

Initial therapies recommended by consensus include the following:

- Administer oxygen and monitor airway and ventilation (particularly if level of consciousness is depressed or seizures develop).
- Provide continuous ECG monitoring and be prepared to treat symptomatic or unstable arrhythmias.
- Perform careful assessment of blood pressure and hemodynamic status.
- Establish vascular access with 2 large-bore catheters.
- If hypotension is present, give a fluid challenge of 500 to 1000 mL of normal saline.[102,103] Monitor closely for signs of myocardial dysfunction and development of pulmonary edema.
- Determine the blood glucose concentration with a bedside rapid test.
- Consider activated charcoal for gastric decontamination in patients who are awake and alert and who present within 1 hour of ingestion with only mild hemodynamic effects.[104,105]
- Orogastric lavage may be useful in patients who have ingested a significant amount of drug within 1 hour of presentation and are symptomatic (eg, seizures, hypotension, bradycardia). Airway protection, with possible rapid sequence intubation, should be performed.

- Whole-bowel irrigation may be considered with polyethylene glycol in persons who have ingested long-acting preparations.
- Perform whole-bowel irrigation when toxic quantities of controlled-release preparations have been consumed, medications may be seen on the abdominal x-ray, and only if bowel sounds are still present.[104]
- Do not give syrup of ipecac, because it has delayed onset and a propensity to worsen bradycardia through vomiting-induced increases in vagal tone. In addition, calcium blockers and β-blockers can cause rapid declines in hemodynamic stability, altered mental status, and seizures before ipecac can take effect.[106]

Specific Therapy for Calcium Channel Blocker Overdose

Immediate vascular access is a priority for the treatment of myocardial dysfunction and hypotension.

Hypotension and Shock

Give a *normal saline* fluid challenge, 1 to 2 boluses, 500 to 1000 mL each. Monitor for development of pulmonary edema. If hemodynamically significant signs and symptoms continue, add the following:

- *Epinephrine* infusion at 2 mcg/min and titrate up to 100 mcg/min. Catecholamine-like vasopressors (norepinephrine is another example) are the first-line drug therapy for hemodynamically significant hypotension or shock caused by calcium channel blocker toxicity.[107,108]
- Consider *calcium chloride* 8 to 16 mg/kg (usually 5 to 10 mL or 0.5 to 1 g of a 10% solution from 10-mL vials with 100 mg/mL) if the shock fails to respond adequately to the fluid challenges and the epinephrine or norepinephrine infusion.
- Additional *IV calcium (*slow IV push or continued infusion) to a total dose of 1 to 3 g IV is appropriate for patients who experience a positive hemodynamic response to the initial calcium infusion. Epinephrine and other α-agonists may sensitize the vasculature to the effects of calcium.

Bradycardia

Refractory hemodynamically significant bradycardia caused by calcium channel blocker toxicity is treated with immediate transcutaneous pacing while preparations are made for transvenous access and pacing.

Additional Therapies to Consider

In specific cases and refractory patients, additional lifesaving measures and supportive therapy have been used. These therapies generally have been published as case reports or are supported only by animal data.

- *Glucose/insulin infusion:* Infusions of glucose and insulin have been used in the treatment of calcium channel blocker overdose.[109,110]
- *Glucagon:* Myocardial toxicity caused by calcium channel blockers has responded to the inotropic agent glucagon.[111] Administer in a dose of 1 to 5 mg IV.
- *Circulatory assist devices:* Devices such as the intra-aortic balloon pump or extracorporeal membrane oxygenation[112] should be considered if available for patients refractory to *maximal* medical therapy.
- *There is good evidence* that calcium salts may be beneficial in cases of mild to moderate calcium channel blocker poisoning. Stimulation of the α- and β-adrenergic receptors is believed to increase intracellular levels of calcium and to help reduce calcium channel blocker toxicity. Patients with severe, refractory calcium channel blocker–induced shock may benefit from modest doses of calcium salts.

Specific Therapy for β-Blocker Overdose

General measures are the same as those for calcium channel blocker overdose. Immediate vascular access is a priority for the treatment of myocardial dysfunction and hypotension. The following treatment sequence for hypotension and hemodynamic instability can be individualized and requires continual assessment and reassessment.

Hypotension and Shock

Give a *normal saline* fluid challenge, 1 to 2 boluses, 500 to 1000 mL each. Monitor for development of pulmonary edema. If hemodynamically significant signs and symptoms continue, add the following:

- *Vasopressors:* If hemodynamically significant hypotension is present, treat with a vasopressor with moderate to high α-adrenergic activity, such as *epinephrine* infused at 0.1 to 0.5 mcg/kg per minute.
- *Glucagon:* In patients with mild to moderate shock unresponsive to vasopressors, glucagon can be administered at a dose of 1 to 5 mg IV. One method of administration is to give a 3 mg IV bolus and then initiate a continuous infusion at 3 mg/h, with titration as necessary. For severe cardiovascular instability, the recommended dose of glucagon is a bolus of 3 to 10 mg, administered slowly over 3 to 5 minutes, followed by an infusion of 3 to 5 mg/h (0.05 to 0.15 mg/kg followed by an infusion of 0.05 to 0.10 mg/kg per hour) (Class IIb, LOE C).[113]
- *Isoproterenol:* Isoproterenol can be used carefully as an adjunct with an epinephrine infusion or in combination with other agents, although significant improvement is rare. Do not use isoproterenol as a first-line agent.
- *Calcium:* Calcium infusions (8 to 16 mg/kg, usually 5 to 10 mL or 0.5 to 1 g of a 10% solution from 10-mL vials with 100 mg/mL) may be of benefit in β-blocker–induced shock that is unresponsive to glucagon and epinephrine. However, calcium cannot be recommended specifically because of data from conflicting clinical case reports.[114,115]

Bradycardia

- *Refractory, hemodynamically significant bradycardia:* If hemodynamically significant bradycardia is present, add pacing (either transvenous or transcutaneous).
- Additional therapies to consider:
  - *Atropine:* Although not harmful, atropine is rarely effective in β-blocker–induced bradycardia or in reversal of symptomatic AV block.
  - *Circulatory assist devices:* As with calcium channel blocker overdose, circulatory assist devices or extracorporeal circulation may be effective for drug-induced shock that fails to respond to maximal medical therapy, but this approach must be started before irreversible end-organ damage has occurred.
  - *Glucose-insulin infusion:* This therapy may produce hypokalemia unless potassium is monitored and supplementation provided.

Digitalis and Cardiac Glycoside Overdose

Digitalis-induced cardiac toxicity may develop in acute overdose or in long-term users of this widely prescribed medication.

Signs and Symptoms of Digitalis Toxicity

Many of the early symptoms of digitalis intoxication are nonspecific signs of CNS and gastrointestinal toxicity. Fatigue, visual symptoms, weakness, nausea, vomiting, and abdominal pain are common. Cardiac arrhythmias occur in patients with digitalis toxicity. The most common arrhythmias are ventricular ectopy and bradycardia, often in association with various degrees of AV block. The following rhythm disturbances should immediately suggest digitalis intoxication: atrial tachycardia with high-degree AV block, nonparoxysmal accelerated junctional tachycardia, multifocal VT, new-onset bigeminy, and regularized atrial fibrillation.

Cardiac Toxicity of Digitalis

The cardiac toxicity of digitalis is caused by the combination of its inhibitory effects on nodal conduction and its excitatory effects on individual atrial and ventricular fibers. Life-threatening digitalis toxicity most often is caused by

- Bradyarrhythmias with resultant congestive heart failure
- Malignant ventricular arrhythmias
- Hyperkalemia that results from digitalis poisoning of the sodium-potassium adenosine triphosphatase pump

General Approach to Treatment of Digitalis Toxicity

The treatment of arrhythmias caused by digitalis toxicity is determined by the acuity of the overdose and the patient's hemodynamic function.

Management of Digitalis Toxicity Associated With Chronic Therapy

Digitalis intoxication in long-term users generally develops in association with hypokalemia, hypomagnesemia, dehydration, declining renal function, or loss of muscle mass. Cardiotoxicity in these patients is initially treated by

- Replenishing total body potassium
- Replenishing total body magnesium stores[116]
- Replacing volume with normal saline

If the patient with digitalis toxicity is hypokalemic, assume that he is also hypomagnesemic until proven otherwise. Rapid replacement of potassium, magnesium, and volume will usually correct most arrhythmias in long-term digitalis users within a few hours. For severe toxicity consider use of digoxin-specific antibody (Fab fragments).

Management of Acute Digitalis Overdose

Gastric Decontamination With Activated Charcoal

Emergency physicians should consider decontamination with activated charcoal in all patients with an acute digitalis overdose who present within 1 hour of ingestion.[105,117] Syrup of ipecac is not useful in the hospital care of patients with digitalis overdose; other gastric emptying techniques are available.[106]

Life-Threatening Digitalis Overdose

Digoxin-specific antibodies (Fab) should be administered to patients with severe life-threatening cardiac glycoside toxicity (Class I, LOE B).[95-97,118-124]

Precautions

Patients with digitalis toxicity are more prone to pacemaker-induced ventricular rhythm disturbances. Use of transvenous pacemakers should be highly selective,[125] if not contraindicated. It is advisable to seek expert guidance.

When arrhythmias develop, perform cardioversion or defibrillation when indicated. However, patients with digitalis toxicity may develop malignant ventricular arrhythmias or asystole after cardioversion. For this reason a lower initial cardioversion dose is used. (see "Critical Concept: Synchronized Cardioversion in Unstable VT Associated With Digitalis Toxicity").

Patients with digitalis toxicity develop high levels of intracellular calcium, so do not give them additional calcium salts.[126] The use of calcium may delay depolarization and be proarrhythmic. Hypokalemia and hypomagnesemia are risk factors for development of digitalis toxicity, although hyperkalemia may be present with acute severe toxicity (see below).

Management of Digitalis-Induced Symptomatic Bradycardias

Atropine

Patients with symptomatic bradycardia and AV block should initially receive atropine in doses starting at 0.5 mg IV. Because of the vagally mediated effects of digitalis, atropine may temporarily reverse digitalis intoxication associated with bradycardia.[116,127]

Digoxin-Specific Antibody (Fab) Fragment Therapy

The availability of digoxin-specific antibodies (Fab) fragments to treat severe chronic and acute toxicity has dramatically reduced morbidity and mortality from digitalis intoxication. Fab fragments bind to free digoxin, which results in an inactive compound that is excreted in the urine. Effects begin in minutes; complete reversal of digitalis-mediated effects most often occurs within 30 minutes of administration.[128]

Indications for Fab Fragment Therapy

The indications for Fab fragment therapy are digoxin toxicity in association with

- Cardiac arrest
- Life-threatening arrhythmias refractory to conventional therapy
- Shock or congestive heart failure
- Hyperkalemia (K^+ more than 5 mEq/L) in the setting of acute ingestion
- Steady-state serum digoxin levels above 10 ng/mL more than 6 hours after ingestion or more than 15 ng/mL in adults at any time
- Acute ingestions of more than 10 mg in adults, 4 mg or 0.1 mg/kg in children
- Postdistribution serum digoxin levels greater than 5 ng/mL

Dosing of Fab Fragments

One vial of digoxin-specific antibodies is standardized to neutralize 0.5 mg of digoxin. Although the ideal dose is unknown, a reasonable strategy is as follows:

- If the ingested dose of digoxin is known, administer 2 vials of Fab for every milligram of digoxin ingested.
- In cases of chronic digoxin toxicity or when the ingested dose is not known, calculate the number of vials to administer by using the following formula: Number of vials = serum digoxin concentration (ng/mL) × weight (kg)/100.
- In critical cases in which therapy is required before a serum digoxin level can be obtained or in cases of life-threatening toxicity caused by cardiac glycosides, empirically administer 10 to 20 vials. However, in most adults with symptomatic toxicity, 6 vials will often be an adequate starting dose. Doses should ordinarily be rounded up to the next whole vial.
- Hyperkalemia is a marker of severity in acute cardiac glycoside poisoning and is associated with poor prognosis.[129] Digoxin-specific antibody (Fab) may be administered empirically to patients with acute poisoning from digoxin or related cardiac glycosides whose serum potassium levels exceed 5.0 mEq/L.[130]

Management of Digitalis-Induced Ventricular Arrhythmias

Most episodes of digitalis toxicity–induced ventricular ectopy respond to simple administration of potassium, magnesium, and isotonic crystalloid.

Fab Fragment Antibodies

When digitalis toxicity induces stable VT, Fab fragment antibodies combined with rapidly active antiarrhythmics are the treatment of choice.[116]

Lidocaine

Lidocaine is the antiarrhythmic of choice if ventricular arrhythmias persist after administration of potassium, magnesium,

Critical Concept **Synchronized Cardioversion in Unstable VT Associated With Digitalis Toxicity**	• Once digitalis-induced VT becomes clinically unstable, the treatment priorities are – Synchronized cardioversion – Immediate administration of 10 to 20 vials of Fab fragments – Lidocaine – Magnesium sulfate • If the patient is rapidly deteriorating and hemodynamically unstable, give an immediate shock using defibrillation doses. • Synchronized cardioversion attempts are preferable to unsynchronized shocks if the clinical situation allows the slightly longer time required to perform this procedure. • When performing immediate cardioversion, start at low energy levels of 25 to 50 J. The likelihood of postcountershock rhythm deterioration is increased in patients with digitalis toxicity. • If no response, immediately reattempt cardioversion using defibrillation doses. • When possible, sedate the patient before giving shocks.

and normal saline. Lidocaine acts rapidly and rarely causes acute toxicity when used in the recommended dose of 1 to 1.5 mg/kg.[116,127,131] If the patient responds, begin a lidocaine infusion of 1 to 4 mg/min until the Fab fragment therapy is effective. Observe closely for early signs of lidocaine toxicity when placing elderly patients with congestive heart failure or renal impairment on a lidocaine maintenance infusion.

Magnesium

Magnesium has been suggested as the initial drug of choice for digitalis-induced ventricular tachyarrhythmias.[132,133] A dose of 1 to 2 g of magnesium sulfate diluted in 10 mL of D_5W and given by IV push over 1 to 2 minutes may be used as first-line therapy. Some providers use magnesium only in patients with ventricular tachyarrhythmias unresponsive to lidocaine. A continuous magnesium infusion of 1 to 2 g (8 to 16 mEq) of magnesium diluted in 50 to 100 mL of D_5W given over 1 hour and then 0.5 to 1 g per hour may be required for continued arrhythmia suppression.

Hypomagnesemia increases myocardial digoxin uptake and decreases cellular sodium/potassium-ATPase activity. Patients may become cardiotoxic even with therapeutic digitalis levels as a result of hypomagnesemia or hypokalemia. An intravenous dose of 1 to 2 g/hour with serial monitoring of serum magnesium levels, potassium levels, telemetry, respiratory rate, deep tendon reflexes, and blood pressure is advised. **Caution: Magnesium is contraindicated in bradycardia or AV nodal block and should be used cautiously in patients with renal failure.**

Management of Digitalis-Induced VF

There are no data to support the use of specific antidotes in the setting of cardiac arrest due to digoxin overdose. Resuscitation from cardiac arrest should follow standard BLS and ACLS algorithms, with specific antidotes used in the post–cardiac arrest phase if severe cardiotoxicity is encountered.

Drug-Induced Impaired Conduction

Poisonings with sodium channel antagonists (eg, flecainide, procainamide) and TCAs can result in prolonged ventricular conduction.

Treatment

Hypertonic Saline and Systemic Alkalinization

Hypertonic saline and systemic alkalinization may prevent or terminate ventricular tachycardia (VT) secondary to poisoning from sodium channel blocking agents (eg, flecainide, procainamide), TCAs, and cocaine.[60,134,135] *Hypertonic sodium bicarbonate* provides both hypertonic saline and systemic alkalinization.

Calcium channel antagonist and β-adrenergic antagonist overdose may lead to seriously impaired conduction. These patients may require chronotropic adrenergic agents such as epinephrine or high-dose glucagon,[136] or possibly pacing.[108]

Treatment Goals for Systemic Alkalinization for Arrhythmias and Hypotension

In severe poisonings the goal of alkalinization therapy is an arterial pH of 7.45 to 7.55.

- Induction of respiratory alkalosis may provide a temporizing measure.
- Use repeated boluses of 1 to 2 mEq/kg of sodium bicarbonate to reach target pH.
- Maintain alkalinization by infusion of an alkaline solution that consists of 3 ampules of sodium bicarbonate (150 mEq) plus 30 mEq of KCl mixed in 850 mL of D_5W.

Local Anesthetic Toxicity

Inadvertent intravascular administration of local anesthetics, such as bupivacaine, mepivacaine, or lidocaine, can produce refractory seizures and rapid cardiovascular collapse that leads to cardiac arrest.

Clinical case reports[137-141] and controlled animal studies[142-146] have suggested that rapid IV infusion of lipids may reverse this toxicity either by redistributing the local anesthetic away from its site of action or by augmenting metabolic pathways within the cardiac myocyte. Case reports have shown return of spontaneous circulation in patients with prolonged cardiac arrest unresponsive to standard ACLS measures,[147,148] which suggests a role for administration of IV lipids during cardiac arrest. Although ideal dosing has not been determined because dosage varied across all studies, it may be reasonable to consider 1.5 mL/kg of 20% long-chain fatty acid emulsion as an initial bolus, repeated every 5 minutes until cardiovascular stability is restored (Class IIb, LOE C).[149]

After the patient is stabilized, some literature suggests a maintenance infusion of 0.25 mL/kg per minute for at least 30 to 60 minutes. A maximum cumulative dose of 12 mL/kg has been proposed.[149] Some animal data suggest that lipid infusion alone may be more effective than standard doses of epinephrine or vasopressin.[143,146] Although there is limited evidence to change routine care for severe cardiotoxicity, several professional societies advocate the use of clinical protocols.[150-152]

Because this is a rapidly evolving clinical area,[153,154] prompt consultation with a medical toxicologist, anesthesiologist, or other specialist with up-to-date knowledge is strongly recommended.

Tricyclic Antidepressants

When taken in excess, the TCAs are among the most cardiotoxic agents in medicine. Although TCAs rarely cause cardiovascular side effects when taken in therapeutic amounts, they are the number one cause of death from overdose in patients who arrive at the hospital alive.[155]

The toxic side effects of TCAs are caused by the interplay of their 4 major pharmacologic properties. Tricyclics

- Stimulate catecholamine release and then block reuptake at postganglionic synapses
- Have central and peripheral anticholinergic actions
- Inhibit potassium channels in myocardium and fast (voltage-dependent) sodium channels in brain and myocardium
- Have direct α-blocking actions

Major Signs of TCA Toxicity

As a toxic dose of a tricyclic begins to take effect, the following signs appear:

- Alterations in mental status, including agitation, irritability, confusion, delirium, hallucinations, hyperactivity, seizures, and hyperpyrexia
- Sinus tachycardia (especially in association with a rightward QRS axis); wide-complex tachycardia in conjunction with the terminal positive QRS in lead aVR is characteristic of serious TCA toxicity
- Supraventricular tachycardia and hypertension may develop early after ingestion; prolongation of the QT interval
- Anticholinergic effects, such as delirium, mydriasis, urinary retention, and gastric atony

More ominous signs that require immediate therapy include coma, seizures, QRS widening, wide-complex arrhythmias, ventricular arrhythmias, preterminal sinus bradycardia and AV block, and hypotension acidosis. This progression is highly variable and may take minutes to hours. It is often unpredictable. Patients may suddenly deteriorate into cardiac arrest.

The signs of significant TCA overdose may be recalled by the memory aid "Three C's and an A." Note that these may occur in later stages:

- **C**oma
- **C**onvulsions (seizures)
- **C**ardiac arrhythmias
- **A**cidosis

Time Course of TCA Toxicity

Most, but not all, patients will manifest some sign of toxicity within 2 to 4 hours of ingestion of an excessive amount. Patients who are asymptomatic after 6 hours of continuous monitoring, with no QT prolongation on the 12-lead ECG, are at essentially low risk for toxicity.[156,157]

General Management of TCA Overdose

- Activated charcoal may be considered in patients with significant ingestions. Patients with TCA overdose may deteriorate rapidly. Airway protection, oxygen, and IV access are essential. All patients suspected of TCA overdose should be monitored closely. Induction of emesis is contraindicated.
- Patients with decreased mental status, seizures, or inability to control the airway should receive rapid sequence intubation before orogastric lavage.

Bicarbonate for TCA Overdose

Alkalinization With Sodium Bicarbonate

Alkalinization with sodium bicarbonate is the mainstay of therapy for severe TCA overdose.[156,158-160] Alkalinization

- Decreases the free, non–protein-bound form of the tricyclic molecule and overrides the tricyclic-induced sodium channel blockade of phase 0 of the action potential[157]
- Is not required in patients who have only a mild resting tachycardia or stable prolongation of the QT interval
- Is indicated for patients with
  - Prolongation or increase of the QRS to more than 100 milliseconds
  - Ventricular arrhythmias
  - Hypotension unresponsive to a saline bolus of 500 to 1000 mL

Alkalinization for the Unstable Patient With TCA Overdose

- Provide immediate hyperventilation to a pH of 7.50 to 7.55 for patients who present with seizures or inadequate respiratory function.[161]
- Give *sodium bicarbonate* 1 to 2 mEq/kg over 1 to 2 minutes.
- Follow with a *sodium bicarbonate* infusion of 3 ampules (150 mEq) plus 30 mEq of KCl mixed in 850 mL of D_5W, at an initial rate of 150 to 200 mL/h, titrated to keep pH at 7.50 to 7.55.
- The initial goal of therapy is to raise the pH to 7.50 to 7.55 and then to maintain that pH, confirmed by measurement of venous and arterial pH on a regular basis.

Critical Concept **Emergency Treatment for Acute Decompensation**	Boluses of sodium bicarbonate are used without prior determination of serum pH for acute decompensation if the QRS duration is more than 100 milliseconds or if hypotension develops.

- Continue to infuse sodium bicarbonate until the patient's condition stabilizes.

Magnesium for TCA Overdose

Some patients may develop arrhythmias because of tricyclic actions on phase 2 of the action potential.

- The phase 2 effects are initially manifested by a prolongation of the QT interval. They may result in the torsades de pointes variant of VT.[19,162-165]
- Magnesium sulfate is the drug of choice for this select group of patients.[19,163-165]
- The dose of magnesium is 1 to 2 g diluted in 10 mL D_5W IV push in unstable patients (a total of 5 to 10 g IV may be used). Give this dose more slowly (over 1 to 5 minutes) in hemodynamically stable patients.[19,163,166]

TCA-Induced Cardiac Arrest

Cardiac arrest caused by cyclic antidepressant toxicity should be managed by current BLS and ACLS treatment guidelines. A small case series of cardiac arrest patients-demonstrated improvement with sodium bicarbonate and epinephrine,[167] but the concomitant use of physostigmine in the prearrest period in this study reduces the ability to generalize about the results. Administration of sodium bicarbonate for cardiac arrest due to cyclic antidepressant overdose may be considered (Class IIb, LOE C).

TCA-Induced Seizures and Hypotension

Seizures caused by TCA overdose should be terminated immediately with benzodiazepines. Uncontrolled seizure activity results in hypoxia, acidosis, tachycardia, hypotension, and electrolyte fluxes. These responses increase morbidity and mortality from TCA overdose.

- Hypotension usually responds to infusions of 500 to 1000 mL of normal saline.
- Alkalinization with sodium bicarbonate is recommended for nonresponders.
- Patients with refractory hypotension may be treated with dopamine or norepinephrine.[28,62,125,168]

Summary of Symptom-Based Therapy: Management of Cardiovascular Compromise Caused by Drugs or Toxins

In treatment of acute poison-induced shock and cardiac arrest, the standard ACLS protocols may not be effective.[88] Care of severely poisoned patients can be enhanced by urgent consultation with a medical toxicologist. The following alternative approaches may be needed for treatment of poisonings:

- The use of *higher doses* of drugs than usual
- The use of *drugs rarely given in cardiac arrest,* such as inamrinone, calcium, esmolol, glucagon, insulin, labetalol, phenylephrine, physostigmine, and sodium bicarbonate
- More frequent use of *heroic measures* such as prolonged CPR and circulatory assist devices
- *Earlier consideration of organ donation* when resuscitative efforts from a critical poisoning are unsuccessful and brain death is expected

When evaluating patients with cardiovascular emergencies, differentiate patients according to toxidromes, consider vital signs, and assess the 12-lead ECG. These steps will assist in the formulation of a differential diagnosis that can initially drive a therapy or treatment strategy while avoiding contraindicated drugs or interventions (Table 47). When a toxidrome is suspected, the cardiotoxicity of the specific drug or drug class can be evaluated and therapeutic recommendations considered (Table 49).

Central Nervous System Changes and Respiratory Depression

There are many medications and chemicals that cause central nervous system (CNS) changes and respiratory depression. Supportive and protective care and time will often be adequate to correct these problems.

Seizures

Seizures or convulsions occur after exposure or overdose from a large variety of toxins and medications, including some antibiotics, cocaine and amphetamines, TCAs, and local anesthetics. CNS excitability is often seen in drug withdrawal states after chronic use, such as ethanol withdrawal. Seizures that occur because of toxicologic emergencies may be followed by hemodynamic compromise or collapse that will require specialized management for successful resuscitation. For example, an inadvertent overdose of local anesthetic may be indicated by neurologic symptoms, followed by seizures before cardiovascular collapse occurs. Knowledge of the cause and initiation of specific therapy, in this case lipid emulsion, early during the resuscitation may lead to a more rapid recovery. Recognition of seizures that are caused by a toxicologic emergency can provide an early warning that hemodynamic collapse is imminent.

Opiate Poisoning

The hallmarks of opiate poisoning are CNS depression, respiratory depression, and miosis (small pupils). Heroin, morphine, oxycodone, and fentanyl are examples of agents in the opioid class. People can experience life-threatening overdose through "recreational" use, through intentional overdose, and accidentally through self-administration or iatrogenic overdose.

Poisoned patients can deteriorate rapidly. Frequent assessment of the airway, breathing, and circulation is required. Opiate poisoning eliminates airway protective reflexes and directly suppresses respiratory drive. Respiratory failure is the most common cause of death in cases of opiate overdose and poisoning.

Opiate Reversal

Opiate poisoning commonly causes respiratory depression followed by respiratory insufficiency and arrest. Noncardiac pulmonary edema can also complicate narcotic overdose, particularly if a large bolus of opiates has been administered. The respiratory effects of opiates are reversed rapidly by the opiate antagonist naloxone.

Naloxone has been used successfully in the hospital setting without the need for advanced airway placement in otherwise healthy adults with no chronic exposure and a normal cardiovascular system.[169] If the patient's airway can be maintained and ventilation provided with a bag-mask device and the patient is otherwise stable, naloxone can be titrated to achieve an adequate respiratory rate and level of consciousness.

Specific ACLS recommendations for naloxone administration, endotracheal intubation, and support of ventilation for opiate toxicity include the following:

- When patients with suspected opiate overdose have *respiratory insufficiency and are not in cardiac arrest,* support ventilation with a bag and mask while preparing to administer naloxone (Class I, LOE A).[1,170-174]
- If naloxone therapy is not effective, proceed with placement of an advanced airway.
- Existing evidence does not justify withholding naloxone until endotracheal intubation is performed. In the United States, opiates are associated with more drug-induced cardiopulmonary arrests than any other drug, but the incidence of severe complications after opiate reversal is less than 2%.[175]
- Naloxone is the preferred reversal agent for opiate toxicity even though it has a shorter duration of action (45 to 70 minutes) than heroin (4 to 5 hours).

End Points for Opiate Reversal

- The end-point objectives for opiate reversal are adequate airway reflexes and ventilation, not complete arousal.
- Acute, abrupt opiate withdrawal increases the likelihood of severe complications such as pulmonary edema, ventricular arrhythmias, and severe agitation and hostility.

Naloxone: Dose and Route

- Naloxone can be administered by a number of routes: intravenously (IV),[7,172,176,177] intramuscularly (IM),[7,170,172] subcutaneously,[178] intranasally,[170,176] or into the trachea.[179]
- Naloxone can cause fulminate opioid withdrawal for individuals with opioid dependence. Therefore, the recommended initial dose of naloxone is 0.04 to 0.4 mg IV or 0.4 mg[180] IM or subcutaneously. Repeat dosing or dose escalation to 2 mg may be required if the initial response is not adequate.
- For intranasal administration, an initial dose of 2 mg (1 mg in each nostril) may be effective.[170,176] An additional intranasal dose of 2 mg can be given in 5 minutes if respiratory depression persists.
- The clinical effects of naloxone may not last as long as those of the opioid, which can make repeated dosing necessary.
- Atypical opioid or massive overdose ingestions may require higher doses of naloxone to reverse the intoxication.[181,182]
- Higher doses of naloxone may also be necessary when a propoxyphene compound has been ingested.
- When opiate overdose is strongly suspected or in locations where "China white" (ie, fentanyl and its derivatives) abuse is prevalent, titration to total naloxone doses of 6 to 10 mg over a short period of time may be necessary.

Benzodiazepines

Flumazenil is a potent antagonist of the binding of benzodiazepines to their CNS receptors. Administration of flumazenil can reverse CNS and respiratory depression caused by benzodiazepine overdose; however, the administration of flumazenil to patients with undifferentiated coma confers risk and is not recommended (Class III, LOE B). Flumazenil administration can precipitate seizures in benzodiazepine-dependent patients and has been associated with seizures, arrhythmias, and hypotension in patients with coingestion of certain medications, such as tricyclic antidepressants (TCAs).[185,186] Flumazenil may be used safely to reverse the excessive sedation known to be caused by the

Critical Concept Evaluation and Management After Naloxone Administration	• It is recommended that opiate-intoxicated patients aroused with naloxone be observed for recurrence of respiratory depression. Some EMS systems, especially in Europe, allow selected patients aroused with naloxone to refuse to be transported to the hospital. – Although the incidence of severe complications after opiate reversal is less than 2%, the duration of action of naloxone is shorter than the duration of action of many opiates. In poisonings with long-acting opioids (eg, methadone) or sustained-release preparations, failure to continue care has occasionally led to serious consequences, such as severe renarcotization or delayed pulmonary edema.[183,184] – It is recommended that all patients be observed after arousal beyond the duration of the naloxone effect (typically 45 to 70 minutes) to ensure their safety.

Critical Concept

Benzodiazepine Reversal and Flumazenil

- Reversal of benzodiazepine intoxication with flumazenil is associated with significant toxicity in patients with benzodiazepine dependence or coingestion of proconvulsant medications such as tricyclic antidepressants.
- Flumazenil is not recommended for routine use or inclusion in a "coma cocktail." It may be useful for reversal of respiratory depression when benzodiazepines have been used for procedural sedation.

use of benzodiazepines in a patient without known contraindications (eg, procedural sedation).[187]

Carbon Monoxide

Apart from complications from deliberate drug abuse, carbon monoxide is the leading cause of unintentional poisoning death in the United States.[188] In addition to reducing the ability of hemoglobin to deliver oxygen, carbon monoxide causes direct cellular damage to the brain and myocardium. Survivors of carbon monoxide poisoning are at risk for lasting neurologic injury.[189] Several studies have suggested that very few patients who develop cardiac arrest from carbon monoxide poisoning survive to hospital discharge, regardless of treatment administered after return of spontaneous circulation.[190-192] Routine care of patients in cardiac arrest and severe cardiotoxicity from carbon monoxide poisoning should comply with standard BLS and ACLS recommendations.

Hyperbaric Oxygen

Two studies suggested that neurologic outcomes were improved in patients with carbon monoxide toxicity of all levels of severity (with the exclusion of "moribund" patients)[193] and of mild to moderate severity (with the exclusion of loss of consciousness and cardiac instability)[194] who received hyperbaric oxygen therapy. Other studies found no difference in neurologically intact survival.[195,196] A systematic review[197,198] and a recent evidence-based clinical policy review[199] concluded that on the basis of the available evidence, improvement in neurologically intact survival after treatment for carbon monoxide poisoning with hyperbaric oxygen is possible but unproven. Hyperbaric oxygen therapy is associated with a low incidence of severe side effects. Available data suggest that hyperbolic oxygen treatment confers little risk; it may be helpful in the treatment of acute carbon monoxide poisoning in patients with severe toxicity (Class IIb, LOE C). Patients with carbon monoxide poisoning who develop a cardiac injury have an increased risk of cardiovascular and all-cause mortality for at least 7 years after the event, even if hyperbaric oxygen is administered.[200,201] Although data about effective interventions in this population are lacking, it is reasonable to advise enhanced follow-up for these patients. On the basis of this conflicting evidence, the routine transfer of patients to a hyperbaric treatment facility after resuscitation from severe cardiovascular toxicity should be considered carefully, with the risk of transport weighed against the possible improvement in neurologically intact survival.

Methemoglobinemia

Methemoglobinemia is a clinical syndrome caused by an increase in the blood levels of methemoglobin or hemoglobin in which the iron is oxidized from its ferrous (Fe_2^+) to its ferric (Fe_3^+) state. Methemoglobin does not carry oxygen and shifts the normal HbO_2 dissociation curve to the left, thereby limiting the release of oxygen to the tissues. It can be congenital from altered hemoglobin (Hb) synthesis or metabolism, or acquired from exposure to medications or chemical agents. Its prevalence is unknown because mild cases are often undiagnosed. Central cyanosis unresponsive to the administration of oxygen is the main characteristic of methemoglobinemia.[202-206]

There are 2 causes of the congenital form: (1) a defect in the body's systems to reduce methemoglobin to hemoglobin; and (2) a mutant form of hemoglobin called hemoglobin M that cannot bind to oxygen. Both of these forms are typically benign but may make exposure to oxidizing agents more dangerous.

Acquired methemoglobinemia is caused by exposure to certain drugs or chemicals (oxidizing agents) that accelerate the oxidation of Hb by 10 to 100 times normal and eventually overwhelm the capacity of reducing endogenous systems. This creates an imbalance in reduction and oxidation reactions that can overwhelm the body's systems of reducing methemoglobin to hemoglobin, which results in a high level of methemoglobin.

Normally, 5 g/dL of deoxyhemoglobin (compared with 1.5 g/dL (10% to 15%) of methemoglobin) produces noticeable cyanosis. Methemoglobin levels below 30% in a healthy person produce minimal symptoms (fatigue, lightheadedness, and headache) or no symptoms; whereas levels from 30% to 50% produce moderate depression of the cardiovascular and central nervous systems (weakness, headache, tachycardia, tachypnea, and mild dyspnea).

Methemoglobin levels between 50% and 70% cause severe symptoms (stupor, bradycardia, respiratory depression, convulsions, dysrhythmias, and acidosis). Levels above

60% can be lethal, and levels above 70% usually are not compatible with life.

The typical arterial blood gas analysis (ABG) calculates values for hemoglobin oxygen saturation and actual oxygen content from the partial pressure of oxygen (PO_2). If other hemoglobins are suspected or present, co-oximetery testing is necessary.

Co-oximetry uses light absorption at different wavelengths to calculate the percentage of hemoglobin to the total content of all hemoglobin and gives values for oxyhemoglobin (normal), carboxyhemoglobin (carbon monoxide poisoning), and methemoglobin (methemoglobinemia).

Patients with mild methemoglobinemia most often have asymptomatic cyanosis. Stopping the causative drug or chemical exposure is often sufficient.

The signs and symptoms of significant methemoglobinemia are those of tissue hypoxia and may include confusion, angina, and myalgias. Respiratory alkalosis is often an early finding. The development of metabolic acidosis may occur in later stages or in large acute ingestions.

The decision to treat patients with methemoglobinemia is based on a combination of blood levels and clinical presentation. Treatment is with methylene blue, a reducing agent (1% solution given slowly IV, 1 to 2 mg/kg). In severe cases, exchange transfusion or hyperbaric oxygen may be required. The patient needs to be continually reassessed.

Symptoms generally correlate with the amount of methemoglobin and the presence of underlying medical disease, particularly anemia, coronary artery disease, and pulmonary disease. The onset of methemoglobinemia is usually within 20 to 60 minutes of drug administration, and the half-life of methemoglobin is 55 minutes.

Metabolic Acidosis

Cyanide

Cyanide is a surprisingly common chemical. In addition to industrial sources, cyanide can be found in jewelry cleaners, electroplating solutions, and as a metabolic product of sodium nitroprusside infusions and of the putative antitumor drug amygdalin.

Cyanide is a major component of fires and combustion of certain materials, such as plastics. Cyanide poisoning must be considered in victims of smoke inhalation who have hypotension, CNS depression, metabolic acidosis, or soot in the nares or respiratory secretions.[207] Chronic cyanide exposure occurs with ingestion of cyanide-containing foods such as cassava root and apricot seeds.

Cyanide poisoning causes rapid cardiovascular collapse, which manifests as hypotension, lactic acidosis, central apnea, and seizures. Patients in cardiac arrest[207-209] or those presenting with cardiovascular instability[207-213] caused by known or suspected cyanide poisoning should receive cyanide antidote therapy with a cyanide scavenger (either IV hydroxocobalamin or a nitrate such as IV sodium nitrite and/or inhaled amyl nitrite), followed as soon as possible by IV sodium thiosulfate.[211,214,215] Both hydroxocobalamin[207-213] and sodium nitrite[211,214,215] serve to rapidly and effectively bind cyanide in the serum and reverse the effects of cyanide toxicity.

Nitrites induce methemoglobin formation[214] and can cause hypotension.[216] Hydroxocobalamin has a safety advantage, particularly in children and victims of smoke inhalation who might also have carbon monoxide poisoning. A detailed comparison of these measures has been published recently.[217] Sodium thiosulfate serves as a metabolic cofactor that enhances the detoxification of cyanide to thiocyanate.

Thiosulfate administration enhances the effectiveness of cyanide scavengers in animal experimentation[218-221] and has been used successfully in humans with both hydroxocobalamin and sodium nitrite.[211,214,215] Sodium thiosulfate is associated with vomiting but has no other significant toxicity.[222] Therefore, on the basis of the best evidence available, a treatment regimen of 100% oxygen and hydroxocobalamin, with or without sodium thiosulfate, is recommended (Class I, LOE B).

Critical Concept

Agents That Can Cause Methemoglobinemia

- Dapsone
- Local anesthetics: Benzocaine, prilocaine, procaine, lidocaine
- Nitrates: Nitrofurantoin, nitroglycerin, isosorbide dinitrate
- Primaquine
- Sulfonamides: Trimethoprim/sulfamethoxazole
- Ciprofloxacin, flutamide, metoclopramide, phenazopyradine, phenelzine, phenobarbital, quinine, aniline dyes
- Benzene derivatives

Salicylates

Salicylate toxicity or salicylism may either be (1) **acute**, resulting from accidental or intentional ingestion of more than 150 mg/kg; or (2) **chronic**, after repeated high therapeutic doses (higher than 100 mg/kg per day) of salicylates. These substances are widely used and easily available as over-the-counter oral and topical analgesics: acetylsalicylic acid (ASA), methyl salicylates, sulfasalazine, bismuth subsalicylate, wart removers, and liniments.[223-228]

Salicylates stimulate medullary respiratory centers leading to hyperventilation and respiratory alkalosis. Intracellularly, saliclylates uncouple oxidative phosphorylation and decrease ATP production. Salicylates also increase the production of endogenous acids, leading to metabolic acidosis.

Acute salicylate toxicity is often diagnosed clinically, with a high index of suspicion in patients presenting with nausea, vomiting, fever, hyperventilation, hearing loss, tinnitus, and decreased level of consciousness. Tachycardia, dehydration, and seizures may also be observed. Because respiratory alkalosis and metabolic acidosis are common manifestations, measurement of arterial blood gases, anion gap, and serum salicylate levels help in establishing the diagnosis. The condition may progress to rhabdomyolysis and multiple organ failure.

Chronic toxicity may be more subtle and present with nonspecific signs and symptoms, such as confusion, altered mental status, dehydration, hypotension, and seizures. It is more common in elderly patients, but is often undiagnosed.

Patients may be treated with activated charcoal, alkaline diuresis, or hemodialysis.

1. Activated charcoal may be given immediately if available and if bowel sounds are present and there are no contraindications. This may be repeated until the patient's condition and laboratory parameters improve.
2. Alkaline diuresis with sodium bicarbonate plus potassium chloride may be used to increase urine pH to facilitate salicylate excretion. It may also help prevent renal failure in patients with rhabdomyolysis. Volume and electrolyte abnormalities should be corrected early.
3. In acute toxicity, salicylate levels should be monitored frequently but this should not delay treatment.
4. Hemodialysis is recommended in severe cases and for chronic toxicity, especially with altered mental status, seizures, and renal or respiratory failure.
5. Glucose should be given if a patient has a significant change in mental status, even with normal serum glucose levels.
6. Supportive therapy, including benzodiapines for seizures and external cooling for fever, should be administered if indicated.
7. Patients with stated or suspected self-harm or who are the victims of a potentially malicious administration of a salicylate, should be referred to an emergency department immediately. This referral should be guided by local poison center procedures. Generally, this should occur regardless of the dose reported.

The prognosis depends on prompt recognition and treatment. Delayed diagnosis results in increased morbidity and mortality, particularly in the elderly.

Dosing Guide for Antidotes in Toxicologic Emergencies

Table 49 presents a quick dosing reference for antidotes to common intoxications and drug overdoses. Note that these doses are often different from doses used in other emergency cardiovascular care situations. The ideal dose has not been determined for many indications; the doses presented may not be ideal. Most antidotes may be repeated as needed to achieve and maintain the desired clinical effect. Whenever possible, consult a medical toxicologist or call a poison center (eg, in USA: 1-800-222-1222) for advice before administering antidotes.

Table 49. Rapid Dosing Guide for Antidotes Used in Emergency Cardiovascular Care for Treatment of Toxic Ingestions

Antidote	Common Indications: Toxicity due to	Adult Dose*	Pediatric Dose* *Do not exceed adult dose.*	Notes
Atropine	• β-Blockers • Calcium channel blockers • Clonidine • Digoxin	• 0.5-1 mg IV every 2-3 minutes	• 0.02 mg/kg IV (minimum dose 0.1 mg) every 2-3 minutes	• Use for hemodynamically significant bradycardia. Higher doses often required for organophosphate or carbamate poisoning.
Calcium	• β-Blockers • Calcium channel blockers	• Calcium chloride (10%): 1-2 g (10-20 mL) IV • Calcium gluconate (10%): 3-6 g (30-60 mL) IV • Follow initial dose with same dose by continuous hourly infusion	• Calcium chloride (10%): 20 mg/kg (0.2 mL/kg) IV • Calcium gluconate (10%): 60 mg/kg (0.6 mL/kg) IV • Follow initial dose with same dose by continuous hourly infusion	• Use for hypotension. Avoid calcium chloride when possible if using peripheral IV, particularly in children. Higher doses may be required for calcium channel blocker overdose (use caution and monitor serum calcium).
Digoxin Immune Fab	• Digoxin and related glycosides	• If amount of digoxin ingested is known: Give 1 vial IV for every 0.5 mg digoxin ingested. • If amount of digoxin ingested is unknown or if chronic intoxication with a known digoxin level: Dose (vials, administered IV) = $\frac{\text{(serum digoxin concentration [ng/mL]} \times \text{weight [kg])}}{100}$ • Unknown dose and level, cardiovascular collapse: 10-20 vials IV		
Flumazenil	• Benzodiazepines	• 0.2 mg IV every 15 seconds, up to 3 mg total dose	• 0.01 mg/kg IV every 15 seconds, up to 0.05 mg/kg total dose	• Do not use for unknown overdose, suspected TCA overdose, or patients who are benzodiazepine dependent due to risk of precipitating seizures.
Glucagon	• β-Blockers • Calcium channel blockers	• 3-10 mg IV bolus, followed by 3-5 mg per hour IV infusion	• 0.05-0.15 mg/kg IV bolus, followed by 0.05-0.10 mg/kg per hour IV infusion	• Bolus often causes vomiting.
Hydroxocobalamin	• Cyanide	• 5 g IV	• 70 mg/kg IV	• Dilute in 100 mL normal saline; infuse over 15 minutes. • Toxicologist or other specialist may follow with sodium thiosulfate (separate IV).
Lipid Emulsion	• Local anesthetics • Calcium channel blockers • β-Blockers • Other drugs	• 1.5 mL/kg of 20% long-chain fatty acid solution IV bolus, followed by 0.25 mL/kg per minute IV infusion for 30-60 minutes		

(continued)

(continued)

Insulin	• β-Blockers • Calcium channel blockers	• 1 unit/kg IV bolus, then 0.5-1 units/kg per hour IV infusion, titrated to blood pressure		• Give dextrose 0.5 g/kg with insulin. Start dextrose infusion 0.5 g/kg per hour and check blood sugar frequently. Replace potassium to maintain serum potassium 2.5-2.8 mEq/L.
Naloxone	• Opioids	• 0.04-0.4 mg IV; repeat every 2-3 minutes and escalate dose as needed to maximum 10 mg	• 0.1 mg/kg IV (up to 2 mg per dose). Repeat every 2-3 minutes. For partial reversal of respiratory depression (eg, procedural sedation), 0.001-0.005 mg/kg (1-5 mcg/kg) IV. Titrate to effect.	• Use only for respiratory depression or loss of airway reflexes. May also be given by IM, IO, intranasal, or endotracheal routes.
Sodium Bicarbonate	• Cyclic antidepressants	• 1 mEq/kg IV (1 mL/kg of 8.4% solution); consider infusion following initial dose		• Repeat as needed until QRS narrows. Avoid sodium >155 mEq/L or pH >7.55. Dilute before administration in small children.
Sodium Nitrite	• Cyanide	• 300 mg IV over 3-5 minutes (10 mL of 3% solution)	• 10 mg/kg (0.33 mL/kg of 10% solution) IV over 3-5 minutes	• Hydroxocobalamin preferred to sodium nitrite, if available. May give inhaled amyl nitrite as temporizing measure while establishing vascular access. Follow with sodium thiosulfate administration. Reduced dose required for children with anemia.
Sodium Thiosulfate	• Cyanide	• 12.5 g (50 mL of 25% solution) IV over 10 minutes	• 400 mg/kg (1.65 mL/kg of 25% solution) IV over 10 minutes	• Use separate IV from hydroxocobalamin. Consider expert consultation.

*These doses are often different from doses used in other emergency cardiovascular care situations. The ideal dose has not been determined for many indications; the doses above may not be ideal. Most antidotes may be repeated as needed to achieve and maintain the desired clinical effect. Unless otherwise noted, IV doses may also be given via the IO route. Contact medical toxicologist, call poison center (eg, in USA: 1-800-222-1222), or refer to written treatment guidance for specific dosing advice.

References

1. Vanden Hoek TL, Morrison LJ, Shuster M, Donnino M, Sinz E, Lavonas EJ, Jeejeebhoy FM, Gabrielli A. Part 12: cardiac arrest in special situations: 2010 American Heart Association Guidelines for Cardiopulmonary Resuscitation and Emergency Cardiovascular Care. *Circulation*. 2010;122:S829-S861.
2. Vale JA, Kulig K. Position paper: gastric lavage. *J Toxicol Clin Toxicol*. 2004;42:933-943.
3. Position paper: whole bowel irrigation. *J Toxicol Clin Toxicol*. 2004;42:843-854.
4. Position paper: Ipecac syrup. *J Toxicol Clin Toxicol*. 2004;42:133-143.
5. Chyka PA, Seger D, Krenzelok EP, Vale JA. Position paper: single-dose activated charcoal. *Clin Toxicol (Phila)*. 2005;43:61-87.
6. American Academy of Clinical Toxicology; European Association of Poisons Centres and Clinical Toxicologists. Position statement and practice guidelines on the use of multi-dose activated charcoal in the treatment of acute poisoning. *J Toxicol Clin Toxicol*. 1999;37:731-751.
7. Leach M. Naloxone: a new therapeutic and diagnostic agent for emergency use. *J Amer Coll Emerg Phys*. 1973;2:21-23.
8. Adelson L. Poison and the pathologist. *JAMA*. 1964;187:918-920.
9. Burkhart KK. Intravenous propranolol reverses hypertension after sympathomimetic overdose: two case reports. *J Toxicol Clin Toxicol*. 1992;30:109-114.
10. Durward A, Guerguerian AM, Lefebvre M, Shemie SD. Massive diltiazem overdose treated with extracorporeal membrane oxygenation. *Pediatr Crit Care Med*. 2003;4:372-376.

11. Ramsay ID. Survival after imipramine poisoning. *Lancet*. 1967;2:1308-1309.
12. Southall DP, Kilpatrick SM. Imipramine poisoning: survival of a child after prolonged cardiac massage. *Br Med J*. 1974;4:508.
13. Holzer M, Behringer W, Schorkhuber W, Zeiner A, Sterz F, Laggner AN, Frass M, Siostrozonek P, Ratheiser K, Kaff A. Mild hypothermia and outcome after CPR. Hypothermia for Cardiac Arrest (HACA) Study Group. *Acta Anaesthesiol Scand Suppl*. 1997;111:55-58.
14. Hebert MJ, Boucher A, Beaucage G, Girard R, Dandavino R. Transplantation of kidneys from a donor with carbon monoxide poisoning. *N Engl J Med*. 1992;326:1571.
15. Kolecki PF, Curry SC. Poisoning by sodium channel blocking agents. *Critical Care Clinics*. 1997;13:829-848.
16. Mayron R, Ruiz E. Phenytoin: does it reverse tricyclic-antidepressant-induced cardiac conduction abnormalities? *Ann Emerg Med*. 1986;15:876-880.
17. Callaham M, Schumaker H, Pentel P. Phenytoin prophylaxis of cardiotoxicity in experimental amitriptyline poisoning. *J Pharmacol Exp Ther*. 1988;245:216-220.
18. Citak A, Soysal DD, Ucsel R, Karabocuoglu M, Uzel N. Efficacy of long duration resuscitation and magnesium sulphate treatment in amitriptyline poisoning. *Eur J Emerg Med*. 2002;9:63-66.
19. Knudsen K, Abrahamsson J. Effects of magnesium sulfate and lidocaine in the treatment of ventricular arrhythmias in experimental amitriptyline poisoning in the rat. *Crit Care Med*. 1994;22:494-498.
20. Lange RA, Cigarroa RG, Flores ED, McBride W, Kim AS, Wells PJ, Bedotto JB, Danziger RS, Hillis LD. Potentiation of cocaine-induced coronary vasoconstriction by β-adrenergic blockade. *Ann Intern Med*. 1990;112:897-903.
21. Sand IC, Brody SL, Wrenn KD, Slovis CM. Experience with esmolol for the treatment of cocaine-associated cardiovascular complications. *Am J Emerg Med*. 1991;9:161-163.
22. Dattilo PB, Hailpern SM, Fearon K, Sohal D, Nordin C. Beta-blockers are associated with reduced risk of myocardial infarction after cocaine use. *Ann Emerg Med*. 2008;51:117-125.
23. Vongpatanasin W, Mansour Y, Chavoshan B, Arbique D, Victor RG. Cocaine stimulates the human cardiovascular system via a central mechanism of action. *Circulation*. 1999;100:497-502.
24. McCord J, Jneid H, Hollander JE, de Lemos JA, Cercek B, Hsue P, Gibler WB, Ohman EM, Drew B, Philippides G, Newby LK. Management of cocaine-associated chest pain and myocardial infarction: a scientific statement from the American Heart Association Acute Cardiac Care Committee of the Council on Clinical Cardiology. *Circulation*. 2008;117:1897-1907.
25. Wood DM, Dargan PI, Hoffman RS. Management of cocaine-induced cardiac arrhythmias due to cardiac ion channel dysfunction. *Clin Toxicol (Phila)*. 2009;47:14-23.
26. Gowda RM, Khan IA, Wilbur SL, Vasavada BC, Sacchi TJ. Torsade de pointes: the clinical considerations. *Int J Cardiol*. 2004;96:1-6.
27. Yap YG, Camm AJ. Drug induced QT prolongation and torsades de pointes. *Heart*. 2003;89:1363-1372.
28. Vernon D, Banner W, Dean M. Dopamine and norepinephrine are equally effective for treatment of shock in amitriptyline intoxication. *Crit Care Med*. 1990;18:S239.
29. Vernon DD, Banner W Jr, Garrett JS, Dean JM. Efficacy of dopamine and norepinephrine for treatment of hemodynamic compromise in amitriptyline intoxication. *Crit Care Med*. 1991;19:544-549.
30. Wenzel V, Lindner KH. Employing vasopressin during cardiopulmonary resuscitation and vasodilatory shock as a lifesaving vasopressor. *Cardiovasc Res*. 2001;51:529-541.
31. Kollef MH. Labetalol overdose successfully treated with amrinone and α-adrenergic receptor agonists. *Chest*. 1994;105:626-627.
32. Wolf LR, Spadafora MP, Otten EJ. Use of amrinone and glucagon in a case of calcium channel blocker overdose. *Ann Emerg Med*. 1993;22:1225-1228.
33. Love JN, Hanfling D, Howell JM. Hemodynamic effects of calcium chloride in a canine model of acute propranolol intoxication. *Ann Emerg Med*. 1996;28:1-6.
34. Love JN, Sachdeva DK, Bessman ES, Curtis LA, Howell JM. A potential role for glucagon in the treatment of drug-induced symptomatic bradycardia. *Chest*. 1998;114:323-326.
35. Hollander JE, Hoffman RS, Gennis P, Fairweather P, DiSano MJ, Schumb DA, Feldman JA, Fish SS, Dyer S, Wax P, Whelan C, Schwarzwald E. Nitroglycerin in the treatment of cocaine associated chest pain—clinical safety and efficacy. *J Toxicol Clin Toxicol*. 1994;32:243-256.
36. Baumann BM, Perrone J, Hornig SE, Shofer FS, Hollander JE. Randomized, double-blind, placebo-controlled trial of diazepam, nitroglycerin, or both for treatment of patients with potential cocaine-associated acute coronary syndromes. *Acad Emerg Med*. 2000;7:878-885.
37. Brogan WC III, Lange RA, Kim AS, Moliterno DJ, Hillis LD. Alleviation of cocaine-induced coronary vasoconstriction by nitroglycerin. *J Am Coll Cardiol*. 1991;18:581-586.
38. Lange RA, Cigarroa RG, Yancy CW Jr, Willard JE, Popma JJ, Sills MN, McBride W, Kim AS, Hillis LD. Cocaine-induced coronary-artery vasoconstriction. *N Engl J Med*. 1989;321:1557-1562.
39. Lange RA, Cigarroa RG, Flores ED, McBride W, Kim AS, Wells PJ, Bedotto JB, Danziger RS, Hillis LD. Potentiation of cocaine-induced coronary vasoconstriction by beta-adrenergic blockade. *Ann Intern Med*. 1990;112:897-903.
40. Sand IC, Brody SL, Wrenn KD, Slovis CM. Experience with esmolol for the treatment of cocaine-associated cardiovascular complications. *Am J Emerg Med*. 1991;9:161-163.
41. Tracey JA, Cassidy N, Casey PB, Ali I. Bupropion (Zyban) toxicity. *Ir Med J*. 2002;95:23-24.
42. Lange RA, Hillis LD. Cardiovascular complications of cocaine use [published correction appears in *N Engl J Med*. 2001;345:1432]. *N Engl J Med*. 2001;345:351-358.
43. Lange RA, Willard JE. The cardiovascular effects of cocaine. *Heart Dis Stroke*. 1993;2:136-141.
44. Burns MJ, Linden CH, Graudins A, Brown RM, Fletcher KE. A comparison of physostigmine and benzodiazepines for the treatment of anticholinergic poisoning. *Ann Emerg Med*. 2000;35:374-381.
45. Hollander JE. Cocaine intoxication and hypertension. *Ann Emerg Med*. 2008;51:S18-20.
46. Cregler LL, Mark H. Medical complications of cocaine abuse. *N Engl J Med*. 1986;315:1495-1500.
47. Jekel JF, Allen DF, Podlewski H, Clarke N, Dean-Patterson S, Cartwright P. Epidemic free-base cocaine abuse. Case study from the Bahamas. *Lancet*. 1986;1:459-462.

48. Farrar HC, Kearns GL. Cocaine: clinical pharmacology and toxicology. *J Pediatr*. 1989;115(pt 1):665-675.
49. Lowenstein DH, Massa SM, Rowbotham MC, Collins SD, McKinney HE, Simon RP. Acute neurologic and psychiatric complications associated with cocaine abuse. *Am J Med*. 1987;83:841-846.
50. Gradman AH. Cardiac effects of cocaine: a review. *Yale J Biol Med*. 1988;61:137-147.
51. Barth CW III, Bray M, Roberts WC. Rupture of the ascending aorta during cocaine intoxication. *Am J Cardiol*. 1986;57:496.
52. Brody SL, Slovis CM, Wrenn KD. Cocaine-related medical problems: consecutive series of 233 patients. *Am J Med*. 1990;88:325-331.
53. Derlet RW, Albertson TE. Emergency department presentation of cocaine intoxication. *Ann Emerg Med*. 1989;18:182-186.
54. Rich JA, Singer DE. Cocaine-related symptoms in patients presenting to an urban emergency department. *Ann Emerg Med*. 1991;20:616-621.
55. Kloner RA, Hale S, Alker K, Rezkalla S. The effects of acute and chronic cocaine use on the heart. *Circulation*. 1992;85:407-419.
56. Isner JM, Estes NA III, Thompson PD, Costanzo-Nordin MR, Subramanian R, Miller G, Katsas G, Sweeney K, Sturner WQ. Acute cardiac events temporally related to cocaine abuse. *N Engl J Med*. 1986;315:1438-1443.
57. Wood DM, Dargan PI, Hoffman RS. Management of cocaine-induced cardiac arrhythmias due to cardiac ion channel dysfunction. *Clinical Toxicology (Phila)*. 2009;47:14-23.
58. Hoffman JR, Votey SR, Bayer M, Silver L. Effect of hypertonic sodium bicarbonate in the treatment of moderate-to-severe cyclic antidepressant overdose. *Am J Emerg Med*. 1993;11:336-341.
59. Koppel C, Wiegreffe A, Tenczer J. Clinical course, therapy, outcome and analytical data in amitriptyline and combined amitriptyline/chlordiazepoxide overdose. *Hum Exp Toxicol*. 1992;11:458-465.
60. Brown TC. Tricyclic antidepressant overdosage: experimental studies on the management of circulatory complications. *Clin Toxicol*. 1976;9:255-272.
61. Hedges JR, Baker PB, Tasset JJ, Otten EJ, Dalsey WC, Syverud SA. Bicarbonate therapy for the cardiovascular toxicity of amitriptyline in an animal model. *J Emerg Med*. 1985;3:253-260.
62. Knudsen K, Abrahamsson J. Epinephrine and sodium bicarbonate independently and additively increase survival in experimental amitriptyline poisoning. *Crit Care Med*. 1997;25:669-674.
63. Nattel S, Mittleman M. Treatment of ventricular tachyarrhythmias resulting from amitriptyline toxicity in dogs. *J Pharmacol Exp Ther*. 1984;231:430-435.
64. Pentel P, Benowitz N. Efficacy and mechanism of action of sodium bicarbonate in the treatment of desipramine toxicity in rats. *J Pharmacol Exp Ther*. 1984;230:12-19.
65. Sasyniuk BI, Jhamandas V, Valois M. Experimental amitriptyline intoxication: treatment of cardiac toxicity with sodium bicarbonate. *Ann Emerg Med*. 1986;15:1052-1059.
66. Kerns W II, Garvey L, Owens J. Cocaine-induced wide complex dysrhythmia. *J Emerg Med*. 1997;15:321-329.
67. Wang RY. pH-dependent cocaine-induced cardiotoxicity. *Am J Emerg Med*. 1999;17:364-369.
68. Williams RG, Kavanagh KM, Teo KK. Pathophysiology and treatment of cocaine toxicity: implications for the heart and cardiovascular system. *Can J Cardiol*. 1996;12:1295-1301.
69. Noel B. Cardiovascular complications of cocaine use. *N Engl J Med*. 2001;345:1575; author reply 1576.
70. Hsue PY, McManus D, Selby V, Ren X, Pillutla P, Younes N, Goldschlager N, Waters DD. Cardiac arrest in patients who smoke crack cocaine. *Am J Cardiol*. 2007;99:822-824.
71. Gay GR. Clinical management of acute and chronic cocaine poisoning. *Ann Emerg Med*. 1982;11:562-572.
72. Silverstein W, Lewin NA, Goldfrank L. Management of the cocaine-intoxicated patient. *Ann Emerg Med*. 1987;16:234-235.
73. Gay GR, Loper KA. The use of labetalol in the management of cocaine crisis. *Ann Emerg Med*. 1988;17:282-283.
74. Briggs RS, Birtwell AJ, Pohl JE. Hypertensive response to labetalol in phaeochromocytoma. *Lancet*. 1978;1:1045-1046.
75. Hollander JE, Carter WA, Hoffman RS. Use of phentolamine for cocaine-induced myocardial ischemia. *N Engl J Med*. 1992;327:361.
76. Mody CK, Miller BL, McIntyre HB, Cobb SK, Goldberg MA. Neurologic complications of cocaine abuse. *Neurology*. 1988;38:1189-1193.
77. Hoffman CK, Goodman PC. Pulmonary edema in cocaine smokers. *Radiology*. 1989;172:463-465.
78. Cucco RA, Yoo OH, Cregler L, Chang JC. Nonfatal pulmonary edema after "freebase" cocaine smoking. *Am Rev Respir Dis*. 1987;136:179-181.
79. Amin M, Gabelman G, Karpel J, Buttrick P. Acute myocardial infarction and chest pain syndromes after cocaine use. *Am J Cardiol*. 1990;66:1434-1437.
80. Hollander JE, Hoffman RS. Cocaine-induced myocardial infarction: an analysis and review of the literature. *J Emerg Med*. 1992;10:169-177.
81. Mittleman MA, Mintzer D, Maclure M, Tofler GH, Sherwood JB, Muller JE. Triggering of myocardial infarction by cocaine. *Circulation*. 1999;99:2737-2741.
82. Nademanee K, Gorelick DA, Josephson MA, Ryan MA, Wilkins JN, Robertson HA, Mody FV, Intarachot V. Myocardial ischemia during cocaine withdrawal. *Ann Intern Med*. 1989;111:876-880.
83. Kimura T, Yasue H, Sakaino N, Rokutanda M, Jougasaki M, Araki H. Effects of magnesium on the tone of isolated human coronary arteries. Comparison with diltiazem and nitroglycerin. *Circulation*. 1989;79:1118-1124.
84. Woods KL, Fletcher S, Roffe C, Haider Y. Intravenous magnesium sulphate in suspected acute myocardial infarction: results of the second Leicester Intravenous Magnesium Intervention Trial (LIMIT-2). *Lancet*. 1992;339:1553-1558.
85. Gitter MJ, Goldsmith SR, Dunbar DN, Sharkey SW. Cocaine and chest pain: clinical features and outcome of patients hospitalized to rule out myocardial infarction. *Ann Intern Med*. 1991;115:277-282.
86. Hollander JE, Hoffman RS, Gennis P, Fairweather P, DiSano MJ, Schumb DA, Feldman JA, Fish SS, Dyer S, Wax P, Whelan C, Schwarzwald E. Prospective multicenter evaluation of cocaine-associated chest pain. Cocaine Associated Chest Pain (COCHPA) Study Group. *Acad Emerg Med*. 1994;1:330-339.
87. Hollander JE, Shih RD, Hoffman RS, Harchelroad FP, Phillips S, Brent J, Kulig K, Thode HC Jr. Predictors of coronary

artery disease in patients with cocaine-associated myocardial infarction. Cocaine-Associated Myocardial Infarction (CAMI) Study Group. *Am J Med*. 1997;102:158-163.

88. 2005 American Heart Association Guidelines for Cardiopulmonary Resuscitation and Emergency Cardiovascular Care. *Circulation*. 2005;112:IV1-IV203.
89. Hoffman RS, Hollander JE. Evaluation of patients with chest pain after cocaine use. *Crit Care Clin*. 1997;13:809-828.
90. Freemantle N, Cleland J, Young P, Mason J, Harrison J. β-Blockade after myocardial infarction: systematic review and meta regression analysis. *BMJ*. 1999;318:1730-1737.
91. Heesch CM, Wilhelm CR, Ristich J, Adnane J, Bontempo FA, Wagner WR. Cocaine activates platelets and increases the formation of circulating platelet containing microaggregates in humans. *Heart*. 2000;83:688-695.
92. Negus BH, Willard JE, Hillis LD, Glamann DB, Landau C, Snyder RW, Lange RA. Alleviation of cocaine-induced coronary vasoconstriction with intravenous verapamil. *Am J Cardiol*. 1994;73:510-513.
93. Dusenberry SJ, Hicks MJ, Mariani PJ. Labetalol treatment of cocaine toxicity. *Ann Emerg Med*. 1987;16:235.
94. Karch SB. Managing cocaine crisis. *Ann Emerg Med*. 1989;18:228-229.
95. Antman EM, Wenger TL, Butler VP Jr, Haber E, Smith TW. Treatment of 150 cases of life-threatening digitalis intoxication with digoxin-specific Fab antibody fragments. Final report of a multicenter study. *Circulation*. 1990;81:1744-1752.
96. Lapostolle F, Borron SW, Verdier C, Taboulet P, Guerrier G, Adnet F, Clemessy JL, Bismuth C, Baud FJ. Digoxin-specific Fab fragments as single first-line therapy in digitalis poisoning. *Crit Care Med*. 2008;36:3014-3018.
97. Eddleston M, Rajapakse S, Rajakanthan, Jayalath S, Sjostrom L, Santharaj W, Thenabadu PN, Sheriff MH, Warrell DA. Anti-digoxin Fab fragments in cardiotoxicity induced by ingestion of yellow oleander: a randomised controlled trial. *Lancet*. 2000;355:967-972.
98. Dasgupta A, Szelei-Stevens KA. Neutralization of free digoxin-like immunoreactive components of oriental medicines Dan Shen and Lu-Shen-Wan by the Fab fragment of antidigoxin antibody (Digibind). *Am J Clin Pathol*. 2004;121:276-281.
99. Bosse GM, Pope TM. Recurrent digoxin overdose and treatment with digoxin-specific Fab antibody fragments. *J Emerg Med*. 1994;12:179-185.
100. Pearigen PD, Benowitz NL. Poisoning due to calcium antagonists: experience with verapamil, diltiazem and nifedipine. *Drug Saf*. 1991;6:408-430.
101. Jackson CD, Fishbein L. A toxicological review of β-adrenergic blockers. *Fundam Appl Toxicol*. 1986;6:395-422.
102. Erickson FC, Ling LJ, Grande GA, Anderson DL. Diltiazem overdose: case report and review. *J Emerg Med*. 1991;9:357-366.
103. Weinstein RS. Recognition and management of poisoning with beta-adrenergic blocking agents. *Ann Emerg Med*. 1984;13:1123-1131.
104. Kulig K, Bar-Or D, Cantrill SV, Rosen P, Rumack BH. Management of acutely poisoned patients without gastric emptying. *Ann Emerg Med*. 1985;14:562-567.
105. Park GD, Spector R, Goldberg MJ, Johnson GF. Expanded role of charcoal therapy in the poisoned and overdosed patient. *Arch Intern Med*. 1986;146:969-973.
106. Wrenn K, Rodewald L, Dockstader L. Potential misuse of ipecac. *Ann Emerg Med*. 1993;22:1408-1412.
107. Oe H, Taniura T, Ohgitani N. A case of severe verapamil overdose. *Jpn Circ J*. 1998;62:72-76.
108. Proano L, Chiang WK, Wang RY. Calcium channel blocker overdose. *Am J Emerg Med*. 1995;13:444-450.
109. Kline JA, Tomaszewski CA, Schroeder JD, Raymond RM. Insulin is a superior antidote for cardiovascular toxicity induced by verapamil in the anesthetized canine. *J Pharmacol Exp Ther*. 1993;267:744-750.
110. Yuan TH, Kerns WPI, Tomaszewski CA, Ford MD, Kline JA. Insulin-glucose as adjunctive therapy for severe calcium channel antagonist poisoning. *J Toxicol Clin Toxicol*. 1999;37:463-474.
111. Zaritsky AL, Horowitz M, Chernow B. Glucagon antagonism of calcium channel blocker-induced myocardial dysfunction. *Crit Care Med*. 1988;16:246-251.
112. Holzer M, Sterz F, Schoerkhuber W, Behringer W, Domanovits H, Weinmar D, Weinstabl C, Stimpfl T. Successful resuscitation of a verapamil-intoxicated patient with percutaneous cardiopulmonary bypass. *Crit Care Med*. 1999;27:2818-2823.
113. Fahed S, Grum DF, Papadimos TJ. Labetalol infusion for refractory hypertension causing severe hypotension and bradycardia: an issue of patient safety. *Patient Saf Surg*. 2008;2:13.
114. Snook CP, Sigvaldason K, Kristinsson J. Severe atenolol and diltiazem overdose. *J Toxicol Clin Toxicol*. 2000;38:661-665.
115. Pertoldi F, D'Orlando L, Mercante WP. Electromechanical dissociation 48 hours after atenolol overdose: usefulness of calcium chloride. *Ann Emerg Med*. 1998;31:777-781.
116. Dick M, Curwin J, Tepper D. Digitalis intoxication recognition and management. *J Clin Pharmacol*. 1991;31:444-447.
117. Kulig K. Initial management of ingestions of toxic substances. *N Engl J Med*. 1992;326:1677-1681.
118. Smith TW, Butler VP Jr, Haber E, Fozzard H, Marcus FI, Bremner WF, Schulman IC, Phillips A. Treatment of life-threatening digitalis intoxication with digoxin-specific Fab antibody fragments: experience in 26 cases. *N Engl J Med*. 1982;307:1357-1362.
119. Wenger TL, Butler VP Jr, Haber E, Smith TW. Treatment of 63 severely digitalis-toxic patients with digoxin-specific antibody fragments. *J Am Coll Cardiol*. 1985;5:118A-123A.
120. Woolf AD, Wenger T, Smith TW, Lovejoy FH Jr. The use of digoxin-specific Fab fragments for severe digitalis intoxication in children. *N Engl J Med*. 1992;326:1739-1744.
121. Hickey AR, Wenger TL, Carpenter VP, Tilson HH, Hlatky MA, Furberg CD, Kirkpatrick CH, Strauss HC, Smith TW. Digoxin Immune Fab therapy in the management of digitalis intoxication: safety and efficacy results of an observational surveillance study. *J Am Coll Cardiol*. 1991;17:590-598.
122. Wenger TL. Experience with digoxin immune Fab (ovine) in patients with renal impairment. *Am J Emerg Med*. 1991;9:21-23.
123. Woolf AD, Wenger TL, Smith TW, Lovejoy FH Jr. Results of multicenter studies of digoxin-specific antibody fragments in managing digitalis intoxication in the pediatric population. *Am J Emerg Med*. 1991;9:16-20.
124. Taboulet P, Baud FJ, Bismuth C, Vicaut E. Acute digitalis intoxication—is pacing still appropriate? *J Toxicol Clin Toxicol*. 1993;31:261-273.

125. Teba L, Schiebel F, Dedhia HV, Lazzell VA. Beneficial effect of norepinephrine in the treatment of circulatory shock caused by tricyclic antidepressant overdose. *Am J Emerg Med*. 1988;6:566-568.

126. Davey M, Caldicott D. Calcium salts in management of hyperkalaemia. *Emerg Med J*. 2002;19:92-93.

127. Sharff JA, Bayer MJ. Acute and chronic digitalis toxicity: presentation and treatment. *Ann Emerg Med*. 1982;11:327-331.

128. Smith TW, Butler VP Jr, Haber E, Fozzard H, Marcus FI, Bremner WF, Schulman IC, Phillips A. Treatment of life-threatening digitalis intoxication with digoxin-specific Fab antibody fragments: experience in 26 cases. *N Engl J Med*. 1982;307:1357-1362.

129. Bismuth C, Gaultier M, Conso F, Efthymiou ML. Hyperkalemia in acute digitalis poisoning: prognostic significance and therapeutic implications. *Clin Toxicol*. 1973;6:153-162.

130. Lapostolle F, Borron SW. Digitalis. In: Shannon MW, Borron SW, Burns MJ, eds. *Haddad and Winchester's Clinical Management of Poisoning and Drug Overdose*. Philadelphia, PA: Saunders/Elsevier; 2007:949-962.

131. Antman EM, Smith TW. Digitalis toxicity. *Annu Rev Med*. 1985;36:357-367.

132. Reisdorff EJ, Clark MR, Walters BL. Acute digitalis poisoning: the role of intravenous magnesium sulfate. *J Emerg Med*. 1986;4:463-469.

133. Cohen L, Kitzes R. Magnesium sulfate and digitalis-toxic arrhythmias. *JAMA*. 1983;249:2808-2810.

134. Brown TC, Barker GA, Dunlop ME, Loughnan PM. The use of sodium bicarbonate in the treatment of tricyclic antidepressant-induced arrhythmias. *Anaesth Intensive Care*. 1973;1:203-210.

135. Hoffman JR, McElroy CR. Bicarbonate therapy for dysrhythmia and hypotension in tricyclic antidepressant overdose. *West J Med*. 1981;134:60-64.

136. Bailey PM, Little M, Jelinek GA, Wilce JA. Jellyfish envenoming syndromes: unknown toxic mechanisms and unproven therapies. *Med J Aust*. 2003;178:34-37.

137. Foxall GL, Hardman JG, Bedforth NM. Three-dimensional, multiplanar, ultrasound-guided, radial nerve block. *Reg Anesth Pain Med*. 2007;32:516-521.

138. Shah S, Gopalakrishnan S, Apuya J, Martin T. Use of Intralipid in an infant with impending cardiovascular collapse due to local anesthetic toxicity. *J Anesth*. 2009;23:439-441.

139. Zimmer C, Piepenbrink K, Riest G, Peters J. Cardiotoxic and neurotoxic effects after accidental intravascular bupivacaine administration. Therapy with lidocaine propofol and lipid emulsion [in German]. *Anaesthesist*. 2007;56:449-453.

140. Litz RJ, Roessel T, Heller AR, Stehr SN. Reversal of central nervous system and cardiac toxicity after local anesthetic intoxication by lipid emulsion injection. *Anesth Analg*. 2008;106:1575-1577.

141. Ludot H, Tharin JY, Belouadah M, Mazoit JX, Malinovsky JM. Successful resuscitation after ropivacaine and lidocaine-induced ventricular arrhythmia following posterior lumbar plexus block in a child. *Anesth Analg*. 2008;106:1572-1574.

142. Cave G, Harvey MG, Winterbottom T. Evaluation of the Association of Anaesthetists of Great Britain and Ireland lipid infusion protocol in bupivacaine induced cardiac arrest in rabbits. *Anaesthesia*. 2009;64:732-737.

143. DiGregorio RV, Fung HB. Rapid dosing of critical care infusions: the dopamine and norepinephrine "clocks." *J Emerg Nurs*. 2009;35:165-168.

144. Weinberg GL, VadeBoncouer T, Ramaraju GA, Garcia-Amaro MF, Cwik MJ. Pretreatment or resuscitation with a lipid infusion shifts the dose-response to bupivacaine-induced asystole in rats. *Anesthesiology*. 1998;88:1071-1075.

145. Weinberg G, Ripper R, Feinstein DL, Hoffman W. Lipid emulsion infusion rescues dogs from bupivacaine-induced cardiac toxicity. *Reg Anesth Pain Med*. 2003;28:198-202.

146. Weinberg GL, Di Gregorio G, Ripper R, Kelly K, Massad M, Edelman L, Schwartz D, Shah N, Zheng S, Feinstein DL. Resuscitation with lipid versus epinephrine in a rat model of bupivacaine overdose. *Anesthesiology*. 2008;108:907-913.

147. Litz RJ, Popp M, Stehr SN, Koch T. Successful resuscitation of a patient with ropivacaine-induced asystole after axillary plexus block using lipid infusion. *Anaesthesia*. 2006;61:800-801.

148. Rosenblatt MA, Abel M, Fischer GW, Itzkovich CJ, Eisenkraft JB. Successful use of a 20% lipid emulsion to resuscitate a patient after a presumed bupivacaine-related cardiac arrest. *Anesthesiology*. 2006;105:217-218.

149. Civetta JM, Gabel JC. Flow directed-pulmonary artery catheterization in surgical patients: indications and modifications of technic. *Ann Surg*. 1972;176:753-756.

150. Association of Anaesthetists of Great Britain and Ireland. *Guidelines for the Management of Severe Local Anaesthetic Toxicity.* http://www.aagbi.org/sites/default/files/la_toxicity_2010_0.pdf. Published 2010. Accessed October 8, 2012.

151. United Kingdom Resuscitation Council. Cardiac arrest or cardiovascular collapse caused by local anaesthetic. 2008. http://www.resus.org.uk/pages/caLocalA.htm.

152. Neal JM, Bernards CM, Butterworth JFt, Di Gregorio G, Drasner K, Hejtmanek MR, Mulroy MF, Rosenquist RW, Weinberg GL. ASRA practice advisory on local anesthetic systemic toxicity. *Reg Anesth Pain Med*. 2010;35:152-161.

153. Turner-Lawrence DE, Kerns Ii W. Intravenous fat emulsion: a potential novel antidote. *J Med Toxicol*. 2008;4:109-114.

154. Picard J, Ward SC, Zumpe R, Meek T, Barlow J, Harrop-Griffiths W. Guidelines and the adoption of 'lipid rescue' therapy for local anaesthetic toxicity. *Anaesthesia*. 2009;64:122-125.

155. Litovitz TL, Holm KC, Bailey KM, Schmitz BF. 1991 annual report of the American Association of Poison Control Centers National Data Collection System. *Am J Emerg Med*. 1992;10:452-505.

156. Frommer DA, Kulig KW, Marx JA, Rumack B. Tricyclic antidepressant overdose. A review. *JAMA*. 1987;257:521-526.

157. Callaham M, Kassel D. Epidemiology of fatal tricyclic antidepressant ingestion: implications for management. *Ann Emerg Med*. 1985;14:1-9.

158. Braden NJ, Jackson JE, Walson PD. Tricyclic antidepressant overdose. *Pediatr Clin North Am*. 1986;33:287-297.

159. Marshall JB, Forker AD. Cardiovascular effects of tricyclic antidepressant drugs: therapeutic usage, overdose, and management of complications. *Am Heart J*. 1982;103:401-414.

160. Blackman K, Brown SG, Wilkes GJ. Plasma alkalinization for tricyclic antidepressant toxicity: a systematic review. *Emerg Med (Fremantle)*. 2001;13:204-210.

161. Bessen HA, Niemann JT. Improvement of cardiac conduction after hyperventilation in tricyclic antidepressant overdose. *J Toxicol Clin Toxicol*. 1985;23:537-546.

162. Liberatore MA, Robinson DS. Torsade de pointes: a mechanism for sudden death associated with neuroleptic drug therapy? *J Clin Psychopharmacol*. 1984;4:143-146.

163. Tzivoni D, Banai S, Schuger C, Benhorin J, Keren A, Gottlieb S, Stern S. Treatment of torsade de pointes with magnesium sulfate. *Circulation*. 1988;77:392-397.

164. Perticone F, Adinolfi L, Bonaduce D. Efficacy of magnesium sulfate in the treatment of torsade de pointes. *Am Heart J*. 1986;112:847-849.

165. Keren A, Tzivoni D, Gavish D, Levi J, Gottlieb S, Benhorin J, Stern S. Etiology, warning signs and therapy of torsade de pointes. A study of 10 patients. *Circulation*. 1981;64:1167-1174.

166. Iseri LT, Chung P, Tobis J. Magnesium therapy for intractable ventricular tachyarrhythmias in normomagnesemic patients. *West J Med*. 1983;138:823-828.

167. Pentel P, Peterson CD. Asystole complicating physostigmine treatment of tricyclic antidepressant overdose. *Ann Emerg Med*. 1980;9:588-590.

168. Tran TP, Panacek EA, Rhee KJ, Foulke GE. Response to dopamine vs norepinephrine in tricyclic antidepressant–induced hypotension. *Acad Emerg Med*. 1997;4:864-868.

169. Gill AM, Cousins A, Nunn AJ, Choonara IA. Opiate-induced respiratory depression in pediatric patients. *Ann Pharmacother*. 1996;30:125-129.

170. Kelly AM, Kerr D, Dietze P, Patrick I, Walker T, Koutsogiannis Z. Randomised trial of intranasal versus intramuscular naloxone in prehospital treatment for suspected opioid overdose. *Med J Aust*. 2005;182:24-27.

171. Rupreht J, Dworacek B, Oosthoek H, Dzoljic MR, Valkenburg M. Physostigmine versus naloxone in heroin-overdose. *J Toxicol Clin Toxicol*. 1983;21:387-397.

172. Sporer KA, Firestone J, Isaacs SM. Out-of-hospital treatment of opioid overdoses in an urban setting. *Acad Emerg Med*. 1996;3:660-667.

173. Yealy DM, Paris PM, Kaplan RM, Heller MB, Marini SE. The safety of prehospital naloxone administration by paramedics. *Ann Emerg Med*. 1990;19:902-905.

174. Mills CA, Flacke JW, Flacke WE, Bloor BC, Liu MD. Narcotic reversal in hypercapnic dogs: comparison of naloxone and nalbuphine. *Can J Anaesth*. 1990;37:238-244.

175. Part 8: advanced challenges in resuscitation. Section 2: toxicology in ECC. European Resuscitation Council. *Resuscitation*. 2000;46:261-266.

176. Robertson TM, Hendey GW, Stroh G, Shalit M. Intranasal naloxone is a viable alternative to intravenous naloxone for prehospital narcotic overdose. *Prehosp Emerg Care*. 2009;13:512-515.

177. Evans LE, Swainson CP, Roscoe P, Prescott LF. Treatment of drug overdosage with naloxone, a specific narcotic antagonist. *Lancet*. 1973;1:452-455.

178. Wanger K, Brough L, Macmillan I, Goulding J, MacPhail I, Christenson JM. Intravenous vs subcutaneous naloxone for out-of-hospital management of presumed opioid overdose. *Acad Emerg Med*. 1998;5:293-299.

179. Greenberg MI, Roberts JR, Baskin SI. Endotracheal naloxone reversal of morphine-induced respiratory depression in rabbits. *Ann Emerg Med*. 1980;9:289-292.

180. Clarke SF, Dargan PI, Jones AL. Naloxone in opioid poisoning: walking the tightrope. *Emerg Med J*. 2005;22:612-616.

181. Moore RA, Rumack BH, Conner CS, Peterson RG. Naloxone: underdosage after narcotic poisoning. *Am J Dis Child*. 1980;134:156-158.

182. Schneir AB, Vadeboncoeur TF, Offerman SR, Barry JD, Ly BT, Williams SR, Clark RF. Massive OxyContin ingestion refractory to naloxone therapy. *Ann Emerg Med*. 2002;40:425-428.

183. Vilke GM, Buchanan J, Dunford JV, Chan TC. Are heroin overdose deaths related to patient release after prehospital treatment with naloxone? *Prehosp Emerg Care*. 1999;3:183-186.

184. Moss ST, Chan TC, Buchanan J, Dunford JV, Vilke GM. Outcome study of prehospital patients signed out against medical advice by field paramedics. *Ann Emerg Med*. 1998;31:247-250.

185. Treatment of benzodiazepine overdose with flumazenil. The Flumazenil in Benzodiazepine Intoxication Multicenter Study Group. *Clin Ther*. 1992;14:978-995.

186. Lheureux P, Vranckx M, Leduc D, Askenasi R. Flumazenil in mixed benzodiazepine/tricyclic antidepressant overdose: a placebo-controlled study in the dog. *Am J Emerg Med*. 1992;10:184-188.

187. Pitetti RD, Singh S, Pierce MC. Safe and efficacious use of procedural sedation and analgesia by nonanesthesiologists in a pediatric emergency department. *Arch Pediatr Adolesc Med*. 2003;157:1090-1096.

188. Unintentional poisoning deaths—United States, 1999-2004. *MMWR Morb Mortal Wkly Rep*. 2007;56:93-96.

189. Weaver LK. Clinical practice. Carbon monoxide poisoning. *N Engl J Med*. 2009;360:1217-1225.

190. Hampson NB, Zmaeff JL. Outcome of patients experiencing cardiac arrest with carbon monoxide poisoning treated with hyperbaric oxygen. *Ann Emerg Med*. 2001;38:36-41.

191. Sloan EP, Murphy DG, Hart R, Cooper MA, Turnbull T, Barreca RS, Ellerson B. Complications and protocol considerations in carbon monoxide-poisoned patients who require hyperbaric oxygen therapy: report from a ten-year experience. *Ann Emerg Med*. 1989;18:629-634.

192. Chou KJ, Fisher JL, Silver EJ. Characteristics and outcome of children with carbon monoxide poisoning with and without smoke exposure referred for hyperbaric oxygen therapy. *Pediatr Emerg Care*. 2000;16:151-155.

193. Weaver LK, Hopkins RO, Chan KJ, Churchill S, Elliott CG, Clemmer TP, Orme JF Jr, Thomas FO, Morris AH. Hyperbaric oxygen for acute carbon monoxide poisoning. *N Engl J Med*. 2002;347:1057-1067.

194. Thom SR, Taber RL, Mendiguren II, Clark JM, Hardy KR, Fisher AB. Delayed neuropsychologic sequelae after carbon monoxide poisoning: prevention by treatment with hyperbaric oxygen. *Ann Emerg Med*. 1995;25:474-480.

195. Scheinkestel CD, Bailey M, Myles PS, Jones K, Cooper DJ, Millar IL, Tuxen DV. Hyperbaric or normobaric oxygen for acute carbon monoxide poisoning: a randomised controlled clinical trial. *Med J Aust*. 1999;170:203-210.

196. Raphael JC, Elkharrat D, Jars-Guincestre MC, Chastang C, Chasles V, Vercken JB, Gajdos P. Trial of normobaric and hyperbaric oxygen for acute carbon monoxide intoxication. *Lancet*. 1989;2:414-419.

197. Juurlink DN, Buckley NA, Stanbrook MB, Isbister GK, Bennett M, McGuigan MA. Hyperbaric oxygen for carbon monoxide poisoning. *Cochrane Database Syst Rev*. 2005:CD002041.

198. Buckley NA, Isbister GK, Stokes B, Juurlink DN. Hyperbaric oxygen for carbon monoxide poisoning: a systematic review and critical analysis of the evidence. *Toxicol Rev*. 2005;24:75-92.

199. Wolf SJ, Lavonas EJ, Sloan EP, Jagoda AS. Clinical policy: critical issues in the management of adult patients presenting to the emergency department with acute carbon monoxide poisoning. *J Emerg Nurs*. 2008;34:e19-32.

200. Satran D, Henry CR, Adkinson C, Nicholson CI, Bracha Y, Henry TD. Cardiovascular manifestations of moderate to severe carbon monoxide poisoning. *J Am Coll Cardiol*. 2005;45:1513-1516.

201. Henry CR, Satran D, Lindgren B, Adkinson C, Nicholson CI, Henry TD. Myocardial injury and long-term mortality following moderate to severe carbon monoxide poisoning. *JAMA*. 2006;295:398-402.

202. do Nascimento TS, Pereira RO, de Mello HL, Costa J. Methemoglobinemia: from diagnosis to treatment. *Rev Bras Anestesiol*. 2008;58:651-664.

203. Mansouri A, Lurie AA. Concise review: methemoglobinemia. *Am J Hematol*. 1993;42:7-12.

204. Ash-Bernal R, Wise R, Wright SM. Acquired methemoglobinemia: a retrospective series of 138 cases at 2 teaching hospitals. *Medicine (Baltimore)*. 2004;83:265-273.

205. Guay J. Methemoglobinemia related to local anesthetics: a summary of 242 episodes. *Anesth Analg*. 2009;108:837-845.

206. Wright RO, Lewander WJ, Woolf AD. Methemoglobinemia: etiology, pharmacology, and clinical management. *Ann Emerg Med*. 1999;34:646-656.

207. Baud FJ, Barriot P, Toffis V, Riou B, Vicaut E, Lecarpentier Y, Bourdon R, Astier A, Bismuth C. Elevated blood cyanide concentrations in victims of smoke inhalation. *N Engl J Med*. 1991;325:1761-1766.

208. Borron SW, Baud FJ, Barriot P, Imbert M, Bismuth C. Prospective study of hydroxocobalamin for acute cyanide poisoning in smoke inhalation. *Ann Emerg Med*. 2007;49:794-801, 801 e791-792.

209. Fortin JL, Giocanti JP, Ruttimann M, Kowalski JJ. Prehospital administration of hydroxocobalamin for smoke inhalation-associated cyanide poisoning: 8 years of experience in the Paris Fire Brigade. *Clin Toxicol (Phila)*. 2006;44(suppl 1):37-44.

210. Borron SW, Baud FJ, Megarbane B, Bismuth C. Hydroxocobalamin for severe acute cyanide poisoning by ingestion or inhalation. *Am J Emerg Med*. 2007;25:551-558.

211. Espinoza OB, Perez M, Ramirez MS. Bitter cassava poisoning in eight children: a case report. *Vet Hum Toxicol*. 1992;34:65.

212. Houeto P, Hoffman JR, Imbert M, Levillain P, Baud FJ. Relation of blood cyanide to plasma cyanocobalamin concentration after a fixed dose of hydroxocobalamin in cyanide poisoning. *Lancet*. 1995;346:605-608.

213. Pontal P, Bismuth C, Garnier R. Therapeutic attitude in cyanide poisoning: retrospective study of 24 non-lethal cases *Vet Hum Toxicol*. 1982;24:286-287.

214. Kirk MA, Gerace R, Kulig KW. Cyanide and methemoglobin kinetics in smoke inhalation victims treated with the cyanide antidote kit. *Ann Emerg Med*. 1993;22:1413-1418.

215. Chen KK, Rose CL. Nitrite and thiosulfate therapy in cyanide poisoning. *J Am Med Assoc*. 1952;149:113-119.

216. Kiese M, Weger N. Formation of ferrihaemoglobin with aminophenols in the human for the treatment of cyanide poisoning. *Eur J Pharmacol*. 1969;7:97-105.

217. Hall AH, Saiers J, Baud F. Which cyanide antidote? *Crit Rev Toxicol*. 2009;39:541-552.

218. Hobel M, Engeser P, Nemeth L, Pill J. The antidote effect of thiosulphate and hydroxocobalamin in formation of nitroprusside intoxication of rabbits. *Arch Toxicol*. 1980;46:207-213.

219. Mengel K, Kramer W, Isert B, Friedberg KD. Thiosulphate and hydroxocobalamin prophylaxis in progressive cyanide poisoning in guinea-pigs. *Toxicology*. 1989;54:335-342.

220. Friedberg KD, Shukla UR. The efficiency of aquocobalamine as an antidote in cyanide poisoning when given alone or combined with sodium thiosulfate. *Arch Toxicol*. 1975;33:103-113.

221. Hall AH, Rumack BH. Hydroxycobalamin/sodium thiosulfate as a cyanide antidote. *J Emerg Med*. 1987;5:115-121.

222. Forsyth JC, Mueller PD, Becker CE, Osterloh J, Benowitz NL, Rumack BH, Hall AH. Hydroxocobalamin as a cyanide antidote: safety, efficacy and pharmacokinetics in heavily smoking normal volunteers. *J Toxicol Clin Toxicol*. 1993;31:277-294.

223. Pearlman BL, Gambhir R. Salicylate intoxication: a clinical review. *Postgrad Med*. 2009;121:162-168.

224. Kuzak N, Brubacher JR, Kennedy JR. Reversal of salicylate-induced euglycemic delirium with dextrose. *Clin Toxicol (Phila)*. 2007;45:526-529.

225. Proudfoot AT, Krenzelok EP, Brent J, Vale JA. Does urine alkalinization increase salicylate elimination? If so, why? *Toxicol Rev*. 2003;22:129-136.

226. Chyka PA, Erdman AR, Christianson G, Wax PM, Booze LL, Manoguerra AS, Caravati EM, Nelson LS, Olson KR, Cobaugh DJ, Scharman EJ, Woolf AD, Troutman WG. Salicylate poisoning: an evidence-based consensus guideline for out-of-hospital management. *Clin Toxicol (Phila)*. 2007;45:95-131.

227. Dargan PI, Wallace CI, Jones AL. An evidence based flowchart to guide the management of acute salicylate (aspirin) overdose. *Emerg Med J*. 2002;19:206-209.

228. Position statement and practice guidelines on the use of multi-dose activated charcoal in the treatment of acute poisoning. American Academy of Clinical Toxicology; European Association of Poisons Centres and Clinical Toxicologists. *Clin Toxicol.* 1999;37:731-751.

Chapter 15

Life-Threatening Electrolyte and Acid-Base Abnormalities

This Chapter

- Common Causes of Electrolyte Imbalances
- Early Recognition of Symptoms of Electrolyte and Acid-Base Disorders
- Diagnostic and Therapeutic Equations for Treating Electrolyte Abnormalities
- Rapid Response Interventions for Life-Threatening Electrolyte Imbalances
- Diagnosing Acid-Base Imbalances
- Diabetic Ketoacidosis in Patients *Without* Insulin-Dependent Diabetes?
- The Importance of Potassium in Diabetic Ketoacidosis
- Classic Findings of Nonketotic Hyperosmolar Syndrome

Introduction

Electrolyte and acid-base abnormalities are commonly associated with cardiovascular and neurologic emergencies and may cause or contribute to cardiac arrest, hinder resuscitative efforts, and affect hemodynamic recovery after cardiac arrest. Identified abnormalities probably represent only the tip of the iceberg—the numerator of a much larger, unrecognized denominator.

Conditions that can frequently cause electrolyte and acid-base abnormalities are listed in Table 50.

This chapter refers to electrolyte values that are above or below the normal range. For ease of reference, Table 51 presents the normal range for a number of relevant clinical parameters. Table 51 also contains the various diagnostic and therapeutic equations presented throughout the chapter. But be sure to check the reference ranges for your laboratory because there may be slight variations based on patient demographics and test variability.

Table 50. Examples of Conditions Frequently Associated With Life-Threatening Electrolyte or Acid-Base Abnormalities

Possible Presenting Signs and Symptoms	
• Vomiting • Diarrhea, constipation	• Confusion, lethargy, irritability • Weakness, fatigue
Acute Conditions	
• Use of multiple medications • Alcohol abuse, acute • Pancreatitis • Poor oral intake • Recent seizures	• Recent surgery • Peritonitis • Poisoning and overdose • Diabetic ketoacidosis • Acute respiratory failure • Shock states
Chronic Medical Problems	
• Renal failure • Drug abuse • Metastatic cancer • Immobilization • Alcohol abuse, chronic • Hyperalimentation • Malnutrition • Nephrotic syndrome	• Insulin-dependent diabetes • Hypertension • Cirrhosis • Congestive heart failure • COPD

Abbreviation: COPD, chronic obstructive pulmonary disease.

Table 51. Normal Values of Electrolytes (A) and Diagnostic and Therapeutic Equations (B)

A. Normal Values			
Parameter (Symbol)	**Reference Range (Normal)**	**Parameter (Symbol)**	**Reference Range (Normal)**
Sodium (Na^+)	135 to 145 mEq/L	**Arterial Blood Gases (Room Air)**	
Potassium (K^+)	3.5 to 5 mEq/L	pH	7.35 to 7.45
Chloride (Cl^-)	98 to 108 mEq/L	Pco_2	35 to 45 mm Hg
Carbon dioxide (as HCO_3^-)	22 to 32 mEq/L	Bicarbonate (HCO_3^-)	22 to 32 mEq/L
Anion gap	10 to 15 mEq/L	Base excess	> +2 = Metabolic alkalosis
Glucose	62 to 125 mg/dL	Base deficit	< −2 = Metabolic acidosis
Urea nitrogen (BUN)	8 to 21 mg/dL	Calculated vs measured pH	See below
Creatinine	0.3 to 1.2 mg/dL		
Calcium, total (Ca^{2+})	8.5 to 10.5 mg/dL		
Calcium, ionized	4.2 to 4.8 mg/dL		
Magnesium (Mg^{2+})	1.3 to 2.2 mEq/L		
Urine specific gravity	1.005 to 1.030 mg/mL		
Albumin	3.5 to 5.2 g/dL		
Protein, total	6 to 8.2 g/dL		
Osmolality, serum	275 to 295 mOsm/L		

B. Useful Calculations and Formulae*		
Calculation	**Formula**	**Comments**
Anion gap (serum concentration in mEq/L)	$[Na^+] - ([Cl^-] + [HCO_3^-])$	Normal range: 10 to 15 mEq/L. A gap >15 suggests metabolic acidosis.
Osmolal gap	$\text{Osmolality}_{measured} - \text{Osmolality}_{calculated}$ Normal = <10	Osmolal gap normally <10. If osmolal gap is >10, suspect unknown osmotically active substances.
Calculated osmolality (in mOsm/L)	$(2 \times [Na^+]) + ([\text{Glucose}] \div 18) + ([\text{BUN}] \div 2.8)$	Simplified to give *effective* osmolality. Normal = 272 to 300 mOsm/L.
Total free water deficit (in liters)	$\frac{([Na^+]_{measured} - 140) \times \text{TBW}}{140}$ $\text{TBW}_{in\ L} = (0.6_{men} \text{ or } 0.5_{women}) \times \text{Weight}_{in\ kg}$	Use to calculate quantity of water needed to correct water deficit in hypernatremia.
Sodium deficit (in total mEq)	$([Na^+]_{desired} - [Na^+]_{measured}) \times \text{TBW}_{in\ L}$ $\text{TBW}_{in\ L} = (0.6_{men} \text{ or } 0.5_{women}) \times \text{Weight}_{in\ kg}$	Use to calculate sodium deficit to replace with 3% saline in severe hyponatremia (3% saline contains sodium 513 mEq/L).
Determination of predicted pH	$(40 - Pco_2) \times 0.008 =$ $\pm\Delta$ in pH from 7.4	For every 1 mm Hg change in Pco_2 from 40, pH will change by 0.008. Measured pH less than calculated pH: metabolic acidosis is present. Measured pH greater than predicted pH: metabolic alkalosis is present.

Abbreviations: BUN, blood urea nitrogen; TBW, total body water.

*See text for details. Concentration units are the same as listed above.

Potassium

Maintaining the potassium gradient across cell membranes is critical for muscular and neurologic function. Minor changes in the serum potassium concentration can have major effects on the excitability of the heart and conduction within it. Of all significant electrolyte abnormalities, rapid changes in serum potassium are the most likely to be life threatening.

Hyperkalemia

Normal potassium range: 3.5 to 5 mEq/L

Hyperkalemia is one of the few potentially lethal electrolyte disturbances.

Causes

Table 52 lists the most common causes of hyperkalemia. Hyperkalemia generally is caused by either increased K^+ release from cells or impaired excretion by the kidneys. Acute hyperkalemia may also be iatrogenic caused by rapid or excessive administration of potassium for replacement therapy. Evaluation of serum potassium must include the effects of changes in serum pH. When serum pH falls, serum potassium rises because potassium shifts from the cellular to the vascular space. When serum pH rises, serum potassium falls because potassium shifts from the vascular space into the cells. Remember that *serum potassium changes in a direction opposite to serum pH.*

Early recognition of conditions that cause hyperkalemia may prevent or minimize hyperkalemic cardiac arrhythmias.[1-3] The most common cause of severe, life-threatening hyperkalemia is kidney failure.[4]

Medications are the most frequent *exogenous* cause of hyperkalemia.

- Potassium supplements prescribed to prevent *hypo*kalemia are the most frequent cause of hyperkalemia in hospitalized patients.

Diagnosis

The most common symptoms of hyperkalemia are nonspecific: *weakness, hypotension,* and *paresthesias.* As serum potassium rises, an *ascending flaccid paralysis* may develop. Severe hyperkalemia may also cause paresthesia, depressed tendon reflexes, or respiratory paralysis.[5,6]

The physical examination, the 12-lead electrocardiogram (ECG), and serum potassium concentration provide

Table 52. **Common Causes of Hyperkalemia**

Endogenous Causes
• Chronic renal failure
• Metabolic acidosis (eg, diabetic ketoacidosis)
• Pseudohypoaldosteronism type II (also known as Gordon's syndrome; familial hyperkalemia and hypertension)
• Chemotherapy causing tumor lysis
• Muscle breakdown (rhabdomyolysis)
• Renal tubular acidosis
• Hemolysis
• Hypoaldosteronism (Addison's disease, hyporeninemia)
• Hyperkalemic periodic paralysis
Exogenous Causes
• Medications: K^+-sparing diuretics, ACE inhibitors, nonsteroidal anti-inflammatory drugs, potassium supplements, penicillin derivatives, succinylcholine (in paralyzed patients), β-blockers
• Blood administration (particularly with older "bank" blood)
• Diet (rarely the sole cause), salt substitutes
• Pseudohyperkalemia (due to blood sampling or hemolysis, high white blood cell count, high platelets, tumor lysis syndrome)

Abbreviation: ACE, angiotensin-converting enzyme.

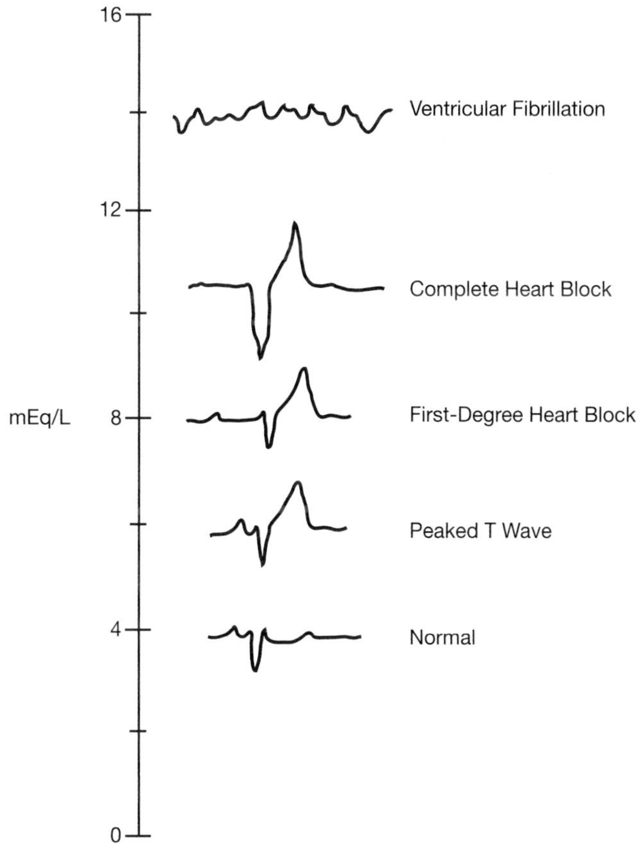

Figure 107. Electrocardiographic changes associated with progressive hyperkalemia. Adapted from Burch and Winsor.[7]

Table 53. Increasing Serum Potassium Levels and Most Frequently Associated ECG Findings

Serum Potassium Range (mEq/L)	Frequent ECG Findings
5.5 to <6	Peaking (tenting) of T waves (most prominent early ECG change)
6 to <6.5	Increasing PR and QT intervals
6.5 to <7	Flattened P waves and ST segments
7 to <7.5	Widened QRS complexes
7.5 to <8	Deepening S waves, merging of S and T waves
8 to <10	Sine-wave-shaped complexes begin; idioventricular complexes and rhythms; VT-like appearance
≥10	PEA (often with a "sine wave" appearance), VF/VT, asystole

Abbreviations: ECG, electrocardiographic; PEA, pulseless electrical activity; VF, ventricular fibrillation; VT, ventricular tachycardia.

important (though indirect) information about the significance of the hyperkalemia. These evaluations must be performed promptly for critically ill patients. As the hyperkalemia worsens, the ECG becomes abnormal. The first indicator of hyperkalemia may be the presence of peaked T waves (tenting) on the ECG. The ECG may progressively develop flattened or absent P waves, a prolonged PR interval, widened QRS complex, deepened S waves, and merging of S and T waves. Table 53 lists these ECG changes in roughly the sequence in which they occur, and Figure 107 illustrates their appearance. The development of widened QRS complexes heralds significant cardiac dysfunction.

Treatment

The first critical action in treating hyperkalemia is to reduce potassium intake as much as possible:

- Stop any potassium supplementation.
- Identify and discontinue any prescribed or over-the-counter drugs that can cause hyperkalemia.

Therapeutic interventions involve treatments that antagonize or inhibit the action of potassium on cell membranes (calcium), induce a transcellular shift of potassium (insulin/dextrose, albuterol, sodium bicarbonate), and enhance clearance (resins, loop diuretics, hemodialysis).

- **Mild hyperkalemia (5 to 6 mEq/L):** Remove potassium from the body by one or more of the following therapies:
  - Diuretics: Furosemide 1 mg/kg (40 to 80 mg), slow intravenous (IV) (Note that dehydration, hypovolemia, hypotension, or other electrolyte imbalance may occur.)
  - Resins: Kayexalate 15 to 50 g in 50 to 100 mL of 20% sorbitol, either orally or by retention enema
  - Dialysis: For patients with chronic renal failure receiving peritoneal or hemodialysis
- **Moderate hyperkalemia (6 to 7 mEq/L):** Initiate a rapid but *temporary* intracellular shift of potassium using the following agents:
  - Sodium bicarbonate: 50 mEq IV or up to 1 mEq/kg IV over 5 minutes (sodium bicarbonate alone is less effective than glucose plus insulin or nebulized albuterol; it is best used in conjunction with these medications)
  - Glucose plus insulin: Mix 10 units regular insulin and 25 g (50 mL of D_{50}) glucose, and give IV over 15 to 30 minutes
  - Nebulized albuterol: 5 to 20 mg over 15 minutes

The Hyperkalemic Patient in Periarrest

Hyperkalemic patients in periarrest usually have renal failure. Hyperkalemia can also complicate systemic acidosis, so therapy must also be directed at reversing the cause of the acidosis. Patients with severe potassium elevation (more than 6.5 mEq/L), especially those with widened QRS complexes, require urgent care.

- **Severe hyperkalemia (more than 6.5 mEq/L with potassium-induced ECG changes):**
  - First and most urgent, give 5 to 10 mL of 10% calcium chloride IV over 2 to 5 minutes or 15 to 30 mL of 10% calcium gluconate IV over 2 to 5 minutes. Calcium will antagonize the toxic effects of potassium at the myocardial cell membrane, lowering the risk of ventricular fibrillation (VF).
  - Second, as described for moderate hyperkalemia, initiate a rapid shift of K^+ into cells with sodium bicarbonate, glucose plus insulin, and nebulized albuterol (as for moderate hyperkalemia; see Table 54). This may need to be repeated.
  - Third, begin removal of K^+ from the body with diuretics, resins, or dialysis as described for mild hyperkalemia. Dialysis is the treatment of choice for patients with renal failure.

If hyperkalemia is left untreated, a sine-wave ECG pattern, idioventricular rhythms, and asystolic cardiac arrest may develop.[8,9] When cardiac arrest occurs secondary to hyperkalemia, it may be reasonable to administer adjuvant IV therapy as outlined above in addition to standard ACLS (Class IIb, Level of Evidence [LOE] C).

Table 54 summarizes the emergency treatments and treatment sequence recommended for hyperkalemia.

Hypokalemia

Normal potassium range: 3.5 to 5 mEq/L

Life-threatening hypokalemia is uncommon but can occur in the setting of gastrointestinal (GI) and renal losses and is associated with hypomagnesemia. Severe hypokalemia will alter cardiac tissue excitability and conduction. Hypokalemia can produce ECG changes such as U waves, T-wave flattening, and arrhythmias (especially if the patient is taking digoxin), particularly ventricular arrhythmias,[10,11] which, if left untreated, deteriorate to pulseless electrical activity (PEA) or asystole. Several studies reported an association with hypokalemia and development of VF,[12-15] whereas a single animal study reported that hypokalemia lowered the VF threshold.[16] However, the management of hypokalemia in the setting of cardiotoxicity, specifically torsades de pointes, is largely based on historical case reports that report slow infusion of potassium over hours.[17]

Causes

The most common causes of low serum potassium are GI loss (diarrhea, laxatives), renal loss (hyperaldosteronism, severe hyperglycemia, potassium-depleting diuretics, carbenicillin, sodium penicillin, amphotericin B), intracellular shift (alkalosis or a rise in pH), and malnutrition (Table 55).

Diagnosis

In 1 survey, severe hypokalemia (potassium less than 3.0 mEq/L) was present in 2.6% of hospitalized patients and was associated with a 21% mortality rate.[18] Hypokalemia in patients hospitalized with acute myocardial infarction is an independent risk factor for VF.[13] Hypokalemia may exist for several reasons. Patients with cardiovascular disease may be taking potassium-wasting diuretics. In addition, stress hormones such as catecholamines can cause a transcellular shift of potassium into cells, causing or aggravating hypokalemia. Patients with cardiac ischemia, heart failure, or ventricular hypertrophy have an increased risk of cardiac arrhythmias even with mild to moderate hypokalemia.[19]

Signs and symptoms of hypokalemia correlate with both the level of serum potassium and the speed of the fall in serum potassium[10]:

- **Mild (3 to 3.5 mEq/L):** Often no symptoms
- **Moderate (2.5 to less than 3.0 mEq/L):** Generalized weakness, fatigue, lassitude, constipation, leg cramps

Table 54. **Emergency Treatments and Treatment Sequence for Hyperkalemia**

Therapy	Dose	Effect/Mechanism	Onset of Effect	Duration of Effect
Calcium	• **Calcium chloride** (10%): 5 to 10 mL IV over 2 to 5 min • **Calcium gluconate** (10%): 15 to 30 mL IV over 2 to 5 min	• Antagonism of toxic effects of hyperkalemia at cell membrane	• 1 to 3 min	• 30 to 60 min
Sodium bicarbonate	• Give 50 mEq IV over 5 min	• Redistribution: intracellular shift	• 5 to 10 min	• 1 to 2 h
Insulin plus glucose (use 2 units insulin per 5 g glucose)	• 10 units regular insulin IV plus 25 g dextrose (50 mL D_{50})	• Redistribution: intracellular shift	• 30 min	• 4 to 6 h
Nebulized albuterol	• 10 to 20 mg over 15 min • May repeat	• Redistribution: intracellular shift	• 15 min	• 15 to 90 min
Diuresis with furosemide	• 40 to 80 mg IV bolus	• Removal from body	• At start of diuresis	• Until end of diuresis
Cation-exchange resin (Kayexalate)	• 15 to 50 g PO or PR plus sorbitol	• Removal from body	• 1 to 2 h	• 4 to 6 h
Peritoneal or hemodialysis	• Per institutional protocol	• Removal from body	• At start of dialysis	• Until end of dialysis

Abbreviation: IV, intravenous.

Table 55. Common Causes of Hypokalemia

Decreased Intake
• Poor dietary intake • Malnutrition
Gastrointestinal and Sweat Losses
• Vomiting (including eating disorders) • Nasogastric suction • Diarrhea (including laxative or enema abuse) • Malabsorption syndromes • Enteric fistula • Ureterosigmoidostomy • Loss through sweating (heavy exercise, heat stroke, febrile illnesses)
Increased Renal Losses
• Diuretic use • Renal tubular acidosis • Primary aldosteronism • Secondary aldosteronism (renal artery stenosis, CHF, cirrhosis plus ascites, excess of ACTH or glucocorticosteroids) • Licorice ingestion • Chewing tobacco • Rare causes of renal loss: – Bartter's syndrome: Disorder of renal tubules causing high aldosterone, low potassium, and metabolic alkalosis – Liddle's syndrome: Autosomal dominant condition of renal tubules causing increased potassium secretion
Medications
• Aminoglycosides • Penicillins (eg, carbenicillin) • Cisplatin, amphotericin B • L-Dopa • Lithium • Thallium • Theophylline
Redistribution: Extracellular to Intracellular Potassium Shifts
• Redistribution with pH changes: – Acidosis (or fall in pH) raises serum K^+ – Alkalosis (or rise in pH) lowers serum K^+ • Treatment of diabetic ketoacidosis • Insulin administration • Hypomagnesemia • β_2-Adrenergic agents (eg, albuterol) • Hypokalemic periodic paralysis (congenital disorder causing intermittent episodes of muscle weakness due to low serum potassium)

Abbreviations: ACTH, adrenocorticotropic hormone; CHF, congestive heart failure.

- **Severe (2.0 to less than 2.5 mEq/L):** Muscle breakdown (rhabdomyolysis), paralytic ileus, bowel obstruction
- **Life threatening (less than 2.0 mEq/L):** Development of ascending paralysis, impairment of respiratory function, unstable cardiac arrhythmias

Hypokalemia is suggested by changes in the ECG (see Table 56).

Treatment

The effect of bolus administration of potassium for cardiac arrest suspected to be secondary to hypokalemia is unknown and ill advised (Class III, LOE C).

Mild and Moderate Hypokalemia

Whereas critical hypokalemia is treated empirically, calculated potassium replacement for mild and moderate hypokalemia should be based on an estimate of the total body potassium deficit:

- As a rule of thumb, for every 1 mEq/L decrease in serum potassium, the total body deficit is 150 to 400 mEq.
- Total body potassium and the estimated deficit are based on age, sex, and body size. For example, the 150 mEq estimated deficit is appropriate for an elderly woman with low muscle mass. But for a young, muscular man, an estimated deficit of 400 mEq for every 1 mEq/L decrease in serum K^+ is more appropriate.
- Because changes in pH affect serum potassium, another rule of thumb has evolved: serum K^+ decreases by about 0.3 mEq/L for every 0.1 unit increase in pH above normal. Consequently, a patient with alkalosis (pH more than 7.45) will have a lower serum potassium than expected on the basis of total body potassium. The astute clinician will decrease the amount of replacement potassium for an alkalotic patient with hypokalemia if the alkalosis is also corrected.
- Base decisions about route (oral versus IV) and speed (fast versus slow) of potassium replacement on the patient's clinical condition. In general, oral potassium

Table 56. Decreasing Potassium Levels and Most Frequently Associated ECG Findings

Serum Potassium Range (mEq/L)	Frequent ECG Findings
2.5 to 3	U waves begin, flattened T waves, low QRS voltage, prominent P waves
2 to <2.5	More prominent U waves, more ST-segment changes
<2	Widened QRS complexes, arrhythmias, PEA, asystole

Abbreviations: ECG, electrocardiographic; PEA, pulseless electrical activity.

replacement is preferable. Rapid correction is appropriate only for clinically unstable patients.

- Stable patients: Limit the potassium replacement dose to approximately 10 to 20 mEq/h.
  - Maximum concentration: Approximately 40 mEq in 1 L of normal saline. Maximum rate: Approximately 40 mEq in 1 hour. An infusion of 40 mEq will acutely raise the serum potassium concentration by approximately 0.5 mEq/L.
  - Monitor the ECG continuously during IV potassium infusion. If potassium is infused through a central line, the tip of the catheter should not be in the right atrium. Potassium infusion into the coronary sinus is thought to contribute to life-threatening arrhythmias.

For more information, see Weaver and Burchell's classic article on ECG changes in hypokalemia.[20]

Sodium

Sodium abnormalities are unlikely to lead to cardiac arrest, and there are no specific recommendations for either checking or treating sodium during cardiac arrest. Disturbances in sodium level are unlikely to be the primary cause of severe cardiovascular instability.

Sodium is the major intravascular ion that influences serum osmolality. An acute increase in serum sodium will produce an acute increase in serum osmolality; an acute decrease in serum sodium will produce an acute fall in serum osmolality. Sodium concentration and osmolality in the intravascular and interstitial spaces equilibrate across the vascular membrane.

Acute changes in serum sodium will produce free water shifts into and out of the vascular space until osmolality equilibrates in these compartments. An acute fall in serum sodium will produce an acute shift of free water from the vascular into the interstitial space and may cause cerebral edema.[21-23] An acute rise in serum sodium will produce an acute shift of free water from the interstitial to the vascular space. Rapid correction of hyponatremia has been associated with development of rhabdomyolysis,[24,25] pontine myelinolysis,[26,27] and cerebral bleeding.[24,26,27] For these reasons, monitor neurologic function closely in the patient with hypernatremia or hyponatremia, particularly during correction of these conditions. Whenever possible, correct serum sodium slowly, carefully controlling the total change in serum sodium over 48 hours and avoiding overcorrection.[28,29]

Under normal conditions the serum sodium concentration and serum osmolality are controlled through the *renin-angiotensin-aldosterone system* and with the *antidiuretic hormone* (ADH, also known as arginine vasopressin, or AVP). Sodium, the most abundant positive ion in the extracellular space, determines the size of the extracellular fluid (ECF) volume. Abnormalities in sodium concentration generally reflect abnormalities of total body water.

Sodium is an extracellular ion. It is present in relatively small concentrations intracellularly and relatively large concentrations extracellularly (in the interstitial space). When the total sodium content of the body increases, ECF will increase, resulting in volume overload. Sodium retention and ECF volume overload occur frequently with congestive heart failure (CHF), congestive cirrhosis of the liver, and the nephrotic syndrome. When the total sodium content decreases, ECF volume also decreases (volume depletion). This causes signs of poor skin turgor, tachycardia, and orthostatic hypotension.

Remember these general rules:

1. High serum sodium concentration generally indicates free water depletion; low serum sodium concentration indicates free water overload.
2. Abnormally high or low serum sodium concentration usually indicates volume-related problems.
3. Clinical problems related to inappropriate intravascular volume (eg, CHF, edema, orthostatic syncope) often reflect problems in sodium concentration.

Hypernatremia

Normal sodium range: 135 to 145 mEq/L

Hypernatremia may be caused by a primary gain in Na^+ or excess loss of water. Hypernatremia may cause neurologic symptoms such as altered mental status, weakness, irritability, focal neurologic deficits, and even coma or seizures. The severity of symptoms is determined by the speed and magnitude of the change in serum sodium concentration.

Causes

Gains in sodium can result from hyperaldosteronism (excess mineralocorticoid), Cushing's syndrome (excess glucocorticoid), or excessive hypertonic saline or sodium bicarbonate administration. Loss of free water can result from GI losses or renal excretion (eg, osmotic diuresis or diabetes insipidus).

Hypernatremia is generally caused by 1 of 3 mechanisms:

1. Insufficient water intake, resulting most often in *normovolemic hypernatremia*
2. Loss of water and sodium (but water loss in excess of sodium loss), resulting most often in *hypovolemic hypernatremia*
3. Gain of water and sodium (but sodium gain exceeds water gain), resulting most often in *hypervolemic hypernatremia*

The most frequent clinical scenario is loss of both water and sodium but more water relative to sodium (hypovolemic hypernatremia). Most hypernatremic patients in periarrest are hypovolemic. Somewhat counterintuitively, patients with hypernatremia usually have an absolute reduction in total body sodium. As serum sodium is lowered to a safe level, these patients will require administration of normal saline to replenish total body stores. Table 57 lists the most common causes of hypernatremia according to these 3 mechanisms. This method of classification helps identify the cause of the hypernatremia and provides guidance for therapy.

Table 57. Common Causes of Hypernatremia

Reduced Intake of Free Water: Normovolemic or Hypovolemic Hypernatremia
• Mild free water loss, such as increased insensible water losses • Conditions that lead to inability to obtain free water: – Infancy – Coma, dementia – Bed confinement, intubation – Injuries – Environmental emergencies (wilderness travel, castaways)
Significant Loss of Free Water (With Moderate Loss of Sodium): Hypovolemic Hypernatremia
• GI losses: vomiting, diarrhea, nasogastric suctioning, fistulas • Renal losses: – Osmotic diuresis such as mannitol administration – Diabetes insipidus with loss of concentrating ability: central (no vasopressin from pituitary gland) or nephrogenic (no renal response to vasopressin) – Postobstructive state • Dermal losses: sweating, burns
Significant Gain of Sodium (With Moderate Gain of Free Water): Hypervolemic Hypernatremia
• Excessive sodium bicarbonate administration • Hypertonic saline administration, salt tablets, errors in formula preparation • Seawater ingestion • Excess mineralocorticoid (primary aldosteronism) • Excess glucocorticoid (Cushing's syndrome, exogenous, ectopic ACTH syndromes)

Abbreviations: ACTH, adrenocorticotropic hormone; GI, gastrointestinal.

Diagnosis

Hypernatremia causes water to shift from the interstitial space into the vascular space. Significant hypernatremia can cause a shift of free water from the cellular space, causing intracellular dehydration. The severity of hypernatremia symptoms depends on the acuteness and severity of the rise in serum sodium.

- **Neurologic symptoms:** An acute free water shift from the interstitial to the vascular space can cause nausea and vomiting, lack of appetite, irritability, and fatigue.
- **Neurologic signs:** Physical signs include confusion, stupor, and coma; seizures; altered mental status; muscle weakness, twitching, or spasticity; tremor or ataxia; or focal neurologic signs such as paresis or abnormal plantar reflexes.

Patients with hypernatremia caused by decreased water intake or excessive water loss in relation to sodium loss (hypovolemic hypernatremia) will have signs and symptoms of dehydration and hypovolemia. These patients will usually report excessive thirst, fatigue, and orthostatic symptoms such as dizziness and lightheadedness.

Treatment

Treatment of hypernatremia includes reduction of ongoing water losses (by treating the underlying cause) and correction of the water deficit. For stable, asymptomatic patients, replacement of fluid by mouth or through a nasogastric tube is effective and safe. In hypovolemic patients the ECF volume is typically restored with normal saline or a solution of 5% dextrose in half-normal saline to prevent a rapid fall in the serum sodium concentration. Avoid D_5W because it will reduce serum sodium too rapidly. During rehydration, monitor serum sodium closely to ensure a gradual fall (and prevent a rapid fall) in serum sodium.

It is important to remember that sodium abnormalities primarily indicate water problems. The major therapeutic approach is *not* to remove excess sodium but to replace the lost water.

- Most patients with hypernatremia are hypovolemic. They have a deficit of free water and sodium, but the free water deficit is more significant than the sodium deficit. Treatment requires careful replacement of both volume and sodium while avoiding a rapid fall in serum sodium and osmolality.
- Too rapid a correction in serum sodium will cause dangerous fluid shifts and risk of cerebral edema or other physiologic derangements.

Calculation of water deficit: Correct the water deficit (usually with normal saline) and stop ongoing water losses by treating the underlying cause. The key step is to calculate the quantity of water needed to correct the water deficit:

Water deficit (in liters) =

$$\frac{\text{plasma Na}^{+}\text{ concentration} - 140}{140} \times \text{total body water}$$

Total body water is approximately 50% of lean body weight in men and 40% of lean body weight in women, so to determine total body water, multiply body weight by 0.5 for men or 0.4 for women. For example, if a 70-kg man has a serum Na^+ level of 160 mEq/L, the estimated free water deficit would be

$$\frac{160 - 140}{140} \times (0.5 \times 70) = 5 \text{ L}$$

Rate of replacement: Once the free water deficit is calculated, administer fluid to lower serum sodium at a rate of 0.5 to 1 mEq/h with a decrease of no more than approximately 12 mEq/L in the first 24 hours and the remainder over the next 48 to 72 hours.

Route of replacement: Select the route of replacement of free water based on the patient's clinical status:

- **Stable, asymptomatic:** Give fluids by mouth or through a nasogastric tube.
- **Symptomatic but not significantly hypovolemic:** Typically use 0.45% sodium chloride (half-normal saline) IV.
- **Symptomatic, significantly hypovolemic:** Use 0.9% sodium chloride (normal saline) IV to correct the hypovolemia; then correct the free water deficit with 0.45% sodium chloride (half-normal saline).

Rapid Response Interventions for Periarrest Hypernatremia

Patients with periarrest hypernatremia will be severely hypovolemic and markedly dehydrated with shock. The key for these patients is rapid volume replacement with normal saline:

- Give normal saline 500 mL wide open as a *medical bolus* and evaluate clinical response. Repeat every 20 to 30 minutes until the patient is hemodynamically stable.
- Alternatively, give 10 to 20 mL/kg over 20 minutes (700 to 1400 mL for a patient weighing 70 kg) and evaluate hemodynamic response.

Calculate and correct the free water deficit as outlined in the text when the patient is hemodynamically stable.

Hyponatremia

Normal sodium range: 135 to 145 mEq/L

Hyponatremia represents an excess of water relative to sodium.[30]

Causes

Most cases of hyponatremia are caused by reduced renal excretion of water with continued water intake or by loss of sodium in the urine.[23] Several conditions can impair renal water excretion, including use of thiazide diuretics, renal failure, ECF depletion (eg, vomiting with continued water intake), the syndrome of inappropriate antidiuretic hormone (SIADH), edematous states (eg, CHF, cirrhosis with ascites), hypothyroidism, and adrenal insufficiency. The most frequent cause of potentially life-threatening hyponatremia is SIADH (Table 58).[31]

Most cases of hyponatremia also are associated with low serum osmolality (so-called hypo-osmolar hyponatremia). The one common exception to this is in uncontrolled diabetes, in which hyperglycemia leads to a hyperosmolar state despite a serum sodium concentration that is below normal (hyperosmolar hyponatremia).

Table 58. Common Causes of Hyponatremia

Increased Retention of Free Water (Inadequate Free Water Excretion): Normovolemic Hyponatremia
• SIADH • Hypoadrenalism (ie, adrenal insufficiency) • Hypothyroidism • Renal failure • Polydipsia (psychogenic)
Significant Retention of Free Water (With Moderate Retention of Sodium): Hypervolemic Hyponatremia

• Edematous states:
  – CHF
  – Hepatic cirrhosis
  – Nephrotic syndrome (renal failure)

Significant Loss of Sodium (With Moderate Loss of Free Water): Hypovolemic Hyponatremia
• GI losses: vomiting, diarrhea, nasogastric suctioning, fistulas • Renal losses • Third space losses • Excessive sweating • Addison's disease
Miscellaneous Causes
• Sampling error • Pseudohyponatremia: hyperlipemia, hyperproteinemia • Redistributive hyponatremia: hyperglycemia, mannitol

Abbreviations: CHF, congestive heart failure; GI, gastrointestinal; SIADH, syndrome of inappropriate antidiuretic hormone secretion.

Syndrome of Inappropriate Antidiuretic Hormone

SIADH can occur in a wide variety of clinical situations common to ACLS patients (Table 59). SIADH is caused by the nonphysiologic release of vasopressin (ADH, also known as arginine vasopressin [AVP]) from either the posterior pituitary or an ectopic source, such as a malignant tumor. ADH stimulates renal retention of normovolemic free water with continued excretion of sodium. This results in multiple abnormalities: normovolemia combined with low sodium and low osmolality in serum but with high sodium and high osmolality (more than 100 mOsm/kg) in urine. The hallmark finding of SIADH is a highly concentrated urine with a urine osmolality that is higher than the serum osmolality.

Table 59. Common Causes of the SIADH

CNS Disease or Injury
• Stroke • Brain injury, infarction, tumor, abscess • Meningitis • Encephalitis
Other
• Pain • Postoperative complications • Hypothyroidism
Nonmalignant Pulmonary Disease
• Acute respiratory distress syndrome • Pneumonia • Lung cancer • Tuberculosis • Lung abscess • Cystic fibrosis • Asthma
Drugs
• Vasopressin (exogenous) • Diuretics • Chlorpropamide • Vincristine • Cyclophosphamide • Thioridazine
Malignancies
• Pancreatic cancer • Duodenal cancer • Oat cell carcinoma • Lymphoma • Hodgkin's disease

Abbreviations: CNS, central nervous system; SIADH, syndrome of inappropriate antidiuretic hormone secretion.

Untreated SIADH can be fatal or can result in significant neurologic complications. SIADH should be ruled out when significant hyponatremia develops. The acronym "CONDM" can be used to recall the major causes of SIADH:

C: Central nervous system disease or injury

O: Other (pain, post-op, hypothyroidism)

N: Nonmalignant pulmonary disease (chronic obstructive pulmonary disease [COPD], pneumonia)

D: Drugs

M: Malignancy

Diagnosis

Hyponatremia is usually asymptomatic unless it is acute or severe (less than 120 mEq/L). An abrupt fall in serum sodium produces a free water shift from the vascular to the interstitial space that can cause cerebral edema. In this case the patient may present with nausea, vomiting, headache, irritability, lethargy, seizures, coma, or even death.

Treatment

Treatment of hyponatremia involves administration of sodium and elimination of intravascular free water. If SIADH is present, the treatment is restriction of fluid intake to 50% to 66% of estimated maintenance fluid requirement. Correction of asymptomatic hyponatremia should be gradual: typically increase Na^+ by 0.5 mEq/L per hour to a maximum change of about 12 mEq/L in the first 24 hours. Rapid correction of hyponatremia can cause coma, which may be associated with osmotic demyelination syndrome or central *pontine myelinolysis,* lethal disorders thought to be caused by rapid fluid shifts into and out of brain tissue.

To calculate the amount of sodium to administer per hour for *asymptomatic* hyponatremia, multiply 0.5 mEq/L by the appropriate weight coefficient (0.6 for men, 0.5 for women) and then by body weight (kilograms).

If the patient develops neurologic compromise, administer 3% saline IV immediately to raise the serum sodium concentration at a rate of 1 mEq/L per hour until neurologic symptoms are controlled (to a maximum of 4 mEq/L over 4 hours). Some experts recommend a faster rate of correction (ie, 2 to 4 mEq/L per hour) when seizures are present. Once neurologic symptoms are controlled, provide 3% saline IV to raise serum sodium at a rate of no more than 0.5 mEq/L per hour.

To calculate the amount of 3% saline to administer to patients with neurologic symptoms, use the following formula:

$$\textbf{Total Na}^+\textbf{ dose} = \textbf{4 mEq/L} \times \textbf{Weight coefficient*} \times \textbf{Body weight (kg)}$$

*Use 0.6 for men and 0.5 for women.

After you calculate the total sodium dose, determine the volume of 3% saline (513 mEq/L Na^+) needed to reach this dose (divide total dose by 513 mEq/L). Then administer the 3% saline at the appropriate rate (divide the volume of 3% saline by the number of hours over which you wish to administer a total of 4 mEq/L, which is generally 4). Check serum sodium frequently and monitor neurologic status. Switch to the lower rate (0.5 mEq/L per hour or lower) once neurologic symptoms are controlled.

A stepwise approach taking into account the patient's volume status can be helpful in determining the rapidity and degree of sodium replacement.

1. **Assess intravascular volume.** Determine if the patient is hypervolemic (edematous states), hypovolemic, or normovolemic.
   - Signs of hypervolemia with volume overload: CHF, peripheral edema, elevated jugular veins, rales, weight gain, S_3 heart sound.
   - Signs of hypovolemia with volume depletion: Tachycardia, resting and orthostatic hypotension, dry mucous membranes, poor peripheral perfusion, poor skin turgor.
2. **Plan treatment based on the severity of symptoms and volume status.**
   - Volume depletion: Replace volume with normal saline.
   - Volume overload: Restrict water and initiate diuresis with furosemide. *Note:* Some researchers have reported superior outcomes with IV normal saline or 3% saline administration instead of fluid restriction.
   - Normal or near-normal ECF volume (eg, with SIADH, hypothyroidism, adrenal insufficiency): Restrict fluid intake to one half to one third maintenance fluid requirements and treat underlying cause.
   - Asymptomatic: Aim for gradual restoration of serum sodium, limiting the increase in Na^+ to no more than 0.5 mEq/L per hour (maximum increase of 12 mEq/L in the first 24 hours).
   - *Note:* Rapid increases in Na^+ can lead to a higher plasma osmolality that can dehydrate and injure the brain. This life-threatening condition, called *osmotic demyelination syndrome* or *central pontine myelinolysis,* is caused by rapid fluid shifts in the brain.

The Periarrest Patient With Hyponatremia

Patients with hyponatremia will often present with alarming neurologic symptoms, such as seizures or coma, with increased intracranial pressure that can lead to cardiac arrest. Rapid deterioration is more likely with rapid development of hyponatremia.

Rapid Response Interventions for Life-Threatening Hyponatremia

If neurologic compromise is present, administer 3% saline IV immediately to correct (raise) the serum sodium concentration at a rate of 1 mEq/L per hour until neurologic symptoms are controlled.

- After neurologic symptoms are controlled, correct the serum sodium concentration at a rate of no more than 0.5 mEq/L per hour.
- Gradual correction is particularly important for treatment of chronic hyponatremia.

Use 3% Saline With Great Caution

Overly aggressive treatment with hypertonic saline can be lethal. Do not use hypertonic saline to *normalize* Na^+; use it only to raise the serum sodium concentration sufficiently to control neurologic symptoms.

Recommended Steps for Using 3% Saline

1. Calculate the amount of 3% saline to administer to increase the sodium concentration to the desired level (generally 1 mEq/L per hour over 4 hours,* for a total increase of 4 mEq/L):

   Total Na^+ dose = 4 mEq/L × Weight coefficient* × Body weight (kg)

   *Use 0.6 for men, 0.5 for women.

2. Calculate the volume of 3% saline (513 mEq Na^+/L) needed to reach this total dose:

   Volume of 3% saline = Total Na^+ dose ÷ 513 mEq/L Na^+

3. Administer the required volume of 3% saline at the appropriate rate (generally 1 mEq/L per hour over 4 hours*):

   Administration rate = Volume of 3% saline ÷ Number of hours

   *Some experts recommend more aggressive correction if the patient is obtunded or comatose (2 mEq/L per hour) or demonstrating seizures (2 to 4 mEq/L per hour). This would require administration of the amount of 3% saline calculated above over 1 to 2 hours instead of over 4 hours.

Calcium (Ca^{2+})

Calcium abnormality as an etiology of cardiac arrest is rare. There are no studies evaluating the treatment of hypercalcemia or hypocalcemia during arrest. However, empirical use of calcium (calcium chloride [10%] 5 to 10 mL OR calcium gluconate [10%] 15 to 30 mL IV over 2 to 5 minutes) may be considered when hyperkalemia or hypermagnesemia is suspected as the cause of cardiac arrest (Class IIb, LOE C).

Calcium is the most abundant mineral in the body. Many processes depend on intracellular calcium, such as enzymatic reactions, receptor activation, muscle contraction, cardiac contractility, and platelet aggregation. Calcium is essential for bone strength and neuromuscular function. Half of all calcium in the ECF is bound to albumin; the other half is in the biologically active, ionized form. The calcium concentration is normally regulated by parathyroid hormone (PTH) and vitamin D.

Total serum calcium is directly related to the serum albumin concentration. The total serum calcium will increase 0.8 mg/dL for every 1 g/dL rise in serum albumin and will fall 0.8 mg/dL for every 1 g/dL fall in serum albumin.

Although total serum albumin is directly related to total serum calcium, ionized calcium is *inversely* related to serum albumin. The lower the serum albumin, the higher the portion of the total calcium that is present in ionized form. In the presence of hypoalbuminemia, the total calcium level may be low, but the ionized calcium level may be normal. If the patient is unstable or if symptoms of hypocalcemia are present, request a specific measurement of ionized calcium. Often the widely used "metabolic panels" that present findings of multiple laboratory tests report total serum calcium but not ionized calcium. But the more comprehensive panels include both.

To calculate the true total calcium adjusted for the hypoalbuminemia, use the following formula:

$$\textbf{True calcium}_{total} = \textbf{Measured calcium}_{total} + [(0.8) \times (\textbf{Protein}_{normal} - \textbf{Protein}_{measured})]$$

Calcium is primarily an extracellular ion. Calcium and sodium are actively pumped out of cells. Because calcium antagonizes the effects of both potassium and magnesium at the cell membrane, it is the agent of choice for treating both severe hyperkalemia and hypermagnesemia. Indications include

- Known or suspected hyperkalemia
- Ionized hypocalcemia (eg, multiple blood transfusions)
- Antidote for toxic effects of calcium channel blocker overdose

Because of the critical role of calcium, the serum calcium concentration is controlled within a narrow range. This control is chiefly exerted by secretion of PTH from the parathyroid gland in response to low ionized calcium levels. Figure 108 depicts the body's typical response to a low level of ionized serum calcium. The opposite response occurs with elevated calcium.

Hypercalcemia

Normal total calcium range: 8.5 to 10.5 mg/dL

Normal ionized calcium range: 4.2 to 4.8 mg/dL

In most forms of hypercalcemia, release of calcium from the bones and intestines is increased, and renal clearance may be compromised.

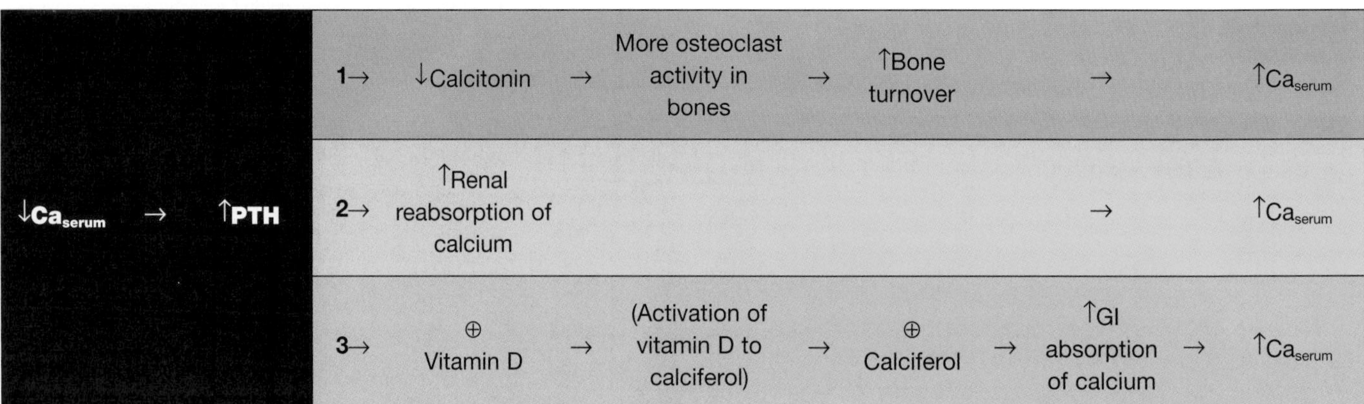

Figure 108. Regulation of serum calcium concentration. This figure illustrates the body's response to an abnormally low level of calcium. Low ionized serum calcium results in increased release of PTH, which has 3 major effects: (**1**) PTH decreases calcitonin. Because calcitonin inhibits the activity of bone osteoclasts, a decrease in calcitonin allows more bone turnover, resulting in an increase in serum calcium; (**2**) PTH increases calcium resorption in the kidneys, resulting in a rapid rise in serum calcium; (**3**) PTH activates vitamin D to the more active metabolite, calciferol, which causes increased GI absorption of calcium. PTH also has a direct effect on calcium absorption in the GI tract.

GI symptoms of hypercalcemia include dysphagia, constipation, peptic ulcer, and pancreatitis. Effects on the kidney include diminished ability to concentrate urine; diuresis, leading to loss of sodium, potassium, magnesium, and phosphate; and a vicious cycle of calcium reabsorption that worsens hypercalcemia.

Causes

The overall incidence of hypercalcemia in the general population is 0.3% to 6.0%, making it much more common than hypocalcemia. More than 90% of reported cases of hypercalcemia are caused by malignancy or hyperparathyroidism.[32] Some malignancies secrete a PTH-like substance, causing increased calcium release from the bone. Primary hyperparathyroidism causes increased gut resorption of calcium. Table 60 presents the common causes of hypercalcemia.

Diagnosis

Hypercalcemia is defined as a total calcium concentration of 10.5 mg/dL or higher or an ionized calcium concentration higher than 4.8 mg/dL. Symptoms of hypercalcemia usually develop when the total serum calcium concentration is 12 to 15 mg/dL or higher. At these levels depression, weakness, fatigue, and confusion may occur. At higher levels (more than 15 to 20 mg/dL) patients may experience hallucinations, disorientation, hypotonicity, seizures, and coma. Hypercalcemia interferes with renal concentration of urine; the diuresis can cause dehydration. A classic *memory aid* for frequent signs and symptoms of hypercalcemia is *"Stones, bones, moans and groans, and psychologic overtones":*

- Stones: Renal lithiasis
- Bones: Osteolysis releasing calcium (metastatic disease)
- Moans and groans: Abdominal pain in general, plus pancreatitis, peptic ulcers
- Psychologic overtones: Apathy, depression, stupor and coma, irritability, hallucinations

Myocardial contractility may initially increase until the calcium level reaches more than 15 mg/dL. Above this level myocardial depression occurs. Automaticity is decreased and ventricular systole is shortened. Arrhythmias occur because the refractory period is shortened. Hypercalcemia can worsen digitalis toxicity and may cause hypertension. In addition, many patients with hypercalcemia develop hypokalemia. Both of these conditions contribute to cardiac arrhythmias.[33] The QT interval typically shortens when serum calcium is more than 13 mg/dL and the PR and QRS intervals are prolonged. Atrioventricular (AV) block may develop and progress to complete heart block and even cardiac arrest when the total serum calcium concentration is more than 15 to 20 mg/dL.

Table 60. **Common Causes of Hypercalcemia**

Primary Hyperparathyroidism and Malignancy (>90% of Cases)
• Cancers causing osteolytic bone metastases: lung, breast, kidney, myeloma, leukemia • Paraneoplastic tumors: PTH–related proteins, bone-resorbing substances, ectopic production of calciferol
Pulmonary and Granulomatous Diseases
• Berylliosis • Adult respiratory distress syndrome • Histoplasmosis • Coccidioidomycosis • Tuberculosis • Sarcoidosis
Drugs
• Lithium • Thiazide diuretics • Hormonal therapy for breast cancer (estrogens) • Hypervitaminosis A and D • Calcium ingestion
Endocrine Disorders (Nonparathyroid)
• Hyperthyroidism • Adrenal insufficiency • Pheochromocytoma • Acromegaly • Vasoactive polypeptide-producing tumors (intestinal)
Miscellaneous Causes
• Immobilization • Paget's disease of bone • Milk-alkali syndrome • Acute renal failure, recovery phase

Treatment

Treatment for hypercalcemia is required if the patient is symptomatic or if the calcium level is more than 15 mg/dL. Immediate therapy is directed at restoring intravascular volume with normal saline with simultaneous administration of calcitonin and a bisphosphonate.[34] In patients with adequate cardiovascular and renal function, this is accomplished with infusion of 0.9% saline at 300 to 500 mL/h (saline diuresis) until any fluid deficit is replaced and diuresis occurs (urine output 200 to 300 mL/h or higher). The rate of saline infusion should be adjusted based on patient factors, including the severity of hypercalcemia and the presence of comorbidities, especially cardiac or renal insufficiency. Once adequate rehydration has occurred, the saline infusion rate is reduced to 100 to 200 mL/h. During this therapy, monitor and maintain potassium and magnesium concentrations closely because the diuresis can reduce potassium and magnesium concentrations.

Calcitonin reduces serum calcium concentration by decreasing bone resorption of osteoclasts and increasing renal calcium excretion. Although not particularly potent, it works rapidly and is relatively safe and nontoxic.[35] The bisphosphonates inhibit calcium release by interfering with osteoclast-mediated bone resorption.[36] Pamidronate and zoledronic acid are the 2 drugs in this class that are commonly used for severe hypercalcemia.[37,38] These drugs are relatively nontoxic and have a higher potency and duration of effect than calcitonin. Because the peak effect of these agents is between 2 to 4 days, they are often given in conjunction with calcitonin, which has a faster onset.

Hemodialysis is the treatment of choice to rapidly decrease serum calcium in patients with heart failure or renal insufficiency.[39] Chelating agents (eg, 50 mmol PO_4 over 8 to 12 hours or ethylenediaminetetraacetic acid (EDTA) 10 to 50 mg/kg over 4 hours) have been used for extreme conditions.

If the hypercalcemia is due to malignancy, progressive hypercalcemia will inevitably accompany tumor progression. If the underlying disease cannot be treated, the patient may be given maintenance therapy to prevent recurrent hypercalcemia. When these patients develop hypercalcemia, carefully consider the patient's prognosis and wishes before starting acute therapy. A patient dying of cancer may need no treatment. In all other cases aggressive treatment is needed.

A stepwise approach to hypercalcemia based on serum level and symptoms is useful when treating these patients:

- **Total calcium concentration is 12 to less than 15 mg/dL:** Begin the treatment outlined below for symptomatic patients.
- **Total calcium concentration is 15 mg/dL:** Begin treatment whether the patient is symptomatic or not. There are 4 components to hypercalcemia therapy. ACLS providers will seldom be responsible for more than the first 2 of these components: volume restoration and starting calcium elimination through the kidneys.

Treatment Sequence

1. **Restore volume:**
    - Establish vascular access with a large-bore IV.
    - Infuse normal saline (0.9% sodium chloride) at 300 to 500 mL/h until fluid deficits are replaced. Volume replacement promotes increased excretion of calcium by the kidneys.
    - Decrease infusion rate to 100 to 200 mL/h once you have established adequate rehydration.
2. **Increase renal calcium elimination:**
    - The saline diuresis induced by volume restoration will usually decrease the serum calcium concentration by 1.5 to 2.5 mg/dL.
    - Consider furosemide 1 mg/kg, especially for patients in heart failure. But do *not* administer loop diuretics until you have restored intravascular volume. *Note:* The use of furosemide in hypercalcemia is controversial because it can foster reuptake of calcium ions, worsening the hypercalcemia.
    - Some experts recommend empirically adding magnesium (15 mg/h) and potassium (up to 10 mEq/h) during volume restoration because they are excreted during saline diuresis.
3. **Reduce calcium release from bones** by administering drugs that inhibit osteoclast activity. These drugs do not work immediately (onset of action and peak effect may take several hours).
    - Calcitonin inhibits osteoclast activity and promotes calcium deposition in bone, but it produces only modest reductions in serum calcium concentration.
    - Bisphosphonates decrease serum calcium levels by interfering with osteoclast activity and stimulating osteoclast *apoptosis*.[40] Commonly used bisphosphonates include pamidronate and zoledronic acid.
    - Glucocorticoids, indomethacin, gallium nitrate, and oral phosphates are other options.
4. **Treat the primary disorder** causing the hypercalcemia. For example, discontinue any causative medications; perform parathyroidectomy for hyperparathyroidism due to excess PTH or with vitamin D deficiency and provide specific treatment for paraneoplastic syndromes, nonparathyroid endocrine disorders, or granulomatous diseases.

Hypocalcemia

Normal total calcium range: 8.5 to 10.5 mg/dL

Normal ionized calcium range: 4.2 to 4.8 mg/dL

Causes

The incidence of hypocalcemia in the general population is 0.6%. Hypocalcemia may develop with toxic shock syndrome, with abnormalities in serum magnesium, after thyroid surgery, with fluoride poisoning, and with tumor lysis syndrome (rapid cell turnover with resultant hyperkalemia, hyperphosphatemia, and hypocalcemia). The most important and frequent causes of hypocalcemia are acute pancreatitis, lack of vitamin D, and medications (see Table 61).

Diagnosis

Clinically significant hypocalcemia is defined as a serum calcium concentration of less than 8.5 mg/dL (or ionized calcium less than 4.2 mg/dL). Symptoms usually occur when ionized levels fall to less than 2.5 mg/dL and include

Table 61. Common Causes of Hypocalcemia

Insufficient Parathyroid Hormone
• Post-parathyroidectomy for hyperparathyroidism • Neck surgery (eg, thyroidectomy) • Post–neck irradiation • Destruction of parathyroid glands by metastatic carcinoma, infiltrative diseases
Insufficient Vitamin D
• Malnutrition, dietary abnormalities • Malabsorption • Congenital rickets • Chronic liver disease • Chronic renal disease • Sunlight deficiency • Hypo- or hypermagnesemia • Advanced bone disease
Medications
• Cimetidine (most frequent cause of drug-induced hypocalcemia) • Phosphates (from enemas, laxatives) • Phenytoin, phenobarbital • Gentamicin, tobramycin, actinomycin • Calcitonin, mithramycin • EDTA (citrate from blood administration) • Heparin, protamine • Theophylline • Glucagon • Norepinephrine • Loop diuretics • Nitroprusside • Bisphosphonates
Miscellaneous Causes
• Pancreatitis • Shock or sepsis • Burns • Toxic shock syndrome • Magnesium deficiency • Citrate toxicity

Abbreviation: EDTA, ethylenediaminetetraacetic acid.

paresthesias of the extremities and face, followed by muscle cramps, carpopedal spasm, laryngospasm, stridor, tetany, seizures, or coma. Patients with hypocalcemia show hyperreflexia and positive Chvostek (a tap over the facial nerve in front of the ear produces a twitch in the eyelid or a corner of the mouth) and Trousseau signs (carpal spasm of hand and fingers after the blood pressure cuff has been inflated above systolic pressure for 3 minutes; this spasm occurs because cuff inflation induces ischemia of the ulnar nerve). Cardiac effects include decreased myocardial contractility, acute CHF, and heart failure. Hypocalcemia can exacerbate digitalis toxicity. ECG changes may include prolongation of the QT interval, terminal T-wave inversion, bradycardias, AV block, and ventricular tachycardia (VT).

Treatment

Treatment of hypocalcemia requires administration of calcium. Calcium exchange depends on adequate serum concentrations of potassium and magnesium. Effective treatment of hypocalcemia often requires administration of all 3 electrolytes.

Treat acute, symptomatic hypocalcemia with calcium chloride (10%) 5 to 10 mL *or* calcium gluconate (10%) 15 to 30 mL IV over 2 to 5 minutes. Aim to maintain the total serum calcium concentration at 7 to 9 mg/dL. Correct abnormalities in magnesium, potassium, and pH simultaneously. Note that untreated hypomagnesemia will often make hypocalcemia refractory to therapy. For this reason, evaluate serum magnesium when hypocalcemia is present, particularly if the hypocalcemia is refractory to initial calcium therapy.

Magnesium

Magnesium is the fourth most common mineral and the second most abundant intracellular cation (after potassium) in the human body. Because approximately half of total body magnesium resides in bone and because extracellular magnesium is bound to serum albumin, magnesium levels do not reliably reflect total body magnesium stores. Magnesium is necessary for the movement of sodium, potassium, and calcium into and out of cells, and it plays an important role in stabilizing excitable membranes. Low potassium in combination with low magnesium is a risk factor for severe arrhythmias. Magnesium balance is closely tied to sodium, calcium, and potassium balance.

Hypermagnesemia

Normal magnesium range: 1.3 to 2.2 mEq/L

Causes

ACLS providers will rarely encounter hypermagnesemia. When hypermagnesemia does occur, it is almost always associated with significant renal failure because normally functioning kidneys easily excrete large amounts of magnesium. Table 62 lists the most common causes of hypermagnesemia.

Symptoms and Diagnosis

Hypermagnesemia causes neurologic symptoms of muscular weakness, paralysis, ataxia, drowsiness, and confusion. Nausea and vomiting are common GI symptoms. Other symptoms include flushing, hypotension, transient

Table 62. Common Causes of Significant Hypermagnesemia

Renal Failure (Acute or Chronic) or Increased Magnesium Load
• Laxatives, antacids, or enemas containing magnesium • Treatment of pre-eclampsia or eclampsia (may affect both mother and neonate) • Rhabdomyolysis • Tumor lysis syndrome
Impaired Elimination of Magnesium From GI Tract
• Anticholinergics • Narcotics • Chronic constipation • Bowel obstruction • Gastric dilatation
Increased Magnesium Absorption by Kidneys
• Hyperparathyroidism • Hypothyroidism • Adrenal insufficiency • Mineralocorticoid deficiency • Lithium therapy

Abbreviation: GI, gastrointestinal.

tachycardia followed by bradycardia, hypoventilation, and cardiorespiratory arrest.[41-44] ECG changes of hypermagnesemia include increased PR and QT intervals, increased QRS duration, decrease in P-wave voltage, variable degree of T-wave peaking, complete AV block, and asystole.

Symptoms will become more severe as the serum magnesium concentration rises:

- **3 to less than 4 mEq/L:** Neuromuscular irritability, somnolence, and loss of deep tendon reflexes
- **4 to less than 5 mEq/L:** Increasing muscle weakness
- **5 to less than 8 mEq/L:** Onset of severe vasodilation and hypotension
- **8 mEq/L or higher:** Onset of cardiac conduction abnormalities, neuromuscular paralysis, hypotension, ventilation failure, and cardiac arrest

Treatment

Hypermagnesemia is treated with administration of calcium, which removes magnesium from serum. It is important to eliminate sources of ongoing magnesium intake. Cardiorespiratory support may be needed until magnesium levels are reduced.

Administration of calcium (calcium chloride [10%] 5 to 10 mL or calcium gluconate [10%] 15 to 30 mL IV over 2 to 5 minutes) may be considered during cardiac arrest associated with hypermagnesemia (Class IIb, LOE C).

In the pregnant patient, hypermagnesemia may be caused by iatrogenic overdose of magnesium sulfate, particularly if she becomes oliguric. Empirical calcium administration may be lifesaving in this case.[45-47]

Treatment Details

- Dialysis is ultimately the treatment of choice, but ready availability is a problem in some clinical settings.
- **General treatment for hypermagnesemia:**
  - Stop any oral or parenteral sources of magnesium.
  - Support the ABCDs of ACLS.
  - Dilute the serum magnesium concentration with administration of IV fluids.
  - Antagonize the cellular effects of elevated magnesium with calcium gluconate or calcium chloride.
  - Remove excess magnesium from the body.
- **Antagonize the effects of hypermagnesemia:**
  - Administer *either* calcium gluconate or calcium chloride as stated above.
- **Remove excess magnesium from the body:**
  - Induce diuresis with normal saline IV at 500 mL/h plus furosemide 1 mg/kg if renal function is normal. Saline diuresis will hasten magnesium excretion by the kidneys.

    Note: Saline diuresis may increase calcium excretion, making signs and symptoms of hypermagnesemia worse. Be prepared to administer calcium chloride 10% solution IV.

Hypomagnesemia

Normal magnesium range: 1.3 to 2.2 mEq/L

Hypomagnesemia, defined as a serum magnesium concentration of less than 1.3 mEq/L, is far more common than hypermagnesemia. Hypomagnesemia interferes with the effects of PTH, resulting in hypocalcemia. It may also lead to hypokalemia. Symptoms of low serum magnesium are muscular tremors and fasciculations, ocular nystagmus, tetany, altered mental state, and cardiac arrhythmias such as torsades de pointes (multifocal VT). Other possible symptoms are ataxia, vertigo, seizures, and dysphagia.

Causes

Hypomagnesemia occurs in 11% of all hospitalized patients and in up to 65% of severely ill patients.[48] Hypomagnesemia usually results from decreased absorption or increased loss of magnesium from either the kidneys or intestines (diarrhea). Alterations in thyroid hormone function and certain medications (eg, pentamidine, diuretics, alcohol) can also induce hypomagnesemia. Multiple neurohumoral mechanisms become activated in patients with decompensated CHF, leading to hypomagnesemia and other acid-base and electrolyte disturbances. These patients face a high risk of deleterious arrhythmias (see Table 63).

Table 63. Common Causes of Hypomagnesemia

Decreased Intake
• Alcoholism • Malnutrition • Starvation
Increased Loss
• GI loss: bowel resection, pancreatitis, diarrhea • Burns • Lactation • Renal disease
Miscellaneous Causes
• Drugs: diuretics, pentamidine, gentamicin, digoxin • Parathyroid abnormalities • Hypothermia • Hypercalcemia • Diabetic ketoacidosis • Hyper- or hypothyroidism • Phosphate deficiency

Abbreviation: GI, gastrointestinal.

Diagnosis

Most patients with hypomagnesemia are asymptomatic. Patients with symptomatic hypomagnesemia most commonly present with one or more of the following symptoms: muscular tremors, fasciculations, vertigo, ataxia, altered mentation, Chvostek's or Trousseau's sign, and various paresthesias. Many of the symptoms indicate the presence of hypocalcemia. Other possible symptoms are ocular nystagmus, tetany, dysphagia, and seizures.

Hypomagnesemia is often associated with hypokalemia or hypocalcemia. Providers should always check potassium and calcium levels in patients with low serum magnesium.

ECG changes of hypomagnesemia include prolonged QT and PR intervals, ST depression and T-wave inversion, flattening or inversion of precordial P waves, widening of the QRS interval, torsades de pointes, treatment-resistant VF (and other arrhythmias), and worsening of digitalis toxicity.

Treatment

Treatment of hypomagnesemia depends on its severity and the patient's clinical status. In patients with renal insufficiency, replace magnesium cautiously; there is a significant risk of life-threatening hypermagnesemia.[49]

- **Mild or chronic hypomagnesemia:**
  - Oral replacement is the preferred route for mild hypomagnesemia. (Parenteral magnesium administration is indicated if symptoms are present even if hypomagnesemia is mild.)
  - Give magnesium oxide 400 mg PO once or twice a day.
  - Several weeks of therapy may be required to replenish total body magnesium stores.
- **Moderate hypomagnesemia:**
  - Give $MgSO_4$ IV at a rate of 1 to 2 g over 15 minutes, then 6 g in IV fluid over 24 hours. This problem may require 3 to 7 days for correction.
  - Monitor magnesium level and deep tendon reflexes.
- **Significant symptomatic hypomagnesemia:**
  - Start with $MgSO_4$ 1 to 2 g IV over 15 minutes.
  - Add 6 g magnesium to daily IV fluids for the next 3 to 7 days.
  - Check the patient's magnesium levels and reflexes daily.
- **Cardiac arrest and severe cardiotoxicity due to hypomagnesemia:**
  - Hypomagnesemia can be associated with polymorphic VT, including torsades de pointes, a pulseless form (polymorphic) of VT.
  - For cardiotoxicity and cardiac arrest, IV magnesium 1 to 2 g of $MgSO_4$ bolus IV push is recommended (Class I, LOE C).
  - For cardiac arrest, repeat the dose in 10 to 15 minutes if the patient remains unstable or in refractory arrest.

Life-Threatening Acid-Base Abnormalities

Physiology and Definitions

The healthy human body closely regulates serum pH between 7.35 and 7.45. When pH falls below 7.35, *acidosis* is present. When pH rises above 7.45, *alkalosis* is present.

There are 4 main types of acid-base imbalances:

- Metabolic acidosis
- Metabolic alkalosis
- Respiratory acidosis
- Respiratory alkalosis

This classification is actually an oversimplification because there are mixed acid-base disturbances as well. Whenever acid-base imbalances occur, the body attempts to correct the abnormality and bring the pH back toward the normal range. But in mixed disorders the compensatory mechanisms never completely correct the imbalance, so a primary abnormality is offset by a secondary compensation.

Diagnostic Approaches to Acid-Base Abnormalities

Using the ABG: pH, Pco_2, Bicarbonate

To assess a patient's acid-base status, obtain an arterial blood gas (ABG) analysis. The ABG is critical for identifying acid-base abnormalities and the degree of any compensation. In addition to PO_2 and O_2 saturation, the following variables appear on a typical ABG report (normal range follows variable):

- pH: 7.35 to 7.45
- PCO_2 (partial pressure of carbon dioxide): 35 to 45 mm Hg
- Bicarbonate (HCO_3): 22 to 32 mEq/L
- Base deficit or base excess: –2 to +2

An average PCO_2 value of 40 mm Hg is used in calculations to compare the *predicted pH* with the *measured pH*. The magnitude and direction of any difference between predicted and measured pH provide a rough estimate of whether a metabolic or respiratory acidosis or alkalosis is present.

Comparing Predicted pH With Measured pH

When interpreting the ABG, you must evaluate both the PCO_2 and the pH to identify any acid-base disorder and metabolic and respiratory components. You make this assessment by first predicting the pH from the PCO_2:

- Step 1: Determine if the pH is acidotic (less than 7.35), alkalotic (more than 7.45), or normal (7.35 to 7.45), and note if the patient is hypercarbic (PCO_2 more than 45) or hypocarbic (PCO_2 less than 35). Hypocarbia indicates a respiratory alkalosis, and hypercarbia indicates a respiratory acidosis. To identify the primary problem and any compensation, you now need to determine the contribution of the PCO_2 to any acidosis or alkalosis.
- Step 2: Subtract the patient's measured PCO_2 from 40 (estimated normal PCO_2). The result will be either positive (if the patient's PCO_2 is low) or negative (if PCO_2 is high).
- Step 3: Multiply the result of Step 2 by 0.008. Note that the product may be a positive or negative number because Step 2 may result in a positive or a negative number.
- Step 4: Add the positive or negative product obtained in Step 3 to 7.4. This will result in either the addition of a number to 7.4 or subtraction of a number from 7.4. The resulting number is the pH predicted from the PCO_2. Every 1 mm Hg uncompensated rise in PCO_2 above 40 mm Hg (more hypercarbic) is predicted to make the pH fall by 0.008 (more acidotic).
- Overall, $(40 - PCO_2) \times 0.008 = \pm\Delta$ in pH from 7.4.

If the patient's measured pH is higher than the calculated pH, *metabolic alkalosis* must be associated with the hypocarbia or hypercarbia. If the measured pH is lower than the calculated pH, *metabolic acidosis* must be associated with the hypocarbia or hypercarbia.

Example

ABG: pH 7.30, PCO_2 30 mm Hg

Perform the calculation steps noted above:

- Step 1: The pH is acidotic (less than 7.35). You also note that the PCO_2 of 30 mm Hg is hypocarbic, so the patient has a respiratory alkalosis.
- Step 2: Subtract the measured PCO_2 (30) from 40. The difference is +10.
- Step 3: Multiply the +10 difference from Step 2 by 0.008. The product is +0.08.
- Step 4: Add the product of Step 3 (0.08) to 7.4. This represents the change in pH predicted from the PCO_2 alone. Adding +0.08 to 7.4 yields a predicted pH of 7.48.

Interpretation: On the basis of the PCO_2 level of 30, this patient's predicted pH is 7.48. But this patient's measured pH is 7.30, which is quite acidotic. The conclusion is that the much lower measured pH is due to the presence of a *primary metabolic acidosis*. The respiratory alkalosis represents partial compensation (the pH is still acidotic), so your conclusion is primary metabolic acidosis with partial respiratory compensation.

Compensation in Acid-Base Disturbances

In the previous example, why is the patient's PCO_2 less than the normal range of 35 to 45 mm Hg? The patient is attempting to compensate for the metabolic acidosis by increased ventilation, or "blowing off CO_2." As the CO_2 is "blown off" and the PCO_2 falls, the pH rises—what is called a *compensatory respiratory alkalosis*. Provided the patient is alert and has no compromise of the airway, respiratory compensation will be almost immediate. If the acidosis were respiratory, the kidneys would attempt to compensate by retaining bicarbonate (a base). Unlike respiratory compensation, which is immediate, metabolic compensation for underlying respiratory acid-base problems takes 8 to 48 hours to occur. Note that a compensatory mechanism is terminated when the pH approaches normal (see "The Overcompensation Rule").

Primary Respiratory Acidosis With Compensatory Metabolic Alkalosis

A common example of a primary respiratory acid-base disturbance occurs in COPD with CO_2 retention (see "Case Scenario"). As the PCO_2 rises, the pH falls, leading to a *primary respiratory acidosis.* Over time the kidneys will retain extra bicarbonate (HCO_3) to neutralize the acid created by the retained CO_2 in an attempt to restore the pH to near-normal. This response is called a *compensatory metabolic alkalosis,* or *metabolic compensation.*

Using the Measured Base Deficit or Base Excess

Another factor to use in interpreting the acid-base balance from the ABG is the base deficit or base excess. It is normally between –2 and +2.

- If the base deficit is more negative than –2, a *metabolic acidosis* is present (base deficit less than –2 indicates metabolic acidosis).
- If a base excess is more positive than +2, *metabolic alkalosis* is present.

The Overcompensation Rule

An additional useful rule to keep in mind with acid-base disturbances is that *compensatory mechanisms are unlikely to **overcompensate** in acid-base abnormalities.* As the pH approaches normal, the compensatory mechanisms shut off.

If a patient with chronic respiratory failure presents with an *alkalotic* pH, this does not represent metabolic compensation because a compensatory mechanism for respiratory acidosis will not overcorrect the pH to the alkalotic range. You should look for a condition responsible for a metabolic alkalosis. For example, hypochloremic or hypokalemic metabolic alkalosis can develop in patients with chronic respiratory failure. This can occur during diuretic (eg, furosemide) therapy if the patient does not receive adequate potassium chloride supplementation.

Keeping this rule in mind, the ACLS provider can determine which is the primary acid-base disturbance and which is the compensatory mechanism.

Anion Gap

The *anion gap* is another calculated value that can help identify the underlying cause of an acid-base disturbance. The number of positive ions in the body (eg, sodium and potassium) should be approximately equal to the number of negative ions (chloride and bicarbonate). But this balance never occurs because there is always a difference (the gap) caused by unmeasured negative ions such as ketones and lactic acid. This anion gap quantifies the difference between the serum sodium concentration and the serum chloride plus bicarbonate concentrations:

$$\textbf{Anion gap} = [Na^+] - ([Cl^-] + [HCO_3^-])$$

Normal anion gap: 7 ± 4 mEq/L*

*The normal value of the anion gap was originally listed as 12 ± 4 mEq/L. Newer automated systems are more accurate, and the revised normal value has decreased.

With an anion gap in the normal range (7 ± 4 mEq/L), any existing acidosis will be due to the negative ions in the equation, chloride and bicarbonate. A *normal anion gap acidosis* occurs with diarrhea because a fall in serum bicarbonate is balanced by a rise in serum chloride (hyperchloremic metabolic acidosis). With an anion gap that is abnormally high (more than 11 mEq/L), any existing acidosis is caused by an accumulation of unmeasured negative ions, such as ketones or lactic acid, or a fall in serum bicarbonate that is not balanced by a rise in serum chloride. The classic example of a high anion gap acidosis is diabetic ketoacidosis.

Diabetic Ketoacidosis

Pathophysiology

Diabetic ketoacidosis (DKA) is a life-threatening complication of diabetes that ACLS providers may encounter. A relative insulin deficiency is the primary cause of DKA. It is important to understand the major abnormalities in the pathophysiology of DKA because these problems define the therapeutic approach:

- **Hyperglycemia:** Without sufficient insulin, glucose cannot enter the cells, so it reaches higher and higher concentrations in the blood (hyperglycemia). The blood glucose is further elevated by the effects of the hormone *glucagon,* which is released by the liver during insulin deficiency, and catecholamines, which stimulate gluconeogenesis (the formation of glucose).
- **Dehydration:** The hyperglycemia causes an osmotic diuresis (polyuria), with excretion of glucose-containing urine (glucosuria). Significant volume can be lost during this osmotic diuresis. This volume loss leads to severe dehydration, worsening acidosis, and hypotension.
- **Ketoacidosis:** Without intracellular glucose, the body begins to metabolize existing lipids (fat stores). These lipids are partially oxidized into free fatty acids and acetoacetic acids. The free fatty acids accumulate and the acetoacetic acid is converted into ketones. These processes result in the development of ketoacidosis. These ketones and free fatty acids account for the high-anion-gap metabolic acidosis invariably present in DKA.
- **Hypokalemia:** Total body potassium stores decrease during the osmotic diuresis and dehydrating volume loss of DKA. The serum potassium, however, may be normal or even slightly elevated when the patient presents with DKA. *The ketoacidosis (low pH) results in an acute shift of potassium from the intracellular to the extracellular (including the vascular) space. This explains how the serum potassium may be normal or even elevated despite the total body loss of potassium.* During treatment of DKA and correction of the acidosis, the potassium returns to the intracellular space (from the vascular space). This can result in severe hypokalemia if the ACLS provider fails to anticipate the shift and initiate potassium replacement.

Causes of DKA

Although DKA can develop in patients with insulin-dependent diabetes, it can be the presenting sign of diabetes. If the patient has no history of insulin-dependent diabetes, clinicians can lose valuable time under the mistaken assumption that DKA is a diagnostic impossibility. DKA can be the initial presentation of a person with undiagnosed diabetes. Furthermore, patients with non–insulin-dependent diabetes may develop insulin dependency that is not recognized until they experience an episode of DKA.[50]

DKA frequently results when a patient with insulin-dependent diabetes stops or reduces insulin therapy. The clinical history of many patients with insulin-dependent diabetes

Critical Concept DKA Often the Presenting Sign of Diabetes	If a patient with DKA has no history of insulin-dependent diabetes, do not automatically assume that DKA is a diagnostic impossibility: • DKA can be the initial presentation of a person with undiagnosed diabetes. • Patients with non–insulin-dependent diabetes may develop insulin dependency that is not recognized until they experience an episode of DKA.[50]

qualifies them as "brittle diabetics." The reason for frequent episodes of DKA is unclear: the DKA may develop despite uninterrupted insulin therapy. The risk factors for DKA are well known for most patients with insulin-dependent diabetes. One commonly used memory aid for the more common precipitants of DKA is the so-called "6 I's":

infection, infarction, ignorance, ischemia, intoxication, and implantation.

- **Infection:** Pneumonia and urinary tract infections are the infections that most commonly precipitate an episode of DKA.
- **Infarction** (brain): Stroke syndromes, especially those leading to coma, are often associated with rapid deterioration in persons with insulin-dependent diabetes.
- **Ignorance:** Noncompliance with insulin regimens or dietary restrictions and errors of commission and omission in insulin therapy may occur due to a poor understanding of diabetes.
- **Ischemia:** Acute myocardial infarction, with its associated stress and hyper-adrenaline state, will often induce DKA.
- **Intoxication:** Excessive alcohol consumption is a common precipitant of DKA.
- **Implantation:** This "I" refers to the many complications that women with diabetes can experience during pregnancy.

Signs and Symptoms of DKA

The clinical presentation of DKA is highly variable and often nonspecific. All healthcare professionals must maintain the stereotypical "high index of suspicion" in emergency settings, especially when a person with insulin-dependent diabetes presents with virtually any complaint. The most common symptoms associated with DKA are nausea, vomiting, and vague abdominal pain. The widely repeated clinical axiom that *"any GI complaint in a person with insulin-dependent diabetes is DKA until proven otherwise"* merits both compliance and repetition.

Treatment of DKA

DKA is a life-threatening condition. The ACLS provider must be able to recognize and treat it effectively. First, begin general assessment and therapy following the Systematic Approach of ACLS:

- **Airway patency and breathing effectiveness:** If the obtunded patient demonstrates hypoventilation, intubation may be necessary for airway maintenance and protection and for oxygenation and ventilation. Careful monitoring and appropriate adjustment of mechanical ventilation settings are warranted.
- **Circulation:** Dehydration and hypovolemia are virtually always present.
- **Differential diagnosis:** Initially order a 12-lead ECG, measurement of serum electrolytes, ABG, and urinalysis.
- **Assess vital signs:** Evaluate temperature, blood pressure, heart rate and rhythm, respirations (rate and pattern), and oxygen saturation (on room air and in response to low-flow oxygen).
- **Oxygen-IV-monitor-fluids:** Provide oxygen (if indicated), start an IV, attach a cardiac monitor, and initiate fluids.

Then assess the 4 major pathophysiologic abnormalities that may be present in DKA, organize therapy, and plan a strategy. Providers should address the abnormalities in the following order of priority and correct

1. Dehydration
2. Hypokalemia
3. Hyperglycemia
4. Ketoacidosis

Correct Dehydration

Begin with administration of normal saline (0.9% sodium chloride) IV. Establish IV access with a large-bore catheter and infuse 1 L rapidly; follow with 1 to 2 L over the first and second hours. When volume status is stable, give half-normal saline (0.45% sodium chloride) IV at 150 to 300 mL/h. Ideally urine output should be at least 1 mL/kg per hour after initial fluid resuscitation. If urine output fails to reach this level by the second hour, more aggressive fluid therapy will be needed, provided the patient has normal renal function. Rather than change to half-normal saline, continue with normal saline at higher rates.

- When serum glucose falls to less than 300 mg/dL, provide dextrose 5% with half-normal saline at 150 to 300 mL/h. This switch to glucose-containing solutions will help prevent the patient from developing hypoglycemia from the IV insulin.
- Determine the effectiveness of fluid resuscitation by close observation of hourly urine output. Most patients with DKA will require insertion of a urinary catheter.

Correct Hypokalemia

First, DKA patients have severe depletion of total body potassium stores. Because these patients are severely acidotic, they often initially have a false "normal" potassium (as pH falls, potassium moves from intracellular to extracellular space). A normal serum potassium level of 3.6 mEq/L in a patient with DKA is likely to represent severe depletion of total body potassium stores. Second, as therapy corrects the acidosis, the serum potassium will fall because the potassium returns to the intracellular spaces (from the extracellular spaces, including from the vascular space). This shift can lead to life-threatening hypokalemia. ACLS providers should anticipate this shift and start IV potassium therapy early.

Add KCl to the above IV fluids at a rate of 10 to 20 mEq/L. Exceptions will be patients with initial hyperkalemia (more than 6 mEq/L or with ECG signs of high potassium), patients with renal failure, or patients who are not producing urine as confirmed by hourly urine output.

- For patients with documented hypokalemia on presentation, add KCl at a rate of 40 mEq per *hour*—not per liter!
- The clinical goal is to maintain potassium levels in the normal range while recognizing 2 major caveats: that patients with DKA have severe depletion of total body potassium stores and that as therapy corrects the acidosis, serum potassium will fall (see above).

Treat Hyperglycemia

In the past, treatment algorithms recommended giving an initial IV bolus of regular insulin (0.1 unit per kilogram) followed by an infusion of 0.1 unit per kilogram per hour. Current consensus recommendations now cite recent studies, which have shown that a bolus dose of insulin is not necessary if patients receive an infusion of 0.14 unit per kilogram per hour (10 units per hour in a 70-kg patient).[51-53]

It is important to reduce the serum glucose concentration gradually. Aim for a gradual reduction at a rate of 50 to 75 mg/dL per hour. If the serum glucose does not decrease by at least 10% or 50 to 75 mg/dL from the initial value in the first hour, the dose of insulin should be increased until a steady glucose decline is achieved. When the serum glucose reaches 200 mg/dL, the insulin infusion rate may be decreased to 0.02 to 0.05 units per kilogram per hour, and dextrose may be added to the IV fluids. This switch to glucose-containing solutions will help prevent the development of hypoglycemia from the IV insulin. The concentration of dextrose and the rate of insulin infusion should be adjusted to maintain serum glucose levels between 150 and 200 mg/dL until the DKA is resolved.[53]

Correct Ketoacidosis

Bicarbonate administration is *not* routine therapy for DKA. The increase in pH from bicarbonate can be severely deleterious, shifting potassium into cells and producing life-threatening hypokalemia[54,55] and cerebral edema, especially in children.[56,57] In addition, the sodium bicarbonate will increase serum osmolality that is already high from the hyperglycemia.

The generally accepted indications for administration of bicarbonate in DKA are

- Hyperkalemia producing ECG changes
- Severe acidosis: pH less than 7.1 (some experts recommend no bicarbonate until pH is less than 7.0)
- Severe depletion of buffering reserve: bicarbonate less than 5 mEq/L
- Shock or coma
- Acidosis-induced cardiac or pulmonary dysfunction

If indicated, administer sodium bicarbonate by adding 50 to 100 mEq to 1 L of 0.45% sodium chloride and infusing the 1 L over 30 to 60 minutes. To avoid hypokalemia, some experts recommend the addition of 10 mEq potassium to the 1 L of 0.45% sodium chloride.

- If bicarbonate therapy is initiated, do not try to normalize pH. Just raise the pH enough to *get the patient out of trouble.*

The Periarrest Patient With DKA

Be particularly alert for life-threatening problems in patients with DKA. These problems may include cardiac arrhythmias from hypokalemia or hyperkalemia, shock and lactic acidosis, and cerebral edema (osmotic encephalopathy).

Cardiac Arrhythmias From Hypokalemia or Hyperkalemia

Beware of the false "normal" potassium level in patients with DKA as therapy begins. Volume replacement with normal saline and insulin infusion will begin a rapid shift of potassium into the cells. You should expect that the serum potassium will fall as the serum pH rises.

Critical Concept

False "Normal" Potassium Levels in Patients With DKA

Patients with DKA have severe depletion of total body potassium stores. Because these patients are severely acidotic, they often initially have a false "normal" potassium level (as pH falls, potassium moves from intracellular to extracellular space).

- A normal serum potassium level of 3.6 mEq/L in a patient with DKA is likely to represent severe depletion of total body potassium stores.

With profound acidosis, potassium can shift outside the cells to such a degree that life-threatening arrhythmias from hyperkalemia may develop before the DKA is treated. In such an event, follow the treatment sequence for hyperkalemia. Generally the patient will require only urgent addition of calcium chloride or calcium gluconate plus sodium bicarbonate because IV insulin and high levels of glucose are already in place.

Shock and Lactic Acidosis

Shock and lactic acidosis causing tissue hypoxia and abnormalities of cellular metabolism can occur from prolonged dehydration and volume depletion, hypotension, and tissue hypoxia: Suspect these problems in patients with DKA who have a persistent anion gap and metabolic acidosis despite appropriate initial therapy. These patients need aggressive fluid resuscitation, and as noted earlier, some may receive sodium bicarbonate administration.

Cerebral Edema (Osmotic Encephalopathy)

The precise mechanism of this complication is not known, but it has been theorized to include rapid correction of hyperglycemia (more than 100 mg/dL per hour) and a fall in serum osmolality. Suspect the development of cerebral edema in patients with DKA who show signs of increasing intracranial pressure, such as headache, altered mental status, or pupil dilation. Hyponatremia provides an important clue to imminent overhydration and pending cerebral edema. Patients with DKA will initially have a low serum sodium concentration, which may be normal in the presence of hyperglycemia.

For every increase in serum glucose of 100 mg/dL above 180 mg/dL, the serum sodium concentration will be reduced by 1.6 mEq/L below 135 mEq/L. For this reason, you should watch for a matching rise in serum sodium (ie, 1.6 mEq/L rise for every 100 mg/dL fall in serum glucose) as hyperglycemia is corrected. Failure of serum sodium to rise appropriately as the glucose falls, or an actual fall, is a red flag for cerebral edema. Urgent computed tomographic (CT) scanning can establish this diagnosis, which should be treated urgently with IV mannitol.

Nonketotic Hyperosmolar Syndrome

Pathophysiology

The nonketotic hyperosmolar syndrome (NKHS) is a life-threatening acid-base abnormality that occurs in patients with diabetes.[58] DKA occurs predominantly in insulin-dependent (type 1) diabetes mellitus; NKHS occurs almost exclusively in non–insulin-dependent (type 2) diabetes mellitus. NKHS is nonketotic because residual insulin secretion, although insufficient to prevent hyperglycemia, effectively inhibits the breakdown of lipids and the production of free fatty acids and ketones *(ketogenesis)*.

Other than ketoacidosis, all the pathophysiologic abnormalities of DKA occur with NKHS: hyperglycemia with osmotic diuresis develops, leading to dehydration and volume loss and depletion of potassium through increased renal output.

Causes

Most of the same processes that initiate DKA also precipitate NKHS. Patients with NKHS often omit or are unable to take their regular oral antidiabetic agents. Other precipitating factors include infection, infarction (stroke), and indiscretions with medications or diet. NKHS often develops in patients who are manifestly ill and debilitated with near-obtundation.

Diagnosis

Providers should suspect NKHS in any patient who appears to be ill and is known to have type 2 diabetes. Patients will frequently be severely dehydrated and may be obtunded. The syndrome has often been called "nonketotic hyperosmolar coma" because so many of these patients are unconscious and unresponsive on presentation. The laboratory findings are classic and diagnostic:

- Hyperglycemia, often with blood sugar higher than 600 mg/dL
- Hyperosmolality, with plasma osmolality higher than 320 mOsm/L
- Absence of acidosis
- Absence of ketones in the urine and blood

Treatment

For the ACLS provider, the initial treatment approach for NKHS is the same as the approach for DKA. These treatment measures include volume replacement with normal saline, potassium replacement, treatment of hyperglycemia with insulin, and close monitoring of electrolytes and pH, and response to therapy.

The Periarrest Patient With NKHS

Life-threatening NKHS is most likely to occur in elderly patients with known type 2 diabetes. On presentation these patients are often comatose with severe hypotension or overt shock. The mainstay of treatment for the unstable patient with NKHS is rapid volume replacement and consideration of pressor agents for shock.

By definition NKHS patients rarely have the ketoacidosis of DKA with the associated intracellular to extracellular shift of potassium, so the patients are not as likely to develop the intracellular potassium shift (and fall in serum potassium) during therapy.[58] For this reason, these patients are less prone to the life-threatening cardiac arrhythmias that may develop in patients with DKA.

The same recommendations noted above for periarrest patients with DKA apply to these patients with NKHS. Although cerebral edema can occur in NKHS, it seems to be diagnosed less often. Children with NKHS, like children with DKA, are much more likely than adults to develop cerebral edema during resuscitation.[59,60]

Summary: Life-Threatening Electrolyte and Acid-Base Abnormalities

Electrolyte abnormalities can cause severe physiologic and metabolic derangements, including cardiac arrhythmias and other types of cardiovascular decompensation.

Clinicians should maintain a high index of suspicion for possible electrolyte disturbances. Prompt diagnosis and aggressive treatment can often prevent life-threatening complications.

References

1. Jackson MA, Lodwick R, Hutchinson SG. Hyperkalaemic cardiac arrest successfully treated with peritoneal dialysis. *BMJ*. 1996;312:1289-1290.
2. Voelckel W, Kroesen G. Unexpected return of cardiac action after termination of cardiopulmonary resuscitation. *Resuscitation*. 1996;32:27-29.
3. Niemann JT, Cairns CB. Hyperkalemia and ionized hypocalcemia during cardiac arrest and resuscitation: possible culprits for postcountershock arrhythmias? *Ann Emerg Med*. 1999;34:1-7.
4. Allon M. Hyperkalemia in end-stage renal disease: mechanisms and management. *J Am Soc Nephrol*. 1995;6:1134-1142.
5. Weiner ID, Wingo CS. Hyperkalemia: a potential silent killer. *J Am Soc Nephrol*. 1998;9:1535-1543.
6. Weiner M, Epstein FH. Signs and symptoms of electrolyte disorders. *Yale J Biol Med*. 1970;43:76-109.
7. Burch GE, Winsor TA. *A Primer of Electrocardiography*. 5th ed. Philadelphia, PA: Lea & Febiger; 1966:143.
8. Mattu A, Brady WJ, Robinson DA. Electrocardiographic manifestations of hyperkalemia. *Am J Emerg Med*. 2000;18:721-729.
9. Frohnert PP, Giuliani ER, Friedberg M, Johnson WJ, Tauxe WN. Statistical investigation of correlations between serum potassium levels and electrocardiographic findings in patients on intermittent hemodialysis therapy. *Circulation*. 1970;41:667-676.
10. Gennari FJ. Hypokalemia. *N Engl J Med*. 1998;339:451-458.
11. Slovis C, Jenkins R. ABC of clinical electrocardiography: conditions not primarily affecting the heart. *BMJ*. 2002;324:1320-1323.
12. Clausen TG, Brocks K, Ibsen H. Hypokalemia and ventricular arrhythmias in acute myocardial infarction. *Acta Med Scand*. 1988;224:531-537.
13. Higham PD, Adams PC, Murray A, Campbell RW. Plasma potassium, serum magnesium and ventricular fibrillation: a prospective study. *Q J Med*. 1993;86:609-617.
14. Nordrehaug JE. Malignant arrhythmia in relation to serum potassium in acute myocardial infarction. *Am J Cardiol*. 1985;56:20D-23D.
15. Nordrehaug JE, von der Lippe G. Hypokalaemia and ventricular fibrillation in acute myocardial infarction. *Br Heart J*. 1983;50:525-529.
16. Obeid AI, Verrier RL, Lown B. Influence of glucose, insulin, and potassium on vulnerability to ventricular fibrillation in the canine heart. *Circ Res*. 1978;43:601-608.
17. Curry P, Fitchett D, Stubbs W, Krikler D. Ventricular arrhythmias and hypokalaemia. *Lancet*. 1976;2:231-233.
18. Paltiel O, Salakhov E, Ronen I, Berg D, Israeli A. Management of severe hypokalemia in hospitalized patients: a study of quality of care based on computerized databases. *Arch Intern Med*. 2001;161:1089-1095.
19. Schulman M, Narins RG. Hypokalemia and cardiovascular disease. *Am J Cardiol*. 1990;65:4E-9E.
20. Weaver WF, Burchell HB. Serum potassium and the electrocardiogram in hypokalemia. *Circulation*. 1960;21:505-521.
21. Adrogue HJ, Madias NE. Aiding fluid prescription for the dysnatremias. *Intensive Care Med*. 1997;23:309-316.
22. Fraser CL, Arieff AI. Epidemiology, pathophysiology, and management of hyponatremic encephalopathy. *Am J Med*. 1997;102:67-77.
23. Adrogue HJ, Madias NE. Hyponatremia. *N Engl J Med*. 2000;342:1581-1589.
24. Gross P, Reimann D, Neidel J, Doke C, Prospert F, Decaux G, Verbalis J, Schrier RW. The treatment of severe hyponatremia. *Kidney Int Suppl*. 1998;64:S6-S11.
25. Menashe G, Borer A, Gilad J, Horowitz J. Rhabdomyolysis after correction of severe hyponatremia. *Am J Emerg Med*. 2000;18:229-230.
26. Laureno R, Karp BI. Myelinolysis after correction of hyponatremia. *Ann Intern Med*. 1997;126:57-62.
27. Soupart A, Decaux G. Therapeutic recommendations for management of severe hyponatremia: current concepts on pathogenesis and prevention of neurologic complications. *Clin Nephrol*. 1996;46:149-169.
28. Brunner JE, Redmond JM, Haggar AM, Kruger DF, Elias SB. Central pontine myelinolysis and pontine lesions after rapid correction of hyponatremia: a prospective magnetic resonance imaging study. *Ann Neurol*. 1990;27:61-66.
29. Ayus JC, Krothapalli RK, Arieff AI. Treatment of symptomatic hyponatremia and its relation to brain damage: a prospective study. *N Engl J Med*. 1987;317:1190-1195.
30. Anderson RJ, Chung HM, Kluge R, Schrier RW. Hyponatremia: a prospective analysis of its epidemiology and the pathogenetic role of vasopressin. *Ann Intern Med*. 1985;102:164-168.
31. Miller M. Syndromes of excess antidiuretic hormone release. *Crit Care Clin*. 2001;17:11-23, v.
32. Barri YM, Knochel JP. Hypercalcemia and electrolyte disturbances in malignancy. *Hematol Oncol Clin North Am*. 1996;10:775-790.
33. Aldinger KA, Samaan NA. Hypokalemia with hypercalcemia. Prevalence and significance in treatment. *Ann Intern Med*. 1977;87:571-573.

34. Stewart AF. Clinical practice. Hypercalcemia associated with cancer. *N Engl J Med*. 2005;352:373-379.
35. Silva OL, Becker KL. Salmon calcitonin in the treatment of hypercalcemia. *Arch Intern Med*. 1973;132:337-339.
36. Carano A, Teitelbaum SL, Konsek JD, Schlesinger PH, Blair HC. Bisphosphonates directly inhibit the bone resorption activity of isolated avian osteoclasts in vitro. *J Clin Invest*. 1990;85:456-461.
37. Gucalp R, Ritch P, Wiernik PH, Sarma PR, Keller A, Richman SP, Tauer K, Neidhart J, Mallette LE, Siegel R, et al. Comparative study of pamidronate disodium and etidronate disodium in the treatment of cancer-related hypercalcemia. *J Clin Oncol*. 1992;10:134-142.
38. Major P, Lortholary A, Hon J, Abdi E, Mills G, Menssen HD, Yunus F, Bell R, Body J, Quebe-Fehling E, Seaman J. Zoledronic acid is superior to pamidronate in the treatment of hypercalcemia of malignancy: a pooled analysis of two randomized, controlled clinical trials. *J Clin Oncol*. 2001;19:558-567.
39. Edelson GW, Kleerekoper M. Hypercalcemic crisis. *Med Clin North Am*. 1995;79:79-92.
40. Berenson JR. Treatment of hypercalcemia of malignancy with bisphosphonates. *Semin Oncol*. 2002;29:12-18.
41. Higham PD, Adams PC, Murray A, Campbell RW. Plasma potassium, serum magnesium and ventricular fibrillation: a prospective study. *Q J Med*. 1993;86:609-617.
42. Mordes JP, Swartz R, Arky RA. Extreme hypermagnesemia as a cause of refractory hypotension. *Ann Intern Med*. 1975;83:657-658.
43. McDonnell NJ, Muchatuta NA, Paech MJ. Acute magnesium toxicity in an obstetric patient undergoing general anaesthesia for caesarean delivery. *Int J Obstet Anesth*. 2010;19:226-231.
44. James MF. Cardiopulmonary arrest in pregnancy. *Br J Anaesth*. 2010;104:115.
45. Poole JH, Long J. Maternal mortality: a review of current trends. *Crit Care Nurs Clin North Am*. 2004;16:227-230.
46. Munro PT. Management of eclampsia in the accident and emergency department. *J Accid Emerg Med*. 2000;17:7-11.
47. McDonnell NJ. Cardiopulmonary arrest in pregnancy: two case reports of successful outcomes in association with perimortem caesarean delivery. *Br J Anaesth*. 2009;103:406-409.
48. Elisaf M, Milionis H, Siamopoulos KC. Hypomagnesemic hypokalemia and hypocalcemia: clinical and laboratory characteristics. *Miner Electrolyte Metab*. 1997;23:105-112.
49. al-Ghamdi SM, Cameron EC, Sutton RA. Magnesium deficiency: pathophysiologic and clinical overview. *Am J Kidney Dis*. 1994;24:737-752.
50. Faich GA, Fishbein HA, Ellis SE. The epidemiology of diabetic acidosis: a population-based study. *Am J Epidemiol*. 1983;117:551-558.
51. Kitabchi AE, Murphy MB, Spencer J, Matteri R, Karas J. Is a priming dose of insulin necessary in a low-dose insulin protocol for the treatment of diabetic ketoacidosis? *Diabetes Care*. 2008;31:2081-2085.
52. Goyal N, Miller JB, Sankey SS, Mossallam U. Utility of initial bolus insulin in the treatment of diabetic ketoacidosis. *J Emerg Med*. 2010;38:422-427.
53. Kitabchi AE, Umpierrez GE, Miles JM, Fisher JN. Hyperglycemic crises in adult patients with diabetes. *Diabetes Care*. 2009;32:1335-1343.
54. Viallon A, Zeni F, Lafond P, Venet C, Tardy B, Page Y, Bertrand JC. Does bicarbonate therapy improve the management of severe diabetic ketoacidosis? *Crit Care Med*. 1999;27:2690-2693.
55. Kannan CR. Bicarbonate therapy in the management of severe diabetic ketoacidosis. *Crit Care Med*. 1999;27:2833-2834.
56. Glaser N, Barnett P, McCaslin I, Nelson D, Trainor J, Louie J, Kaufman F, Quayle K, Roback M, Malley R, Kuppermann N. Risk factors for cerebral edema in children with diabetic ketoacidosis. The Pediatric Emergency Medicine Collaborative Research Committee of the American Academy of Pediatrics. *N Engl J Med*. 2001;344:264-269.
57. Dunger DB, Edge JA. Predicting cerebral edema during diabetic ketoacidosis. *N Engl J Med*. 2001;344:302-303.
58. Magee MF, Bhatt BA. Management of decompensated diabetes. Diabetic ketoacidosis and hyperglycemic hyperosmolar syndrome. *Crit Care Clin*. 2001;17:75-106.
59. Gottschalk ME, Ros SP, Zeller WP. The emergency management of hyperglycemic-hyperosmolar nonketotic coma in the pediatric patient. *Pediatr Emerg Care*. 1996;12:48-51.
60. Ellis EN. Concepts of fluid therapy in diabetic ketoacidosis and hyperosmolar hyperglycemic nonketotic coma. *Pediatr Clin North Am*. 1990;37:313-321.

Chapter 16

Cardiac Arrest Associated With Asthma

This Chapter

- Pathophysiology of Severe, Life-Threatening Asthma Attacks
- Asthma Severity Scores
- Patient Deterioration and Immediate Actions to Take Before Imminent Respiratory and Cardiac Arrest
- Mechanical Ventilation and Avoiding Auto-PEEP
- Post-Treatment/Postarrest Care

Overview and Epidemiology

In 2010, an estimated 25.7 million people in the United States had asthma. The prevalence of asthma increased from 7.3% in 2001 to 8.4% in 2010. Children aged 0 to 17 years had higher prevalence of asthma (7 million children, or 9.5%) than adults aged 18 and over (18.7 million adults, or 7.7%) for the period 2008-2010, and females had a higher prevalence than males (9.2% compared with 7.0%).

From 2001 to 2009, rates for emergency department (ED) visits and hospitalizations per 100 persons with asthma remained stable, while rates for asthma visits in primary care settings (physician offices or hospital outpatient departments) and asthma deaths declined. In 2010, there were 3388 deaths due to asthma in the US. Asthma death rates per 1000 persons with asthma were more than 30% higher for females than males, 75% higher for blacks than whites, and almost 7 times higher for adults than children. The highest rate was for adults aged 65 and over (0.58 per 1000 persons with asthma).[1] This disease is responsible for more than 2 million ED visits per year, and approximately 25% of these visits results in a hospital admission.[2] Severe asthma accounts for approximately 2% to 20% of admissions to intensive care units (ICUs), with up to one third of these patients requiring intubation and mechanical ventilation.[3] Some experts think that as many as 50% of asthma-related deaths are attributed to other causes such as upper respiratory infection and influenza, especially in adult victims.[4] Most acute episodes resulting in death are related to severe underlying disease, inadequate baseline management, and acute exacerbations of inflammation. Although asthma death rates per 1000 persons with asthma declined from 2001 to 2009,[1] these potentially preventable deaths often strike the young, and they can be very painful for families, friends, and healthcare providers.

The *2010 American Heart Association Guidelines for Cardiopulmonary Resuscitation and Emergency Cardiovascular Care* do not discuss care for chronic asthma or typical exacerbations. However, the guidelines do make recommendations for the management of *acute, severe, life-threatening asthma attacks.* Near-fatal,[5] severe, life-threatening asthma,[6] and status asthmaticus are the most common types. Status asthmaticus refers to attacks that fail to respond to continuous, aggressive treatment after a specified amount of time (eg, 4 hours).

The Global Initiative for Asthma and the National Asthma Education and Prevention Program of the National Heart, Lung, and Blood Institute have developed guidelines for the assessment of the severity of acute asthma exacerbations in the emergency care setting.[7] On the basis of the patient's symptoms, physical examination findings, and functional assessment, the patient may be classified as having a mild, moderate, or severe exacerbation, or as being in imminent respiratory arrest (Table 64). This evaluation may be applied to children, adolescents, and adults.

Table 64. Asthma Severity Score: Classification of Mild, Moderate, and Severe Asthma

FORMAL EVALUATION OF ASTHMA EXACERBATION SEVERITY IN THE URGENT OR EMERGENCY CARE SETTING

	Mild	Moderate	Severe	Subset: Respiratory Arrest Imminent
Symptoms				
Breathlessness	While walking Can lie down	While at rest (infant—softer, shorter cry, difficulty feeding) Prefers sitting	While at rest (infant—stops feeding) Sits upright	
Talks in	Sentences	Phrases	Words	
Alertness	May be agitated	Usually agitated	Usually agitated	Drowsy or confused
Signs				
Respiratory rate	Increased	Increased Guide to rates of breathing in awake children: *Age* <2 months 2–12 months 1–5 years 6–8 years	Often >30/minute *Normal rate* <60/minute <50/minute <40/minute <30/minute	
Use of accessory muscles; suprasternal retractions	Usually not	Commonly	Usually	Paradoxical thoracoabdominal movement
Wheeze	Moderate, often only end expiratory	Loud; throughout exhalation	Usually loud; throughout inhalation and exhalation	Absence of wheeze
Pulse/minute	<100	100–120 Guide to normal pulse rates in children:: *Age* 2–12 months 1–2 years 2–8 years	>120 *Normal rate* <160/minute <120/minute <110/minute	Bradycardia
Pulsus paradoxus	Absent <10 mmHg	May be present 10–25 mmHg	Often present >25 mmHg (adult) 20–40 mmHg (child)	Absence suggests respiratory muscle fatigue
Functional Assessment				
PEF percent predicted or percent personal best	≥70 percent	Approx. 40–69 percent or response lasts <2 hours	<40 percent	<25 percent Note: PEF testing may not be needed in very severe attacks
PaO_2 (on air)	Normal (test not usually necessary)	≥60 mmHg (test not usually necessary)	<60 mmHg: possible cyanosis	
and/or PCO_2	<42 mmHg (test not usually necessary)	<42 mmHg (test not usually necessary)	≥42 mmHg: possible respiratory failure (See pages 393–394, 399.)	
SaO_2 percent (on air) at sea level	>95 percent (test not usually necessary) Hypercapnia (hypoventilation) develops more readily in young children than in adults and adolescents.	90–95 percent (test not usually necessary)	<90 percent	

Key: PaO_2, arterial oxygen pressure; PCO_2, partial pressure of carbon dioxide; PEF, peak expiratory flow; SaO_2, oxygen saturation

Notes:

- The presence of several parameters, but not necessarily all, indicates the general classification of the exacerbation.
- Many of these parameters have not been systematically studied, especially as they correlate with each other. Thus, they serve only as general guides (Cham et al. 2002; Chey et al. 1999; Gorelick et al. 2004b; Karras et al. 2000; Kelly et al. 2002b and 2004; Keogh et al. 2001; McCarren et al. 2000; Rodrigo and Rodrigo 1998b; Rodrigo et al. 2004; Smith et al. 2002).
- The emotional impact of asthma symptoms on the patient and family is variable but must be recognized and addressed and can affect approaches to treatment and followup (Ritz et al. 2000; Strunk and Mrazek 1986; von Leupoldt and Dahme 2005).

Reproduced from the National Heart, Lung, and Blood Institute.[7]

Life-Threatening and Fatal Asthma

Pathophysiology

The pathophysiology of asthma consists of 3 key abnormalities:

- Bronchoconstriction
- Airway inflammation
- Mucous impaction

Severe exacerbations of asthma can lead rapidly to death. Cardiac arrest in patients with bronchial asthma has been linked to a variety of pathophysiologic mechanisms complicating exacerbations of asthma, but the most likely cause is thought to be bronchospasm with subsequent plugging of the narrowed airways by mucus (Figure 109).[8] At autopsy these patients display marked mucous plugging, airway edema, exudation of plasma proteins, hypertrophy of airway smooth muscle, and cellular activation with increased production and activation of inflammatory mediators.[9-11] Some patients experience a sudden onset of severe bronchospasm that responds rapidly to inhaled β_2-agonists.[12] This observation suggests that marked bronchiolar smooth muscle spasm is the major component in some cases of fatal asthma.

Bronchoconstriction and airway obstruction from mucous plugging cause hyperinflation and increased airway resistance (Figure 109). As a consequence, the work of breathing increases dramatically. Some patients who receive mechanical ventilation develop *auto-PEEP* (positive end-expiratory pressure). A simple explanation of auto-PEEP is that the inspiratory tidal volume is greater than the expiratory tidal volume (see below). This net and ever-increasing volume leads to an increase in intrathoracic pressure (the auto-PEEP), which decreases venous return to the heart. Hemodynamic compromise rapidly follows, largely as a result of inadequate cardiac output.

Severe asthma attacks are prone to be fatal when combined with one or more asthma-related complications. These complications include tension pneumothorax (often bilateral), pneumomediastinum, pneumonia, lobar atelectasis (from mucous plugging, often of larger airways), cardiac dysfunction, and pulmonary edema.

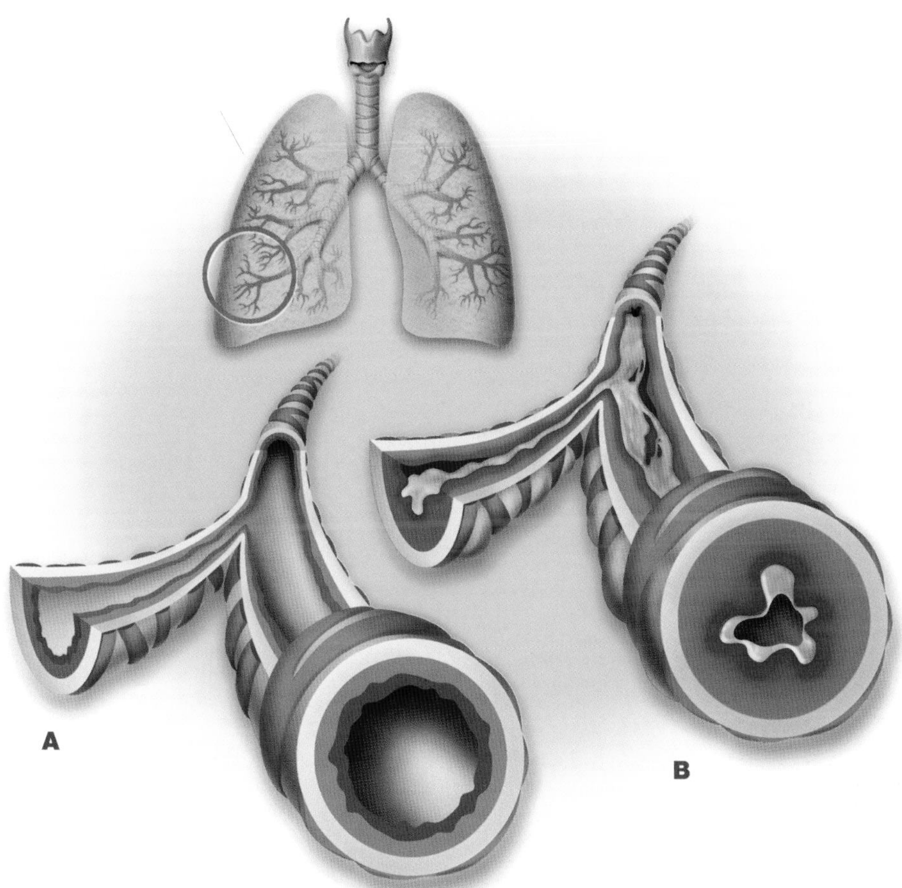

Figure 109. Asthma occurs in the setting of underlying inflammation. Diffuse bronchospasm occurs, causing air passages to constrict. Hypersecretion of mucus leads to a partial or full mucous plug, which blocks oxygenation and ventilation. **A,** Normal healthy bronchiole. **B,** Bronchiole during an asthma attack.

Signs and Symptoms

Fatal, near-fatal,[5] or life-threatening asthma[6] occurs more frequently in the following groups of patients with asthma:

- Black men
- Inner-city residents
- Patients who:
  - Were recently hospitalized for asthma[13]
  - Are steroid dependent
  - Were recently intubated for asthma[13]
  - Delay seeking care for attacks and whose condition deteriorates at home
  - Do not recognize the severity of their attack
  - Try to treat themselves during attacks without notifying their primary provider about exacerbations
  - Were diagnosed with asthma when they were 5 years of age or younger

The number of patients with severe asthma attacks who present to the ED at night is about 10 times greater than the number who present during the day.

Severe, life-threatening asthma (Table 60) will present to ACLS providers in 1 of 2 ways:

- Clinical deterioration despite hours of therapy
- Periarrest

Asthma Triggers

Patient profiles and risk factors for asthma can be identified, as can triggers for attacks in many persons (Table 65). Some triggers are unavoidable, but they should be identified if possible. Others can be avoided in the future, or medical care can be sought early if patients and their families are aware of them. In some cases the trigger needs to be treated concomitantly with the asthma attack.

A case-control study showed that nearly half of near-fatal and fatal attacks occurred suddenly and unexpectedly, outside the hospital, in stable, younger, atopic patients who were reportedly compliant with their medical plan of care and used inhaled corticosteroids daily.[14]

Table 65. Triggers of Fatal and Near-Fatal Asthma

1. Environment
   - Extremes of temperature
   - High humidity and dew points
   - Episodic contaminants (smoke, cigarette smoke)
2. Upper respiratory infections (viruses and bacteria)
3. Allergens (pollens and molds)
4. Exercise (cold-induced)
5. Other medical conditions (COPD, gastroesophageal reflux)
6. Drugs (aspirin, β-blockers, nonsteroidal antiinflammatory medications)

Abbreviation: COPD, chronic obtrusive pulmonary disease.

Signs and Symptoms: Assessing Severity

The patient's report of subjective symptoms is an inaccurate gauge of the severity of asthma.

- Reported severity correlates poorly with objective severity scores.
- Some patients with severe, life-threatening asthma have an impaired response to hypercapnia and hypoxia. Their perception of dyspnea appears to be blunted. These patients may present with severe abnormalities of oxygenation and respiratory acidosis.[15]

In severe asthma, the severity of wheezing is a poor indicator of airflow or adequacy of gas exchange.

- A patient with severe bronchospasm and obstruction may not move air and may not wheeze at all.[16,17]
- The silent asthmatic chest is an ominous sign. Treatment that results in the return of wheezes on auscultation is effective treatment.

A patient with asthma who is sitting upright to breathe, using accessory inspiratory muscles in the neck and chest, is at risk for sudden respiratory failure. Somnolence, mental confusion, and a moribund or exhausted appearance are ominous signs that respiratory arrest is imminent.

The key to assessing severity is to use asthma severity scores (Table 60). These scores are based on objective evaluation of clinical signs, airway obstruction and work of breathing, oxygenation (with oximetry) and ventilation, and either FEV_1 (forced expiratory volume in 1 second) or peak expiratory flow (PEF). Clinical severity scores are much more reliable than observations of healthcare providers.[17]

A peak flow meter provides a quick, accurate, and reproducible measure of PEF in cooperative adults that is not influenced by the person supervising the test.[18] EDs should consider PEF as a vital sign for a person with asthma.

Differential Diagnosis

When a patient presents with wheezing, the ACLS provider must determine if the patient has acute asthma. When a patient presents with extreme dyspnea, you may be unable to confirm a history of asthma.

Other conditions may cause patients to wheeze and to be acutely short of breath, including

- Cardiac disease (congestive heart failure [CHF] or myocarditis)
- Emphysema
- Pneumonia
- Upper airway obstruction (structural or psychogenic, due to vocal cord dysfunction)

Critical Concept Oxygen Saturation Can Be Misleading	• Oxygen saturation (SaO_2) levels may not reflect progressive alveolar hypoventilation, particularly if O_2 is being administered. • SaO_2 may initially fall during therapy because β-agonists produce both bronchodilation and vasodilation and may initially increase intrapulmonary shunting.

- Acute allergic bronchospasm or anaphylaxis[19] (aspirin, foods, or idiopathic)
- Pulmonary embolism
- Pulmonary edema[20]
- Chronic obtrusive pulmonary disease (COPD)

If urticaria and multisystem abnormalities are present with wheezing, anaphylaxis could be the cause.

Bronchospasm also may be caused by medications, such as β-blockers,[21] or by drugs such as cocaine and opiates.[22,23] Abrupt discontinuation of corticosteroids may lead to life-threatening asthma. Long-term use of corticosteroids may produce a relative adrenal insufficiency because endogenous cortisol secretion is suppressed.

Prehospital Clinical Deterioration, Imminent Respiratory Arrest, and Cardiopulmonary Arrest

ACLS providers will most often treat people with severe, life-threatening asthma attacks and those who are deteriorating despite therapy and may stop breathing within minutes. The immediate goal is to prevent deterioration to respiratory or cardiopulmonary arrest.

Immediate Actions

If supplementary **oxygen** has not been initiated, start it at once; use a nonrebreathing mask with high-flow oxygen or a bag and mask. Immediately administer a **selective inhaled short-acting β_2-agonist** by nebulizer or metered-dose inhaler (MDI) (with spacer), whichever can be assembled more quickly. Administer every 20 minutes or continuously for 1 hour.

Combining several doses of ipratropium bromide (0.5 mg every 20 minutes for 3 doses, then as needed) with an inhaled selective **β_2-agonist** improves bronchodilation and is recommended for severe exacerbation in the ED, but its use is not recommended after admission to the hospital.

Systemic corticosteroids are recommended for most patients with moderate or severe exacerbations or patients who don't respond completely to initial **β_2-agonist** therapy.

Systemic **β_2-agonist** can be administered subcutaneously or intravenously if inhaler therapy is not possible because the patient is unable to use the equipment effectively or if the inhaler equipment is not readily available. **Epinephrine** 0.3 to 0.5 mg or terbutaline 0.25 mg can be administered subcutaneously every 20 minutes up to 3 doses.

For severe exacerbations that do not respond to these initial therapies, consider magnesium sulfate or heliox as adjunct treatments.

Evaluate Immediate Response

Evaluate how well the patient responds in the first 10 to 20 minutes to initial therapy. There should be unequivocal and significant objective improvement (eg, improvement in oxygenation and clinical appearance, a change in PEF from a severe degree of obstruction of less than 100 L/min to 150 to 200 L/min).

If the patient's condition deteriorates, proceed immediately to rapid sequence intubation (RSI) if resources and skilled personnel are available. Support ventilations with a bag-mask device while preparations are made.

Primary Therapy and Reassessment in the ED

Primary Therapy

Patients with severe, life-threatening asthma require urgent and aggressive treatment with simultaneous administration of oxygen, bronchodilators, and steroids. Healthcare providers must monitor these patients closely for deterioration. Only bronchoconstriction and inflammation are amenable to drug treatment. If the patient does not respond to therapy, early consultation or transfer to a pulmonologist or intensivist is appropriate.

Critical Concept Do Not Hyperventilate	**Critical Action** • Do not hyperventilate the patient during bag-mask ventilation. • Hyperventilation can exacerbate auto-PEEP, compromising cardiac output. • Auto-PEEP from breaths given too rapidly causes increased intrathoracic pressure and inadequate exhalation in some patients.

Oxygen

- Start oxygen at 4 L/min for all patients with acute severe asthma. The immediate treatment goal according to the National Heart, Lung, and Blood Institute guidelines is to achieve an oxygen saturation (SaO_2) of 90% or higher.
- Start supplementary oxygen before or simultaneously with initial inhaled β_2-agonists. Give oxygen to all patients with asthma, including those with normal oxygen saturation.
  - Without administration of supplementary oxygen, a paradoxical worsening of hypoxemia could follow administration of inhaled bronchodilators.
  - β-Agonists may induce both pulmonary vasodilation and bronchodilation. This condition may produce a right-to-left shunt (shunting of systemic venous blood through the lungs so that it is desaturated when it returns to the left atrium), which will contribute to worsening of hypoxemia.
- Some patients may require high-flow oxygen by mask.

Inhaled β_2-Agonists

Albuterol and **levalbuterol** are equivalent β_2-selective β-agonists that act by relaxing bronchial smooth muscles. These drugs provide rapid, dose-dependent, short-acting reduction in bronchospasm with minimal adverse effects. Albuterol has gained almost universal acceptance as the therapeutic cornerstone for acute asthma. Inhaled albuterol, delivered through a nebulizer or an MDI, has proved to be much more effective than IV albuterol. Because the administered dose depends on lung volume and inspiratory flow rates, the same dose can be used in most adult patients regardless of age or size. Levalbuterol has been shown to provide the same efficacy and safety as albuterol when administered at half the milligram dose.

MDIs Versus Nebulizers

Although studies have shown no difference in the effects of continuous versus intermittent administration of nebulized albuterol, continuous administration was more effective in patients with severe exacerbations of asthma,[24,25] and it was more cost-effective in a pediatric trial.[26] A Cochrane meta-analysis showed no overall difference between the effects of albuterol delivered by MDI with spacer or nebulizer.[27] Delivery by nebulizer has become the most common ED treatment for acute asthma attacks. Some studies suggest that MDIs with spacers have several advantages over nebulizers.[28-31]

The recommended dose of albuterol by nebulizer is 2.5 to 5 mg every 20 minutes for 3 doses or continuous nebulization in a dose of 10 to 15 mg/h. Aggressive dosing for more severe cases calls for higher amounts of the agent at shorter intervals. The typical dose of albuterol by MDI-with spacer (90 mcg per puff) is 4 to 8 puffs every 20 minutes for up to 4 hours, then every 1 to 4 hours as needed.

Corticosteroids

Systemic corticosteroids are the only proven treatment for the inflammatory component of asthma, but the onset of their anti-inflammatory effects is 6 to 12 hours after administration. Early use of systemic steroids reduced rates of admission to the hospital.[32] In addition, reduction of inflammation and bronchial edema reduces length of hospital stay, in-hospital complications, readmissions, and return visits to the ED.[33,34]

Healthcare providers should administer steroids as early as possible to all patients with asthma but should not expect effects for several hours. The IV route is preferable because patients with severe, near-fatal asthma may vomit or be unable to swallow. The typical initial IV dose for methylprednisolone is 125 mg (dose range: 40 to 250 mg). Then the dose for methylprednisolone, prednisone, and prednisolone is 40 to 80 mg/d in 1 or 2 divided doses until PEF is 70% or more of predicted value.

Inhaled Steroids

Incorporation or substitution of inhaled steroids into this scheme remains controversial. There is insufficient evidence to conclude that inhaled corticosteroids alone are as effective as systemic steroids.[33]

Adjunctive Therapy

Anticholinergics

Ipratropium bromide is an anticholinergic bronchodilator that is pharmacologically related to atropine. It can produce a clinically modest improvement in lung function compared with albuterol alone.[35,36] The nebulizer dose is 0.5 mg. Ipratropium bromide has a slow onset of action (approximately 20 minutes), with peak effectiveness at 60 to 90 minutes and no systemic side effects. It is typically given only once because of its prolonged onset of action, but some studies have shown clinical improvement only with repeated doses.[37] Given the few side effects, ipratropium should be considered an adjunct to albuterol. The National Institutes of Health Expert Panel on the Management of Asthma endorses the combination of β_2-agonists plus an inhaled anticholinergic agent for asthma patients with a PEF or FEV_1 lower than 80% of the predicted normal value.[38]

Pharmacology

Ipratropium bromide is an anticholinergic (parasympatholytic) bronchodilator that is pharmacologically related to atropine. Ipratropium inhibits vagally mediated constriction of bronchial smooth muscles. Ipratropium bromide produces less bronchodilation than inhaled β_2-agonists,[36,39] and it has a slower onset (about 20 minutes longer).[40]

Use in Severe, Life-Threatening Asthma

There does appear to be a role for ipratropium bromide *in combination* with selective inhaled β-agonists for cases of severe, life-threatening asthma. A meta-analysis of randomized, controlled trials limited to adults with asthma observed a modest benefit from ipratropium combined with β_2-agonists.[41] Ipratropium bromide is not recommended for use after hospital admission.

Dose

Ipratropium bromide is usually mixed 0.5 mg in 2.5 mL of normal saline in a nebulizer with the first dose of albuterol and administered every 4 to 6 hours. There is evidence that repeat doses of 250 mcg or 500 mcg every 20 minutes can be beneficial.[37] Patients with severe asthma appear to benefit the most.[42]

Magnesium Sulfate

IV magnesium sulfate can modestly improve pulmonary function in patients with asthma when combined with nebulized β-adrenergic agents and corticosteroids.[43]

Pharmacology

When combined with nebulized β-adrenergic agents and corticosteroids, IV magnesium sulfate can improve pulmonary function moderately in patients with asthma.[43] Magnesium causes relaxation of bronchial smooth muscle independent of serum magnesium level, with only minor side effects (flushing, lightheadedness). A Cochrane meta-analysis of 7 studies concluded that IV magnesium sulfate improves pulmonary function and reduces hospital admissions, particularly for patients with the most severe exacerbations of asthma.[44] The use of nebulized magnesium sulfate as an adjunct to nebulized β-adrenergic agents has been reported in a small case series to improve FEV_1 and SpO_2,[45] although a prior meta-analysis demonstrated only a trend toward improved pulmonary function with nebulized magnesium.[46] For those with severe refractory asthma, providers may consider IV magnesium at the standard adult dose of 2 g administered over 20 minutes.

Dose

The standard adult dose of magnesium sulfate 2 g IV given over 20 minutes when used with conventional therapy has been shown to reduce hospitalization rates for ED patients with severe exacerbations but did not improve pulmonary function in patients whose initial FEV_1 was 25% or more of predicted value.[47] When given with a β_2-agonist, nebulized magnesium sulfate improved pulmonary function during acute asthma.[48]

Heliox

Heliox is a mixture of helium and oxygen (usually a helium-to-oxygen ratio of 70:30) that is less viscous than ambient air. Heliox has been shown to improve the delivery and deposition of nebulized albuterol and may decrease the likelihood of intubation.[47,49] Although a meta-analysis of 4 clinical trials did not support the use of heliox in the initial treatment of patients with acute asthma,[50] it may be useful for asthma that is refractory to conventional therapy.[51] The heliox mixture requires at least 70% helium for effect, thereby limiting the percentage of supplemental oxygen that can be provided concurrently.

Parenteral Epinephrine or Terbutaline

Epinephrine and terbutaline are adrenergic agents that can be given subcutaneously to patients with acute severe asthma. Epinephrine is an effective bronchial smooth muscle dilator with a rapid onset of action. The dose of subcutaneous epinephrine (concentration of 1:1000, 1 mg/mL, total dose 0.01 mg/kg) is divided into 3 doses of approximately 0.3 to 0.5 mg given at 20-minute intervals. Terbutaline is given in a dose of 0.25 mg subcutaneously and can be repeated every 20 minutes for 3 doses. These drugs are more commonly administered to children with acute asthma. There is no evidence that subcutaneous epinephrine or terbutaline has advantages over inhaled β_2-agonists. Epinephrine has been administered IV (initiated at 0.25 mcg/min to 1 mcg/min continuous infusion) in severe asthma; however, 1 retrospective investigation indicated a 4% incidence of serious side effects. There is no evidence of improved outcomes with IV epinephrine compared with selective inhaled β_2-agonists.[52]

Epinephrine

Pharmacology

Epinephrine is a nonselective β-agonist that requires parenteral (subcutaneous or IV) administration. Epinephrine also produces tachycardia, acute blood pressure elevation, and increased myocardial oxygen demand.

Indications

Adverse properties and side effects cause many experts to limit the use of epinephrine in acute asthma to patients younger than 35 years who are unable to use inhalers.[53] However, subcutaneous epinephrine is well tolerated and effective for the treatment of older adults with asthma.

Use in Severe, Life-Threatening Asthma

Subcutaneous epinephrine can be administered to patients who are "too tight to wheeze" and cannot effectively inhale β_2-agonists through an MDI or a nebulizer. As the patient's condition deteriorates, the inspiratory flow rate decreases and compromises delivery of inhaled medications.

Terbutaline

Pharmacology

Terbutaline is a selective β_2-agonist with pharmacologic and adverse effects similar to those of albuterol. In the ED terbutaline is given by subcutaneous injection or IV infusion.

Use in Severe, Life-Threatening Asthma?

Compared with epinephrine, terbutaline has a slower onset of action (5 to 30 minutes), longer time to peak effects (1 to 2 hours), and a much longer duration of action (3 to 6 hours). As an alternative to epinephrine, terbutaline has little role to play in adults with severe, life-threatening asthma because of the slow onset of action and longer time to peak effects. But in children, at least 1 ED study has found terbutaline to be more efficacious than epinephrine for reversal of wheezing.

Dose

The dose of terbutaline is 0.25 mg subcutaneously. This dose can be administered every 20 minutes for 3 doses.

Other Agents

Ketamine

Ketamine is a parenteral, dissociative anesthetic with bronchodilatory properties that also can stimulate copious bronchial secretions. One case series[54] suggested substantial efficacy, whereas 2 published randomized trials in children[55,56] found no benefit of ketamine when compared with standard care. Ketamine has sedative and analgesic properties that may be useful if intubation is planned.

Methylxanthines

Although previously a mainstay in the treatment of acute asthma, methylxanthines are infrequently used because of questionable efficacy, erratic pharmacokinetics, and known side effects and are no longer recommended for managing acute exacerbations of asthma.

Leukotriene Receptor Antagonists

Leukotriene receptor antagonists (LTRAs) improve lung function and decrease the need for short-acting β-agonists during long-term asthma therapy. One study showed improvement in lung function with the addition of IV montelukast to standard therapy,[57] but further research is needed.

Inhaled Anesthetics

Case reports in adults[58] and children[59] suggest a benefit of inhalation anesthetics (sevoflurane and isoflurane) for patients with status asthmaticus unresponsive to maximal conventional therapy. These anesthetic agents may work directly as bronchodilators and may have indirect effects by enhancing patient-ventilator synchrony and reducing oxygen demand and carbon dioxide production.

Post-Treatment and Postresuscitation Care

Response to Initial Treatment: Severity Scoring System

To aid decision making, use the severity scoring system (Table 64). In addition, you can place patients into 1 of the following categories after first-line treatment:

- Clinical improvement and FEV_1 or PEF 70% or more of predicted value after 1 to 3 hours of treatment: consider discharge home
- Some clinical improvement and FEV_1 or PEF 40% to 69% of predicted value after 4 hours of intensive treatment: "incomplete responder"
- Inadequate clinical improvement and FEV_1 or PEF less than 40% of predicted value after 4 hours of intensive treatment: hospital admission plus noninvasive assisted ventilation
- No clinical improvement and FEV_1 or PEF less than 25% of predicted value after 4 hours of intensive treatment: ICU admission plus assisted ventilation

Clinical Improvement

FEV_1 or PEF 70% or More of Predicted Value After 1 to 3 Hours of Treatment: Consider Discharge Home

Most patients who improve clinically and are breathing room air with adequate oxygenation (oxyhemoglobin saturation 95% or higher) and FEV_1 or PEF 70% or more of predicted value after receiving 1 to 3 hours of inhaled short-acting β_2-agonists, anticholinergics, and oral corticosteroids can be discharged home. You may need to modify this disposition on the basis of known risk factors.

- Observe these patients for at least 1 hour after they reach 70% or higher of predicted FEV_1 or PEF to ensure their stability.
- Review the discharge medications closely. Studies confirm the value of continued inhaled or oral steroids and of inhaled β_2-agonists *after* an acute exacerbation. These medications significantly reduce the need for return visits to the ED.

Some Clinical Improvement

FEV_1 or PEF 40% to 69% of Predicted Value After 4 Hours of Intensive Treatment: Incomplete Responders

Risk stratification for incomplete responders: Patients who achieve some clinical improvement but have persistent signs of moderate to severe asthma with improved oxygenation (oxyhemoglobin saturation of 90% to 95%) and FEV_1 or PEF 40% to 69% of predicted value after 4 hours of intensive treatment are classified as *incomplete responders*. They require careful triage. Concurrent comorbidity, such as insulin-dependent diabetes, coronary artery disease, cerebrovascular disease, COPD, or acute pneumonia, adds to the risk.

Low-risk incomplete responders: Some incomplete responders are at low risk for continued deterioration and may be discharged conditionally. Appropriate discharge requires that patients have adequate discharge medications, home resources, access to follow-up care, and a detailed discharge care plan.

High-risk incomplete responders: Incomplete responders with 1 or more of the following risk factors should be hospitalized (with occasional individual exceptions):

- History of intubation and mechanical ventilation for acute, life-threatening asthma
- Recent (within 2 to 4 weeks) hospitalization for asthma
- Bounce-back ED visits (ie, patient was evaluated and treated in an ED in the previous 24 to 48 hours)
- Duration of attack is 1 week or longer
- Current use of oral steroids (steroid dependent); studies have not yet established whether patients currently using inhaled steroids should be stratified as high risk
- Inadequate home care resources
- Known or suspected poor compliance

Inadequate Clinical Improvement

FEV_1 or PEF 25% to 40% of Predicted Value After 4 Hours of Intensive Treatment: Hospital Admission Plus Noninvasive Assisted Ventilation

Emergency physicians should admit these patients to the hospital for continued treatment and close monitoring. Noninvasive positive-pressure ventilation (NIPPV) is often an effective technique for respiratory support and may avert the need for endotracheal intubation. Bronchodilator therapy should continue with NIPPV.

No Clinical Improvement

FEV_1 or PEF Less Than 25% of Predicted Value After 4 Hours of Intensive Treatment: ICU Admission Plus Assisted Ventilation

These patients need not only hospital admission but also intensive monitoring and care. Endotracheal intubation and mechanical ventilation may be necessary if the patient continues to be unresponsive to therapy.

Indications for ICU admission: In addition to an FEV_1 or PEF less than 25% of predicted value, other objective signs and clinical symptoms indicate the need for ICU admission and probable intubation:

- Pa_{O_2} less than 65 mm Hg with 40% inspired oxygen (oxyhemoglobin saturation less than 90%)
- Pa_{CO_2} greater than 40 mm Hg (especially if rising during treatment in the ED)
- Altered level of consciousness
- Breathlessness that makes talking difficult
- Inability to lie supine
- Increasing fatigue and tiredness

Noninvasive Assisted Ventilation

The decision to intubate a patient with asthma is difficult. NIPPV may offer short-term support to patients with acute respiratory failure and may delay or eliminate the need for endotracheal intubation.[60,61] This therapy requires an alert patient with adequate spontaneous respiratory effort.

Description

NIPPV uses a mechanical ventilation device to deliver positive-pressure ventilation through a sealed mask to assist the patient's spontaneous respiratory efforts. The mask may cover a patient's nose, nose and mouth, or entire face. Bilevel positive airway pressure, the most common way of delivering NIPPV, allows for separate control of inspiratory and expiratory pressures.

Benefits

These devices are intended for patients suffering from severe, life-threatening asthma that is refractory to bronchodilators and steroids. By eliminating the need for intubation, these techniques convey numerous benefits.

NIPPV can enable support of ventilation without the need for and hazards of endotracheal tube placement (Table 66). This technique tends to be more comfortable for the patient and avoids the need for sedation. Morbidity and mortality are reduced for the patient, and the costs and technical difficulty are decreased with this method of ventilatory support.

Table 66. **Initial Steps to Follow for NIPPV**[61,62]

1. Secure a full face mask with head straps over the nose and mouth. Avoid a tight fit.
2. Connect the ventilator to the face mask. Use either a conventional mechanical ventilator or a ventilator specially made for NIPPV.
3. Start with CPAP set to 0 cm H_2O. Slowly increase CPAP to maintain PEEP even during spontaneous inspiration.
4. Set positive-pressure support (inspiratory pressure) of ventilation at 10 cm H_2O. Adjust on the basis of arterial blood gases, but do not exceed 25 cm H_2O.
5. Set tidal volume at 500 mL (7 mL/kg).
6. Set ventilation rate at <25 breaths/min.
7. Continue to administer nebulized medications through the system.

Abbreviations: CPAP, continuous positive airway pressure; PEEP, positive end-expiratory pressure.

Requirements and Contraindications

Experienced clinicians often recommend NIPPV for patients who do not respond satisfactorily to aggressive first-line therapy. However, patients must

- Be alert and able to protect the airway
- Be cooperative
- Demonstrate effective spontaneous respirations

Contraindications: Noninvasive assisted ventilation techniques are contraindicated for patients who are

- Severely hypoxemic: Pao_2 less than 60 mm Hg or O_2 saturation less than 90% on rebreathing mask
- A rising $Paco_2$ (greater than 40 mm Hg) with a falling pH
- Deteriorating steadily or rapidly
- Confused, somnolent, moribund, or uncooperative
- Unable to protect the airway
- Hypotensive (blood pressure less than 90 mm Hg)
- Known to have ischemic heart disease
- Having ventricular arrhythmias

Bilevel Positive Airway Pressure

Bilevel positive airway pressure has proved to be the most effective type of NIPPV for life-threatening asthma. Intermittent assisted ventilation with a bilevel positive airway pressure ventilator may help to delay or eliminate the need for endotracheal intubation. Carefully selected settings allow this type of ventilator to counteract the effects of auto-PEEP. Bilevel positive airway pressure devices reduce the work of breathing (more than any other noninvasive respiratory support technique) by reducing the force required for exhalation and assisting the work of inspiration. Most experts begin with an inspiratory positive airway pressure of 8 to 10 cm H_2O and an expiratory positive airway pressure of 3 to 5 cm H_2O.

Endotracheal Intubation for Life-Threatening Asthma

Endotracheal intubation does not solve the problem of small airway constriction in patients with severe asthma. In addition, intubation and positive-pressure ventilation can trigger further bronchoconstriction and complications such as breath stacking (auto-PEEP) and barotrauma. Although endotracheal intubation introduces risks, elective intubation should be performed if the condition of the patient with asthma deteriorates despite aggressive management.

RSI is the technique of choice. The provider should use the largest endotracheal tube available (usually 8 or 9 mm) to decrease airway resistance. Immediately after intubation, confirm endotracheal tube placement by clinical examination and continuous waveform capnography followed by a chest radiograph.

Indications

The major indications for rapid endotracheal intubation in life-threatening asthma are

- Failure to improve with NIPPV
- Continued deterioration despite aggressive first-line therapy
- Association with anaphylaxis (see Chapter 17)
- Deterioration with fatigue and exhaustion
- Onset of altered level of consciousness, confusion, or somnolence
- A rising $Paco_2$ (higher than 40 mm Hg) with a falling pH. These values are particularly worrisome when associated with clinical signs of obtundation, somnolence, and poor muscle tone. Note that isolated hypercarbia does not require immediate endotracheal intubation. *Treat the patient, not the numbers.*
- Pao_2 less than 50 mm Hg on a nonrebreathing mask, especially when associated with clinical signs of hypoxemia. These signs include severe agitation, confusion, and fighting against the oxygen mask.

RSI/Intubation

Precautions

RSI is the technique of choice for endotracheal intubation in patients with severe, life-threatening asthma.[62,63] However, one must be mindful that the combination of pre-existing volume depletion, air trapping, and strong sedatives may lead to marked hypotension or even cardiac arrest.

- Select the most experienced laryngoscopist to perform the procedure.
- It may be impossible to provide effective bag-mask ventilation when status asthmaticus is present.
- Use the largest endotracheal tube (8 to 9 mm) possible. The larger the tube diameter, the less the airway resistance. Suctioning the airway secretions can be handled better with large-diameter tubes. Immediately after intubation, proper endotracheal tube placement should be confirmed by clinical examination and continuous waveform capnography. A radiograph of the chest should then be performed.

Premedications

The most critical of the **LOAD** premedications (lidocaine, opioids, atropine, defasciculating agent) is lidocaine.

- Give lidocaine 1 to 2 mg/kg (maximum: 100 mg) IV 3 minutes before administration of opioids, sedatives, or paralytics. This dose will reduce bronchospasm induced by laryngoscopy and intubation.

Sedation and Anesthesia

Several intravenous anesthetics are powerful bronchodilators, especially propofol and ketamine.[64,65]

Propofol is a sedative with bronchodilator properties.[66] It is effective for both intubation and maintenance of sedation during mechanical ventilation. A dose of 1 to 2 mg/kg induces anesthesia in approximately 1 minute or less and lasts 5 to 10 minutes. This drug may cause hypotension.

Etomidate is an acceptable hypnotic to use, although it lacks bronchodilator properties.[67] Etomidate is short acting and has a safer hemodynamic profile than propofol. A dose of 0.2 to 0.4 mg/kg induces anesthesia in less than 60 seconds and lasts 5 to 10 minutes. This drug has no analgesic effects.

Ketamine is an effective sedative, analgesic, and dissociative anesthetic. Many experts recommend ketamine as the IV anesthetic of choice for patients with status asthmaticus. Ketamine possesses strong bronchodilator properties.[55] Ketamine potentiates catecholamines and relaxes bronchiolar smooth muscle. It does not cause vasodilatation, circulatory collapse, or myocardial depression. A dose of 1 to 2 mg/kg ketamine IV induces anesthesia in 30 to 60 seconds and lasts 10 to 20 minutes. Because ketamine increases bronchial secretions, many experts also premedicate with **atropine** (0.01 mg/kg; minimum dose of 0.1 mg; maximum single dose: 0.5 mg).

Paralysis

Succinylcholine, at a dose of 1 to 1.5 mg/kg, is the clear paralytic agent of choice for RSI in patients with severe asthma and no contraindications to the drug. **Rocuronium,** at a dose of 0.6 to 1.2 mg/kg, is the second paralytic of choice. Its rapid onset of action is similar to that of succinylcholine, but it has a longer duration of action. Vecuronium, at a dose of 0.1 to 0.2 mg/kg, has a slower onset (1 to 3 minutes) and longer duration of action than succinylcholine.

Airway Obstruction: A Persistent Problem

Endotracheal intubation enables use of external mechanical power to assist the patient's failing ventilation efforts. It does not solve the problem of airway obstruction. In addition, hypercarbia may create a respiratory acidosis. These problems with oxygenation and ventilation may persist even once the tube is in place.

- **Continue inhaled β_2-agonists:** Because breathing efforts may be inadequate, the patient may not have had adequate distribution of β_2-agonists before intubation. Immediately after intubation, administer 2.5 to 5 mg of albuterol via the endotracheal tube.
- **Ventilate the patient slowly with 100% oxygen:** When severe asthma is present, significant obstruction to air flow persists even after intubation.

Anyone performing manual ventilation for patients with severe asthma after intubation should ventilate *slowly* at a rate of only 6 to 10 breaths/min with smaller tidal volumes (eg, 6 to 8 mL/kg),[63] shorter inspiration time (eg, adult inspiratory flow rate 80 to 100 L/min), and longer expiratory time (eg, inspiratory to expiratory ratio 1:4 or 1:5) than generally would be provided to patients without asthma.[68] This slow respiratory rate and adequate exhalation time can minimize the development of auto-PEEP and its serious consequences of severe hypotension and pneumothorax. Prevention of hyperventilation and auto-PEEP is preferable to treatment of the complications.

Table 67 summarizes the steps needed to insert an endotracheal tube and begin mechanical ventilatory support for patients with severe, life-threatening asthma.

Mechanical Ventilation in Patients With Severe Asthma

Mechanical ventilation in patients with severe, life-threatening asthma is challenging, and the associated risks require careful management.

Table 67. Sample Summary of Steps to Initiate Mechanical Ventilatory Support for Severe Life-Threatening Asthma[62]

This sequence is one example. Variations are acceptable.

1. Place the patient in an upright position if comfortable.
2. Administer *lidocaine* 1.5 to 2 mg/kg 3 minutes before administration of anesthesia.
3. Administer *ketamine* 2 mg/kg.
4. *Immediately* follow with *succinylcholine* 1.5 mg/kg.
5. As the patient loses consciousness, gently place the patient in the supine position.
6. Perform *laryngoscopy* and *endotracheal intubation.* Use an 8- to 9-mm tube if possible.
7. Confirm correct placement of the endotracheal tube with clinical assessment and continuous waveform capnography. Begin mechanical ventilator support.
8. Begin maintenance sedation *(benzodiazepine or propofol)* and paralysis *(rocuronium or vecuronium).* Continue for 4 to 6 hours.
9. Adjust mechanical ventilation parameters as recommended in Table 66.
10. Provide additional *ketamine* as needed.
11. Administer bronchodilator agents via the endotracheal tube.
12. Monitor airway pressures to evaluate patient response to therapy.
13. Administer fluids (eg, normal saline) if needed to counteract the fall in blood pressure from auto-PEEP.

Abbreviation: PEEP, positive end-expiratory pressure.

Critical Concept
Sudden Deterioration in a Ventilated Patient

If the condition of the patient with asthma deteriorates or if it is difficult to ventilate the patient, verify endotracheal tube position, eliminate tube obstruction (any mucous plugs and kinks), and rule out (or decompress) a pneumothorax. Only experienced providers should perform needle decompression or insertion of a chest tube for pneumothorax.

Check the ventilator circuit for leaks or malfunction. High end-expiratory pressure can be quickly reduced by separating the patient from the ventilator circuit; this will allow PEEP to dissipate during passive exhalation.

- To minimize auto-PEEP if present, decrease inhalation time (this increases exhalation time), decrease respiratory rate by 2 breaths/min, and reduce tidal volume.
- Continue treatment with inhaled albuterol.

Troubleshooting Problems in the Intubated, Ventilator-Dependent Patient With Asthma

Auto-PEEP

Clinicians who provide mechanical ventilatory support for patients with severe asthma must understand the concept of auto-PEEP. Although patients with asthma experience some obstruction of inspiration, they experience *marked* obstruction of expiration. As resistance to exhalation increases, the inevitable result will be air trapping and "breath stacking" (inspired air enters and then cannot exit).

With severe airway obstruction, the duration of spontaneous expiration increases. If the ventilator settings are such that expiratory time is inadequate, this can lead to "self-produced" or "auto-produced" PEEP. In this case end-expiratory pressure increases above the PEEP settings to the mechanical ventilatory circuit. Increased intrathoracic pressure from auto-PEEP can reduce venous return to the heart. This reduced venous return can lead to reduced cardiac output, hemodynamic compromise, and hypotension. Note that hyperinflation and increased intrathoracic pressure can also produce barotrauma, such as a tension pneumothorax.

When severe bronchoconstriction is present, breath stacking (auto-PEEP) can develop during positive-pressure ventilation, leading to complications such as hyperinflation (Figure 110), tension pneumothorax, and hypotension. During manual or mechanical ventilation, use a slower respiratory rate (6 to 10 breaths/min) with smaller tidal

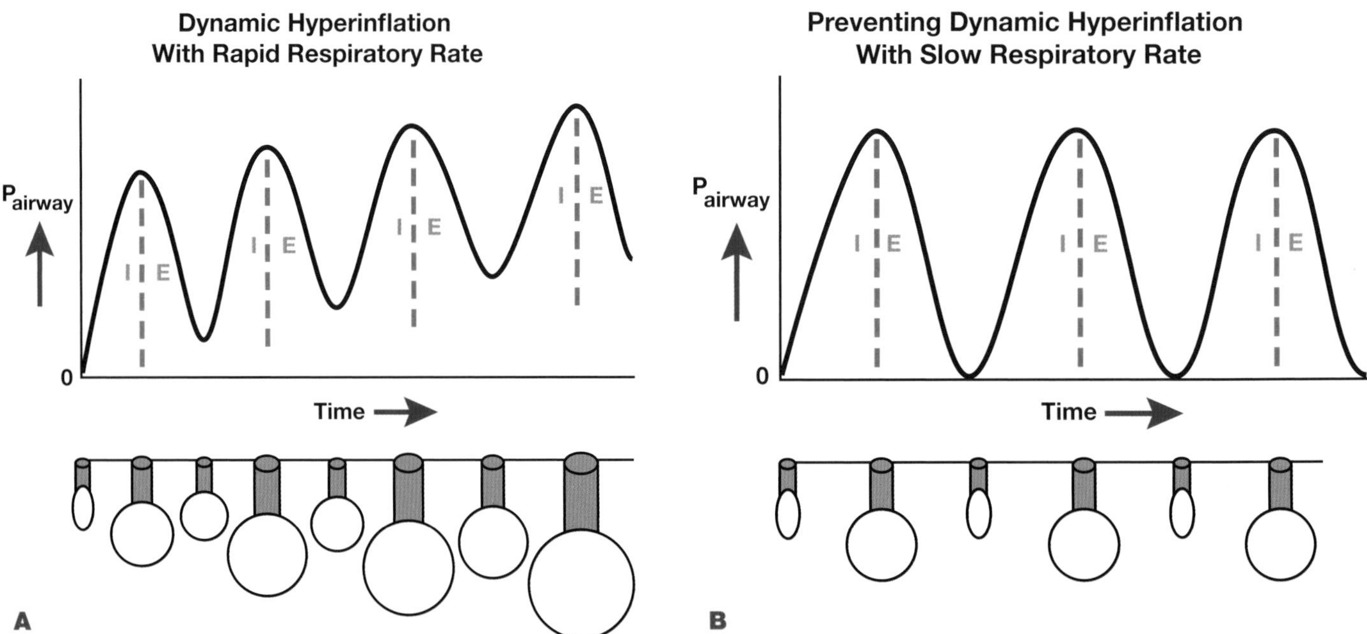

Figure 110. Dynamic hyperinflation. Bronchospasm and endobronchiole secretions delay alveolar emptying. Increased ventilatory rates cause air trapping (**A**) and increased alveolar volume, leading to decreased compliance or lung stiffness. Use of a slower ventilation rate and lower volume (**B**) allows the alveolus more time to empty. Abbreviations: I, inspiration; E, expiration.

volumes (6 to 8 mL/kg),[63] shorter inspiratory time (adult inspiratory flow rate 80 to 100 mL/min), and longer expiratory time (inspiratory to expiratory ratio 1:4 or 1:5) than those typical for patients without asthma.

Ventilation With "Permissive Hypercapnia"

Adequate oxygenation is relatively easy to achieve with mechanical ventilation in patients with severe asthma. The problem is ventilation or getting rid of the carbon dioxide. Mild hypoventilation reduces the risk of barotrauma from significant levels of auto-PEEP and is typically well tolerated.[69-71] This concept of controlled hypoventilation, using ventilator settings that result in a mild elevation of $Paco_2$, is referred to as *permissive hypercapnia* or *permissive hypercarbia*.

To prevent the development of significant levels of auto-PEEP, set the mechanical ventilator to low tidal volume, low respiratory rate, and long expiratory time (Table 68). These settings will lead to a mild increase in $Paco_2$, but because ventilatory support is controlled, hypercapnia develops gradually ($Paco_2$ levels may rise to 70 to 90 mm Hg over 3 to 4 hours). Acidemia also develops, with pH values in the range of 7.2 to 7.3, but the level is controlled by managing the rise in $Paco_2$. Within 24 to 48 hours the patient's serum pH will be restored to a near-normal level because the kidneys will reabsorb bicarbonate to compensate for the respiratory acidosis.

In addition to setting the ventilator for reduced tidal volume and slower respiratory rates, you should increase the inspiratory flow rate to 80 to 120 L/min. To tolerate such settings, patients usually require heavy sedation with narcotics and occasionally complete paralysis. Closely monitor the patient's tolerance of the respiratory acidosis, particularly during the first 24 to 48 hours of therapy, before renal compensation has occurred. In some patients arrhythmias may develop when acidosis is present, and this may limit the level of permissive hypercapnia used. It may be necessary to allow the $Paco_2$ to rise in smaller increments over a longer period of time.

Table 68. Sample of Initial Settings for Ventilation After Endotracheal Intubation[62]

1. Calculate the patient's **ideal body weight.**
2. **Tidal volume:** Set to 6 to 8 mL/kg.
3. **Respiratory rate:** Set to 8 to 10 breaths/min.
4. **Inspiratory flow rate:** Set to 80 to 100 L/min. The objective is to achieve a ratio of inspired to expired air (I:E) of 1:4 to 1:5.
5. **Positive inspiratory pressure:** Start at 10 cm H_2O. Do not set at >25 cm H_2O. Keep the **peak inspiratory pressure (PIP)** under 40 cm H_2O. This level will reduce the occurrence of barotrauma and hemodynamic compromise. Sudden increases in the inspiratory pressures may indicate a pneumothorax, obstructed endotracheal tube, or mucous plugging. Conversely a precipitous fall in PIP may indicate extubation. Investigate any sudden change in PIP.
6. **Permissive hypercarbia:** Titrate tidal volume and respiratory rate to allow the gradual development of hypercarbia. It often will occur if inspiratory pressure is maintained at <25 cm H_2O.
7. **Continue sedation:** Maintain continuous sedation with propofol or a benzodiazepine and a narcotic.
8. **Maintain paralysis if needed:** Maintain paralysis with a longer-acting, nondepolarizing muscle relaxant.
9. **Administer inhaled bronchodilators:** Continue to provide (as indicated) the first-line asthma therapies (inhaled β_2-agonists, anticholinergics, and corticosteroids) by nebulizer delivery of drugs through the ventilator and endotracheal tube.

Patient Is Difficult to Ventilate

When ventilation is difficult or inadequate, clinical assessment and evaluation may be difficult and elusive in patients with severe refractory asthma. A lack of audible breath sounds comes from poor airflow and hyperinflation of the chest wall.

Four common causes of acute deterioration in any intubated patient can be recalled by using the mnemonic DOPE:

1. **D**isplacement (tube)
2. **O**bstruction (tube)
3. **P**neumothorax
4. **E**quipment failure

If the patient is extremely "tight" (with airway constriction) and difficult to ventilate, perform the following procedures *in order* until ventilation is adequate:

1. Ensure that the patient is adequately sedated and paralyzed so that there is a passive patient-ventilator interaction.
2. Check the endotracheal tube for patency. Look for obstruction from kinking, mucous plugging, or biting. Suction the tube.
3. Change to a *square-wave pattern* of airflow. You may need to increase the time for exhalation, shorten the time for inhalation, and markedly increase the limit of peak inspiratory pressure to ensure that the patient is receiving the set tidal volume.
4. Reduce the respiratory rate to 6 to 8 breaths/min to reduce auto-PEEP to 15 mm Hg or less.

5. Reduce the tidal volume to 3 to 5 mL/kg to reduce auto-PEEP to 15 mm Hg or less.
6. Increase peak flow to more than 60 L/min (90 to 120 L/min is commonly used) to further shorten inspiratory time and increase exhalation time.

Hypoxia or Hypotension Occurs After Intubation

There are 4 common causes of significant hypoxia or hypotension immediately after intubation: incorrect placement of the endotracheal tube, obstruction of the endotracheal tube, significant auto-PEEP buildup, and tension pneumothorax.

Incorrect Placement of the Endotracheal Tube

With any drop in oxygen saturation or exhaled CO_2, reconfirm tube position immediately. If you suspect incorrect placement of the endotracheal tube, evaluate tube placement *immediately by using primary and secondary confirmation techniques* (eg, waveform capnography). Do not take time to obtain a chest radiograph. It is appropriate to obtain a chest radiograph after intubation, but it may not confirm tube misplacement. Spontaneous extubation or tube migration into a main bronchus is always a respiratory emergency. The patient cannot tolerate the delay that would occur with a confirmatory radiograph.

Note that patients with status asthmaticus can demonstrate false-negative results with the esophageal detector device. When the endotracheal tube is in the esophagus of a patient with severe asthma, the detector bulb may reexpand immediately, suggesting endotracheal tube placement. Providers must be aware that severe asthma may cause erroneous results with the esophageal detector device. Continuous waveform capnography is the most reliable means of monitoring endotracheal tube placement.

Obstruction of the Endotracheal Tube

If it is difficult to ventilate the patient manually, check for patency of the tube. If the tube is patent, attempt to suction the tube and check for tube obstructions from kinking, mucous plugging, or biting.

Massive Auto-PEEP Buildup

The most common cause of profound hypotension after intubation is a massive buildup of auto-PEEP. If auto-PEEP is suspected, first stop ventilating the patient for a brief time (20 to 40 seconds). This pause allows the auto-PEEP to dissipate. Monitor the patient's oxygenation and resume ventilation after auto-PEEP dissipates or if the patient develops significant hypoxemia or clinical signs of further deterioration.

Tension Pneumothorax

Evidence of a tension pneumothorax includes decreased chest expansion and decreased breath sounds on the side of the pneumothorax, shifting of the trachea away from the side of the pneumothorax, or development of subcutaneous emphysema. The immediate lifesaving treatment is *needle decompression* to release air from the pleural space. This procedure is often followed by placement of a chest tube. Slowly insert a 16-gauge cannula (over-the-needle catheter) in the second intercostal space along the midclavicular line. Be careful to avoid direct puncture of the lung. Hearing or feeling the venting of compressed air is diagnostic. You can use other commercially available devices after relief of a tension pneumothorax to prevent further buildup of pneumatic tension. Nonetheless, patients often require a chest tube.

Final Interventions to Consider

ACLS providers may encounter a patient with severe asthma and progressive hypoxia and hypercapnia refractory to the therapy described above. If at all possible, a pulmonologist or critical care specialist should be consulted. The following "interventions of desperation" have occasionally met with some success.

Empiric Bilateral Needle Decompression for Bilateral Pneumothoraxes

Unrecognized bilateral tension pneumothoraxes may underlie some cases of fatal asthma. There are insufficient published data to support a recommendation for empiric attempts at bilateral needle decompression in all severely compromised patients with asthma. The critical point is *to consider* whether unrecognized pneumothoraxes may have precipitated an asthmatic cardiac arrest.

Critical Concept **Needle Decompression: Use Extreme Caution!**	An attempt at needle decompression or insertion of a chest tube in a patient with severe, refractory asthma without a pneumothorax can be a life-threatening error. • The visceral pleura of the hyperinflated lung can be punctured, producing an iatrogenic pneumothorax. • Air would be released through the needle catheter or thoracostomy tube, just as occurs with relief of a tension pneumothorax. • The high pressures in the contralateral, mechanically ventilated lung plus the coexisting auto-PEEP could generate a contralateral tension pneumothorax.

Intravenous β-Agonist (Isoproterenol)

Isoproterenol given by IV infusion over 60 to 90 minutes has been effective for severely ill patients unable to tolerate inhalational therapy. Start with 0.1 mcg/kg per minute; increase to a maximum of 6 mcg/kg per minute. Titrate according to heart rate.

Inhaled Volatile Anesthetics

Volatile anesthetics are powerful bronchial smooth muscle relaxants. Use these agents with extreme caution because they are also vasodilators and myocardial depressants. Some of these anesthetics sensitize the myocardium to catecholamines, leading to life-threatening arrhythmias. Only providers with extensive experience and knowledge of their side effects, precautions, and contraindications should use inhaled anesthetic agents for treating patients with severe, life-threatening asthma.

Extracorporeal Membrane Oxygenation

In rare circumstances, aggressive treatment for acute respiratory failure due to severe asthma will not provide adequate gas exchange. There are case reports that describe successful use of extracorporeal membrane oxygenation (ECMO) in adult and pediatric patients[72-75] with severe asthma after other aggressive measures have failed to reverse hypoxemia and hypercarbia.

Additional Information on Asthma

Several consensus groups have developed excellent practice guidelines for the diagnosis and treatment of asthma. These groups include the National Asthma Education and Prevention Program of the National Institutes of Health,[38,76,77] the Global Initiative for Asthma,[78] the Canadian Association of Emergency Physicians and the Canadian Thoracic Society,[79] and the British Thoracic Society Scottish Intercollegiate Guidelines Network.[80] The following websites are useful:

- National Asthma Education and Prevention Program: http://www.nhlbi.nih.gov/about/naepp/
- Global Initiative for Asthma: http://www.ginasthma.com/
- British Thoracic Society Scottish Intercollegiate Guidelines Network: http://www.brit-thoracic.org.uk/guidelines/asthma-guidelines.aspx

References

1. Akinbami LJ, Moorman JM, Bailey C, Zahran HS, King M, Johnson CA, Liu X. Trends in asthma prevalence, health care use, and mortality in the United States, 2001–2010. NCHS data brief, Number 94.2012.
2. Kenyon N, Albertson TE. Status asthmaticus. From the emergency department to the intensive care unit. *Clin Rev Allergy Immunol*. 2001;20:271-292.
3. McFadden ER Jr. Acute severe asthma. *Am J Respir Crit Care Med*. 2003;168:740-759.
4. McCoy L, Redelings M, Sorvillo F, Simon P. A multiple cause-of-death analysis of asthma mortality in the United States, 1990-2001. *J Asthma*. 2005;42:757-763.
5. Mitchell I, Tough SC, Semple LK, Green FH, Hessel PA. Near-fatal asthma: a population-based study of risk factors. *Chest*. 2002;121:1407-1413.
6. Kolbe J, Fergusson W, Vamos M, Garrett J. Case-control study of severe life threatening asthma (SLTA) in adults: psychological factors. *Thorax*. 2002;57:317-322.
7. National Heart, Lung, and Blood Institute. *Expert Panel Report 3: Guidelines for Diagnosis and Management of Asthma: Full Report 2007*. Bethesda, MD: National Heart, Lung, and Blood Institute, US Department of Health and Human Services; 2007. NIH Publication 07-4051.
8. Molfino NA, Nannini LJ, Martelli AN, Slutsky AS. Respiratory arrest in near-fatal asthma. *N Engl J Med*. 1991;324:285-288.
9. Reid LM. The presence or absence of bronchial mucus in fatal asthma. *J Allergy Clin Immunol*. 1987;80:415-416.
10. Robin ED, McCauley R. Sudden cardiac death in bronchial asthma, and inhaled β-adrenergic agonists. *Chest*. 1992;101:1699-1702.
11. Robin ED, Lewiston N. Unexpected, unexplained sudden death in young asthmatic subjects. *Chest*. 1989;96:790-793.
12. Kallenbach JM, Frankel AH, Lapinsky SE, Thornton AS, Blott JA, Smith C, Feldman C, Zwi S. Determinants of near fatality in acute severe asthma. *Am J Med*. 1993;95:265-272.
13. McFadden ER Jr, Warren EL. Observations on asthma mortality. *Ann Intern Med*. 1997;127:142-147.
14. Hannaway PJ. Demographic characteristics of patients experiencing near-fatal and fatal asthma: results of a regional survey of 400 asthma specialists. *Ann Allergy Asthma Immunol*. 2000;84:587-593.
15. Kikuchi Y, Okabe S, Tamura G, Hida W, Homma M, Shirato K, Takishima T. Chemosensitivity and perception of dyspnea in patients with a history of near-fatal asthma. *N Engl J Med*. 1994;330:1329-1334.
16. Nowak RM, Pensler MI, Sarkar DD, Anderson JA, Kvale PA, Ortiz AE, Tomlanovich MC. Comparison of peak expiratory flow and FEV1 admission criteria for acute bronchial asthma. *Ann Emerg Med*. 1982;11:64-69.
17. Shim CS, Williams MH Jr. Evaluation of the severity of asthma: patients versus physicians. *Am J Med*. 1980;68:11-13.
18. Levin E, Gold MI. The mini-Wright expiratory peak flow meter. *Can Anaesth Soc J*. 1981;28:285-287.
19. Rainbow J, Browne GJ. Fatal asthma or anaphylaxis? *Emerg Med J*. 2002;19:415-417.
20. Jorge S, Becquemin MH, Delerme S, Bennaceur M, Isnard R, Achkar R, Riou B, Boddaert J, Ray P. Cardiac asthma in elderly patients: incidence, clinical presentation and outcome. *BMC Cardiovasc Disord*. 2007;7:16.
21. Odeh M, Oliven A, Bassan H. Timolol eyedrop-induced fatal bronchospasm in an asthmatic patient. *J Fam Pract*. 1991;32:97-98.
22. Weitzman JB, Kanarek NF, Smialek JE. Medical examiner asthma death autopsies: a distinct subgroup of asthma deaths with implications for public health preventive strategies. *Arch Pathol Lab Med*. 1998;122:691-699.
23. Levenson T, Greenberger PA, Donoghue ER, Lifschultz BD. Asthma deaths confounded by substance abuse: an assessment of fatal asthma. *Chest*. 1996;110:604-610.

24. Lin RY, Sauter D, Newman T, Sirleaf J, Walters J, Tavakol M. Continuous versus intermittent albuterol nebulization in the treatment of acute asthma. *Ann Emerg Med*. 1993;22:1847-1853.
25. Rudnitsky GS, Eberlein RS, Schoffstall JM, Mazur JE, Spivey WH. Comparison of intermittent and continuously nebulized albuterol for treatment of asthma in an urban emergency department. *Ann Emerg Med*. 1993;22:1842-1846.
26. Khine H, Fuchs SM, Saville AL. Continuous vs intermittent nebulized albuterol for emergency management of asthma. *Acad Emerg Med*. 1996;3:1019-1024.
27. Newman KB, Milne S, Hamilton C, Hall K. A comparison of albuterol administered by metered-dose inhaler and spacer with albuterol by nebulizer in adults presenting to an urban emergency department with acute asthma. *Chest*. 2002;121:1036-1041.
28. Bowton DL. Metered-dose inhalers versus hand-held nebulizers: some answers and new questions. *Chest*. 1992;101:298-299.
29. Bowton DL, Goldsmith WM, Haponik EF. Substitution of metered-dose inhalers for hand-held nebulizers: success and cost savings in a large, acute-care hospital. *Chest*. 1992;101:305-308.
30. Colacone A, Afilalo M, Wolkove N, Kreisman H. A comparison of albuterol administered by metered dose inhaler (and holding chamber) or wet nebulizer in acute asthma. *Chest*. 1993;104:835-841.
31. Idris AH, McDermott MF, Raucci JC, Morrabel A, McGorray S, Hendeles L. Emergency department treatment of severe asthma: metered-dose inhaler plus holding chamber is equivalent in effectiveness to nebulizer. *Chest*. 1993;103:665-672.
32. Gibbs MA, Camargo CA Jr, Rowe BH, Silverman RA. State of the art: therapeutic controversies in severe acute asthma. *Acad Emerg Med*. 2000;7:800-815.
33. Rowe BH, Spooner CH, Ducharme FM, Bretzlaff JA, Bota GW. Early emergency department treatment of acute asthma with systemic corticosteroids. *Cochrane Database Syst Rev*. 2000:CD002178.
34. Rowe BH, Keller JL, Oxman AD. Effectiveness of steroid therapy in acute exacerbations of asthma: a meta-analysis. *Am J Emerg Med*. 1992;10:301-310.
35. Aaron SD. The use of ipratropium bromide for the management of acute asthma exacerbation in adults and children: a systematic review. *J Asthma*. 2001;38:521-530.
36. Rodrigo G, Rodrigo C. Ipratropium bromide in acute asthma: small beneficial effects? [letter]. *Chest*. 1999;115:1482.
37. Plotnick LH, Ducharme FM. Acute asthma in children and adolescents: should inhaled anticholinergics be added to beta(2)-agonists? *Am J Respir Med*. 2003;2:109-115.
38. Keahey L, Bulloch B, Becker AB, Pollack CV Jr, Clark S, Camargo CA Jr. Initial oxygen saturation as a predictor of admission in children presenting to the emergency department with acute asthma. *Ann Emerg Med*. 2002;40:300-307.
39. Rodrigo G, Rodrigo C, Burschtin O. A meta-analysis of the effects of ipratropium bromide in adults with acute asthma. *Am J Med*. 1999;107:363-370.
40. Karpel JP, Schacter EN, Fanta C, Levey D, Spiro P, Aldrich T, Menjoge SS, Witek TJ. A comparison of ipratropium and albuterol vs albuterol alone for the treatment of acute asthma. *Chest*. 1996;110:611-616.
41. Stoodley RG, Aaron SD, Dales RE. The role of ipratropium bromide in the emergency management of acute asthma exacerbation: a metaanalysis of randomized clinical trials. *Ann Emerg Med*. 1999;34:8-18.
42. Rodrigo GJ, Castro-Rodriguez JA. Anticholinergics in the treatment of children and adults with acute asthma: a systematic review with meta-analysis. *Thorax*. 2005;60:740-746.
43. Silverman RA, Osborn H, Runge J, Gallagher EJ, Chiang W, Feldman J, Gaeta T, Freeman K, Levin B, Mancherje N, Scharf S. IV magnesium sulfate in the treatment of acute severe asthma: a multicenter randomized controlled trial. *Chest*. 2002;122:489-497.
44. Rowe BH, Bretzlaff JA, Bourdon C, Bota GW, Camargo CA Jr. Magnesium sulfate for treating exacerbations of acute asthma in the emergency department. *Cochrane Database Syst Rev*. 2000:CD001490.
45. Gallegos-Solórzanó MC, Pérez-Padilla R, Hernández-Zenteno RJ. Usefulness of inhaled magnesium sulfate in the coadjuvant management of severe asthma crisis in an emergency department. *Pulm Pharmacol Ther* 2010;23:432-437.
46. Blitz M, Blitz S, Hughes R, Diner B, Beasley R, Knopp J, Rowe BH. Aerosolized magnesium sulfate for acute asthma: a systematic review. *Chest*. 2005;128:337-344.
47. Trestrail JH. *Criminal Poisoning: Investigational Guide for Law Enforcement, Toxicologists, Forensic Scientists, and Attorneys*. Totowa, NJ: Humana Press; 2007.
48. Blitz M, Blitz S, Beasely R, Diner BM, Hughes R, Knopp JA, Rowe BH. Inhaled magnesium sulfate in the treatment of acute asthma. *Cochrane Database Syst Rev*. 2005:CD003898.
49. Hess DR, Acosta FL, Ritz RH, Kacmarek RM, Camargo CA Jr. The effect of heliox on nebulizer function using a beta-agonist bronchodilator. *Chest*. 1999;115:184-189.
50. Rodrigo GJ, Rodrigo C, Pollack CV, Rowe B. Use of helium-oxygen mixtures in the treatment of acute asthma: a systematic review. *Chest*. 2003;123:891-896.
51. Reuben AD, Harris AR. Heliox for asthma in the emergency department: a review of the literature. *Emerg Med J*. 2004;21:131-135.
52. Putland M, Kerr D, Kelly AM. Adverse events associated with the use of intravenous epinephrine in emergency department patients presenting with severe asthma. *Ann Emerg Med*. 2006;47:559-563.
53. Safdar B, Cone DC, Pham KT. Subcutaneous epinephrine in the prehospital setting. *Prehosp Emerg Care*. 2001;5:200-207.
54. Petrillo TM, Fortenberry JD, Linzer JF, Simon HK. Emergency department use of ketamine in pediatric status asthmaticus. *J Asthma*. 2001;38:657-664.
55. Howton JC, Rose J, Duffy S, Zoltanski T, Levitt MA. Randomized, double-blind, placebo-controlled trial of intravenous ketamine in acute asthma. *Ann Emerg Med*. 1996;27:170-175.
56. Allen JY, Macias CG. The efficacy of ketamine in pediatric emergency department patients who present with acute severe asthma. *Ann Emerg Med*. 2005;46:43-50.
57. Camargo CA Jr, Smithline HA, Malice MP, Green SA, Reiss TF. A randomized controlled trial of intravenous montelukast in acute asthma. *Am J Respir Crit Care Med*. 2003;167:528-533.
58. Schultz TE. Sevoflurane administration in status asthmaticus: a case report. *AANA J*. 2005;73:35-36.

59. Wheeler DS, Clapp CR, Ponaman ML, Bsn HM, Poss WB. Isoflurane therapy for status asthmaticus in children: a case series and protocol. *Pediatr Crit Care Med*. 2000;1:55-59.

60. Soroksky A, Stav D, Shpirer I. A pilot prospective, randomized, placebo-controlled trial of bilevel positive airway pressure in acute asthmatic attack. *Chest*. 2003;123:1018-1025.

61. Meduri GU, Cook TR, Turner RE, Cohen M, Leeper KV. Noninvasive positive pressure ventilation in status asthmaticus. *Chest*. 1996;110:767-774.

62. Schneider R. Asthma and COPD. In: Walls RM, Luten RC, Murphy MF, Schneider RE, eds. *Manual of Emergency Airway Management*. Philadelphia, Pa: Lippincott Williams & Wilkins; 2000:164-168.

63. Marik PE, Varon J, Fromm R Jr. The management of acute severe asthma. *J Emerg Med*. 2002;23:257-268.

64. Maltais F, Sovilj M, Goldberg P, Gottfried SB. Respiratory mechanics in status asthmaticus: effects of inhalational anesthesia. *Chest*. 1994;106:1401-1406.

65. Rooke GA, Choi JH, Bishop MJ. The effect of isoflurane, halothane, sevoflurane, and thiopental/nitrous oxide on respiratory system resistance after tracheal intubation. *Anesthesiology*. 1997;86:1294-1299.

66. Eames WO, Rooke GA, Wu RS, Bishop MJ. Comparison of the effects of etomidate, propofol, and thiopental on respiratory resistance after tracheal intubation. *Anesthesiology*. 1996;84:1307-1311.

67. Bergen JM, Smith DC. A review of etomidate for rapid sequence intubation in the emergency department. *J Emerg Med*. 1997;15:221-230.

68. Brenner B, Corbridge T, Kazzi A. Intubation and mechanical ventilation of the asthmatic patient in respiratory failure. *J Emerg Med*. 2009;37:S23-S34.

69. Mazzeo AT, Spada A, Pratico C, Lucanto T, Santamaria LB. Hypercapnia: what is the limit in paediatric patients? A case of near-fatal asthma successfully treated by multipharmacological approach. *Paediatr Anaesth*. 2004;14:596-603.

70. Darioli R, Perret C. Mechanical controlled hypoventilation in status asthmaticus. *Am Rev Respir Dis*. 1984;129:385-387.

71. Tuxen DV. Permissive hypercapnic ventilation. *Am J Respir Crit Care Med*. 1994;150:870-874.

72. Mikkelsen ME, Woo YJ, Sager JS, Fuchs BD, Christie JD. Outcomes using extracorporeal life support for adult respiratory failure due to status asthmaticus. *ASAIO J*. 2009;55:47-52.

73. Leiba A, Bar-Yosef S, Bar-Dayan Y, Weiss Y, Segal E, Paret G, Vardi A. Early administration of extracorporeal life support for near fatal asthma. *Isr Med Assoc J*. 2003;5:600-602.

74. Conrad SA, Green R, Scott LK. Near-fatal pediatric asthma managed with pumpless arteriovenous carbon dioxide removal. *Crit Care Med*. 2007;35:2624-2629.

75. Elliot SC, Paramasivam K, Oram J, Bodenham AR, Howell SJ, Mallick A. Pumpless extracorporeal carbon dioxide removal for life-threatening asthma. *Crit Care Med*. 2007;35:945-948.

76. Emond SD, Camargo CA Jr, Nowak RM. 1997 National Asthma Education and Prevention Program guidelines: a practical summary for emergency physicians. *Ann Emerg Med*. 1998;31:579-589.

77. Expert Panel Report 3 (EPR-3): Guidelines for the Diagnosis and Management of Asthma-Summary Report 2007. *J Allergy Clin Immunol*. 2007;120:S94-S138.

78. Alvey Smaha D. Asthma emergency care: national guidelines summary. *Heart Lung*. 2001;30:472-474.

79. Beveridge RC, Grunfeld AF, Hodder RV, Verbeek PR. Guidelines for the emergency management of asthma in adults. CAEP/CTS Asthma Advisory Committee. Canadian Association of Emergency Physicians and the Canadian Thoracic Society. *CMAJ*. 1996;155:25-37.

80. British Thoracic Society, Scottish Intercollegiate Guidelines Network. *British Guideline on the Management of Asthma: Quick Reference Guide.* http://www. www.brit-thoracic.org.uk/Portals/0/Guidelines/AsthmaGuidelines/qrg101%202011.pdf. Published May 2011. Accessed October 3, 2012.

Chapter 17

Cardiac Arrest Associated With Anaphylaxis

This Chapter

- Differential Diagnosis of Anaphylaxis
- Dosing and Use of Epinephrine in Life-Threatening Anaphylaxis
- Priorities for Airway Management in Angioedema
- Special Attention to Volume Status for Cardiovascular Instability

Definitions

Anaphylaxis is a severe, systemic allergic reaction characterized by multisystem involvement, including the skin, airway, vascular system, and gastrointestinal (GI) tract. Severe cases may result in complete obstruction of the airway, cardiovascular collapse, and death.

Immunologic Definitions

The term *classic anaphylaxis* refers to hypersensitivity reactions mediated by the subclass of antibodies, immunoglobulins IgE and IgG. Prior sensitization to an allergen has occurred, producing antigen-specific immunoglobulins. Subsequent reexposure to the allergen provokes the anaphylactic reaction. Many anaphylactic reactions, however, occur without a documented prior exposure.

Anaphylactoid reactions are similar to anaphylactic reactions, but they are triggered by materials such as radiocontrast material and certain parenteral medications and are not mediated by an IgE antibody response. The clinical presentation and management of anaphylactic and anaphylactoid reactions are similar, so it is unnecessary to distinguish between them when determining treatment for an acute attack.

Clinical Definitions

Some authors define *anaphylaxis* as a generalized, rapid-onset allergic reaction (including urticaria) with laryngeal edema, angioedema, or bronchospasm from increased bronchial smooth muscle tone, which causes shortness of breath.[1] Anaphylaxis is graded as severe if loss of consciousness (syncope) or hypotension occurs. These effects are produced by the release of mediators, including histamine, leukotriene C_4, prostaglandin D_2, and tryptase.

Incidence

Anaphylactic reactions occur even when no documented prior exposure exists. Thus, patients may appear to react to their initial exposure to an antibiotic or insect sting. As we age, we all are exposed to potential allergens that can create sensitivity. Therefore, the elderly are at the greatest risk of developing anaphylaxis.

A population-based study from the state of Minnesota estimated the annual rate of *occurrence* of anaphylaxis to be 30 per 100 000 person-years (95% confidence interval [CI]). Because some people had more than 1 episode of anaphylaxis, the average annual rate of *incidence* of anaphylaxis was lower, at 21 per 100 000 person-years (95% CI, 17 to 25).[2] Anaphylaxis is estimated to cause 500 to 1000 deaths per year in the United States alone.[3]

Etiology

Insect stings, drugs, contrast media, and some foods (eg, milk, eggs, and fish in children and shellfish in adults) are the most common causes of anaphylaxis.

Any antigen capable of activating IgE can be a trigger for anaphylaxis. Exercise-induced anaphylaxis (especially after ingestion of certain foods) has been reported. Some allergens such as dust, pollen, and dander are inhaled. Anaphylaxis may even be idiopathic. Without a known allergen, these patients must be managed with long-term oral steroid therapy. β-Blockers may increase the severity of anaphylaxis, blocking the response to endogenous catecholamines and exogenous epinephrine.

Pharmacologic Agents

Antibiotics (especially parenteral penicillins and other β-lactams), aspirin, nonsteroidal anti-inflammatory drugs, and intravenous (IV) contrast agents are the medications most frequently associated with life-threatening anaphylaxis.

Latex

Much attention has focused on latex-induced anaphylaxis, but it is actually rare.[4,5]

Stinging Insects

Fatal anaphylaxis has long been associated with stings from Hymenoptera (membrane-winged insects), including ants, bees, hornets, wasps, and yellow jackets. When a person with IgE antibodies induced by a previous sting is stung again, a fatal reaction can occur within 10 to 15 minutes. Cardiovascular collapse is the most common mechanism.[6-8]

Foods

Peanuts, tree-grown nuts, seafood, and wheat are the foods most frequently associated with life-threatening anaphylaxis.[9] Allergies to peanuts and tree nuts (Brazil, almond, hazel, and macadamia nuts) have recently been recognized as particularly dangerous.[10]

Pathophysiology

The manifestations of anaphylaxis are related to release of chemical mediators from mast cells. These mediators are released when antigens (allergens) bind to antigen-specific IgE attached to previously sensitized basophils and mast cells. In an anaphylactoid reaction, exposure to an antigen causes direct release of mediators, a process that is not mediated by IgE.

The most important mediators of anaphylaxis are histamines, leukotrienes, prostaglandins, thromboxanes, and bradykinins. These mediators contribute to vasodilation, increased capillary permeability, and airway constriction and produce the clinical signs of hypotension, angioedema, and bronchospasm. The sooner the reaction occurs after exposure, the more likely it is to be severe.

Signs and Symptoms

Signs and symptoms can be cutaneous, cardiovascular, respiratory, and gastrointestinal. Consider anaphylaxis when responses from 2 or more body systems (cutaneous, respiratory, cardiovascular, neurologic, or gastrointestinal) are noted. The shorter the interval between exposure and reaction, the more likely the reaction will be severe. Signs and symptoms include the following:

Respiratory

Serious upper airway (laryngeal) edema, lower airway edema (asthma), or both may develop, causing stridor and wheezing. Rhinitis is often an early sign of respiratory involvement.

Cardiovascular

Cardiovascular collapse is the most common periarrest manifestation. Vasodilation produces a relative hypovolemia. Increased capillary permeability contributes to further intravascular volume loss. The patient may be agitated or anxious and may appear either flushed or pale. Additional cardiac dysfunction may result from underlying disease or the development of myocardial ischemia from administration of epinephrine.[6-8]

Gastrointestinal

Gastrointestinal signs and symptoms of anaphylaxis include abdominal pain, vomiting, and diarrhea.

Cutaneous

These symptoms may include diffuse urticaria and conjunctivitis. The patient may appear either flushed or pale.

Differential Diagnosis

Patients with anaphylaxis can present with a wide variety of signs and symptoms. No single finding is pathognomonic. The ACLS provider must recognize the following frequently encountered anaphylaxis "look-alikes":

- **Urticaria** is characterized by distinctive small skin eruptions *(hives)* with well-defined borders and pale centers surrounded by patches of red skin *(wheal-and-flare reaction)*. Typically these red areas are intensely itchy *(pruritus)*.
- **Angioedema** and urticaria are variable manifestations of the same pathologic process. This response is mediated by vasoactive substances, which cause the arterioles to dilate. Capillary fluid leak and edema develop in both conditions. Angioedema involves vessels in the subdermal skin layers. Urticaria is localized in skin layers superficial to the dermis. Angioedema results in areas of well-demarcated, localized, nonpitting edema.

- **Hereditary angioedema** does not cause urticaria but does cause gastrointestinal edema, which can lead to severe abdominal pain, or respiratory mucosal edema, which can lead to airway compromise. Angioedema is treated with C1 esterase inhibitor replacement concentrate if available. Otherwise fresh frozen plasma may be used**.**
- **Severe, life-threatening asthma.** Although bronchospasm is often a component of anaphylaxis, asthma and anaphylaxis are 2 distinct entities that require very different treatment. Failure to identify and treat either anaphylaxis or asthma could be fatal for the patient.[11]
- **Functional vocal cord dysfunction.** Change in voice or loss of voice can lead to a suspicion of angioedema in the pharynx that occurs with allergic/anaphylactic reactions.
- **Scombroid poisoning.** This food-related illness often develops within 30 minutes of eating spoiled tuna, mackerel, or dolphin (mahi-mahi). Ingestion typically causes urticaria, nausea, vomiting, diarrhea, and headache. These symptoms are caused by histamine produced by bacteria on the fish. Antihistamines (H_1 and H_2 blockers) are safe and are often effective in reducing or eliminating these symptoms.
- **Angiotensin-converting enzyme (ACE) inhibitors** are associated with a reactive angioedema predominantly of the upper airway. This reaction can develop as late as days or years after ACE inhibitors are first used.
- **Panic disorder and panic attacks.** In some forms of panic attacks, functional stridor develops from forced adduction of the vocal cords.
- **Vasovagal reactions.** Patients with classic "fainting" may appear to be either flushed or pale when they collapse or lose consciousness.

Treatment of Anaphylaxis

The treatment of anaphylaxis has not been standardized, and recommendations to prevent cardiopulmonary arrest are difficult to standardize because etiology, clinical presentation (including severity and course), and organ involvement vary widely.[13]

Interventions to Prevent Cardiac Arrest

The following therapies are commonly used and widely accepted but are based more on consensus than evidence.

Oxygen: Administer at High Flow Rates

Administer oxygen to all patients, and administer a high concentration of oxygen to patients with respiratory distress. Titrate oxygen administration based on pulse oximetry evaluation of oxyhemoglobin saturation. Be prepared to intubate the patient and provide mechanical ventilatory support if laryngeal edema produces severe upper airway obstruction or if bronchospasm causes severe respiratory distress.

Epinephrine

Absorption and subsequent achievement of maximum plasma concentration after subcutaneous administration are slower and may be significantly delayed with shock.[14,15] The intramuscular (IM) administration of epinephrine (epinephrine autoinjectors) in the anterolateral aspect of the middle third of the thigh provides the highest peak blood levels (Figures 111 and 112).[14] Close monitoring is critical to avoid a fatal overdose of epinephrine.[6,16]

- Administer epinephrine by IM injection early to all patients with signs of a systemic reaction, especially hypotension, airway swelling, or definite difficulty breathing.
- Use an IM dose of 0.2 to 0.5 mg (1:1000) repeated every 5 to 15 minutes if there is no clinical improvement (Class I, LOE C).[17]
- The adult and pediatric epinephrine IM autoinjector will deliver 0.3 mg and 0.15 mg of epinephrine, respectively. In both anaphylaxis and cardiac arrest the immediate use of an epinephrine autoinjector is recommended if available (Class I, LOE C).

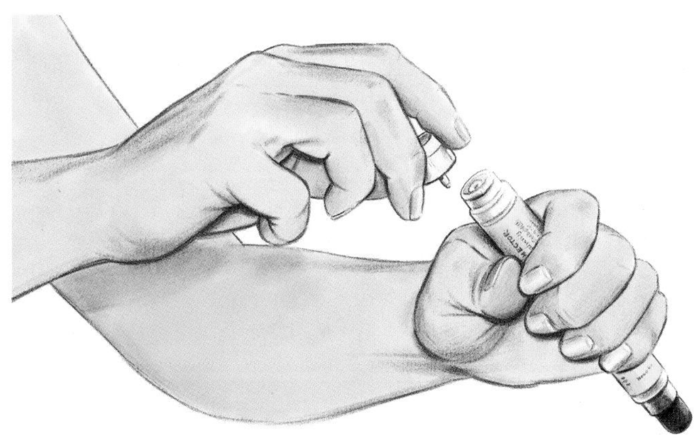

Figure 111. Epinephrine pen.

Critical Concept **Exclude Anaphylaxis First**	A number of disease processes produce some of the signs and symptoms of anaphylaxis. • Only after the clinician eliminates anaphylaxis as a diagnosis should the other conditions be considered, because failure to identify and appropriately treat anaphylaxis can be fatal.[11,12]

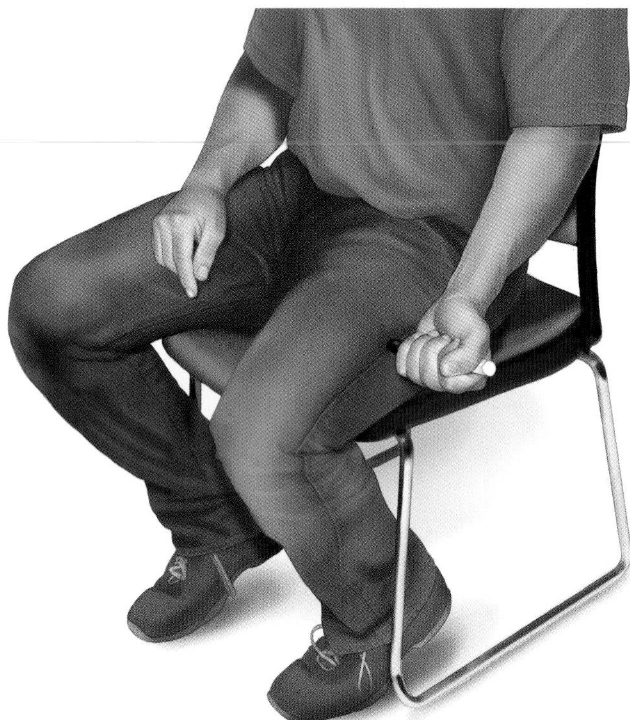

Figure 112. Self-administered epinephrine pen (autoinjector) into the left thigh.

Patients who are taking β-blockers have increased incidence and severity of anaphylaxis and can develop a paradoxical response to epinephrine.[18]

IV Epinephrine

- For patients not in cardiac arrest, IV epinephrine 0.05 to 0.1 mg (5% to 10% of the epinephrine dose used routinely in cardiac arrest) has been used successfully in patients with anaphylactic shock.[20] Because fatal overdose of epinephrine has been reported,[6,16,19,21] close hemodynamic monitoring is recommended (Class I, LOE B). Careful titration of a continuous infusion of IV epinephrine (5 to 15 mcg/min), based on severity of reaction and in addition to crystalloid infusion, may be considered in treatment of anaphylactic shock.[19]
- IV infusion of epinephrine is a reasonable alternative to IV boluses for treatment of anaphylaxis in patients not in cardiac arrest (Class IIa, LOE C) and may be considered in postarrest management (Class IIb, LOE C).

Aggressive Fluid Resuscitation

Give isotonic crystalloid (eg, normal saline) if hypotension is present and does not respond rapidly to epinephrine. A rapid infusion of 1 to 2 L or even 4 L may be needed initially. Titrate to a systolic blood pressure higher than 90 mm Hg. Monitor for the development of pulmonary edema and be prepared to support oxygenation and ventilation.

Other Interventions

There are no prospective randomized clinical studies evaluating the use of other therapeutic agents in anaphylactic shock or cardiac arrest. Adjuvant use of antihistamines (H_1 and H_2 antagonist),[22,23] inhaled β-adrenergic agents,[24] and IV corticosteroids[25] has been successful in management of the patient with anaphylaxis and may be considered in cardiac arrest due to anaphylaxis (Class IIb, LOE C).

Antihistamines

Antihistamines may be given slowly IV or IM (eg, 25 to 50 mg of diphenhydramine). H_2 blockers like cimetidine may be given 300 mg orally, IM, or IV.[26]

Inhaled β-Adrenergic Agents

Provide inhaled albuterol if bronchospasm is a major feature. Inhaled ipratropium may be especially useful for treatment of bronchospasm in patients taking β-blockers. Note that some patients treated for near-fatal asthma actually had anaphylaxis, so they received repeated doses of conventional bronchodilators rather than epinephrine.[27]

Corticosteroids

Infuse high-dose IV corticosteroids early in the course of therapy. Beneficial effects are delayed at least 4 to 6 hours.

Potential Therapies

Potential additional therapies based on limited case reports or pathophysiologic mechanisms include vasopressin, atropine, and glucagon.

- **Vasopressin.** There are case reports that vasopressin may benefit severely hypotensive patients.[28,29]
- **α-Agonists.** Other small case studies reported successful results with alternative α-agonists such as norepinephrine,[30] methoxamine,[31] and metaraminol.[32]
- **Atropine.** Case reports also suggest that when relative or severe bradycardia is present, there may be a role for administration of atropine.[12]
- **Glucagon.** For patients who are unresponsive to epinephrine, especially those receiving β-blockers, glucagon may be effective. This agent is short acting (1 to 2 mg every 5 minutes, IM or IV). Nausea, vomiting, and hyperglycemia are common side effects.

Critical Concept **Administration of Epinephrine**	• IM injection (0.2 to 0.5 mg) of epinephrine can be easily performed with an autoinjector. • IV epinephrine (0.05 to 0.1 mg) can be given as a bolus or continuous infusion with careful monitoring. Epinephrine given subcutaneously may be poorly absorbed, and achievement of maximum plasma concentration may be delayed when systemic perfusion is poor.

Alternative vasoactive drugs (vasopressin, norepinephrine, methoxamine, and metaraminol) may be considered in cardiac arrest secondary to anaphylaxis that is unresponsive to epinephrine (Class IIb, LOE C).

Post-Treatment Management

Patients who respond to therapy require observation. Symptoms may recur in some patients (up to 20%) within 1 to 8 hours (biphasic response) despite an intervening asymptomatic period. Biphasic responses have been reported to occur up to 36 hours after the initial reaction.[2,18,21,33-35] A patient who remains symptom free for 4 hours after treatment may be discharged.[36]

Cardiac Arrest

Cardiac arrest from anaphylaxis may be associated with profound vasodilation, total cardiovascular collapse, tissue hypoxia, and asystole. Consensus recommendations have been made following experience with nonfatal cases.

Death from anaphylaxis is usually due to cardiovascular collapse with massive vasodilation, cardiac pump failure, and progressive shock. The major clinical challenge is providing adequate volume replacement into a cardiovascular "tank" undergoing a life-threatening, but unknown, increase in capacity and capillary leak.

Because of limited evidence, the management of cardiac arrest secondary to anaphylaxis should be treated with standard BLS and ACLS. Other therapies to consider are as follows:

- **Aggressive volume expansion.** Near-fatal anaphylaxis produces profound vasodilation that significantly increases intravascular capacity. Massive volume replacement is needed. Use at least 2 large-bore IVs with pressure bags to administer large volumes (typically totals between 4 and 8 L) of isotonic crystalloid as quickly as possible.
- **Antihistamine IV.** Data are sparse about the value of antihistamines in anaphylactic cardiac arrest, but it is reasonable to assume that little additional harm could result.[26]
- **Steroid therapy.** Steroids given during a cardiac arrest will have little effect, but they may have value in the early hours of any postresuscitation period.
- **Cardiac Arrest Algorithm (PEA/Asystole).** The arrest rhythm in anaphylaxis is often asystole or pulseless electrical activity (PEA). See the Cardiac Arrest Algorithm in Chapter 8, Part 2.

Isolated case reports of anaphylaxis followed by cardiac arrest have shown cardiopulmonary bypass to be effective.[37,38] These advanced techniques can be considered in clinical settings in which the required professional skills and equipment are immediately available (Class IIb, LOE C).

Special Considerations in Management of Anaphylaxis

Treatment of Severe Airway Obstruction

Monitor the patient's airway and breathing closely during therapy (see above). Perform early *elective* intubation if the patient develops hoarseness, lingual edema, posterior or oropharyngeal swelling, or severe bronchospasm. Be prepared to perform *semielective* (awake, sedated) endotracheal intubation without paralytic agents when signs of distress develop and before respiratory arrest is imminent.

Early Endotracheal Intubation: Some Precautions

Consider early airway management if initial treatment does not appear to be effective. If intubation is delayed, patients can deteriorate relatively quickly (within minutes to a few hours) with development of progressive stridor, laryngeal edema, massive lingual swelling, facial and neck swelling, and hypoxemia. At this point both endotracheal intubation and cricothyrotomy may be difficult or impossible. Attempts at endotracheal intubation may only further increase laryngeal edema or compromise the airway with bleeding into the oropharynx and narrow glottic opening.

Hypoxia may lead to agitation and combativeness during administration of oxygen. The glottic opening is narrow and difficult to visualize when lingual and oropharyngeal edema are present. If paralyzing agents are administered, the patient will be unable to contribute to ventilation and it may be impossible to provide effective bag-mask ventilation. Laryngeal edema prevents air entry. Facial edema prevents creation of an effective seal between the face and the bag-mask device.

Airway, Oxygenation, and Ventilation in Cardiac Arrest

Cardiac arrest may result from angioedema and upper or lower airway obstruction.

Plans to intubate should include a primary approach; however, 1 or more alternative approaches should be in place. The clinician most experienced in airway management should be involved.

In these desperate circumstances, some alternative airway techniques include

- Fixed or flexible fiberoptic endotracheal intubation
- Blind intubation, such as digital endotracheal intubation or intubation via a laryngeal mask airway
- Emergency surgical airway, such as a cricothyrotomy

References

1. Stewart AG, Ewan PW. The incidence, aetiology and management of anaphylaxis presenting to an accident and emergency department. *Q J Med*. 1996;89:859-864.
2. Yocum MW, Butterfield JH, Klein JS, Volcheck GW, Schroeder DR, Silverstein MD. Epidemiology of anaphylaxis in Olmsted County: a population-based study. *J Allergy Clin Immunol*. 1999;104(pt 1):452-456.
3. Neugut AI, Ghatak AT, Miller RL. Anaphylaxis in the United States: An investigation into its epidemiology. *Arch Intern Med*. 2001;161:15-21.
4. Dreyfus DH, Fraser B, Randolph CC. Anaphylaxis to latex in patients without identified risk factors for latex allergy. *Conn Med*. 2004;68:217-222.
5. Ownby DR. A history of latex allergy. *J Allergy Clin Immunol*. 2002;110:S27-S32.
6. Pumphrey RS. Lessons for management of anaphylaxis from a study of fatal reactions. *Clin Exp Allergy*. 2000;30:1144-1150.
7. Pumphrey RS. Fatal anaphylaxis in the UK, 1992-2001. *Novartis Found Symp*. 2004;257:116-128.
8. Pumphrey RS, Roberts IS. Postmortem findings after fatal anaphylactic reactions. *J Clin Pathol*. 2000;53:273-276.
9. Mullins RJ. Anaphylaxis: risk factors for recurrence. *Clin Exp Allergy*. 2003;33:1033-1040.
10. Ewan PW. Clinical study of peanut and nut allergy in 62 consecutive patients: new features and associations. *BMJ*. 1996;312:1074-1078.
11. Brown AF. Anaphylaxis: quintessence, quarrels, and quandaries. *Emerg Med J*. 2001;18:328.
12. Brown AF. Anaphylaxis gets the adrenaline going. *Emerg Med J*. 2004;21:128-129.
13. Gavalas M, Walford C, Sadana A, O'Donnell C. Medical treatment of anaphylaxis. *J Accid Emerg Med*. 2000;17:152.
14. Simons FE, Gu X, Simons KJ. Epinephrine absorption in adults: intramuscular versus subcutaneous injection. *J Allergy Clin Immunol*. 2001;108:871-873.
15. Simons FER, Chan ES, Gu X, Simons KJ. Epinephrine for the out-of-hospital (first-aid) treatment of anaphylaxis in infants: is the ampule/syringe/needle method practical? *J Allergy Clin Immunol*. 2001;108:1040-1044.
16. Pumphrey R. Anaphylaxis: can we tell who is at risk of a fatal reaction? *Curr Opin Allergy Clin Immunol*. 2004;4:285-290.
17. Korenblat P, Lundie MJ, Dankner RE, Day JH. A retrospective study of epinephrine administration for anaphylaxis: how many doses are needed? *Allergy Asthma Proc*. 1999;20:383-386.
18. Ellis AK, Day JH. Diagnosis and management of anaphylaxis. *CMAJ*. 2003;169:307-311.
19. Brown SG, Blackman KE, Stenlake V, Heddle RJ. Insect sting anaphylaxis: prospective evaluation of treatment with intravenous adrenaline and volume resuscitation. *Emerg Med J*. 2004;21:149-154.
20. Bochner BS, Lichtenstein LM. Anaphylaxis. *N Engl J Med*. 1991;324:1785-1790.
21. Johnston SL, Unsworth J, Gompels MM. Adrenaline given outside the context of life threatening allergic reactions. *BMJ*. 2003;326:589-590.
22. Simons FE. Advances in H1-antihistamines. *N Engl J Med*. 2004;351:2203-2217.
23. Sheikh A, Ten Broek V, Brown SG, Simons FE. H1-antihistamines for the treatment of anaphylaxis: Cochrane systematic review. *Allergy*. 2007;62:830-837.
24. Gibbs MW, Kuczkowski KM, Benumof JL. Complete recovery from prolonged cardio-pulmonary resuscitation following anaphylactic reaction to readministered intravenous cefazolin. *Acta Anaesthesiol Scand*. 2003;47:230-232.
25. Choo KJ, Simons FE, Sheikh A. Glucocorticoids for the treatment of anaphylaxis. *Cochrane Database Syst Rev*. 2010;3:CD007596.
26. Winbery SL, Lieberman PL. Histamine and antihistamines in anaphylaxis. *Clin Allergy Immunol*. 2002;17:287-317.
27. Rainbow J, Browne GJ. Fatal asthma or anaphylaxis? *Emerg Med J*. 2002;19:415-417.
28. Kill C, Wranze E, Wulf H. Successful treatment of severe anaphylactic shock with vasopressin. Two case reports. *Int Arch Allergy Immunol*. 2004;134:260-261.
29. Williams SR, Denault AY, Pellerin M, Martineau R. Vasopressin for treatment of shock following aprotinin administration. *Can J Anaesth*. 2004;51:169-172.
30. Kluger MT. The bispectral index during an anaphylactic circulatory arrest. *Anaesth Intensive Care*. 2001;29:544-547.
31. Rocq N, Favier JC, Plancade D, Steiner T, Mertes PM. Successful use of terlipressin in post-cardiac arrest resuscitation after an epinephrine-resistant anaphylactic shock to suxamethonium. *Anesthesiology*. 2007;107:166-167.
32. Green R, Ball A. Alpha-agonists for the treatment of anaphylactic shock. *Anaesthesia*. 2005;60:621-622.
33. Smith PL, Kagey-Sobotka A, Bleecker ER, Traystman R, Kaplan AP, Gralnick H, Valentine MD, Permutt S, Lichtenstein LM. Physiologic manifestations of human anaphylaxis. *J Clin Invest*. 1980;66:1072-1080.
34. Stark BJ, Sullivan TJ. Biphasic and protracted anaphylaxis. *J Allergy Clin Immunol*. 1986;78:76-83.
35. Brazil E, MacNamara AF. "Not so immediate" hypersensitivity: the danger of biphasic anaphylactic reactions. *J Accid Emerg Med*. 1998;15:252-253.
36. Brady WJ Jr, Luber S, Carter CT, Guertler A, Lindbeck G. Multiphasic anaphylaxis: an uncommon event in the emergency department. *Acad Emerg Med*. 1997;4:193-197.
37. Allen SJ, Gallagher A, Paxton LD. Anaphylaxis to rocuronium. *Anaesthesia*. 2000;55:1223-1224.
38. Lafforgue E, Sleth JC, Pluskwa F, Saizy C. Successful extracorporeal resuscitation of a probable perioperative anaphylactic shock due to atracurium [in French]. *Ann Fr Anesth Reanim*. 2005;24:551-555.

Chapter 18

Cardiac Arrest Associated With Pregnancy

This Chapter

- Two Patients to Consider: Maternal-Fetal Physiology
- Causes of Cardiopulmonary Arrest During Pregnancy: Rapid Response Interventions to Prevent Arrest
- Implications of the Gravid Uterus in Cardiac Arrest
- When to Perform Emergency Hysterotomy

Background

During attempted resuscitation of a pregnant woman, providers have 2 potential patients, the mother and the fetus. The best hope for fetal survival is maternal survival. For the critically ill patient who is pregnant, rescuers must provide appropriate resuscitation with consideration of the physiologic changes due to pregnancy.

Essential Facts

Pregnancy results in a variety of physiologic changes that make the pregnant woman more vulnerable to cardiovascular insult. These changes can complicate attempted resuscitation during cardiac arrest (see "Critical Concept: Physiologic Changes of Pregnancy That May Affect Resuscitation.") For the critically ill pregnant patient, rescuers must provide appropriate resuscitation based on consideration of the physiologic changes caused by pregnancy. There are no randomized controlled trials evaluating the effect of specialized obstetric resuscitation techniques versus standard care in pregnant women. These guidelines have been developed based on the few studies available that are directly relevant to maternal resuscitation,[1,2] taking into consideration maternal physiology, case reports, and expert opinion.

Frequency

Cardiovascular emergencies in pregnant women are uncommon. Death related to pregnancy itself is rare. The Centre for Maternal and Child Enquiries (CMACE) data set represents the largest population-based data set on this group.[3] The overall maternal mortality rate was calculated at 11.39 deaths per 100 000 maternities. The recent observed frequency of cardiac arrest during pregnancy ranges from 0.02 to 0.05 per 1000 live births, or 1:2000 to 1:50 000.[4,5]

The Second Patient

A cardiovascular emergency in a pregnant woman creates a special situation for the ACLS provider. You must always consider the fetus when an adverse cardiovascular event occurs in a pregnant woman. At approximately 20 weeks or more of pregnancy (and possibly earlier), the size of the uterus begins to adversely affect the attempted resuscitation. At approximately 24 to 25 weeks of gestational age, the fetus may survive outside the womb.

Decisions About Cesarean Delivery

The decision about whether to perform an emergency cesarean delivery must be made quickly when the mother is in cardiac arrest. Emergency cesarean delivery—also known as *hysterotomy*—may improve the outcome for both mother and child.

Physiologic Changes of Pregnancy That May Affect Resuscitation

Airway and Pulmonary Function

- The larynx is displaced anteriorly, with increased edema and blood flow.
- Oxygen consumption increases 20%.
- Elevation of the diaphragm causes decreased functional residual capacity and functional residual volume, which predispose to rapid desaturation during hypoxia.
- Tidal volume and minute ventilation are increased to support increased cardiac output and oxygen demand during pregnancy.
- The normal maternal arterial blood gases (ABG) reflect a respiratory alkalosis with a mild compensatory metabolic acidosis. Mild maternal hypocarbia ($Pa{CO_2}$ 28 to 32 mm Hg) is needed to create a gradient in the placenta to facilitate removal of fetal CO_2. Because respiratory alkalosis is already present, the mother's ability to compensate for any new acid load is limited.

Circulation

- During most of the pregnancy there is a 40% increase in cardiac output and plasma volume; late in the third trimester, cardiac output decreases, particularly when the mother is supine.
- Physiologic anemia may reduce arterial oxygen content even if oxyhemoglobin saturation and $Pa{O_2}$ are satisfactory.
- Systemic and pulmonary vascular resistance decrease.
- Beyond 20 weeks of gestation the uterus is known to compress the inferior vena cava and aorta, compromising systemic venous return and systemic blood flow. Aortocaval compression (ACC) may occur at earlier gestational ages.[6] Reduced systemic venous return results in reduced maternal stroke volume and reduced cardiac output.

Gastrointestinal Function

- Hormonal changes contribute to an incompetent gastroesophageal sphincter even under normal conditions.
- An incompetent gastroesophageal sphincter predisposes the mother to regurgitation and the risk of aspiration with loss of consciousness.

—Contributed by Carolyn M. Zelop, MD, St. Francis Hospital and Medical Center, Hartford, CT

Causes of Maternal Cardiopulmonary Arrest

The many causes of cardiac arrest in pregnant women can be grouped into several defining categories (see Table 69 for a detailed list). According to the CMACE data,[3] cardiac disease is the leading cause of maternal deaths overall, exceeding the rates of death from sepsis, hypertension, thrombosis, and amniotic fluid embolism. The number of deaths from cardiac disease has been increasing since the 1991-1993 inquiries. The leading causes of death from cardiac disease in the most recent inquiries include sudden adult/arrhythmic death syndrome, myocardial infarction, aortic dissection, and cardiomyopathy. In the United States, between 1995 and 2006 the rate of postpartum hospitalizations for patients with chronic heart disease tripled.[7] These patients also experienced an increase in severe complications, including ventricular fibrillation (VF) and cardiac arrest.

Key Interventions: Prevention of Cardiac Arrest in Pregnancy

To treat the critically ill pregnant patient

- Place the patient in the left-lateral decubitus position to relieve possible compression of the inferior vena cava. Uterine obstruction of venous return can produce hypotension and could precipitate arrest in the critically ill patient.[8,9]
- Two methods of supporting the patient in the left-lateral decubitus position are (1) to use the angled backs of 2 or 3 chairs or (2) to use the angled thighs of several providers. Overturn a 4-legged chair so that the top of the chair back touches the floor. Align 1 or 2 more overturned chairs on either side of the first so that all are tilted in the same manner. Place the woman on her left side and align her torso parallel with the chair backs (Figure 113). Remember that this position will not be practical if chest compressions are needed.

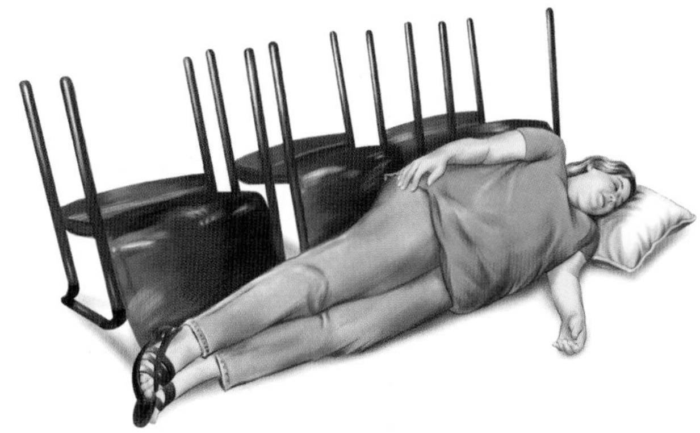

Figure 113. Left-lateral decubitus position for the hypotensive pregnant woman to shift the gravid uterus away from the inferior vena cava and the aorta.

- Give 100% oxygen.
- Establish intravenous (IV) access above the diaphragm and give a fluid bolus.
- Assess for hypotension; maternal hypotension that warrants therapy is defined as a systolic blood pressure less than 100 mm Hg or less than 80% of baseline.[10,11] Maternal hypotension can cause a reduction in placental perfusion.[12-14] In the patient who is not in arrest, both crystalloid and colloid solutions have been shown to increase preload.[15]
- Consider reversible causes of cardiac arrest and identify any preexisting medical conditions that may be complicating the resuscitation.

Table 69. Potential Causes of Maternal Cardiopulmonary Arrest[16,17]

Injury/Trauma
• Homicide • Suicide • Motor vehicle crash • Illicit drug use, unintentional overdose
Obstetric Complications at the Time of Delivery
• Amniotic fluid embolism • Hemorrhagic events: – Placenta previa, accreta, increta, or percreta – Placental abruption – Uterine atony – Disseminated intravascular coagulopathy • Pregnancy-induced malignant hypertension • Idiopathic peripartum cardiomyopathy
Iatrogenic Complications
• Intubation errors • Pulmonary aspiration • Anesthetic overdose (intrathecal, intravascular) • Medication-related errors (overdose, allergies) • Hypermagnesemia
Medical Conditions Related to Pregnancy (increased risk during pregnancy)
• Pulmonary embolism from thrombus, air, or fat (most common nontraumatic cause) • Infection or sepsis
Preexisting Medical Conditions
• Asthma • Cerebral hemorrhage • Cerebral aneurysm • Cerebral thrombosis • Malignant hyperthermia • Cardiac pathology: – Acute coronary syndromes – Arrhythmias – Congenital or vascular heart disease

Changes in Maternal and Fetal Physiology: Relation to Maternal Cardiac Arrest

Uterine-Placental Blood Flow

During pregnancy the mother's cardiac output and plasma volume increase by 40%, and one third of maternal cardiac output flows through the uteroplacental unit. During pregnancy the uterus and placenta form a passive, low-resistance system. Maternal perfusion pressure is the sole determinant of uteroplacental and fetal blood flow. Consequently, any cardiovascular compromise in the mother can severely impair blood flow to the uterus, placenta, and fetus. Restoration and support of maternal systemic perfusion is essential for the mother and the fetus.

Effect of the Enlarging Uterus

By at least the 20th week of pregnancy, the gravid uterus is large enough to significantly compress the inferior vena cava and the aorta. Compression of the inferior vena cava reduces venous return to the heart, and compression of the aorta compromises forward flow. These factors can compromise cardiac output even in a normal pregnancy, particularly when the mother is supine.

If cardiac arrest develops, the gravid uterus can compromise the effectiveness of resuscitation. Because there is obstruction of venous return, you should not administer resuscitation medications through a subdiaphragmatic vein. During cardiac arrest these medications may not reach the mother's heart unless or until the fetus is delivered.

Maternal Physiology

A number of factors can compromise maternal oxygen delivery and ability to compensate for hypoxia and acidosis. If the mother is anemic, arterial oxygen content will be reduced even when oxyhemoglobin saturation and PaO_2 are adequate. By the third trimester the gravid uterus pushes the diaphragm up enough to significantly reduce the functional residual capacity and functional residual volume. The decrease in these lung volumes coupled with the high oxygen consumption that exists during pregnancy can predispose the mother to rapid arterial oxygen desaturation if hypoxia develops. If the mother is supine during cardiac arrest, this reduction in functional residual capacity limits the effectiveness of efforts to oxygenate and ventilate the patient.

Because the pregnant woman maintains a respiratory alkalosis with mild compensatory acidosis, the mother will have limited ability to buffer an acid load. The high level of progesterone during pregnancy reduces the tone of the lower esophageal sphincter. Incompetence of this sphincter increases the risk that positive-pressure ventilation during cardiopulmonary resuscitation (CPR) will cause regurgitation and aspiration of gastric contents. For this reason, the ACLS provider should establish a protected airway early in resuscitation. Maternal laryngeal edema may make intubation more difficult and may require the use of a smaller tracheal tube. Increased laryngeal blood flow increases the risk of bleeding when any tube (orogastric, nasogastric, nasopharyngeal, endotracheal) is inserted into the oropharynx or nasopharynx. As a result of the changes in pulmonary physiology during pregnancy, maternal mortality still occurs from even routine intubation in the nonarrest patient. The incidence of failed intubation in the obstetric population is thought to be higher than in the nonpregnant population, and hypoxia related to failed intubation remains a consistent cause of death.[3] Therefore, the airway of the pregnant patient is always deemed to be a difficult airway, and the most experienced provider should always manage the airway in pregnant patients.

Fetal Physiology

Fetal physiology may offer the fetus some protection during the first minutes of maternal hypoxia or cardiac arrest. Fetal hemoglobin differs from "adult" hemoglobin in that it binds more readily with oxygen. For this reason, it is better saturated at lower arterial oxygen tension. As a result, fetal arterial oxygen content is higher at a given PaO_2. Fetal cardiac output is higher per kilogram of body weight than newborn cardiac output.

The effects of maternal CPR on fetal blood flow have not been studied in humans. Decades-old laboratory research showed that primate fetuses can survive up to 7 minutes of in utero asphyxiation without evidence of neurologic damage after birth. Guidelines have recommended delivery by 5 minutes after the onset of maternal cardiac arrest to reduce the chance of ischemic injury to both the mother and the fetus. The data behind this recommendation are limited. Recent studies have found that the neonate can survive to longer periods after maternal cardiac arrest, even at delivery more than 15 minutes after the cardiac arrest[18,19]; neonatal survival, especially at longer delivery times, is more likely at an older gestational age.[3,18]

Techniques to Improve Maternal Hemodynamics

Shifting the Gravid Uterus

In cardiac arrest, the reduced venous return and cardiac output caused by the gravid uterus put the mother at a hemodynamic disadvantage, thereby most likely reducing the effective coronary and cerebral perfusion produced by standard chest compressions. Therefore, when there is ACC, the effectiveness of the chest compressions may be limited.

A study that used magnetic resonance imaging (MRI) assessment of cardiac output and stroke volume found that at 20 weeks of gestational age there is a 27% increase in maternal stroke volume when the mother is in the full left-lateral tilt compared with the supine position. At 32 weeks of gestational age there is a 35% increase in stroke volume and a 24% increase in cardiac output when the mother is in the full left-lateral tilt compared with the supine position.[20]

Left Lateral Tilt

Reports of noncardiac arrest parturients suggests that left-lateral tilt results in improved maternal hemodynamics of blood pressure, cardiac output, and stroke volume[9,11,21] and improved fetal oxygenation, heart rate, and non–stress test outcomes. If the left-lateral tilt method is used to improve maternal hemodynamics during cardiac arrest, the degree of tilt should be maximized. However, if the tilt is 30° or more, the patient may slide or roll off the inclined plane,[22] so this degree of tilt may not be practical during resuscitation. Although important, the degree of tilt is difficult to estimate reliably; the degree of table tilt is often overestimated.[23] Use of a fixed, hard wedge of a predetermined angle may be beneficial (Figure 114). However, the force of chest compressions performed will be reduced when the patient is tilted.[20]

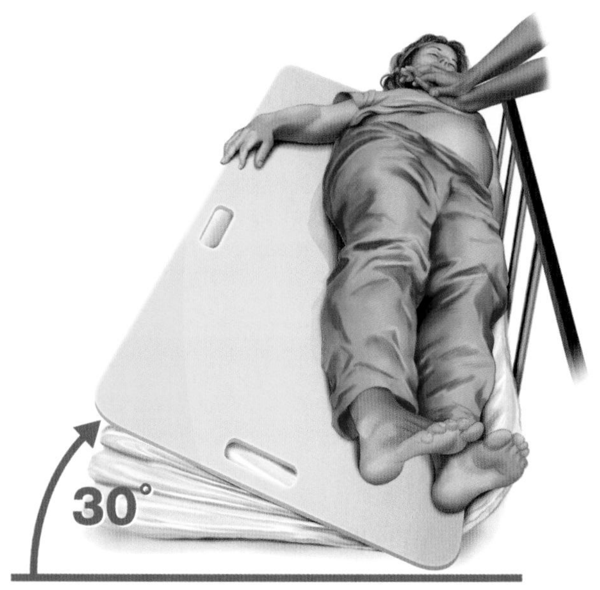

Figure 114. Patient in a 30° left-lateral tilt with a firm wedge to support the pelvis and thorax.

ACC has been documented at 30°[24] and 45°.[25] Therefore, even when left-lateral tilt is used correctly, ACC may still occur. This puts the mother at a hemodynamic disadvantage and reduces the chance of return of spontaneous circulation (ROSC) until there is full relief of the ACC by other methods such as left uterine displacement (LUD) or perimortem delivery.

Manual Displacement

LUD is another method that can be used to relieve ACC. In nonarrest literature, LUD has been found to reduce the incidence of hypotension and ephedrine requirements when compared with 15° left-lateral tilt in patients undergoing cesarean section.[26] Therefore, LUD provides an alternative technique for aortocaval decompression, where at the same time the patient can remain supine and receive concurrent high-quality chest compressions.

Relieve compression of the inferior vena cava and the aorta by shifting the gravid uterus left and upward off the maternal vessels:

- Stand on the left side of the patient, level with the top of the uterus.
- Reach across the midline with both hands (Figure 115) and pull the gravid uterus leftward and upward toward your abdomen.
- If it is not possible to stand to the left of the patient, use one hand to push the gravid uterus (Figure 116) to the patient's left and upward.
- If this technique is unsuccessful and an appropriate wedge is readily available, then you may consider placing the patient in a left-lateral tilt of 27° to 30°,[22] using a firm wedge to support the pelvis and thorax (Figure 114) (Class IIb, LOE C), or consider immediate delivery with perimortem cesarean section.

Chest Compressions in the Left-Lateral Tilt

In cardiac arrest, the reduced venous return caused by the gravid uterus puts the mother at a hemodynamic disadvantage, reducing the cardiac output produced by chest compressions. Therefore, when there is ACC, the effectiveness of the chest compressions may be limited.

Chest compressions performed while the patient is tilted are not ideal. Although it is feasible to perform chest compressions in the tilted patient,[27] it has been found that chest compressions performed in the tilted position are less forceful when compared with the supine position.[22] However, there are no physiologic data available for chest compressions in the tilted position. High-quality chest compressions are essential to maximize the chance of a successful resuscitation. An alternative method of relieving ACC, such as manual displacement, may be more practical and ideal during resuscitation as it allows for continuous and easier delivery of all other aspects of resuscitation, including high-quality chest compressions, defibrillation, IV access, and intubation.

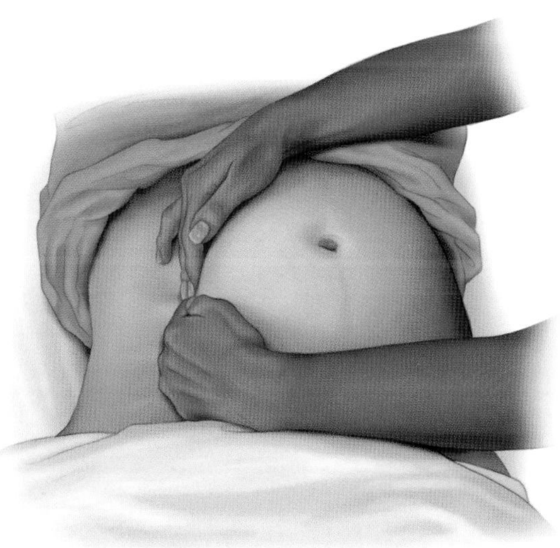

Figure 115. Left uterine displacement with the 2-handed technique.

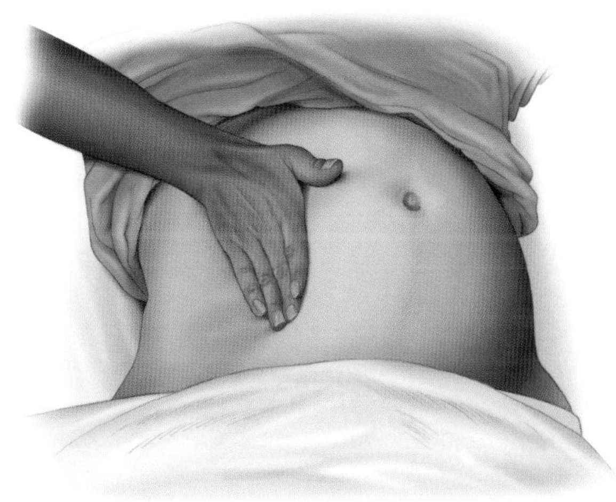

Figure 116. Left uterine displacement with the 1-handed technique.

Maternal Cardiac Arrest

First Responder

- Activate maternal cardiac arrest team
- Document time of onset of maternal cardiac arrest
- Place the patient supine
- Start chest compressions as per BLS algorithm; place hands slightly higher on sternum than usual

Subsequent Responders

Maternal Interventions

Treat per BLS and ACLS Algorithms

- Do not delay defibrillation
- Give typical ACLS drugs and doses
- Ventilate with 100% oxygen
- Monitor waveform capnography and CPR quality
- Provide post–cardiac arrest care as appropriate

Maternal Modifications

- Start IV above the diaphragm
- Assess for hypovolemia and give fluid bolus when required
- Anticipate difficult airway; experienced provider preferred for advanced airway placement
- If patient receiving IV/IO magnesium prearrest, stop magnesium and give IV/IO calcium chloride 10 mL in 10% solution, or calcium gluconate 30 mL in 10% solution
- Continue all maternal resuscitative interventions (CPR, positioning, defibrillation, drugs, and fluids) during and after cesarean section

Obstetric Interventions for Patient With an Obviously Gravid Uterus*

- Perform manual left uterine displacement (LUD)—displace uterus to the patient's left to relieve aortocaval compression
- Remove both internal and external fetal monitors if present

Obstetric and neonatal teams should immediately prepare for possible emergency cesarean section

- If no ROSC by 4 minutes of resuscitative efforts, consider performing immediate emergency cesarean section
- Aim for delivery within 5 minutes of onset of resuscitative efforts

*An obviously gravid uterus is a uterus that is deemed clinically to be sufficiently large to cause aortocaval compression

Search for and Treat Possible Contributing Factors (BEAU-CHOPS)

Bleeding/DIC
Embolism: coronary/pulmonary/amniotic fluid embolism
Anesthetic complications
Uterine atony
Cardiac disease (MI/ischemia/aortic dissection/cardiomyopathy)
Hypertension/preeclampsia/eclampsia
Other: differential diagnosis of standard ACLS guidelines
Placenta abruptio/previa
Sepsis

Figure 117. The Maternal Cardiac Arrest Algorithm. The algorithm is divided into 2 separate columns (maternal and obstetric interventions) to reflect the simultaneous resuscitation interventions of both the maternal resuscitation team and the obstetrical/neonatal team in an effort to improve team performance, efficiency, and success.

Resuscitation of the Pregnant Woman in Cardiac Arrest

Basic Life Support

Several modifications to standard BLS approaches are appropriate for the pregnant woman in cardiac arrest (Figure 117).

Airway

Airway management is more difficult during pregnancy, and placing the patient in a tilt may increase the difficulty. In addition, altered airway anatomy increases the risks of aspiration and rapid desaturation. Therefore, optimal use of bag-mask ventilation and suctioning while preparing for advanced airway placement is critical.

Breathing

Pregnant patients can develop hypoxemia quickly due to decreased functional residual capacity and increased oxygen demand. Ventilation volumes may need to be reduced due to the elevated position of the mother's diaphragm. Therefore, providers should be prepared to support oxygenation and ventilation and monitor oxygen saturation closely.

Circulation: Chest Compressions

Perform chest compressions higher on the sternum. This shift in hand placement will adjust for the elevation of the diaphragm and abdominal contents by the gravid uterus. Clear guidelines on how far the compression point should be shifted are lacking. Use the pulse check during chest compressions to adjust the sternal compression point.

Defibrillation

Use of an automated external defibrillator (AED) on a pregnant victim has not been studied but is reasonable. Transthoracic impedance in the pregnant patient has been found to be the same as that in the nonpregnant patient. Therefore, the current energy requirements for adult defibrillation are appropriate in pregnancy.[28] Although there may be a small risk of inducing fetal arrhythmias, cardioversion and defibrillation on the external chest are considered safe at all stages of pregnancy.[29-31]

If the pregnant woman has VF, deliver defibrillation shocks at the doses recommended in the ACLS guidelines. There is no evidence that shocks from a direct-current defibrillator have adverse effects on the heart of the fetus. If internal or external fetal monitors are attached during cardiac arrest in a pregnant woman, it is reasonable to remove them (Class IIb, LOE C). This helps avoid the potential for electrical arcing and expedites preparation for perimortem cesarean section in the case of unsuccessful resuscitation. However, defibrillation should not be delayed significantly in order to remove fetal monitors as the risk of electrical arcing is theoretical and not proven.

Advanced Cardiovascular Life Support

The treatments listed in the Maternal Cardiac Arrest Algorithm include recommendations for defibrillation, medications, and intubation (Figure 117). There are important considerations to keep in mind, however, about airway, breathing, circulation, and the differential diagnosis.

Airway

Secure the airway early in resuscitation. Pregnancy causes changes in airway mucosa, including edema, friability, hyperemia, and hypersecretion.[32,33] Hormonal changes promote insufficiency of the gastroesophageal sphincter and increase the risk of regurgitation. There are reports of failed intubation in obstetric anesthesia as a major cause of maternal morbidity and mortality.[34,35] Providers should be aware of the increased risk for pregnancy-related complications in airway management.

- A provider experienced in intubation should perform the procedure.
- Edema and swelling may narrow the woman's airway. It may be necessary to use an endotracheal tube that is slightly smaller (0.5 to 1 mm smaller ID [internal diameter]) than that used for a nonpregnant woman of similar size. The provider must be aware that a smaller tube will increase resistance to airflow and work of breathing during spontaneous ventilation.
- Effective preoxygenation before each intubation attempt is especially important because the decrease in functional residual capacity and functional residual volume predispose to rapid development of hypoxia.
- Rapid sequence intubation (RSI) with continuous cricoid pressure is the preferred technique. Etomidate or thiopental is preferred for anesthesia or deep sedation.
- Blood flow to the larynx increases during pregnancy. Watch for excessive bleeding in the airway following insertion of any tube in the oropharynx or nasopharynx.

Breathing

Verify correct endotracheal tube placement with primary and secondary confirmation techniques, including continuous waveform capnography.

Pregnancy decreases functional residual capacity and functional residual volume, but the tidal volume and minute ventilation are increased. As a result, you must tailor ventilatory support based on evaluation of oxygenation and ventilation.

Circulation

Follow the ACLS guidelines for choice of resuscitation medications. Vasopressor agents such as epinephrine, vasopressin, and dopamine will significantly decrease blood flow to the uterus. But there are no alternatives to using all indicated medications in recommended doses. Recall the

Critical Concept **Use of Sodium Bicarbonate in Prolonged Resuscitation**	The ACLS guidelines do not recommend routine use of sodium bicarbonate. The use of sodium bicarbonate creates particular problems in attempted resuscitation during pregnancy. It is unlikely to buffer the fetal pH but may temporarily buffer maternal pH, so it may mask the severity of the fetal acidosis.

Critical Concept Emergency Cesarean Section	• When there is an obvious gravid uterus, the emergency cesarean section team should be activated at the onset of maternal cardiac arrest (Class I, LOE B). • An emergency cesarean section may be considered at 4 minutes after onset of maternal cardiac arrest (with a goal of delivery within 5 minutes after maternal cardiac arrest) if there is no ROSC.

time-honored clinical aphorism that maternal resuscitation is the best method for fetal resuscitation.

Differential Diagnosis

Providers should be familiar with pregnancy-specific diseases and procedural complications (Table 70). Providers should try to identify these common and reversible causes of cardiac arrest in pregnancy during resuscitation attempts. The use of abdominal ultrasound by a skilled operator should be considered in detecting pregnancy and possible causes of the cardiac arrest, but this should not delay other treatments.

Excess magnesium sulfate. Patients with magnesium toxicity can present with cardiac effects ranging from electrocardiographic (ECG) interval changes at magnesium levels of 2.5 to 5 mmol/L to atrioventricular (AV) nodal conduction block, bradycardia, hypotension, and cardiac arrest at concentrations of 6 to 10 mmol/L. Neurologic effects, such as loss of tendon reflexes, sedation, severe muscular weakness, and respiratory depression, are seen at magnesium levels of 4 to 5 mmol/L. Other signs of magnesium toxicity include gastrointestinal (GI) symptoms (nausea and vomiting), skin changes (flushing), and electrolyte/fluid abnormalities (hypophosphatemia, hyperosmolar dehydration). Iatrogenic overdose is possible in women with eclampsia who receive magnesium sulfate, particularly if the woman becomes oliguric. If the woman is receiving magnesium at the time of the arrest, discontinue the magnesium infusion. Empirically administer calcium (calcium chloride [10%] 5 to 10 mL or calcium gluconate [10%] 15 to 30 mL IV over 2 to 5 minutes). Calcium is the treatment of choice for magnesium toxicity and may be lifesaving for these patients.[36,37]

Congenital heart disease. It is estimated that 85% of neonates born with congenital heart disease will survive to adulthood. Therefore, more women with congenital heart disease will have children. These pregnancies may be associated with a higher risk for severe complications, including cardiac arrest.

Sepsis. Sepsis is the leading direct cause of maternal deaths, and the mortality rate is still on the rise.[3] Recognition and aggressive treatment of sepsis are essential during resuscitation of the patient with sepsis.

Acute coronary syndromes. Women are deferring pregnancy to older ages, increasing the chance that they will have atherosclerotic heart disease. Because fibrinolytics are relatively contraindicated in pregnancy, percutaneous coronary intervention is the reperfusion strategy of choice for ST-segment elevation myocardial infarction.[38] But there are reports of successful use of fibrinolytics for massive, life-threatening pulmonary embolism in pregnant women.[39]

Hemorrhage. Hemorrhage remains an important cause of death during pregnancy and in the postpartum period.[3,40] Postpartum hemorrhage (PPH) can go underrecognized until the mother becomes critically ill.[3] Oxytocin is used as a uterotonic agent to prevent and treat PPH.[41,42] However, oxytocin is also associated with significant maternal adverse effects that could precipitate hemodynamic instability[41] and even maternal death.[43] Maternal adverse effects of oxytocin include cardiovascular changes such as hypotension, tachycardia, myocardial ischemia, and arrhythmias. Large doses of oxytocin can cause water retention, hyponatremia, seizures, and coma. A recent report found a reduction in cardiac output in patients with preeclampsia who received oxytocin. A maternal death has been reported following administration of 10 international units of oxytocin during the resuscitation of a hypovolemic patient undergoing cesarean delivery.[43] Recognition of PPH and treatment for PPH with oxytocin must be carefully considered in the unstable patient, the patient with arrest, or the postarrest patient.

Cardiomyopathy. Cardiomyopathy, mainly in the form of peripartum cardiomyopathy is a leading cause of pregnancy-related mortality.[3] However, it should be recognized that deaths related to peripartum cardiomyopathy can occur late after delivery, up to 6 months postpartum.

Preeclampsia/eclampsia. Preeclampsia/eclampsia develops after the 20th week of gestation and can produce severe hypertension and ultimate diffuse organ system failure. If untreated it may result in maternal and fetal morbidity and mortality.

Aortic dissection. The physiologic changes to the aorta during pregnancy place pregnant women at increased risk for spontaneous aortic dissection, which is another major cause of cardiac death in this population.[3] In addition to women with an underlying enlargement of the aorta, those with conditions like Marfan syndrome or Ehlers-Danlos syndrome are at significantly increased risk for aortic dissection during pregnancy.

Table 70. The Emergency Hysterotomy (Cesarean Delivery) Decision: Factors to Consider Upon Maternal Arrest

Factors to Consider	Comments
Arrest Factors • If the uterus is gravid enough to cause ACC, especially if it is palpated at or above the umbilicus and therefore at about ≥20 wk of gestational age, ask that personnel and equipment be assembled for emergency hysterotomy. • Immediately prepare for possible PMCS at first recognition of maternal arrest. This will allow simultaneous continuation of resuscitative efforts and preparation for the cesarean delivery. • Is the mother receiving appropriate BLS and ACLS care, including – CPR with compressions performed with the mother slightly higher on the sternum than for a nonpregnant woman? – Manual LUD (for patients with a gravid uterus) to relieve ACC? – Early intubation with verification of proper placement of the endotracheal tube? – Administration of indicated IV medications to a venous site above the diaphragm? – If defibrillation is appropriate, it should not be delayed. • Has the mother responded to arrest interventions? • Are there any potentially reversible causes of arrest?	**Arrest Factors** • Survival probabilities for the mother and fetus decrease as the interval from maternal arrest increases. • Aim for an interval of ≤5 min from maternal arrest to delivery of the fetus. This goal requires efficient assembly of personnel and equipment. • Do *not* wait until 5 min of unsuccessful resuscitation have passed before you begin to consider the need to deliver the fetus emergently. You should consider the need for hysterotomy immediately to enable assembly of personnel and equipment. If there is no ROSC by 4 min of resuscitative efforts, consider performing an immediate emergency cesarean section. • Ensure that the mother has received superior resuscitative efforts. She cannot be declared "refractory" to CPR and ACLS unless all interventions have been implemented effectively, including PMCS when appropriate. No mother should die with a fetus left undelivered when there is ACC.
Mother-Infant Factors • Is the fetus old enough to survive? • Is the mother's cardiac arrest due to a chronic hypoxic state? • What is the status of the fetus at the time of the mother's cardiac arrest?	**Mother-Infant Factors** • This question recognized the critical importance of gestational age. Survival is unlikely for the infant born at less than approximately 24-25 wk of gestational age. • Do not lose site of the goal of this dramatic event: a live, neurologically intact infant and mother. • Even if the fetus is unlikely to survive (20-23 wk of gestational age), the mother may benefit from emergency hysterotomy. • A recent systematic review found that a crash hysterotomy occurring <10 min after maternal cardiac arrest was a predictor of maternal survival.[19]
Setting and Personnel • Are appropriate equipment and supplies[71] available? • Is hysterotomy within the rescuer's skill "comfort zone"? • Is the airway being managed by the most skilled personnel available? • Are skilled neonatal or pediatric support personnel available to care for the infant, especially if it is not at full term? • Are obstetric personnel immediately available to support the mother after delivery? • In both in-hospital and out-of hospital settings, is there adequate staff and equipment support? In out-of hospital settings, is bystander support available?	**Setting and Personnel** • One predictor of maternal survival for those patients undergoing crash hysterotomy is an in-hospital arrest location. • Availability of a neonatal ICU increases the newborn's chance of survival. • The maternal airway is always a difficult airway.
Differential Diagnosis • Consider whether persistent arrest is due to an immediately reversible problem (eg, excess anesthesia, reaction to analgesia, magnesium toxicity, preeclampsia/eclampsia, severe bronchospasm, hemorrhage or hypovolemia, pulmonary embolism, cardiac ischemia). If it is, correct the problem, and there may be no need for hysterotomy. • Consider whether persistent arrest is due to a fatal, untreatable problem (eg, massive trauma). If it is, an immediate hysterotomy may save the fetus.	

Abbreviations: ACC, aortocaval compression; ACLS, advanced cardiovascular life support; BLS, basic life support; CPR, cardiopulmonary resuscitation; ICU, intensive care unit; IV, intravenous; LUD, left uterine displacement; PMCS, perimortem cesarean section; ROSC, return of spontaneous circulation.

Life-threatening pulmonary embolism and stroke. Successful use of fibrinolytics for a massive, life-threatening pulmonary embolism[44-46] and ischemic stroke[47] have been reported in pregnant women. Pregnant women in cardiac arrest with suspected pulmonary embolism should be treated in accordance with the ACLS section of the *2010 AHA Guidelines for CPR and ECC* (see Part 12.5: "Cardiac Arrest Associated With Pulmonary Embolism").[48]

Anesthetic complications. Anesthesia-related maternal morbidity and mortality have led to the development of specialized obstetric anesthesia techniques.[35] Cardiac arrest can occur from spinal shock as a result of regional anesthesia. Induction of general anesthesia may lead to loss of airway control or pulmonary aspiration, and emergence from anesthesia can be associated with hypoventilation or airway obstruction.[49-54] These conditions can ultimately lead to cardiac arrest.

Amniotic fluid embolism. Clinicians have reported successful use of cardiopulmonary bypass for women with a life-threatening amniotic fluid embolism during labor and delivery.[55] Maternal and neonatal survival have been achieved through the use of perimortem cesarean section.[55]

Trauma and drug overdose. Pregnant women are not exempt from the accidents and mental illnesses that afflict much of society. Domestic violence also increases during pregnancy; in fact, homicide and suicide are leading causes of mortality during pregnancy[16] as well as in the early postpartum period. The majority of suicides associated with pregnancy occur following childbirth, some as late as 6 months after.[3]

Emergency Hysterotomy (Cesarean Delivery) for the Pregnant Woman in Cardiac Arrest

Maternal Cardiac Arrest Persists/Not Immediately Reversed by BLS and ACLS

Clinicians treating a pregnant woman in cardiac arrest must never forget the second patient, the unborn child. With the mother in cardiac arrest, the blood supply to the fetus becomes hypoxic and acidotic. This will prove fatal to the fetus without rapid restoration of the mother's spontaneous circulation. *The key to resuscitation of the infant is resuscitation of the mother.* After approximately 20 weeks of gestation, however, the *key to resuscitation of the mother is possibly removal of the fetus from the gravid uterus.* By this time, the gravid uterus obstructs the inferior vena cava, preventing venous return to the heart, and compresses the aorta, threatening arterial blood flow to critical organs.

The emergency hysterotomy, or perimortem cesarean section (PMCS), has gained general acceptance as a way of resuscitating a pregnant woman who remains in cardiac arrest after the initial few minutes of BLS and ACLS. Although PMCS offers the best chance of resuscitating the gestationally advanced fetus, it also mandates sacrifice of a fetus less than 20 to 23 weeks of gestational age. On the basis of a small number of case reports, the AHA Guidelines for CPR and ECC first recommended PMCS in 1992. Since then, several case reports of emergency cesarean section in maternal cardiac arrest have shown ROSC or improvement in maternal hemodynamic status only after the uterus has been emptied.[8,9,18,55-62]

Recommendations Based on Gestational Age

Hysterotomy allows access to the infant so that newborn resuscitation can begin. It also leads to immediate correction of much of the abnormal physiology of the full-term mother. The critical point to remember is that *both mother and infant will die if you cannot restore blood flow to the mother's heart.*[56]

Once the fetus is delivered, the uterus is decompressed and the abdominal incision may enable direct massage of the mother's heart through the diaphragm. Internal cardiac compression through a thoracotomy may also be attempted. Evidence to support these interventions is lacking.

The gravid uterus reaches a size that will begin to compromise aortocaval blood flow at approximately 20 weeks of gestation for the single fetus.[63] Fetal viability is estimated to begin at approximately 24 to 25 weeks. Consequently there is general acceptance of the following recommendations:

- **Attempt to determine gestational age from history and examination:** Fundal height is often used to estimate gestational age. In a singleton gestation, by 20 weeks fundal height is approximately at the level of the umbilicus[64]; however, the fundus may reach the umbilicus between 15 and 19 weeks of gestation.[65] Fundal height may also be skewed by other factors such as abdominal distention[64] and increased body mass index; therefore, fundal height may be a poor predictor of gestational age. The higher the fundal height, especially when at or above the umbilicus, the greater the likelihood that there is ACC.
- **Gestational age less than 24 weeks:** Perform emergency hysterotomy and deliver the fetus to save the life of the mother. If the mother remains in cardiac arrest and unresponsive to BLS and ACLS by 4 minutes, delivery of the fetus by 5 minutes will relieve the obstruction on the inferior vena cava and the aorta and may enable successful resuscitation of the mother. At less than 20 weeks of gestation, the size of the uterus is less likely to significantly compromise maternal

venous return and cardiac output. But if there is more than 1 fetus, the uterus may compromise maternal blood flow, and PMCS may be advisable. Although resuscitation protocols should focus on the mother, it is important to involve the neonatal team in all maternal resuscitations. There have been cases of neonatal survival at 23 and 24 weeks of gestational age.[4]

- **Gestational age approximately more than 24 to 25 weeks:** After consideration of the factors listed in Table 70, perform emergency hysterotomy to save the life of both the mother and the fetus. The best survival rate for the infant occurs when the infant is delivered no more than 5 minutes after the mother's heart stops beating.[39,66-68] Typically this requires that the provider begin the hysterotomy about 4 minutes after cardiac arrest.
- **Consider factors that influence infant survival:** Although the mother is the primary patient, consider factors that influence the newborn's chance of survival:
  - Short interval between the mother's cardiac arrest and delivery of the infant; however, infant survival has been observed even when delivery occurred more than 5 minutes from onset of maternal cardiac arrest[16,18] and especially at later gestational ages.[3,17] Neonatal survival has been documented when delivery occurred within 30 minutes after onset of maternal cardiac arrest.[50]
  - Maternal cardiac arrest is not associated with sustained prearrest hypoxia.[18,56]
  - Minimal or no signs of fetal distress are present at the time of maternal cardiac arrest.
  - The resuscitation of the mother is conducted effectively and aggressively.
  - Hysterotomy is performed in a medical center with a neonatal intensive care unit.

The Importance of Timing With Emergency Cesarean Section

The 5-minute window that providers have to determine if cardiac arrest can be reversed by BLS and ACLS was first described in 1986 and has been perpetuated in specialty guidelines.[18,57] The rescue team is not required to wait 5 minutes before initiating emergency hysterotomy, and there are circumstances that support an earlier start.[64] For instance, in an obvious nonsurvivable injury,[18,69-71] when the maternal prognosis is grave and resuscitative efforts appear futile, moving straight to an emergency cesarean section may be appropriate, especially if the fetus is viable.

The decision to perform hysterotomy should be made early in the resuscitation. Achieving the 5-minute goal requires that the provider begin the hysterotomy about 4 minutes after cardiac arrest. However, recent studies have found few if any PMCS procedures that are done within the recommended 5-minute time frame.[17,50] There have been reports of long intervals between the urgent decision for PMCS and actual delivery of the infant, which exceeded the obstetric guideline of 30 minutes for patients not in arrest.[72,73] Survival of the mother has been reported with PMCS performed up to 15 minutes after the onset of maternal cardiac arrest.[56,74-76] Assessment of the effectiveness of current guidelines has been lacking.[18,19,56] The most recent systematic review found that the predictors of maternal survival for those patients undergoing PMCS include in-hospital arrest location and PMCS occurring less than 10 minutes after maternal cardiac arrest.[19] However, after approximately 4 minutes without adequate maternal perfusion, ischemic damage occurs. Therefore, the goal to deliver by 5 minutes makes the most physiologic sense for maternal prognosis. The literature consistently demonstrates that this goal is difficult to achieve, and therefore delivery by 5 minutes should not be deemed a standard of care but a goal of care. If delivery does not occur within 5 minutes, teams should work toward the earliest possible delivery of the fetus while simultaneously continuing high-quality resuscitative efforts.

Systems of Care

Table 69 lists the many factors to consider in a very short time during a maternal cardiac arrest and attempted resuscitation.

Every department potentially involved in caring for maternal arrest, including the intensive care unit (ICU), emergency department (ED), and obstetrical (OB) unit, should be prepared[77] and should rehearse the plan of action for this type of event, including location of supplies, sources of extra equipment, and best methods for obtaining subspecialty assistance. Team planning should be done in collaboration with the obstetric, neonatal, emergency, anesthesiology, intensive care, and cardiac arrest services (Class I, LOE C). Implementation strategies can be used by institutions to aid in emergency preparedness and knowledge translation. The code team composition for a maternal cardiac arrest should include the adult resuscitation team, anesthesia, adult respiratory therapy, obstetrics, obstetrical nursing, neonatology, and neonatal respiratory therapy. Systems should be in place to emergently notify all these team members in the event of a maternal cardiac arrest so that all are available during the resuscitation and post–cardiac arrest period.[77]

Post–Cardiac Arrest Care

Therapeutic hypothermia needs to be considered in the pregnant post–cardiac arrest patient. One case study showed that post–cardiac arrest hypothermia can be used safely and effectively in early pregnancy without emergency cesarean section (with fetal heart monitoring), with favorable maternal and fetal outcome after a term delivery.[78] There was 1 case of fetal death after therapeutic hypothermia; however, emergency medical services (EMS) did not arrive until 22 minutes after the onset of maternal cardiac arrest.[79]

A more recent case report demonstrates successful use of therapeutic hypothermia after maternal cardiac arrest with excellent immediate and long-term maternal and fetal neurologic, cardiac, and developmental outcomes.[80] It should be noted that successful resuscitation occurred in this case with usual ACLS measures and without PMCS at 20 weeks of gestational age. Pregnancy should not be a contraindication to therapeutic hypothermia following cardiac arrest. The ethical ideology of beneficence toward the pregnant woman should allow her to receive known beneficial therapy. Impaired coagulation with hypothermia is a concern, although bleeding risk is unknown after cesarean section. Therapeutic hypothermia can be considered on an individual basis after cardiac arrest in a comatose pregnant patient based on current recommendations for the nonpregnant patient (Class IIb, LOE C). During therapeutic hypothermia of the pregnant patient, it is recommended that the fetus be continuously monitored for the potential complication of bradycardia, and obstetric and neonatal consultation should be sought (Class I, LOE C).

It is important that institutions develop training programs for maternal resuscitation. The knowledge and skill for the management of cardiac arrest in pregnancy has been found to be poor.[19,81-83] Simulation-based training is a useful tool for staff to improve skills, knowledge, and confidence in the management of cardiac arrest in pregnancy.[84]

References

1. Jeejeebhoy FM, Zelop CM, Windrim R, Carvalho JC, Dorian P, Morrison LJ. Management of cardiac arrest in pregnancy: a systematic review. *Resuscitation*. 2011;82:801-809.
2. Jeejeebhoy FM, Zelop CM. Worksheet for evidence-based review of science for emergency cardiac care. 2010.
3. Cantwell R, Clutton-Brock T, Cooper G, Dawson A, Drife J, Garrod D, Harper A, Hulbert D, Lucas S, McClure J, Millward-Sadler H, Neilson J, Nelson-Piercy C, Norman J, O'Herlihy C, Oates M, Shakespeare J, de Swiet M, Williamson C, Beale V, Knight M, Lennox C, Miller A, Parmar D, Rogers J, Springett A. Saving mothers' lives: reviewing maternal deaths to make motherhood safer: 2006-2008. The Eighth Report of the Confidential Enquiries into Maternal Deaths in the United Kingdom. *BJOG*. 2011;118(suppl 1):1-203.
4. Allen MC, Donohue PK, Dusman AE. The limit of viability—neonatal outcome of infants born at 22 to 25 weeks' gestation. *N Engl J Med*. 1993;329:1597-1601.
5. Lennox C, Marr L. *Scottish Confidential Audit of Severe Maternal Morbidity.* 8th Annual Report: NHS Quality Improvement Scotland. 2010.
6. McLellan C. Antecubital and femoral venous pressure in normal and toxemia pregnancy. *Am J Obstet Gynecol.* 1943;45:568.
7. Kuklina E, Callaghan W. Chronic heart disease and severe obstetric morbidity among hospitalisations for pregnancy in the USA: 1995-2006. *BJOG*. 2011;118:345-352.
8. Page-Rodriguez A, Gonzalez-Sanchez JA. Perimortem cesarean section of twin pregnancy: case report and review of the literature. *Acad Emerg Med*. 1999;6:1072-1074.
9. Cardosi RJ, Porter KB. Cesarean delivery of twins during maternal cardiopulmonary arrest. *Obstet Gynecol*. 1998;92:695-697.
10. Rees SG, Thurlow JA, Gardner IC, Scrutton MJ, Kinsella SM. Maternal cardiovascular consequences of positioning after spinal anaesthesia for Caesarean section: left 15 degree table tilt vs. left lateral. *Anaesthesia*. 2002;57:15-20.
11. Mendonca C, Griffiths J, Ateleanu B, Collis RE. Hypotension following combined spinal-epidural anaesthesia for Caesarean section. Left lateral position vs. tilted supine position. *Anaesthesia*. 2003;58:428-431.
12. Alahuhta S, Jouppila P. How to maintain uteroplacental perfusion during obstetric anaesthesia. *Acta Anaesthesiol Scand Suppl*. 1997;110:106-108.
13. Tamas P, Szilagyi A, Jeges S, Vizer M, Csermely T, Ifi Z, Balint A, Szabo I. Effects of maternal central hemodynamics on fetal heart rate patterns. *Acta Obstet Gynecol Scand*. 2007;86:711-714.
14. Abitbol MM. Supine position in labor and associated fetal heart rate changes. *Obstet Gynecol*. 1985;65:481-486.
15. Tamilselvan P, Fernando R, Bray J, Sodhi M, Columb M. The effects of crystalloid and colloid preload on cardiac output in the parturient undergoing planned cesarean delivery under spinal anesthesia: a randomized trial. *Anesth Analg*. 2009;109:1916-1921.
16. Johnson MD, Luppi CJ, Over DC. Cardiopulmonary resuscitation. In: Gambling DR, Douglas MJ, eds. *Obstetric Anesthesia and Uncommon Disorders.* Philadelphia, PA: WB Saunders; 1998:51-74.
17. Datner EM, Promes SB. Resuscitation issues in pregnancy. In: Rosen P, Barkin R, eds. *Emergency Medicine: Concepts and Clinical Practice*. St Louis, MO: Mosby; 1998:71-76.
18. Katz V, Balderston K, DeFreest M. Perimortem cesarean delivery: were our assumptions correct? *Am J Obstet Gynecol*. 2005;192:1916-1920.
19. Einav S, Kaufman N, Sela HY. Maternal cardiac arrest and perimortem caesarean delivery: evidence or expert-based? *Resuscitation*. 2012;83:1191-1200.
20. Rossi A, Cornette J, Johnson MR, Karamermer Y, Springeling T, Opic P, Moelker A, Krestin GP, Steegers E, Roos-Hesselink J, van Geuns RJ. Quantitative cardiovascular magnetic resonance in pregnant women: cross-sectional analysis of physiological parameters throughout pregnancy and the impact of the supine position. *J Cardiovasc Magn Reson*. 2011;13:31.
21. Bamber JH, Dresner M. Aortocaval compression in pregnancy: the effect of changing the degree and direction of lateral tilt on maternal cardiac output. *Anesth Analg*. 2003;97:256-258.
22. Rees GA, Willis BA. Resuscitation in late pregnancy. *Anaesthesia*. 1988;43:347-349.
23. Jones SJ, Kinsella SM, Donald FA. Comparison of measured and estimated angles of table tilt at Caesarean section. *Br J Anaesth*. 2003;90:86-87.
24. Kinsella SM, Whitwam JG, Spencer JA. Aortic compression by the uterus: identification with the Finapres digital arterial pressure instrument. *Br J Obstet Gynaecol*. 1990;97:700-705.
25. Archer TL, Suresh P, Shapiro AE. Cardiac output measurement, by means of electrical velocimetry, may be able to determine optimum maternal position during gestation, labour and caesarean delivery, by preventing vena caval compression and maximising cardiac output

and placental perfusion pressure. *Anaesth Intensive Care*. 2011;39:308-311.

26. Kundra P, Khanna S, Habeebullah S, Ravishankar M. Manual displacement of the uterus during Caesarean section. *Anaesthesia*. 2007;62:460-465.
27. Goodwin AP, Pearce AJ. The human wedge. A manoeuvre to relieve aortocaval compression during resuscitation in late pregnancy. *Anaesthesia*. 1992;47:433-434.
28. Nanson J, Elcock D, Williams M, Deakin CD. Do physiological changes in pregnancy change defibrillation energy requirements? *Br J Anaesth*. 2001;87:237-239.
29. Brown O, Davidson N, Palmer J. Cardioversion in the third trimester of pregnancy. *Aust N Z J Obstet Gynaecol*. 2001;41:241-242.
30. Goldman RD, Einarson A, Koren G. Electric shock during pregnancy. *Can Fam Physician*. 2003;49:297-298.
31. Adamson DL, Nelson-Piercy C. Managing palpitations and arrhythmias during pregnancy. *Heart*. 2007;93:1630-1636.
32. Elkus R, Popovich J Jr. Respiratory physiology in pregnancy. *Clin Chest Med*. 1992;13:555-565.
33. Lapinsky SE, Kruczynski K, Slutsky AS. Critical care in the pregnant patient. *Am J Respir Crit Care Med*. 1995;152:427-455.
34. Vasdev GM, Harrison BA, Keegan MT, Burkle CM. Management of the difficult and failed airway in obstetric anesthesia. *J Anesth*. 2008;22:38-48.
35. Marx GF, Berman JA. Anesthesia-related maternal mortality. *Bull N Y Acad Med*. 1985;61:323-330.
36. Poole JH, Long J. Maternal mortality—a review of current trends. *Crit Care Nurs Clin North Am*. 2004;16:227-230.
37. Munro PT. Management of eclampsia in the accident and emergency department. *J Accid Emerg Med*. 2000;17:7-11.
38. Doan-Wiggins L. Resuscitation of the pregnant patient suffering sudden death. In: Paradis NA, Halperin HR, Nowak RM, eds. *Cardiac Arrest: The Science and Practice of Resuscitation Medicine*. Baltimore, MD: Williams & Wilkins; 1997:812-819.
39. Strong THJ, Lowe RA. Perimortem cesarean section. *Am J Emerg Med*. 1989;7:489-494.
40. World Health Organization. *The World Health Report 2005.* Make every mother and child count. 2005.
41. Dyer RA, Butwick AJ, Carvalho B. Oxytocin for labour and caesarean delivery: implications for the anaesthesiologist. *Curr Opin Anaesthesiol*. 2011;24:255-261.
42. Clark SL, Simpson KR, Knox GE, Garite TJ. Oxytocin: new perspectives on an old drug. *Am J Obstet Gynecol*. 2009;200:35 e31-e36.
43. Thomas TA, Cooper GM. Maternal deaths from anaesthesia. An extract from Why mothers die 1997-1999, the Confidential Enquiries into Maternal Deaths in the United Kingdom. *Br J Anaesth*. 2002;89:499-508.
44. Turrentine MA, Braems G, Ramirez MM. Use of thrombolytics for the treatment of thromboembolic disease during pregnancy. *Obstet Gynecol Surv*. 1995;50:534-541.
45. Thabut G, Thabut D, Myers RP, Bernard-Chabert B, Marrash-Chahla R, Mal H, Fournier M. Thrombolytic therapy of pulmonary embolism: a meta-analysis. *J Am Coll Cardiol*. 2002;40:1660-1667.
46. Patel RK, Fasan O, Arya R. Thrombolysis in pregnancy. *Thromb Haemost*. 2003;90:1216-1217.
47. Dapprich M, Boessenecker W. Fibrinolysis with alteplase in a pregnant woman with stroke. *Cerebrovasc Dis*. 2002;13:290.
48. Kuklina EV, Tong X, Bansil P, George MG, Callaghan WM. Trends in pregnancy hospitalizations that included a stroke in the United States from 1994 to 2007: reasons for concern? *Stroke*. 2011;42:2564-2570.
49. Mhyre JM, Riesner MN, Polley LS, Naughton NN. A series of anesthesia-related maternal deaths in Michigan, 1985-2003. *Anesthesiology*. 2007;106:1096-1104.
50. D'Angelo R. Anesthesia-related maternal mortality: a pat on the back or a call to arms? *Anesthesiology*. 2007;106:1082-1084.
51. Hawkins JL, Koonin LM, Palmer SK, Gibbs CP. Anesthesia-related deaths during obstetric delivery in the United States, 1979-1990. *Anesthesiology*. 1997;86:277-284.
52. Fisher RS, Roberts GS, Grabowski CJ, Cohen S. Altered lower esophageal sphincter function during early pregnancy. *Gastroenterology*. 1978;74:1233-1237.
53. Dodds WJ, Dent J, Hogan WJ. Pregnancy and the lower esophageal sphincter. *Gastroenterology*. 1978;74:1334-1336.
54. Baron TH, Ramirez B, Richter JE. Gastrointestinal motility disorders during pregnancy. *Ann Intern Med*. 1993;118:366-375.
55. Stanten RD, Iverson LI, Daugharty TM, Lovett SM, Terry C, Blumenstock E. Amniotic fluid embolism causing catastrophic pulmonary vasoconstriction: diagnosis by transesophageal echocardiogram and treatment by cardiopulmonary bypass. *Obstet Gynecol*. 2003;102:496-498.
56. Dijkman A, Huisman CM, Smit M, Schutte JM, Zwart JJ, van Roosmalen JJ, Oepkes D. Cardiac arrest in pregnancy: increasing use of perimortem caesarean section due to emergency skills training? *BJOG*. 2010;117:282-287.
57. McDonnell NJ. Cardiopulmonary arrest in pregnancy: two case reports of successful outcomes in association with perimortem Caesarean delivery. *Br J Anaesth*. 2009;103:406-409.
58. McCartney CJ, Dark A. Caesarean delivery during cardiac arrest in late pregnancy. *Anaesthesia*. 1998;53:310-311.
59. Lurie S, Mamet Y. Caesarean delivery during maternal cardiopulmonary resuscitation for status asthmaticus. *Emerg Med J*. 2003;20:296-297.
60. O'Connor RL, Sevarino FB. Cardiopulmonary arrest in the pregnant patient: a report of a successful resuscitation. *J Clin Anesth*. 1994;6:66-68.
61. Finegold H, Darwich A, Romeo R, Vallejo M, Ramanathan S. Successful resuscitation after maternal cardiac arrest by immediate cesarean section in the labor room. *Anesthesiology*. 2002;96:1278.
62. Parker J, Balis N, Chester S, Adey D. Cardiopulmonary arrest in pregnancy: successful resuscitation of mother and infant following immediate caesarean section in labour ward. *Aust N Z J Obstet Gynaecol*. 1996;36:207-210.
63. Ueland K, Novy MJ, Peterson EN, Metcalfe J. Maternal cardiovascular dynamics. IV. The influence of gestational age on the maternal cardiovascular response to posture and exercise. *Am J Obstet Gynecol*. 1969;104:856-864.
64. Stallard TC, Burns B. Emergency delivery and perimortem C-section. *Emerg Med Clin North Am*. 2003;21:679-693.
65. Mackway-Jones K. Towards evidence based emergency medicine: best BETs from the Manchester Royal Infirmary. *Emerg Med J*. 2003;20:362.
66. Katz VL, Dotters DJ, Droegemueller W. Perimortem cesarean delivery. *Obstet Gynecol*. 1986;68:571-576.

67. Oates S, Williams GL, Rees GA. Cardiopulmonary resuscitation in late pregnancy. *BMJ*. 1988;297:404-405.

68. Boyd R, Teece S. Towards evidence based emergency medicine: best BETs from the Manchester Royal Infirmary. Perimortem caesarean section. *Emerg Med J*. 2002;19:324-325.

69. Lanoix R, Akkapeddi V, Goldfeder B. Perimortem cesarean section: case reports and recommendations. *Acad Emerg Med*. 1995;2:1063-1067.

70. Tang G, Nada W, Gyaneshwar R, Crooke D. Perimortem Caesarean section: two case reports and a management protocol. *Aust N Z J Obstet Gynaecol*. 2000;40:405-408.

71. Lopez-Zeno JA, Carlo WA, O'Grady JP, Fanaroff AA. Infant survival following delayed postmortem cesarean delivery. *Obstet Gynecol*. 1990;76:991-992.

72. MacKenzie IZ, Cooke I. What is a reasonable time from decision-to-delivery by caesarean section? Evidence from 415 deliveries. *BJOG*. 2002;109:498-504.

73. Helmy WH, Jolaoso AS, Ifaturoti OO, Afify SA, Jones MH. The decision-to-delivery interval for emergency caesarean section: is 30 minutes a realistic target? *BJOG*. 2002;109:505-508.

74. Kazandi M, Mgoyi L, Gundem G, Hacivelioglu S, Yucebilgin S, Ozkinay E. Post-mortem Caesarean section performed 30 minutes after maternal cardiopulmonary arrest. *Aust N Z J Obstet Gynaecol*. 2004;44:351-353.

75. Kupas DF, Harter SC, Vosk A. Out-of-hospital perimortem cesarean section. *Prehosp Emerg Care*. 1998;2:206-208.

76. Kam CW. Perimortem caesarean sections (PMCS). *J Accid Emerg Med*. 1994;11:57-58.

77. Hui D, Morrison LJ, Windrim R, Lausman AY, Hawryluck L, Dorian P, Lapinsky SE, Halpern SH, Campbell DM, Hawkins P, Wax RS, Carvalho JC, Dainty KN, Maxwell C, Jeejeebhoy FM. The American Heart Association 2010 guidelines for the management of cardiac arrest in pregnancy: consensus recommendations on implementation strategies. *J Obstet Gynaecol Can*. 2011;33:858-863.

78. Rittenberger JC, Kelly E, Jang D, Greer K, Heffner A. Successful outcome utilizing hypothermia after cardiac arrest in pregnancy: a case report. *Crit Care Med*. 2008;36:1354-1356.

79. Wible EF, Kass JS, Lopez GA. A report of fetal demise during therapeutic hypothermia after cardiac arrest. *Neurocrit Care*. 2010;13:239-242.

80. Chauhan A, Musunuru H, Donnino M, McCurdy MT, Chauhan V, Walsh M. The use of therapeutic hypothermia after cardiac arrest in a pregnant patient. *Ann Emerg Med*. 2012;60:786-789

81. Lipman SS, Daniels KI, Carvalho B, Arafeh J, Harney K, Puck A, Cohen SE, Druzin M. Deficits in the provision of cardiopulmonary resuscitation during simulated obstetric crises. *Am J Obstet Gynecol*. 2010;203:179 e171-e175.

82. Einav S, Matot I, Berkenstadt H, Bromiker R, Weiniger CF. A survey of labour ward clinicians' knowledge of maternal cardiac arrest and resuscitation. *Int J Obstet Anesth*. 2008;17:238-242.

83. Cohen SE, Andes LC, Carvalho B. Assessment of knowledge regarding cardiopulmonary resuscitation of pregnant women. *Int J Obstet Anesth*. 2008;17:20-25.

84. Fisher N, Eisen LA, Bayya JV, Dulu A, Bernstein PS, Merkatz IR, Goffman D. Improved performance of maternal-fetal medicine staff after maternal cardiac arrest simulation-based training. *Am J Obstet Gynecol*. 2011;205:239 e231-e235.

Chapter 19

Drowning

This Chapter

- Drowning Outcomes
- The Most Important Treatment for the Drowning Patient: Immediate Ventilation
- Removing Water From the Airway: Is It Necessary? How Should It Be Done?
- Grading and Reporting Drowning Events
- Whom to Transport to the Hospital

Overview

Drowning is most common in children and young adults. This can be traumatic for the relatives and loved ones of patients and for emergency providers.

Epidemiology

Drowning accounts for more than 500 000 deaths annually.[1] Drowning is a leading preventable cause of unintentional morbidity and mortality. Reports from many parts of the world emphasize that drowning is a leading cause of cardiopulmonary arrest in children and adolescents.[2-6]

Prevention

Many issues surrounding prevention of drownings are complex and controversial, such as

- Appropriate targets for prevention efforts[7]
- Siblings bathing together without adult supervision[8]
- Pediatric "drownproofing" is an unproven concept.[9] Although the American Academy of Pediatrics (AAP) no longer advises against swimming lessons for very young children,[10] it still does not recommend this practice because current evidence is insufficient.[11]

Many drowning incidents that result in death or neurologic impairment are preventable tragedies. Many are the result of poor judgment, alcohol consumption, or inadequate supervision of children. Despite the ACLS emphasis on immediate treatment, the definitive therapy for drowning is *prevention*.

Rescue of drowning victims occurs on or near the water, exposing rescue teams to danger. Never forget the principle of provider safety: make sure the area is safe and avoid becoming a second victim.

Pathophysiology

The drowning process is a continuum that begins when a person's airway lies below the surface of liquid, usually water, at which time the person voluntarily holds his breath. Breath-holding is usually followed by an involuntary period of laryngospasm secondary to the presence of liquid in the oropharynx or larynx.[12] During this period of breath-holding and laryngospasm, the victim is unable to breathe gas. This results in oxygen being depleted and carbon dioxide not being eliminated. The victim then becomes hypercarbic, hypoxemic, and acidotic.[13] During this time the victim will frequently swallow large quantities of water.[14] The victim's respiratory movements may become very active, but there is no exchange of air because of the obstruction at the level of the larynx. As the victim's arterial oxygen tension drops further, laryngospasm abates, and the victim actively breathes liquid.[15] The amount of liquid inhaled varies considerably from victim to victim. Changes occur in the lungs, body fluids, blood-gas tensions, acid-base balance,

Critical Concept Prevention of Drowning	• Keep only a few inches of water in the bathtub when bathing young children. Never leave young children unsupervised in bathtubs. • Never leave children alone in or near a pool even for a moment, regardless of safety precautions such as self-locking gate and pool alarms. • Be sure adults and adolescents are trained in CPR so that they can rescue a child if necessary. • Surround your pool on all 4 sides with a sturdy 5-foot fence. The house should not form one of the barriers to the pool if there is a doorway from the home to the pool area. Be sure that the gates self-close and self-latch at a height that children cannot reach. • Keep rescue equipment—a shepherd's hook (a long pole with a hook on the end) and a life preserver—and a portable telephone near the pool. • Avoid inflatable swimming aids such as "floaties." They are *not* a substitute for approved life vests and can give children a false sense of security. • Generally children are not developmentally ready for swim lessons until after their fourth birthday.[10] Swim programs for children under 4 should *not* be seen as a way to decrease the risk of drowning. • Whenever infants or toddlers are in or around water, an adult should be within arm's length, providing "touch supervision."

and electrolyte concentrations, which are dependent on the composition and volume of the liquid aspirated and duration of submersion.[13,15,16] Surfactant washout, pulmonary hypertension, and shunting also contribute to development of hypoxemia.[17,18] Additional physiological derangements, such as the cold shock response, may occur in victims immersed in cold water. Water that is 10°C (50°F) or colder has pronounced cardiovascular effects, including increased blood pressure and ectopic tachyarrhythmias. The response may also trigger a gasp reflex followed by hyperventilation, which may occur while the victim is underwater.[19]

A victim may recover from the initial resuscitative efforts, with or without subsequent therapy to eliminate hypoxia, hypercarbia, and acidosis and restore normal organ function. If the victim is not ventilated soon enough or does not start to breathe on his or her own, circulatory arrest will ensue. The development of posthypoxic encephalopathy with or without cerebral edema is the most common cause of death in hospitalized drowning patients.[20,21] The duration of hypoxia is the critical determinant of drowning outcome. The duration of hypoxia can be reduced first by early rescue from the water, then by immediate provision of basic and advanced life support.

Providers should be prepared to treat trauma or hypothermia in drowning patients. Although the incidence of cervical spine injury is low, some patients whose drownings are associated with trauma, such as a dive or fall into water,[22] may need cervical spine (C-spine) immobilization. Otherwise, unnecessary C-spine immobilization may delay or interfere with rescue breaths. Primary or secondary hypothermia may develop in drowning patients. *Primary hypothermia* can develop when a drowning occurs in icy water (colder than 5°C or 41°F). In icy water, core body hypothermia may develop before significant hypoxia occurs. It is possible that such cold-water submersion may provide some protection from hypoxia and organ ischemia. *Secondary hypothermia* occurs as a consequence of heat loss through evaporation after rescue from the water and during attempted resuscitation. Hypothermia in these patients offers no known protective effects.

Drowning Outcomes: Research and Reporting

Uniform Definitions of Drowning

To aid in the use of consistent terminology and the uniform reporting of drowning data, the AHA recommends use of the Utstein definitions and style of data reporting[23]:

- **Drowning.** Drowning is a process resulting in primary respiratory impairment from submersion/immersion in a liquid medium. Implicit in this definition is that a liquid/air interface is present at the entrance of the victim's airway, preventing the victim from breathing air. The victim may live or die after this process, but whatever the outcome, he or she has been involved in a drowning incident.
- **Immersion.** Immersion is to be covered in water. For drowning to occur, usually at least the face and airway are immersed.
- **Submersion.** During submersion, the entire body, including the airway, is under water.
- **Water rescue.** Occurs when a person is alert but experiences some distress while swimming. The patient may receive some help from others and displays minimal, transient symptoms, such as coughing, that clear quickly.

The Utstein statement deemphasizes classification based on type of submersion fluid (salt water versus fresh water).

The most important factors that determine outcome of drowning are the duration and severity of the hypoxia.

Drowning Outcome Prediction

The Challenges

Emergency care providers face a number of difficult questions when attempting resuscitation of drowning patients. Accurate outcome prediction would assist providers in recognizing fatal drowning events for which resuscitative efforts should not be started and drowning events for which resuscitative efforts should be stopped in the field.

Research in Outcome Prediction

Retrospective analyses of a large observational database of drownings in children and adolescents (up to 20 years of age) from King County and Seattle, Washington, confirmed duration of submersion as the most powerful predictor of outcome.[24-27] With increasing duration of submersion, the following associations with death or severe neurologic impairment were observed:

- 0 up to 5 minutes: 10%
- 5 up to 10 minutes: 56%
- 10 up to 25 minutes: 88%
- 25 minutes or longer, 100%

Note how 5 more minutes of submersion in the second group (5 up to 10 minutes) increases mortality almost 6-fold compared with the first group (0 up to 5 minutes).

The following factors have been associated with 100% mortality[26]:

- Submersion duration 25 minutes or longer
- Resuscitation duration longer than 25 minutes
- Pulseless cardiac arrest on arrival in the ED
- No return of consciousness (patient was comatose at the scene and on arrival at the hospital)

Drowning patients who have spontaneous circulation and breathing in the field, before arrival at the ED, usually recover with good neurologic outcomes. In the King County database, no deaths occurred among patients who were responsive at the scene or in the ED.[24]

Several classification systems have attempted to use clinical findings as predictors of outcome for drowning patients.[28,29] The most coherent and logical approach derives from a long-term analysis of 1831 drowning episodes from the beaches of Brazil.[28] Unlike other researchers in this area, Szpilman and colleagues[28] derived the classification grades empirically after recognizing that the worse the cardiopulmonary compromise, the worse the mortality rate (Table 71).

Table 71. **Severity Grades for Drowning Events Based on Clinical Findings With Associated Mortality Rates**

Severity Grade	Clinical Findings	Mortality (%)[30]
1	Some coughing, normal auscultation	0
2	Coughing; with abnormal auscultation: rales in some lung fields on one side	0.6
3	Coughing; abnormal auscultation with acute pulmonary edema (bilateral rales); good cardiac function (no hypotension)	5.2
4	Coughing; abnormal auscultation with acute pulmonary edema (bilateral rales) with poor cardiac function (hypotension)	19.4
5	No spontaneous respirations, pulse is present	44
6	Cardiopulmonary arrest: no spontaneous breathing, no pulse	93

Uniform Reporting of Drowning Data: The Utstein Style

The Utstein guidelines recommend core and supplemental data to collect on drownings (Table 72). Most resuscitations begin at the scene of the drowning and not at a hospital, which makes on-scene data extremely important. Furthermore, many, or possibly most, drowning patients have mild symptoms, recover at the scene, and may or may not be transported to a hospital.

Precipitating Events

In each case of drowning, the precipitating event should be reported if known. Drowning is sometimes precipitated by an injury or a medical condition. Seizure is the most common initiating event in all age groups.[30] Loss of consciousness from any cause, however, such as hyperventilation before breath-holding under water, concussion, stroke, or cardiac arrhythmia, may result in drowning. When assessing a drowning incident, it is important to recognize the role of intentional injury, suicide, homicide, and child abuse. Hypothermia, alcohol, and drugs may impair motor function and judgment. Moreover, alcohol may affect the cardiovascular response to submersion.[31,32] Several precipitating events, such as seizures, alcohol use, and hypothermia, are associated with an increased risk of death from drowning.[33,34]

Table 72. Recommended Data to Report for Drownings: The Utstein Style[23]

	Core	Supplemental
Victim information	• Victim identifier • Gender • Age (estimate if necessary) • Date and time of day of incident • Precipitating event: known/unknown (if known, then specify)	• Race or ethnic category • Residence (city, county, state, country) • Preexisting illness: yes/no (If yes, then specify)
Scene information	• Witnessed (submersion is observed): yes/no • Body of water: bathtub, swimming pool, ocean, lake, river, or other bodies of water or containers • Unconscious when removed from water: yes/no • Resuscitation before EMS arrived: yes/no • EMS called: yes/no • Initial vital signs (spontaneous breathing, palpable pulse) • Time of first EMS resuscitation attempt • Neurologic status: ABC or other neurologic assessment (AVPU, GCS)	• Water/liquid type: fresh, salt, chemical, other • Approximate water temperature: nonicy, icy • Time of submersion if known • Time of removal of victim from water if known • Cyanosis • If patient received resuscitation before EMS arrived, who gave CPR? Layperson, lifeguard, etc • Method of CPR: MTM, ventilation alone, MTM-CC, CC only, automated external defibrillation • EMS vehicle dispatched: yes/no • Time of first EMS assessment • Oxygen saturation, temperature, blood pressure, pupillary reaction (optional)
ED evaluation and treatment	• Vital signs: temperature, heart rate, respiratory rate, blood pressure • Oxygen hemoglobin saturation • Arterial blood gas analysis if unconscious or Sao_2 <95% on room air • Initial neurologic status (GCS, AVPU, or ABC) • Airway and ventilation requirements	• Pupillary reaction • Toxicology testing: blood alcohol level and other drugs
Hospital course	• Airway and ventilation requirements	• Serial neurologic function (admission, 6 hours, 24 hours, 72 hours, discharge) • Complicating illnesses
Disposition	• Alive or dead (if dead, report date, place, and time of death) • Date of hospital discharge • Neurologic outcome at hospital discharge	• Quality of life (OPC, CPC, other) • Cause of death: **1.** How was cause of death determined? **2.** Autopsy: yes/no **3.** Forensic information (suicide, homicide?) • Other injuries and morbidities

Abbreviations: ABC, awake, blunted, comatose; AVPU, Alert, responds to Verbal stimuli, responds to Painful stimuli, Unresponsive to all stimuli; CC, chest compression; CPC, cerebral performance category; CPR, cardiopulmonary resuscitation; ED, emergency department; EMS, emergency medical services; GCS, Glasgow Coma Scale; MTM, mouth-to-mouth; OPC, overall performance category.

Time Intervals and Time Points (Events)

The importance of time intervals in resuscitation science is exemplified by the duration of submersion. The number of minutes submersed is a measure of the period of hypoxic insult. Although this information is usually estimated by bystanders and is often inaccurate, it has been correlated with survival.[27,35-38]

Outcome

The primary outcome of a drowning episode should be categorized as either death or survival. *Survival* indicates that the patient remained alive after the acute event and any acute or subacute sequelae. For example, survival is the outcome of drowning patients who were successfully resuscitated from cardiac or respiratory arrest and were then discharged from the hospital or survived initially and subsequently died of other causes. A drowning in which the patient is successfully resuscitated at the scene but succumbs to a condition that is causally related to the drowning should be categorized as a *death due to drowning*.

Following are examples of common sequelae leading to death from drowning. The most common cause of death in hospitalized drowning victims is posthypoxic encephalopathy.

- Brain death attributable to severe hypoxic or ischemic brain injury
- Acute respiratory distress syndrome
- Multiorgan system dysfunction secondary to severe hypoxic or ischemic insult
- Sepsis syndrome attributable to aspiration pneumonia or nosocomial infections

Although differentiating death from survival is usually easy, judgment occasionally is required to determine whether death after illnesses such as aspiration pneumonia or septic shock is causally related to the drowning episode. A death in the first few days or weeks after a drowning episode would generally be judged to be attributable to the drowning because the chain of causation is clear. There is no time limit between the drowning event and death if there is a clear chain of causality.

The survival category can be subclassified in terms of severity and type of morbidities, such as neurologic impairment or respiratory impairment (eg, ventilator dependence).

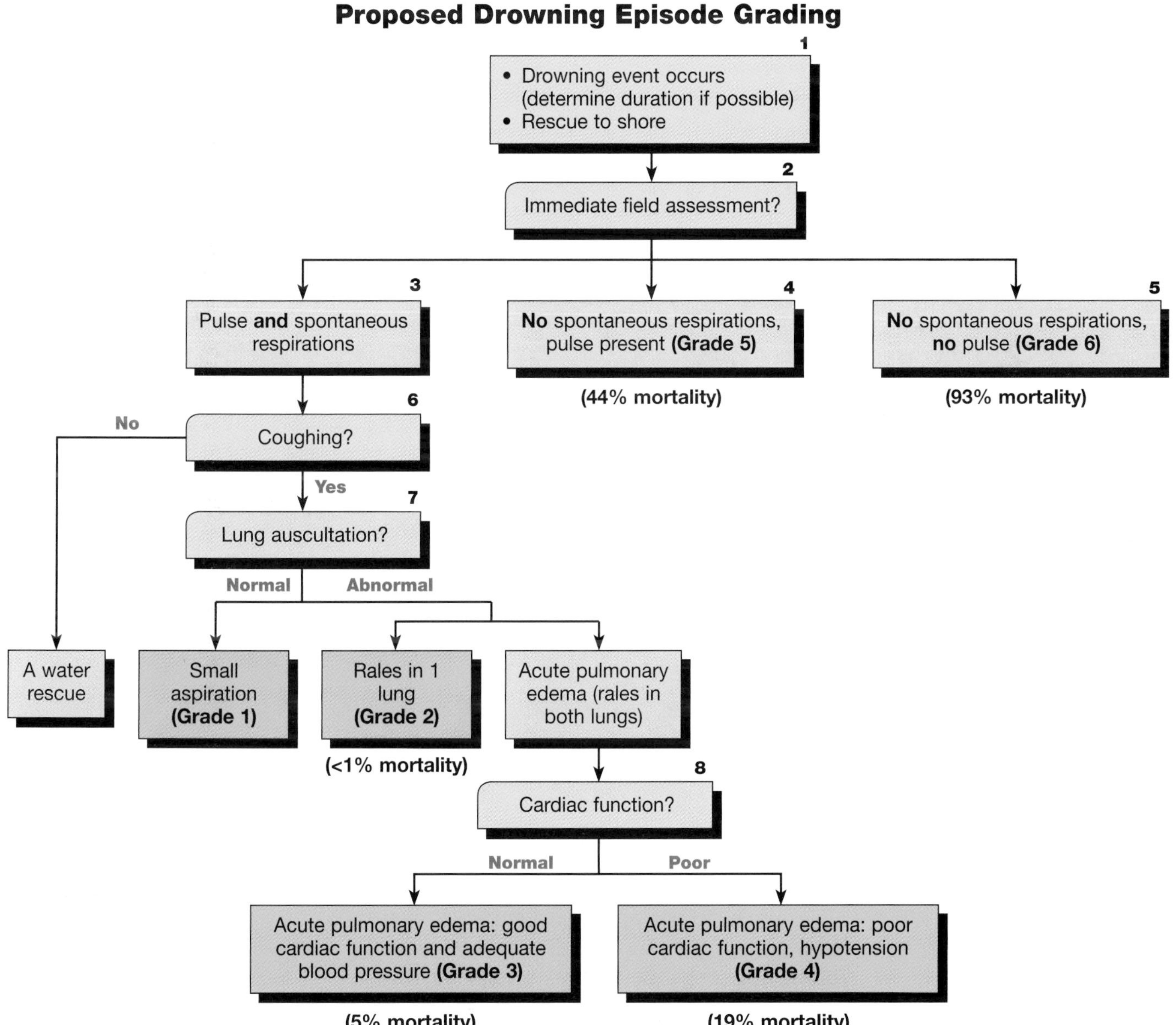

Figure 118. Proposed algorithm for grading of drowning episodes to facilitate uniform international reporting.

Proposed Approach to Grading Drowning Events

To stimulate international discussion of the shortcomings of submersion nomenclature and initiate preliminary solutions, participants in the International Guidelines 2000 Conference on Cardiopulmonary Resuscitation (CPR) and Emergency Cardiovascular Care (ECC) developed an approach to grading drowning episodes (Figure 118). This algorithm can be used by epidemiologists to support a prospective database of drowning cases.

The algorithm is largely derived from the work of Szpilman and his Brazilian collaborators.[28] It has been validated retrospectively, demonstrating a relationship to outcomes (Table 71).

The Proposed Drowning Episode Grading Algorithm: Underlying Concepts

The pathophysiology of drowning represents a continuum from the moment of submersion (head slips under the water), followed by some degree of aspiration, ineffective and then absent breathing, and then progressive hypoxia leading to irreversible apnea, and then asystole (drowning death). An effective grading system needs to reflect the clinical signs demonstrated in patients rescued during the various stages of the drowning process.

- **Submersion:** The initial stage is an actual submersion. The head slips under water (or other liquid), there is no access to air, and some hypoxia develops with some aspiration of fluid into the hypopharynx, trachea, and lungs.
- **Aspiration:** Experienced observers consider entrance of water into the respiratory passages with resultant stimulation of gag and cough reflexes as an essential stage in drowning events. Coughing is a critical dichotomous assessment point (Number 6). If the patient is not coughing and has normal lung auscultation, the patient is classified as a *water rescue*. Modell[29] eloquently presents the range of submersion events that observers describe.
- **Apnea or breathlessness:** Absence of spontaneous breathing is an unambiguous physical sign that also relates to outcomes.
- **Spontaneous circulation:** If the period of hypoxia is prolonged, the heart stops beating.

Algorithm for Drowning Episodes

Number 1

- A drowning event occurs. If possible, determine the duration of submersion.
- If the provider can do so safely, the provider should open the patient's airway and check breathing and provide rescue breaths in the water if needed.
- Proceed with rescue to shore. Pay close attention to safety of both provider and patient. Take C-spine precautions (maintain cervical spine immobilization) *only* as indicated.

Number 2

- After the patient is rescued to shore (or another firm surface), immediately initiate the BLS assessments.
- Immediately initiate all indicated BLS, ACLS, and pediatric resuscitation interventions based on the presence or absence of a patent airway, spontaneous respirations, and spontaneous pulse. These interventions include the following:
  - Send a second provider to phone 911. The lone provider should check for response and breathing almost simultaneously. It is reasonable for the lone provider to administer 5 cycles (about 2 minutes) of CPR before leaving the victim to activate the EMS system.
  - Provide basic life support, including all elements of the primary survey steps. When indicated, provide ventilations and chest compressions. Continue until a defibrillator is available.
  - Once an AED or manual defibrillator is available, check for the presence of VF/VT ("shockable rhythm") and deliver a defibrillatory shock if indicated.
  - Provide advanced adult and pediatric life support, including insertion of airway devices, establishment of IV access, and administration of IV medications.

Number 3

- Drowning patients with spontaneous respirations and a sustained pulse are classified on the basis of 3 criteria:
  - Coughing (Number 6)
  - Lung auscultation (Number 7)
  - Cardiac function, eg, blood pressure (Number 8)

Number 4

- Drowning patients who have no spontaneous respirations but have a detectable pulse are classified as Grade 5. The Brazilian study showed that by using rapid BLS- and ACLS-level response teams, 56% of drowning patients with a severity of Grade 5 survived to hospital discharge.[28]

Critical Concept Lone Provider When To Activate EMS	If hypoxia is the presumed cause of cardiac arrest (such as in a drowning patient), the lone healthcare provider may give about 5 cycles (approximately 2 minutes) of CPR before activating the emergency response system.

- If spontaneous respirations cannot be restored during resuscitative efforts and spontaneous cardiac activity ceases (asystole), treat as Grade 6 (Number 5).

Number 5

- Drowning patients who have no spontaneous respirations and no pulse on initial field assessment are classified as Grade 6. In the Brazilian study, only 7% of these nonbreathing, pulseless drowning patients survived to hospital discharge.[28]
- Patients who fail to respond to initial resuscitative efforts and fail to regain or sustain spontaneous respirations and pulse are classified as *deaths due to drowning*.

Number 6

- Assess whether the patient is coughing. Then auscultate the lungs.
- Coughing in drowning patients implies water aspiration.
- Drowning patients who are not coughing, have clear lungs on auscultation, and have maintained spontaneous circulation and respirations since rescue to shore are classified as *water rescues*.
- Drowning patients who are coughing repeatedly are further classified by the findings on lung auscultation.

Number 7

- The auscultation findings are used to further classify drowning patients with coughing:
  - Grade 1: Normal lung auscultation. Because these patients have been coughing, they are considered to have aspirated only a small amount of water.
  - Grade 2: Lung auscultation reveals some rales but in only one lung.
  - Grades 3 and 4: Lung auscultation reveals *acute pulmonary edema* (rales in both lungs). See Number 8 to separate Grade 3 from Grade 4.

Number 8

- In patients with acute pulmonary edema (rales in both lungs), cardiac function, and blood pressure, distinguish between Grades 3 and 4:
  - Grade 3: Good cardiac function and adequate blood pressure (5% mortality reported in Brazil[28])
  - Grade 4: Impaired cardiac function and hypotension (19% mortality reported in Brazil[28])

Drowning Outcome Prediction: Conclusions

Fate Factors but No System Factors for Drownings

The landmark work of Eisenberg et al[39] on out-of-hospital cardiac arrest identified what he termed *fate factors* and *system factors*.

- *Fate factors* are age, sex, initial arrest rhythm, location of arrest, and whether the arrest was witnessed.
- *System factors* include time to CPR, time to defibrillation, and time to and quality of early advanced care.

Multiple studies have established that drowning outcome is determined largely by a single fate factor—*duration of submersion*.[26-28,35,40] The longer it takes to identify and rescue a drowning person, the worse the outcome.

Immediate bystander CPR can limit the duration of hypoxia to the time of submersion only. Delayed CPR results in a longer period of hypoxia.

Immediate provision of BLS and early ACLS contributes to the best outcome possible, given the duration of submersion. Nonetheless, the relative contributions of these interventions are modest at best. Table 73 shows that early BLS and ACLS significantly improve the chances of survival. But these data also show the greater power that duration of submersion exerts over outcome.

Although survival from drowning episodes has increased in recent years, this increase does not appear to be attributable to improvements in medical treatment.[25]

Table 73. Probability of Neurologically Intact Survival to Hospital Discharge Based on Duration of Submersion and Time to Basic and Advanced Life Support* (Extrapolated From Published Data[26-28,35,40])

Duration of Submersion (minutes)	Probability of Survival With Late BLS and Late ACLS	Probability of Survival With Early BLS and Late ACLS	Probability of Survival With Immediate BLS and ACLS
0 to <5	70%	80%	90%
5 to <10	30%	35%	44%
10 to <25	3%	5%	12%
≥25	0%	0%	0%

**Late* is defined as BLS and ACLS personnel arriving more than 10 minutes after water rescue; early, BLS personnel arrive in less than 10 minutes after water rescue; and *immediate*, BLS and ACLS personnel are present when patient is recovered from the water.

"Do-Not-Start" and "When-to-Stop" Guidelines for Drowning Events

Among drowning patients who are in cardiopulmonary arrest upon rescue from the water (Grade 6 drowning), very few are going to survive. As a rule of thumb, about half of patients submerged for 5 to 10 minutes are pulseless upon water rescue.[26-28] It may seem reasonable to develop do-not-start and when-to-stop guidelines based on objective information on the duration of submersion. However, there have been cases of successful resuscitation after prolonged submersion.

- Virtually all patients who ultimately survive after a Grade 6 drowning (not breathing, no pulse) will demonstrate a pulse in the field after a period of full BLS and ACLS interventions.
- In data from King County, Washington, no one survived to hospital discharge if spontaneous circulation did not return within 25 minutes of the start of resuscitative efforts.[24,25]
- Although survival is uncommon in victims who have undergone prolonged submersion and require prolonged resuscitation,[27,41] successful resuscitation with full neurologic recovery has occurred occasionally after prolonged submersion in icy water[42-45] and, in some instances, warm water.[46,47] For this reason, scene resuscitation should be initiated and the victim transported to the ED unless there is obvious death (eg, rigor mortis, decomposition, hemisection, decapitation, lividity).

BLS Guidelines for Drowning Patients

Provider Safety

A cardinal rule of emergency medicine holds that the provider's primary obligation is to his or her personal safety. The provider must avoid creating "a second patient." Providers should never attempt risky actions that are beyond the scope of their training and experience.

Recovery From the Water

When attempting to rescue a drowning person, the rescuer should get to the person as quickly as possible, preferably by some conveyance (boat, raft, surfboard, or flotation device). Routine stabilization of the cervical spine in the absence of circumstances that suggest a spinal injury is not recommended (Class III, LOE B) (see "Associated Trauma" later in this chapter). Unnecessary cervical spine immobilization can impede adequate opening of the airway and delay delivery of rescue breaths.

The Most Important Treatment for the Drowning Patient: Immediate Ventilation

The most important and detrimental consequence of submersion is hypoxia; therefore, oxygenation, ventilation, and perfusion should be restored as quickly as possible. This will require immediate bystander CPR plus activation of the EMS system. With the updated *2010 AHA Guidelines for CPR and ECC*, the new C-A-B sequence was introduced. However, the guidelines recommend individualization in this sequence based on the presumed etiology of the arrest. CPR for drowning victims should use the traditional A-B-C approach because of the hypoxic nature of the arrest.

The first and most important treatment for the drowning patient is the immediate provision of ventilation. Prompt initiation of rescue breathing increases the patient's chance of survival.[48] Mouth-to-mouth ventilation in the water may be helpful when administered by a trained rescuer (Class IIb, LOE C).[49] However, rescue breathing is usually performed when the unresponsive victim is in shallow water or out of the water. If it is difficult for the rescuer to pinch the victim's nose, support the head, and open the airway in the water, mouth-to-nose ventilation may be used as an alternative to mouth-to-mouth ventilation. Victims with only respiratory arrest usually respond after a few rescue breaths are given. Untrained rescuers should not try to provide care while the victim is still in deep water.

Flotation devices and some appliances can facilitate support of airway and breathing in the water if providers are trained in their use. Providers should not delay rescue breathing for lack of such equipment if they can otherwise provide it safely.

No Need to Drain Water From the Lungs

Management of the drowning patient's airway and breathing is similar to that recommended for any patient in cardiopulmonary arrest. There is no need to clear the airway of aspirated water. Only a modest amount of water is aspirated by the majority of drowning victims, and it is rapidly absorbed into the central circulation, so it does not act as an obstruction in the trachea.[41,50] Some patients aspirate nothing because they develop laryngospasm or breath-holding.[29,41] Most fluid obtained from attempts to drain the lungs comes from the stomach and not from the lungs.[50]

The Heimlich maneuver for submersion patients should be reserved for patients with foreign-body airway obstruction or choking.[51,52] The routine use of abdominal thrusts or

Critical Concept	CPR for drowning victims should use the traditional A-B-C approach because of the hypoxic nature of the arrest.

Critical Concept **Abdominal Thrusts and the Heimlich Maneuver**	• Attempts to remove water from the airway by any means other than suction (eg, abdominal thrusts or the Heimlich maneuver) are unnecessary and potentially dangerous. • The routine use of abdominal thrusts or the Heimlich maneuver is not recommended (Class III, LOE C).

the Heimlich maneuver for drowning victims is not recommended (Class III, LOE C). Such maneuvers may cause injury, vomiting, aspiration, and delay of CPR.[50]

Chest Compressions

As soon as the drowning patient is removed from the water, the rescuer should open the airway, check for breathing, and if there is no breathing, give 2 rescue breaths that make the chest rise (if this was not done in the water). After delivery of 2 effective breaths, the lay rescuer should immediately begin chest compressions and provide cycles of compressions and ventilations according to the BLS guidelines. When rescuing a drowning victim of any age, it is reasonable for the lone healthcare provider to give 5 cycles (about 2 minutes) of CPR before leaving the victim to activate the EMS system.

Chest compressions are difficult to perform in water; they may not be effective and could potentially cause harm to both the rescuer and the victim. In general, providers should attempt chest compressions only on shore or on board a stable vessel or floating surface. External chest compressions can be performed in the water if rigid flotation devices are used or if the patient is extremely small and can be supported on the provider's forearm. Only trained rescuers should try to provide chest compressions in the water.

Vomiting During Resuscitation

The victim may vomit during chest compressions or rescue breathing, complicating efforts to maintain a patent airway. In a 10-year study in Australia, two thirds of patients who received rescue breathing and 86% of those who required compressions and ventilations vomited.[40] If vomiting occurs, turn the patient's mouth to the side and remove the vomitus using a finger, a cloth, or by suction. If spinal cord injury is possible, logroll the patient so that the head, neck, and torso are turned as a unit to protect the cervical spine.

Defibrillation by BLS Providers

Although most drowning patients demonstrate asystole, some patients may demonstrate VF/pulseless VT. Once the patient is out of the water, if the patient is unresponsive and not breathing after the delivery of 2 rescue breaths, rescuers should attach an AED and attempt defibrillation if a shockable rhythm is identified. It is only necessary to dry the chest area before applying the defibrillation pads and using the AED.

You cannot safely attempt defibrillation in standing water. Patients must be moved out of standing water. Dry the patient's chest before attaching electrodes for monitoring or for defibrillation. Deliver up to 5 cycles of CPR (about 2 minutes) and a shock. Then if you suspect hypothermia, evaluate the patient's core body temperature. If the patient's core body temperature is below 30°C (below 86°F) and VF persists, follow the recommendations for ACLS in the presence of hypothermia (Chapter 21).

Associated Trauma

Drowning events may be associated with trauma, and the issue of cervical spine immobilization is a difficult one. If the likelihood of head, neck, or spinal cord injury is significant, the provider should immobilize the head and neck and open the airway with a jaw thrust. But these maneuvers take time and may delay effective provision of rescue breathing.

- Providers should suspect spinal injuries in all drownings associated with diving; body, wind, or board surfing; falls from motorboats or sailboats; hang gliding; parasailing; falls from or crashes of personal watercraft; water slides; and in patients with signs of injury or alcohol intoxication.[22] Providers should immobilize the cervical spine for these patients.
- *Routine stabilization of the cervical spine in the absence of circumstances that suggest a spinal injury is not recommended (Class III, LOE B).* The reported incidence of cervical spine injury in drowning victims is low (0.0009%).[53,54] In a retrospective survey of more than 2244 drownings, only 11 patients (less than 0.5%) had a C-spine injury, and all 11 had obvious trauma from diving, falling from height, or a motor vehicle crash.[22]

First-responding providers who suspect a spinal cord injury should

Critical Concept **Provide CPR**	Providers should give CPR, particularly rescue breathing, as soon as an unresponsive submersion victim is removed from the water (Class I, LOE C).

- Use their hands to stabilize the patient's neck in a neutral position (without flexion or extension).
- Open the airway using a jaw thrust without head tilt or chin lift. This method of airway opening is very difficult to perform in water, so the provider must weigh the likelihood of cervical spine injury against the need for immediate rescue breathing in the water.
- Provide rescue breathing while maintaining the head in a neutral position.
- Float the patient, supine, onto a horizontal back-support device before removing the patient from the water.
- Align and support the head, neck, chest, and body if the patient must be turned.
- If you must move the patient, use a logroll.

Associated Hypothermia

When a patient is hypothermic, respiration and pulse may be slow or difficult to detect.

- Carefully assess breathing and confirm respiratory arrest.
- Check the pulse for 10 seconds.

If the patient fails to respond to initial BLS, providers should evaluate the core temperature as soon as possible to rule out hypothermia. The provider should consider prolonging resuscitation attempts for a Grade 6 drowning patient if the patient's core temperature is below 30°C (86°F). A core temperature at this level is an indication for active internal rewarming. To treat associated hypothermia, remove wet garments, dry the patient as soon as possible, and provide active rewarming. When hypothermia is present, use the following approach *without interrupting CPR:*

- Cover the patient with blankets or other materials to provide passive rewarming and to prevent further heat loss.
- Obtain rectal or tympanic (core body) temperature as soon as practical, and initiate hypothermia protocols as indicated in the Hypothermia Algorithm (Chapter 21).
- If significant hypothermia is thought to be present, resuscitative efforts should continue until core temperature is measured to ensure that hypothermia is not contributing to ineffective resuscitative efforts. Patients should not be considered dead before warming has been provided.
- If the core temperature is above 34°C (93.2°F), passive rewarming is generally adequate.
- If a patient has a core temperature between 30°C (86°F) and 34°C (93.2°F) and a perfusing rhythm, external warming techniques are appropriate.

Consider the potential for hypothermia in all drowning events, especially when the initial immersion occurs in cold water. It is important to recognize that immersion in cold water is more likely to result in hypoxia than in development of protective central hypothermia.[55-57] This occurs because swimming in cold water typically produces a sequence of exhaustion, "swim failure" (inability to maintain horizontal swimming angle, with the body becoming more vertical relative to the water surface), submersion, the beginning of the drowning process, and finally hypoxia. This potentially terminal hypoxia occurs at relatively modest levels of central hypothermia that are insufficient to prevent organ ischemia (Chapter 21).

ACLS Guidelines for Drowning Patients

Airway and Breathing

The submersion patient in cardiac arrest requires ACLS, including an advanced airway.

Early endotracheal intubation is valuable for

- Improved oxygenation and ventilation
- Direct removal of foreign material from the tracheobronchial tree
- Application of continuous positive airway pressure (CPAP) or positive end-expiratory pressure (PEEP)

Circulation and Defibrillation

Patients in cardiac arrest may present with asystole (most common), pulseless electrical activity, or pulseless VF/VT. In children and adolescents, VF/VT on the initial ECG is an extremely poor prognostic sign. Providers should follow the appropriate PALS, BLS, or ACLS guidelines for treatment of these rhythms. Treat drowning patients with hypothermic cardiac arrest according to the recommendations for hypothermia:

- Defibrillation attempts should occur concurrent to rewarming. The value of deferring subsequent defibrillations until a target temperature is reached is uncertain. It may be reasonable to perform further defibrillation attempts according to the standard BLS algorithm.
- It may be reasonable to consider administration of a vasopressor during cardiac arrest according to the standard ACLS algorithm concurrent with rewarming strategies.

Critical Concept **Consider Hypothermia**	Consider the potential for hypothermia in all drowning events. • Immersion in cold water is more likely to result in hypoxia than in development of protective central hypothermia. • Terminal hypoxia occurs at relatively modest levels of central hypothermia that are insufficient to prevent organ ischemia.

Critical Concept **Transport of Drowning Patients**	All victims of drowning who require any form of resuscitation (including rescue breathing alone) should be transported to the hospital for evaluation and monitoring, even if they appear to be alert and demonstrate effective cardiorespiratory function at the scene (Class I, LOE C).

Case reports document the use of surfactant for fresh water–induced respiratory distress,[58,59] but further research is needed. The use of extracorporeal membrane oxygenation in patients with severe hypothermia after submersion has been documented in case reports.[44,45] There is insufficient evidence to support or refute the use of barbiturates, steroids, nitric oxide, therapeutic hypothermia after return of spontaneous circulation (ROSC), or vasopressin.

Summary

- Prevention remains the most powerful therapeutic intervention for drowning.
- *Immediate provision of ventilations is the first and most important treatment for drowning.*
- In 2003 international consensus guidelines for uniform definitions and reporting of data from studies of drowning incidents (the Utstein style) were published.[23]
- Drowning events must be graded by severity. This grading is based on the clinical signs, ranging from simple aspiration with coughing to apnea with a beating heart to cardiopulmonary arrest (no breathing, no pulse).
- When treating drowning patients, providers should consider the possibility of associated trauma and associated hypothermia.
  - A history or strong suspicion of trauma associated with a drowning event is the major indication for C-spine immobilization.
  - Routine C-spine immobilization for all drowning patients is not recommended because it may compromise the delivery of rescue breathing.
  - The neuroprotective value of hypothermia for drowning patients in cardiac arrest is probably exaggerated. This effect is possible only when the hypothermia is severe (core body temperature is below 30°C [86°F]) and body cooling preceded the hypoxia that develops during submersion.
- ACLS personnel should strongly support effective prevention activities, which may at times require legislative and regulatory initiatives. Important prevention activities include
  - Unremitting, responsible, and mature adult supervision for all infants and children when near any source of the 1 to 2 inches of water necessary for a drowning death
  - Safe pool design with self-closing, self-locking gates and fencing that encloses the pool on all sides
  - Trained lifeguards at public pools and beaches
  - Public swim areas fully equipped with rigid backboards, cervical collars, and BLS supplies, including AEDs
  - Swimming and lifesaving classes
  - Lay provider CPR-AED training
  - Widespread availability and appropriate use of personal flotation devices

References

1. Peden MM, McGee K. The epidemiology of drowning worldwide. *Inj Control Saf Promot*. 2003;10:195-199.
2. Weir E. Drowning in Canada. *CMAJ*. 2000;162:1867.
3. Steensberg J. Epidemiology of accidental drowning in Denmark 1989-1993. *Accid Anal Prev*. 1998;30:755-762.
4. Mackie IJ. Patterns of drowning in Australia, 1992-1997. *Med J Aust*. 1999;171:587-590.
5. Mizuta R, Fujita H, Osamura T, Kidowaki T, Kiyosawa N. Childhood drownings and near-drownings in Japan. *Acta Paediatr Jpn*. 1993;35:186-192.
6. Mogayzel C, Quan L, Graves JR, Tiedeman D, Fahrenbruch C, Herndon P. Out-of-hospital ventricular fibrillation in children and adolescents: causes and outcomes. *Ann Emerg Med*. 1995;25:484-491.
7. Quan L, Bennett E, Cummings P, Henderson P, Del Beccaro MA. Do parents value drowning prevention information at discharge from the emergency department? *Ann Emerg Med*. 2001;37:382-385.
8. Jensen LR, Williams SD, Thurman DJ, Keller PA. Submersion injuries in children younger than 5 years in urban Utah. *West J Med*. 1992;157:641-644.
9. Pitt WR, Cass DT. Preventing children drowning in Australia. *Med J Aust*. 2001;175:603-604.
10. Committee on Sports Medicine and Fitness and Committee on Injury and Poison Prevention, American Academy of Pediatrics. Swimming programs for infants and toddlers. *Pediatrics*. 2000;105:868-870.
11. American Academy of Pediatrics Committee on Injury, Violence, and Poison Prevention. Prevention of drowning. *Pediatrics*. 2010;126:178-185.
12. Miller RD, ed. *Anesthesia*. Philadelphia, PA: Churchill Livingstone; 2000:1416-1417.
13. Modell JH, Gaub M, Moya F, Vestal B, Swarz H. Physiologic effects of near drowning with chlorinated fresh water, distilled water and isotonic saline. *Anesthesiology*. 1966;27:33-41.
14. Modell JH, Graves SA, Ketover A. Clinical course of 91 consecutive near-drowning victims. *Chest*. 1976;70:231-238.
15. Modell JH, Moya F. Effects of volume of aspirated fluid during chlorinated fresh water drowning. *Anesthesiology*. 1966;27:662-672.
16. Modell JH, Moya F, Newby EJ, Ruiz BC, Showers AV. The effects of fluid volume in seawater drowning. *Ann Intern Med*. 1967;67:68-80.
17. Halmagyi DF, Colebatch HJ. Ventilation and circulation after fluid aspiration. *J Appl Physiol*. 1961;16:35-40.
18. Giammona ST, Modell JH. Drowning by total immersion. Effects on pulmonary surfactant of distilled water, isotonic saline, and sea water. *Am J Dis Child*. 1967;114:612-616.

19. Tipton MJ. The initial responses to cold-water immersion in man. *Clin Sci (Lond)*. 1989;77:581-588.
20. Conn AW, Montes JE, Barker GA, Edmonds JF. Cerebral salvage in near-drowning following neurological classification by triage. *Can Anaesth Soc J*. 1980;27:201-210.
21. Eriksson R, Fredin H, Gerdman P, Thorson J. Sequelae of accidental near-drowning in childhood. *Scand J Soc Med*. 1973;1:3-6.
22. Watson RS, Cummings P, Quan L, Bratton S, Weiss NS. Cervical spine injuries among submersion victims. *J Trauma*. 2001;51:658-662.
23. Idris AH, Berg RA, Bierens J, Bossaert L, Branche CM, Gabrielli A, Graves SA, Handley AJ, Hoelle R, Morley PT, Papa L, Pepe PE, Quan L, Szpilman D, Wigginton JG, Modell JH. Recommended guidelines for uniform reporting of data from drowning: the "Utstein style." *Circulation*. 2003;108:2565-2574.
24. Cummings P, Quan L. Trends in unintentional drowning: the role of alcohol and medical care. *JAMA*. 1999;281:2198-2202.
25. Quan L. Near-drowning. *Pediatr Rev*. 1999;20:255-259.
26. Quan L, Kinder D. Pediatric submersions: prehospital predictors of outcome. *Pediatrics*. 1992;90:909-913.
27. Quan L, Wentz KR, Gore EJ, Copass MK. Outcome and predictors of outcome in pediatric submersion victims receiving prehospital care in King County, Washington. *Pediatrics*. 1990;86:586-593.
28. Szpilman D. Near-drowning and drowning classification: a proposal to stratify mortality based on the analysis of 1,831 cases. *Chest*. 1997;112:660-665.
29. Modell JH. Drowning. *N Engl J Med*. 1993;328:253-256.
30. Quan L, Cummings P. Characteristics of drowning by different age groups. *Inj Prev*. 2003;9:163-168.
31. Plueckhahn VD. Alcohol and accidental drowning. A 25-year study. *Med J Aust*. 1984;141:22-25.
32. Plueckhahn VD. Alcohol consumption and death by drowning in adults; a 24-year epidemiological analysis. *J Stud Alcohol*. 1982;43:445-452.
33. Diekema DS, Quan L, Holt VL. Epilepsy as a risk factor for submersion injury in children. *Pediatrics*. 1993;91:612-616.
34. Smith GS, Keyl PM, Hadley JA, Bartley CL, Foss RD, Tolbert WG, McKnight J. Drinking and recreational boating fatalities: a population-based case-control study. *JAMA*. 2001;286:2974-2980.
35. Suominen P, Baillie C, Korpela R, Rautanen S, Ranta S, Olkkola KT. Impact of age, submersion time and water temperature on outcome in near-drowning. *Resuscitation*. 2002;52:247-254.
36. Nussbaum E. Prognostic variables in nearly drowned, comatose children. *Am J Dis Child*. 1985;139:1058-1059.
37. Peterson B. Morbidity of childhood near-drowning. *Pediatrics*. 1977;59:364-370.
38. Kruus S, Bergstrom L, Suutarinen T, Hyvonen R. The prognosis of near-drowned children. *Acta Paediatr Scand*. 1979;68:315-322.
39. Eisenberg MS. Who shall live? Who shall die? In: Eisenberg MS, Bergner L, Hallstrom AP, eds. *Sudden Cardiac Death in the Community*. Philadelphia, PA: Praeger Scientific; 1984:44-58.
40. Manolios N, Mackie I. Drowning and near-drowning on Australian beaches patrolled by life-savers: a 10-year study, 1973-1983. *Med J Aust*. 1988;148:165-167, 170-161.
41. Modell JH, Davis JH. Electrolyte changes in human drowning victims. *Anesthesiology*. 1969;30:414-420.
42. Southwick FS, Dalglish PH Jr. Recovery after prolonged asystolic cardiac arrest in profound hypothermia: a case report and literature review. *JAMA*. 1980;243:1250-1253.
43. Siebke H, Rod T, Breivik H, Link B. Survival after 40 minutes; submersion without cerebral sequelae. *Lancet*. 1975;1:1275-1277.
44. Bolte RG, Black PG, Bowers RS, Thorne JK, Corneli HM. The use of extracorporeal rewarming in a child submerged for 66 minutes. *JAMA*. 1988;260:377-379.
45. Gilbert M, Busund R, Skagseth A, Nilsen PA, Solbo JP. Resuscitation from accidental hypothermia of 13.7 degrees C with circulatory arrest. *Lancet*. 2000;355:375-376.
46. Szpilman D, Soares M. In-water resuscitation—is it worthwhile? *Resuscitation*. 2004;63:25-31.
47. Allman FD, Nelson WB, Pacentine GA, McComb G. Outcome following cardiopulmonary resuscitation in severe pediatric near-drowning. *Am J Dis Child*. 1986;140:571-575.
48. Kyriacou DN, Arcinue EL, Peek C, Kraus JF. Effect of immediate resuscitation on children with submersion injury. *Pediatrics*. 1994;94:137-142.
49. Perkins GD. In-water resuscitation: a pilot evaluation. *Resuscitation*. 2005;65:321-324.
50. Rosen P, Stoto M, Harley J. The use of the Heimlich maneuver in near drowning: Institute of Medicine report. *J Emerg Med*. 1995;13:397-405.
51. Heimlich HJ. A life-saving maneuver to prevent food-choking. *JAMA*. 1975;234:398-401.
52. Patrick E. A case report: the Heimlich maneuver. *Emergency*. 1981;13:45-47.
53. Weinstein MD, Krieger BP. Near-drowning: epidemiology, pathophysiology, and initial treatment. *J Emerg Med*. 1996;14:461-467.
54. Watson RS, Cummings P, Quan L, Bratton S, Weiss NS. Cervical spine injuries among submersion victims. *J Trauma*. 2001;51:658-662.
55. Ryan JM. Immersion deaths and swim failure—implications for resuscitation and prevention. *Lancet*. 1999;354:613.
56. Teramoto S, Ouchi Y. Swimming in cold water. *Lancet*. 1999;354:1733.
57. Tipton M, Eglin C, Gennser M, Golden F. Immersion deaths and deterioration in swimming performance in cold water. *Lancet*. 1999;354:626-629.
58. Onarheim H, Vik V. Porcine surfactant (Curosurf) for acute respiratory failure after near-drowning in 12 year old. *Acta Anaesthesiol Scand*. 2004;48:778-781.
59. Cubattoli L, Franchi F, Coratti G. Surfactant therapy for acute respiratory failure after drowning: two children victim of cardiac arrest. *Resuscitation*. 2009;80:1088-1089.

Chapter 20

Cardiac Arrest Associated With Trauma

This Chapter

- **Rapid Scene Survey and Provider Safety First**
- **BLS and ACLS Modifications for Patients With Traumatic Injuries**
- **Emergency Thoracotomy and Penetrating Chest Trauma**
- **Poor Survival Guidelines: When to Withhold or Terminate Resuscitation**

Overview and Epidemiology

In industrialized nations, trauma is the leading cause of death from the age of 6 months through young adulthood,[1-3] and trauma is one of the top 5 causes of death overall.[4] In 2011 there were over 770 000 patients with traumatic injuries who were brought to emergency departments in the US with a mortality rate of 3.8.[5] The total number of deaths attributed to injuries by the CDC was about 175 000, so many victims do not make it to the hospital.[4] When anyone is severely injured, resuscitation must begin as soon as possible, preferably at the scene.[6] Early and effective support of airway, ventilation, oxygenation, and perfusion is vital because survival from out-of-hospital cardiac arrest secondary to blunt trauma is uniformly low in children and adults.[7-9] Following penetrating trauma, rapid transport to a trauma center is associated with better outcomes than prolonged resuscitative attempts in the field.[10]

Despite a rapid and effective out-of-hospital and trauma center response, patients with out-of-hospital cardiac arrest due to trauma rarely survive.[11-14] Those patients with the best outcome from trauma arrest generally are young, have treatable penetrating injuries, have received early (out-of-hospital) endotracheal intubation, and undergo prompt transport (typically in 10 minutes or less) to a trauma care facility.[13-16] Cardiac arrest in the field caused by blunt trauma is almost always fatal in all age groups.[7-9]

BLS and ACLS for the trauma patient are fundamentally the same as the care for a patient with a primary cardiac or respiratory arrest, with focus on support of airway, breathing, and circulation. After completion of the BLS Survey, the provider should perform a more detailed ACLS EP Survey. Use the **SAMPLE** mnemonic to identify important aspects of the patient's history and presenting complaint:

- **S**igns and symptoms
- **A**llergies
- **M**edications
- **P**ast medical history
- **L**ast meal
- **E**vents leading up to the scenario

In the trauma patient, reversible causes of cardiac arrest need to considered. While CPR in the pulseless trauma patient overall has been considered futile in the past, several reversible causes of cardiac arrest in the context of trauma are correctible, and their prompt treatment could be lifesaving.[17]

Potential causes of cardiopulmonary deterioration and arrest include the following:

- Severe central neurologic injury with secondary cardiovascular collapse
- Hypoxia secondary to respiratory insufficiency that results from neurologic injury, airway obstruction, large open pneumothorax, or severe tracheobronchial laceration or crush

- Direct and severe injury to vital structures such as the heart, aorta, or pulmonary arteries
- Underlying medical problems or other conditions that led to the injury, such as sudden cardiac arrest or stroke in the driver of a motor vehicle
- Severely diminished cardiac output from tension pneumothorax or pericardial tamponade
- Exsanguination leading to hypovolemia and severely diminished oxygen delivery
- Injuries in a cold environment (eg, fractured leg) complicated by secondary severe hypothermia

Initial Evaluation and Triage

Extricate and Evaluate

Specially trained providers should rapidly extricate the patient while immobilizing the cervical spine. Provide immediate BLS and ACLS interventions to ensure adequate airway, oxygenation, ventilation, and circulation. Prepare the patient for rapid transport to a facility that provides definitive trauma care. Use lateral neck supports, strapping, and backboards throughout transport to minimize exacerbation of an occult neck or spinal cord injury.

There is considerable evidence that out-of-hospital endotracheal intubation is either harmful or at best ineffective for most EMS patients.[18-21] Researchers and EMS leaders have also questioned the safety and effectiveness of aggressive out-of-hospital IV fluid resuscitation in an urban environment.[10,22-24] In addition, field ACLS interventions unquestionably prolong time at the scene, delay transport to the ED or trauma center, and thereby delay essential interventions such as surgical control of life-threatening bleeding.[24-27]

With the above discussion in mind, the focus of prehospital resuscitation should be to safely extricate and attempt to stabilize the patient and to minimize interventions that will delay transport to definitive care. Strict attention should be paid to stabilizing the spine during care. Patients suspected of having severe traumatic injuries should be transported or

Table 74. Guidelines for Withholding or Terminating Resuscitation in Prehospital Traumatic Cardiopulmonary Arrest[29,30]

A. Specific Criteria and Recommendations by Type of Trauma		
Patient in Cardiac Arrest Associated With Trauma Upon Arrival of EMS Personnel		
Type of Trauma	**Specific Criteria**	**Recommendations**
Blunt	• Thorough primary assessment finds patient to be apneic, pulseless, with no organized ECG activity	• Resuscitative efforts MAY BE WITHHELD
Penetrating	• Further assessment finds **POSITIVE** secondary signs of life (eg, pupillary reflexes, spontaneous movement, agonal respirations, organized ECG activity)	• START resuscitative efforts • TRANSPORT to nearest ED or trauma center
	• Further assessment finds **NO** secondary signs of life (eg, pupillary reflexes, spontaneous movement, agonal respirations, organized ECG activity)	• Resuscitative efforts MAY BE WITHHELD
Blunt or penetrating	• Injuries are obviously incompatible with life (eg, decapitation, hemicorporectomy)	• Resuscitative efforts SHOULD BE WITHHELD
	• Evidence of death (eg, dependent lividity, rigor mortis, decomposition)	
	• Possible nontraumatic cardiac arrest: mechanism of injury does not correlate with clinical condition	• START resuscitative efforts • TRANSPORT to nearest ED or trauma center
	• No signs of life and no ROSC despite appropriate field EMS treatment that includes minimally interrupted CPR*	• Resuscitative efforts MAY BE STOPPED
	• More than 15 minutes transport time to nearest ED or trauma center	

(continued)

(continued)

B. Guideline Elements and Recommendations

Guideline Element	Recommendations
System factors to consider	• Average transport time within EMS system • Definitive care capabilities (trauma centers) within EMS system • Transport time based on accomplishment of IV access and airway management during transport • Resuscitative efforts should not prolong on-scene time
Special resuscitation situations	• Give special consideration (following specific protocols) to victims of drowning, lightning strike, and significant hypothermia
Training	• EMS providers must be thoroughly familiar with all guidelines and protocols for decisions to withhold or stop resuscitative efforts
Medical direction	• EMS medical director should develop and implement all protocols • Online medical control should be available to help determine the appropriateness of withholding or stopping resuscitation • Implementation of termination-of-resuscitation protocols mandates active physician oversight
Notification policies and protocols	• Procedures must include notification of appropriate law enforcement agencies, including medical examiners or coroners, about final disposition of the body
Survivor and provider support	• The family of the deceased should have access to resources (eg, clergy, social workers, counseling personnel) as needed • EMS providers should have access to resources for debriefing and counseling as needed
Quality review	• Policies and protocols for termination or withholding of resuscitation should be monitored through a quality review system

Abbreviations: CPR, cardiopulmonary resuscitation; ECG, electocardiographic; ED, emergency department; EMS, emergency medical services; ROSC, return of spontaneous circulation.

*Protocols should require a specific interval of CPR with other interventions. Past guidance has indicated that up to 15 minutes of CPR should be provided before resuscitative efforts are terminated, but the science in this regard remains unclear. Further research is needed to determine the optimal duration of CPR before terminating resuscitative efforts.

From Hopson et al[30] and National Association of EMS Physicians and American College of Surgeons Committee on Trauma.[29]

receive early transfer to a facility that can provide definitive trauma care. Attempts to stabilize the patient are typically performed during transport to avoid delay.

Multicasualty Triage

When multiple patients have serious injuries, emergency personnel must establish priorities for care. When the number of patients with critical injuries exceeds the capability of the EMS providers at the scene, patients without a pulse are the lowest priority for care.

Withholding or Terminating Resuscitation in Prehospital Traumatic Cardiopulmonary Arrest

In 2003, the National Association of EMS Physicians and the American College of Surgeons Committee on Trauma published a position statement on withholding or terminating resuscitation in prehospital traumatic cardiopulmonary arrest.[28,30] In 2012, the organization reiterated its position on the need for definitive EMS protocols for termination of resuscitative efforts in this setting.[29] These guidelines are summarized in Table 74.

Modifications to BLS for Cardiac Arrest Associated With Trauma

Establish Unresponsiveness

Head trauma, shock, or respiratory arrest may produce loss of consciousness. If spinal cord injury is present, the patient may be conscious but unable to move. Throughout initial assessment and stabilization, the provider should monitor the patient's responsiveness. Deterioration could indicate either neurologic compromise or cardiorespiratory failure.

Airway and Cervical Spine Precautions

When head or neck injury or multisystem trauma is present, providers must immobilize the cervical spine throughout BLS maneuvers. Excessive head and neck movement in patients with an unstable cervical spinal column can cause irreversible injury to the spinal cord or worsen a minor spinal cord injury. Approximately 2% of patients with blunt trauma serious enough to require spinal imaging in the ED have a spinal injury. This risk is tripled if the patient has a head or facial injury. Assume that any patient with multiple trauma, head injury, or facial trauma has a spine injury. Be particularly cautious if a patient has suspected cervical spine injury. Examples are patients who have been involved in a high-speed motor vehicle collision, have fallen from a height, or were injured while diving.

Follow these precautions if you suspect cervical spine trauma:

- Open the airway by using a jaw thrust without head extension. Because maintaining a patent airway and providing adequate ventilation are priorities, use a head tilt–chin lift maneuver if the jaw thrust is not effective.
- Have another team member stabilize the head in a neutral position during airway manipulation. Use manual spinal motion restriction rather than immobilization devices. Manual spinal immobilization is safer. Cervical collars may complicate airway management and may even interfere with airway patency.
- Spinal immobilization devices are helpful during transport.

After opening the airway manually, clear the mouth of blood, vomitus, and other secretions. Remove this material with a (gloved) finger sweep, use gauze or a towel to wipe the mouth, or use suction.

Breathing and Ventilation

Once a patent airway is established, assess for breathing. If breathing is absent, agonal, or slow and extremely shallow, manual ventilation is needed. When ventilation is provided with a barrier device, a pocket mask, or a bag-mask device, the rescuer must still maintain cervical spine stabilization. Deliver breaths slowly to reduce risk of gastric inflation. If the chest does not expand during ventilation despite the presence of an adequate and patent airway, rule out tension pneumothorax or hemothorax. If there is a risk of cervical spine injury, immobilize the spine while providing rescue breathing. Maintain immobilization throughout the rescue attempt.

Circulation

The provider should stop any visible hemorrhage using direct compression and appropriate dressings. After checking for responsiveness and for no breathing or only gasping and activating the emergency response system and getting the AED or sending someone to do so, the healthcare provider should attempt to feel a carotid pulse. If the healthcare provider does not definitely feel a pulse within 10 seconds, the provider should begin chest compressions and provide cycles of compressions and ventilations. During CPR, provide compressions of adequate number and depth (push hard and fast), allow full chest recoil after each compression, and minimize interruptions in chest compressions.

When CPR is provided for a patient with an advanced airway in place, 2 rescuers no longer deliver cycles of compressions interrupted with pauses for ventilation. Instead, the compressing rescuer should deliver at least 100 compressions per minute continuously, without pauses for ventilation. The rescuer delivering the ventilations should give 8 to 10 breaths per minute and should be careful to avoid delivering an excessive number of ventilations. The 2 rescuers should change compressor and ventilator roles approximately every 2 minutes to prevent compressor fatigue and deterioration in quality and rate of chest compressions. When multiple rescuers are present, they should rotate the compressor role about every 2 minutes.

Defibrillation

Sudden cardiac arrest associated with VF/pulseless VT may cause trauma. If the patient develops VF/pulseless VT, the patient will lose consciousness, and this can lead to falls and car crashes. If an AED is available, turn it on and attach it. The AED will evaluate the patient's cardiac rhythm and advise delivery of a shock if appropriate. If VF is present, note that the VF may have been the cause rather than the consequence of the trauma.

Disability

Throughout all interventions, assess the patient's level of consciousness and general neurologic status. Monitor closely for signs of neurologic deterioration during BLS care. The Glasgow Coma Scale is useful and can be calculated in seconds.

Exposure

The patient may lose heat to the environment through conduction, convection, and evaporation. Such heat loss will be exacerbated when the patient's clothes are removed or if the patient is covered in blood or water. Take all practical actions to maintain the patient's temperature.

Modifications to ACLS for Cardiac Arrest Associated With Trauma

ACLS includes continued assessment and support of the airway, oxygenation and ventilation (breathing), circulation, and differential diagnosis. If bag-mask ventilation is inadequate, an advanced airway should be inserted while maintaining cervical spine stabilization. If insertion of an advanced airway is not possible and ventilation remains inadequate, experienced providers should consider a cricothyrotomy. Some of these procedures may be performed only after the patient has arrived at the hospital.

Airway Indications for Intubation in the Injured Patient

Airway indications for intubation in the injured patient include

- Respiratory arrest or apnea
- Respiratory failure, including severe hypoventilation, hypoxemia despite oxygen therapy, or respiratory acidosis
- Shock
- Severe head injury
- Inability to protect the upper airway (eg, loss of gag reflex, depressed level of consciousness, coma)
- Thoracic injuries (eg, flail chest, pulmonary contusion, penetrating trauma)
- Signs of airway obstruction
- Injuries associated with potential airway obstruction (eg, crushing facial or neck injuries)
- Anticipated need for mechanical ventilatory support

Perform endotracheal intubation with cervical spine immobilization. Orotracheal intubation is the preferred method. You should avoid nasotracheal intubation, especially if you suspect cervical spine injury, because nasotracheal intubation is more likely than orotracheal intubation to require excessive manipulation of the cervical spine. Also avoid nasotracheal intubation if you suspect maxillofacial injury or basilar skull fracture. If the maxillofacial injury is associated with a dural tear, a nasogastric or endotracheal tube placed through the nose may migrate intracranially.[31] Nasotracheal intubation also may result in the introduction of bacteria through the dura.

Maintain proper tube placement by use of commercial endotracheal tube holders. Continuously confirm proper tube position by use of pulse oximetry and continuous waveform capnography during transport and after any transfer of the patient (eg, from ambulance to hospital gurney).

The inability to intubate the trachea of the patient with massive facial injury and edema is an indication for a surgical airway. An emergent cricothyrotomy will provide an immediate, secure airway that supports oxygenation, although ventilation may be suboptimal.

Complications

If CPR is needed after endotracheal intubation, provision of simultaneous ventilations and compressions may cause a tension pneumothorax. The patient may require needle decompression and insertion of a 1-way valve. There is a high risk for the development of a tension pneumothorax if lung injury has occurred, especially if the patient has fractured ribs or a fractured sternum.

Stomach Decompression

Insert a gastric tube to decompress the stomach. Insert an orogastric rather than a nasogastric tube in patients with severe head or maxillofacial injuries. If the dura is torn, a nasogastric tube can migrate into sinuses or even into the brain.[31] Always confirm proper orogastric or nasogastric tube placement into the stomach by auscultation over the gastric region while injecting air through a syringe.

Ventilation

Provide high concentrations of oxygen even if the patient's oxygenation appears to be adequate. Once you ensure a patent airway, assess breath sounds and chest expansion.

Complications

Signs of a pneumothorax are a unilateral decrease in breath sounds and inadequate chest expansion during positive-pressure ventilation. Assume that these signs are caused by a *tension pneumothorax* until that complication is either confirmed or ruled out. Perform needle decompression of the pneumothorax immediately and then insert a chest tube. Surgical exploration is indicated if thoracic decompression does not produce immediate hemodynamic improvement or if the patient has a penetrating thoracic wound.[15]

Providers should look for and seal any significant *open pneumothorax*. Tension pneumothorax may develop after sealing of an open pneumothorax, so decompression may be needed.[11] A traumatic *hemothorax* also may interfere with ventilation and chest expansion. Treat significant hemothorax with blood replacement and chest tube insertion. If the hemorrhage is severe and continues, the patient may require surgical exploration.

If the patient has a significant *flail chest,* spontaneous ventilation likely will be inadequate to maintain oxygenation. Flail chest results from multiple fractures of adjacent ribs. These fractures cause instability of a portion of the chest wall. This instability may cause respiratory failure, particularly if the patient is breathing spontaneously. Treat flail chest with positive-pressure ventilation.

Circulation

Once airway, oxygenation, and ventilation are addressed, evaluate and manage circulation. In the setting of trauma and pulseless arrest, the outcome will be poor unless a reversible cause can be immediately identified and treated.

Control external bleeding with pressure. If hypovolemic shock is present, establish vascular access with the largest-bore catheter possible and administer boluses of isotonic crystalloids (see "Volume Resuscitation," below). Note that volume resuscitation is no substitute for manual or surgical control of hemorrhage.[6]

Volume Resuscitation

Volume resuscitation is an important but controversial part of trauma resuscitation. ACLS providers should establish large-bore IV access while en route to the ED or trauma center, limiting attempts to two. Isotonic crystalloid is the resuscitation fluid of choice because research has not clearly established any specific type of solution as superior.[32] When replacement of blood loss is required in the hospital, it is accomplished with a combination of packed red blood cells and isotonic crystalloid.

Recommendations for volume resuscitation in trauma patients with signs of hypovolemic shock are determined by the type of trauma (penetrating vs blunt) and the setting (urban vs rural). A high rate of volume infusion with the therapeutic goal of a systolic blood pressure ≥100 mm Hg is now recommended only for patients with isolated head or extremity trauma, either blunt or penetrating. In the urban setting, aggressive prehospital volume resuscitation for penetrating trauma is no longer recommended because it is likely to increase blood pressure and consequently accelerate the rate of blood loss, delay arrival at the trauma center, and delay surgical interventions to repair or ligate bleeding vessels.[10,14,33] Such delay cannot be justified when the patient can be delivered to a trauma center within a few minutes. In rural settings, transport times to trauma centers will be longer, so volume resuscitation for blunt or penetrating trauma is provided during transport to maintain a systolic blood pressure of 90 mm Hg.

Arrest Rhythms

The most common terminal cardiac rhythms observed in trauma patients are pulseless electrical activity (PEA) and bradyasystolic rhythms. Occasionally VF/VT occurs.

Treatment of PEA requires identification and treatment of reversible causes, such as severe hypovolemia, hypothermia, cardiac tamponade, or tension pneumothorax.[15] Development of bradyasystolic rhythms often indicates the presence of severe hypovolemia, severe hypoxemia, or cardiorespiratory failure. Treat VF/VT with defibrillation. Although epinephrine is typically administered during ACLS treatment of these arrhythmias, it may be ineffective in the presence of severe hypovolemia.

Penetrating Cardiac Injury

Providers should suspect penetrating cardiac injury with any penetrating trauma to the left chest, particularly when the penetrating injury is associated with low cardiac output or signs of tamponade (eg, distended neck veins, hypotension, and decreased heart tones). Remember that bullet and stab wounds may cause thoracic and cardiac injury even when the entrance site is in the right chest, back, or abdomen.

The **F**ocused **A**ssessment **S**onogram in **T**rauma (FAST) is a rapid and accurate method of imaging the heart and the pericardium that can be performed in the emergency department. When used by an experienced operator, the FAST is up to 90% accurate for the diagnosis of pericardial fluid.[6]

Pericardiocentesis can be useful for both diagnosis and treatment of cardiac tamponade. In general, efforts to relieve pericardial tamponade due to penetrating injury should occur in the hospital. Pericardiocentesis can be used to stabilize the patient until exploration, pericardiotomy, and repair of the injury can be accomplished in the operating room.[6]

Cardiac Contusions

Cardiac contusions that cause significant arrhythmias or impair cardiac function are present in approximately 10% to 20% of adult patients with severe blunt chest trauma.[34] You should suspect myocardial contusion if the trauma patient has extreme tachycardia, arrhythmias, and ST-segment or T-wave changes.

The myocardial band fraction of creatine kinase (CK-MB) is frequently elevated in patients with blunt chest injuries, but the elevation has little diagnostic or prognostic significance. Patients with an elevated level are just as likely as others to do well, and patients with a normal level may still have significant cardiac dysfunction. Confirm the diagnosis of myocardial contusion by echocardiography or radionuclide angiography.

Commotio Cordis

Commotio cordis is VF caused by a blow to the anterior chest during a cardiac repolarization.[35,36] Blunt cardiac injury may result in cardiac contusion with injured myocardium and risk of ECG changes and arrhythmias. Even a small blow to the anterior chest during a cardiac repolarization, such as that imparted by the strike of a hockey puck or baseball, can trigger commotio cordis.[37] Events causing commotio cordis are most commonly seen in young people up to 18 years of age who are engaged in sports. Prompt recognition that a precordial blow may cause VF is critical. Rapid defibrillation is often lifesaving for these victims of cardiac arrest. Provision of immediate BLS care with an AED and ACLS for VF in this setting are appropriate.

Indications for Surgical Exploration

Resuscitation may be impossible in the presence of severe, uncontrolled hemorrhage or in the presence of significant cardiac, thoracic, or abdominal injuries. Patients with such injuries require surgical intervention. The following conditions are generally thought to be indications for urgent surgical exploration[3]:

- Hemodynamic instability despite volume resuscitation
- Thoracic injury associated with
  - Excessive chest tube drainage (1.5 to 2 L or more total, or more than 300 mL/h for 3 or more hours)
  - Significant hemothorax on chest x-ray
  - Suspected cardiac or aortic injury. Helical, contrast-enhanced CT of the chest is extremely accurate for diagnosis of aortic injury.[3]
- Gunshot wounds thought to traverse the peritoneal cavity or visceral/vascular retroperitoneum (note that the path of the bullet may be unpredictable)
- Penetrating torso trauma, particularly if associated with
  - Peritoneal perforation or hypotension
  - Bleeding from the stomach, rectum, or genitourinary tract
- Blunt abdominal trauma with the following:
  - Hypotension and clinical evidence of intraperitoneal bleeding
  - Positive diagnostic peritoneal lavage or ultrasound
- Significant solid-organ, diaphragm, or bowel injury or peritonitis:
  - Contrast-enhanced CT indicates a ruptured gastrointestinal tract, intraperitoneal bladder injury, renal pedicle injury, or severe visceral parenchymal injury after blunt or penetrating injury
  - Peritonitis (on presentation or as a later complication)
  - Free air, retroperitoneal air, or rupture of the hemidiaphragm after blunt trauma

Emergency Thoracotomy

Several centers have reported their retrospective observations about resuscitative thoracotomies for patients in traumatic cardiac arrest.[38-41] In one study, none of the patients in cardiac arrest or without signs of life before thoracotomy survived to hospital discharge.[41]

In a database of 959 resuscitative thoracotomies,[40] 22 victims of penetrating trauma and 4 victims of blunt trauma survived to hospital discharge after receiving prehospital CPR (overall survival rate of 3%).

In 2001 the Committee on Trauma of the American College of Surgeons published a systematic review of 42 studies of ED thoracotomies involving nearly 7000 patients.[42] In this database, the survival rate was 7.8% (11.2% for patients with penetrating trauma and 1.6% for patients with blunt trauma).

These studies suggest that there may be a role for open thoracotomy in specific patients or situations. Table 75 describes conditions under which an open thoracotomy may be considered. Open thoracotomy does not improve outcome from out-of-hospital blunt trauma arrest, but it can be lifesaving for patients with penetrating chest trauma if the patient has an arrest immediately before arrival at the ED or while in the ED. During concurrent volume

Table 75. **Suggested Indications for Resuscitative Thoracotomy: Patients With Traumatic Cardiac Arrest**

Type of Injury	Assessment
Blunt trauma	• Patient arrives at ED or trauma center with pulse, blood pressure, and spontaneous respirations, *and* • then experiences witnessed cardiac arrest
Penetrating cardiac trauma	• Patient experiences a witnessed cardiac arrest in ED or trauma center *or* • Patient arrives in ED or trauma center after <5 minutes of out-of-hospital CPR and with positive secondary signs of life (eg, pupillary reflexes, spontaneous movement, organized ECG activity)
Penetrating thoracic (noncardiac) trauma	• Patient experiences a witnessed cardiac arrest in ED or trauma center *or* • Patient arrives in ED or trauma center after <15 minutes of out-of-hospital CPR and with positive secondary signs of life (eg, pupillary reflexes, spontaneous movement, organized ECG activity)
Exsanguinating abdominal vascular trauma	• Patient experiences a witnessed cardiac arrest in ED or trauma center *or* • Patient arrives in ED or trauma center with positive secondary signs of life (eg, pupillary reflexes, spontaneous movement, organized ECG activity) *plus* • Resources available for definitive repair of abdominal-vascular injuries

resuscitation for penetrating trauma, prompt emergency thoracotomy will permit direct massage of the heart, relief of cardiac tamponade, control of thoracic and extrathoracic hemorrhage, and aortic cross-clamping.[12,14]

Practitioners should consult the guidelines for withholding or terminating resuscitation (summarized in Table 74), which were developed for victims of traumatic cardiac arrest by a joint committee of the National Association of EMS Physicians and the American College of Surgeons Committee on Trauma.[29,43,44]

Transfer

If a patient arrives at a facility with limited trauma capability, hospital staff should treat identifiable and reversible injuries to their capability. The patient should then be rapidly transferred to a facility that can provide definitive trauma care.

References

1. Sasser SM, Hunt RC, Faul M, Sugerman D, Pearson WS, Dulski T, Wald MM, Jurkovich GJ, Newgard CD, Lerner EB; Centers for Disease Control and Prevention (CDC). Guidelines for field triage of injured patients. *MMWR Recomm Rep.* 2012;61:1-20.
2. *World Health Statistical Annual, 1994*. Geneva, Switzerland: World Health Organization; 1994.
3. Anderson RN. Deaths: leading causes for 2000. *Natl Vital Stat Rep*. 2002;50:1-85.
4. Murphy SL, Xu J, Kochanek KD. Deaths: preliminary data for 2010. *Natl Vital Stat Rep.* 2012;60:1-51.
5. National Trauma Data Bank 2012 Annual Report. Chicago, IL: American College of Surgeons; 2012.
6. Parks SN, ATLS Subcommittee, American College of Surgeons Committee on Trauma. *Advanced Trauma Life Support, Overview of Changes for 7th Edition*. Chicago, IL: American College of Surgeons; 2001.
7. Rosemurgy AS, Norris PA, Olson SM, Hurst JM, Albrink MH. Prehospital traumatic cardiac arrest: the cost of futility. *J Trauma*. 1993;35:468-473.
8. Hazinski MF, Chahine AA, Holcomb GW III, Morris JA Jr. Outcome of cardiovascular collapse in pediatric blunt trauma. *Ann Emerg Med*. 1994;23:1229-1235.
9. Bouillon B, Walther T, Kramer M, Neugebauer E. Trauma and circulatory arrest: 224 preclinical resuscitations in Cologne in 1987-1990 [in German]. *Anaesthesist*. 1994;43:786-790.
10. Bickell WH, Wall MJ Jr, Pepe PE, Martin RR, Ginger VF, Allen MK, Mattox KL. Immediate versus delayed fluid resuscitation for hypotensive patients with penetrating torso injuries. *N Engl J Med*. 1994;331:1105-1109.
11. Pepe PE. Emergency medical services systems and prehospital management of patients requiring critical care. In: Carlson RW, Geheb MA. *Principles and Practice of Medical Intensive Care.* Philadelphia, PA: Saunders;1993:9-24.
12. Rozycki G, Adams C, Champion H, Kihn R. Resuscitative thoracotomy—trends in outcome. *Ann Emerg Med*. 1990;19:462.
13. Copass MK, Oreskovich MR, Bladergroen MR, Carrico CJ. Prehospital cardiopulmonary resuscitation of the critically injured patient. *Am J Surg*. 1984;148:20-26.
14. Durham LA III, Richardson RJ, Wall MJ Jr, Pepe PE, Mattox KL. Emergency center thoracotomy: impact of prehospital resuscitation. *J Trauma*. 1992;32:775-779.
15. Kloeck W. Prehospital advanced CPR in the trauma patient. *Trauma Emerg Med*. 1993;10:772-776.
16. Schmidt U, Frame SB, Nerlich ML, Rowe DW, Enderson BL, Maull KI, Tscherne H. On-scene helicopter transport of patients with multiple injuries—comparison of a German and an American system. *J Trauma*. 1992;33:548-553.
17. Grasner JT, Wnent J, Seewald S, Meybohm P, Fischer M, Paffrath T, Wafaisade A, Bein B, Lefering R. Cardiopulmonary resuscitation traumatic cardiac arrest—there are survivors. An analysis of two national emergency registries. *Crit Care*. 2011;15:R276.
18. Cummins RO, Hazinski MF. Guidelines based on the principle "First, do no harm." New guidelines on tracheal tube confirmation and prevention of dislodgment. *Resuscitation*. 2000;46:443-447.
19. Katz SH, Falk JL. Misplaced endotracheal tubes by paramedics in an urban emergency medical services system. *Ann Emerg Med*. 2001;37:32-37.
20. Gausche M, Lewis RJ, Stratton SJ, Haynes BE, Gunter CS, Goodrich SM, Poore PD, McCollough MD, Henderson DP, Pratt FD, Seidel JS. Effect of out-of-hospital pediatric endotracheal intubation on survival and neurological outcome: a controlled clinical trial. *JAMA*. 2000;283:783-790.
21. Dutton RP, Mackenzie CF, Scalea TM. Hypotensive resuscitation during active hemorrhage: impact on in-hospital mortality. *J Trauma*. 2002;52:1141-1146.
22. Dretzke J, Sandercock J, Bayliss S, Burls A. Clinical effectiveness and cost-effectiveness of prehospital intravenous fluids in trauma patients. *Health Technol Assess*. 2004;8:1-103.
23. Dula DJ, Wood GC, Rejmer AR, Starr M, Leicht M. Use of prehospital fluids in hypotensive blunt trauma patients. *Prehosp Emerg Care*. 2002;6:417-420.
24. Greaves I, Porter KM, Revell MP. Fluid resuscitation in pre-hospital trauma care: a consensus view. *J R Coll Surg Edinb*. 2002;47:451-457.
25. Koenig KL. Quo vadis: "scoop and run," "stay and treat," or "treat and street"? *Acad Emerg Med*. 1995;2:477-479.
26. Deakin CD, Soreide E. Pre-hospital trauma care. *Curr Opin Anaesthesiol*. 2001;14:191-195.
27. Nolan J. Advanced life support training. *Resuscitation*. 2001;50:9-11.
28. Hopson LR, Hirsh E, Delgado J, Domeier RM, Krohmer J, McSwain NE Jr, Weldon C, Friel M, Hoyt DB. Guidelines for withholding or termination of resuscitation in prehospital traumatic cardiopulmonary arrest. *J Am Coll Surg*. 2003;196:475-481.
29. National Association of EMS Physicians and American College of Surgeons Committee on Trauma. Termination of resuscitation for adult traumatic cardiopulmonary arrest. *Prehosp Emerg Care.* 2012;16:571.
30. Hopson LR, Hirsh E, Delgado J, Domeier RM, McSwain NE, Krohmer J. Guidelines for withholding or termination of resuscitation in prehospital traumatic cardiopulmonary arrest: joint position statement of the National Association of EMS Physicians and the American College of Surgeons Committee on Trauma. *J Am Coll Surg*. 2003;196:106-112.

31. Baskaya MK. Inadvertent intracranial placement of a nasogastric tube in patients with head injuries. *Surg Neurol*. 1999;52:426-427.
32. Moore FA, McKinley BA, Moore EE. The next generation in shock resuscitation. *Lancet*. 2004;363:1988-1996.
33. Solomonov E, Hirsh M, Yahiya A, Krausz MM. The effect of vigorous fluid resuscitation in uncontrolled hemorrhagic shock after massive splenic injury. *Crit Care Med*. 2000;28:749-754.
34. McLean RF, Devitt JH, Dubbin J, McLellan BA. Incidence of abnormal RNA studies and dysrhythmias in patients with blunt chest trauma. *J Trauma*. 1991;31:968-970.
35. Maron BJ, Estes NA III. Commotio cordis. *N Engl J Med*. 2010;362:917-927.
36. Maron BJ, Doerer JJ, Haas TS, Estes NA, Hodges JS, Link MS. Commotio cordis and the epidemiology of sudden death in competitive lacrosse. *Pediatrics*. 2009;124:966-971.
37. Link MS, Maron BJ, Wang PJ, VanderBrink BA, Zhu W, Estes NA III. Upper and lower limits of vulnerability to sudden arrhythmic death with chest-wall impact (commotio cordis). *J Am Coll Cardiol*. 2003;41:99-104.
38. Grove CA, Lemmon G, Anderson G, McCarthy M. Emergency thoracotomy: appropriate use in the resuscitation of trauma patients. *Am Surg*. 2002;68:313-316.
39. Ladd AP, Gomez GA, Jacobson LE, Broadie TA, Scherer LR III, Solotkin KC. Emergency room thoracotomy: updated guidelines for a level I trauma center. *Am Surg*. 2002;68:421-424.
40. Powell DW, Moore EE, Cothren CC, Ciesla DJ, Burch JM, Moore JB, Johnson JL. Is emergency department resuscitative thoracotomy futile care for the critically injured patient requiring prehospital cardiopulmonary resuscitation? *J Am Coll Surg*. 2004;199:211-215.
41. Aihara R, Millham FH, Blansfield J, Hirsch EF. Emergency room thoracotomy for penetrating chest injury: effect of an institutional protocol. *J Trauma*. 2001;50:1027-1030.
42. Practice management guidelines for emergency department thoracotomy. Working Group, Ad Hoc Subcommittee on Outcomes, American College of Surgeons–Committee on Trauma. *J Am Coll Surg*. 2001;193:303-309.
43. Hopson LR, Hirsh E, Delgado J, Domeier RM, McSwain NE, Krohmer J. Guidelines for withholding or termination of resuscitation in pre-hospital traumatic cardiopulmonary arrest: joint position statement of the National Association of EMS Physicians and the American College of Surgeons Committee on Trauma. *J Am Coll Surg*. 2003;196:106-112.
44. *Advanced Trauma Life Support for Doctors*. Chicago, IL: American College of Surgeons; 2004.

Chapter 21

Cardiac Arrest in Accidental Hypothermia and Avalanche Victims

---

This Chapter

- **Hypothermia: Definitions, Signs, and Symptoms**
- **Prearrest Interventions**
- **Cardiac Arrest Interventions**
- **Modifications to BLS and ACLS for Hypothermia**

Introduction

Unintentional or accidental hypothermia is a serious and often preventable health problem. Severe hypothermia (body temperature lower than 30°C [86°F]) is associated with marked depression of critical body functions that may make the patient appear clinically dead during the initial assessment. But in some cases hypothermia may exert a protective effect on the brain and organs in cardiac arrest.[1] Intact neurologic recovery may be possible after hypothermic cardiac arrest, although those with nonasphyxial arrest have a better prognosis than those with asphyxia-associated hypothermic arrest.[2-4] Therefore, lifesaving procedures should be initiated unless the victim is obviously dead (eg, rigor mortis, decomposition, hemisection, decapitation). Patients should be transported as soon as possible to a center where aggressive and monitored rewarming during resuscitation is possible.

Epidemiology

Accidental hypothermia is defined as a decrease in core body temperature below 35°C or 36°C (95°F or 96.8°F). ACLS providers will most often encounter patients in cardiac arrest associated with accidental hypothermia in 1 of 3 clinical settings:

- Cold stress or exposure (often subacute) in persons with thermoregulatory impairment
- Cold weather exposure
- Cold water immersion (with or without submersion)

Cold exposure in persons with impaired thermoregulatory function is surprisingly the most frequent cause of death caused by hypothermia.[3,5-15] *Impaired thermoregulatory function* may develop in many patient groups: the elderly, insulin-dependent diabetics, the malnourished, the alcohol-intoxicated or drug-intoxicated, the chronically ill, and the polymedicated, medically disabled. These patients have decreased basal metabolism, dysfunctional shivering thermogenesis, and impaired vasoconstriction.

Sudden immersion in cold water (usually defined as water temperature below 21°C [70°F]) most often occurs in association with boating or recreational aquatic mishaps.[16] Cooling occurs rapidly during cold water immersion because conductive heat loss is 25 to 35 times faster in water than in air. In water at 4.44°C (40°F), mortality approaches 50% after 1 hour. Victims of cold water immersion also face a high risk of *cold water submersion* with resultant aspiration, asphyxia, hypoxia, and even death. Recent experiments suggest that cold water immersion produces exhaustion (and subsequent submersion) faster than it produces a neurologically protective degree of core hypothermia.[17-19] Nearly all reports of successful resuscitation with full neurologic recovery describe prolonged cold water submersion in icy water (below 5°C [41°F]).

Pathophysiology

Severe hypothermia (body temperature below 30°C [86°F]) is associated with marked depression of cerebral blood flow and oxygen consumption, reduced cardiac output, and decreased arterial pressure.[20] Patients can appear to be clinically dead because of marked depression of brain function.[20-22]

Hypothermia may exert a protective effect on the brain and organs during cardiac arrest if the patient cools rapidly with no hypoxia before the cardiac arrest.[1,23] If the patient cools rapidly, oxygen consumption decreases and metabolism slows before the arrest, which reduces organ ischemia during the arrest.[24]

This protective effect appears to account for the rare occurrence of resuscitation with intact neurologic recovery after hypothermic cardiac arrest.[4] The effects of hypothermia on cerebral oxygen consumption and metabolism are thought to be the mechanism for the therapeutic effects of induced hypothermia. Induced hypothermia for comatose survivors of out-of-hospital VF cardiac arrest has produced marked improvements in survival to hospital discharge,[25] 6-month mortality rate,[26] and neurologic outcomes.[26]

Hypothermia: Definitions, Signs, and Symptoms

The severity of hypothermia is determined from the patient's core body temperature. Table 76 presents the most commonly used definitions of hypothermia severity, based on a range of core body temperatures:

- **Mild hypothermia** (above 34°C or 93.2°F): The clinical hallmark of mild hypothermia is the onset of shivering, which can become severe. Shivering represents a centrally mediated attempt at thermogenesis.[20] The onset of mental confusion and disorientation marks the symptomatic transition from mild to moderate hypothermia.
- **Moderate hypothermia** (30°C to 34°C or 86°F to 93.2°F): The hallmark of moderate hypothermia is progressive loss of higher cognitive functions with onset of marked confusion, disorientation, stupor, and loss of consciousness. With moderate hypothermia, shivering diminishes and eventually disappears completely.
- **Severe hypothermia** (below 30°C or 86°F): The hallmark of severe hypothermia is unconsciousness with immobility and the progressive loss of all signs of life. The vital functions disappear completely in roughly the following order as hypothermia becomes more and more severe:
  - Loss of consciousness and all voluntary movement
  - Loss of papillary light reflexes
  - Loss of deep tendon reflexes
  - Loss of spontaneous respirations
  - Loss of organized cardiac rhythm (onset of VF)
- **Profound hypothermia** (below 20°C or 68°F): Profound hypothermia may be considered as a subcategory of severe hypothermia.[21,22] This category, however, has little clinical utility because it has no therapeutic implications. Profound hypothermia is managed the same way as severe hypothermia.
  - The hallmark of profound hypothermia is the total loss of any sign of life. Cardiac activity is completely lost, and the monitor displays only asystole. The electroencephalogram (EEG) is totally silent, with no detectable brain activity. No distinction can be made from death.
  - There have been rare case reports of patients with profound hypothermia resuscitated with internal rewarming. Few of these patients have demonstrated complete neurologic recovery.[4]

General Care of All Hypothermia Patients

The answers to 2 clinical questions shape the treatment of unintentional hypothermia:

- First, is the patient in cardiopulmonary arrest?
- Second, what is the core temperature?

The Hypothermia Algorithm (Figure 119) shows how the answers to these 2 questions determine the recommended actions for patients with unintentional hypothermia.

Prearrest Interventions

When the patient is extremely cold but has maintained a perfusing rhythm, the provider should focus on interventions that prevent further heat loss and begin to rewarm the patient immediately. These interventions may also help prevent cardiac arrest.

General care includes the following procedures:

- Prevent additional evaporative heat loss by removing wet garments and insulating the patient from further environmental exposure.
- Begin rewarming immediately.
- Begin clinical monitoring, particularly measurement of core temperature and monitoring of cardiac rhythm.
- Provide rapid transport to definitive care.

Try to keep hypothermic patients in a horizontal position from the time of initial rescue and extrication (as feasible). Hypothermic patients are often volume depleted from "cold diuresis" with dysfunctional cardiovascular regulatory mechanisms. Avoid excess movement or rough activity. However, do not delay urgently needed procedures such as rescue breathing, intubation, insertion of a vascular catheter, or even CPR chest compressions. Perform procedures gently, and monitor cardiac rhythm closely. An exaggerated fear of "precipitating VF" and other arrhythmias in hypothermic patients should not cause prehospital personnel to withhold essential interventions. Spontaneous VF or VF secondary to jarring movements becomes a risk at severe levels of hypothermia (below 30°C [86°F]).

Table 76. Hypothermia: Definitions, Signs and Symptoms, and Recommended Therapy

Core Temperature* °C	Core Temperature* °F	Signs and Symptoms	Recommended Therapy		
Mild hypothermia[61] >34°C or >93.2°F					
36°	**96.8°**	Muscle tone increases ("preshivering"). Metabolic rate and blood pressure increase to adjust for heat loss. Shivering begins.	**Passive external rewarming**	**Consider active rewarming**	
35°	**95°**	Shivering continues and reaches maximum thermogenesis level. Victim is still mentally responsive.			
34°	**93.2°**	Extreme subjective coldness; some amnesia and dysarthria. Poor judgment and maladaptive behavior begin. Blood pressure is adequate; tachycardia and then progressive bradycardia occur.			
Moderate hypothermia 30°C to 34°C or 86°F to 93.2°F					
33°	**91.4°**	Mental confusion increases; ataxia; apathy; shivering decreases. Maximum respiratory stimulation with tachypnea, then progressive drop in minute volume.	**Passive external rewarming**	**Active external rewarming**	
32°	**89.6°**	Consciousness is much more clouded; victim may become stuporous. Shivering almost stopped. Oxygen consumption <75% normal. Pupils may be dilated.			
31°	**87.8°**	Thermogenesis through shivering stops. Severe peripheral vasoconstriction; blood pressure is difficult to obtain.			
30°	**86°**	Muscles increasingly rigid; more loss of consciousness; risk of atrial fibrillation and other arrhythmias. Cardiac output drops to <67% of normal.			
Severe hypothermia <30°C or <86°F (purple shading = risk of VF with rough movements, but this concern should not delay necessary interventions)					
29°	**84.2°**	Pulse and respirations slow perceptibly; cardiac arrhythmias become more frequent. Pupils usually dilated. Paradoxical undressing observed.	**Passive external rewarming**	**Active external rewarming**	**Active internal rewarming**
28°	**82.4°**	**High risk of VF if heart is irritated from rough movements. Oxygen consumption <50% normal.**			
27°	**80.6°**	**Consciousness usually lost; all voluntary motion stops.**			

(continued)

(continued)

Core Temperature* °C	°F	Signs and Symptoms	Recommended Therapy		
			Passive external rewarming	Active external rewarming	Active internal rewarming
26°	78.8°	**Deep tendon and pupillary light reflexes usually absent. Victim can appear dead.**			
25°	77°	**VF can occur spontaneously even without irritation.**			
24°	75.2°	**Pulmonary edema, severe hypotension, and severe bradycardia may develop.**			
23°	73.4°	**VF risk very high; deathlike appearance; no corneal or oculocephalic reflexes.**			
22°	71.6°	**VF occurs spontaneously in majority of victims. Oxygen consumption <25% normal.**			
21°	69.8°	VF amplitude diminishes.			
20°	68°	VF becomes very fine, more like "coarse asystole"; EEG signals flatten.			
Profound hypothermia (<20°C or <68°F)					
19°	66.2°	Either PEA or asystole; EEG almost flat.			
18°	64.4°	Almost invariably asystole.			
17°	62.6°	EEG totally silent.			
16°	60.8°	Total irreversible cardiac and brain death (except in rare cases).			
15°	59°	Lowest recorded infant core temperature with intact neurologic recovery from accidental hypothermia.[90]			
13.7°	56.6°	Lowest recorded adult core temperature with full neurologic recovery from accidental hypothermia.[4]			
10°	50°	Oxygen consumption <8% normal.			
9°	48.2°	Lowest recorded core temperature for survival from therapeutic hypothermia.[22]			

*Adapted from Cummins RO, Graves JR. *ACLS Scenarios: Core Concepts for Case-Based Learning.* St Louis, MO: Mosby Lifeline; 1996, with permission from Elsevier. With additional data from references 20-22.

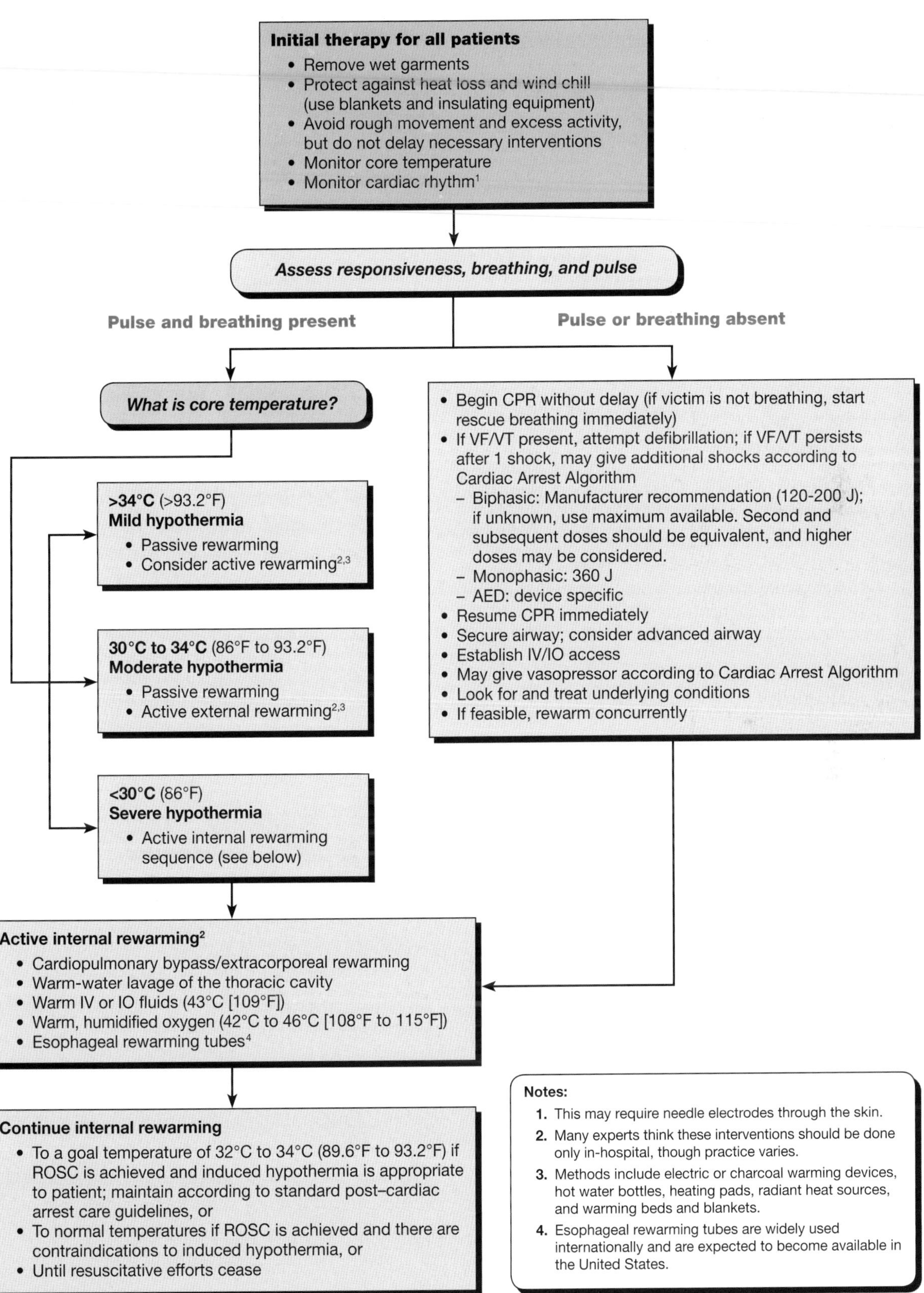
Initial therapy for all patients
• Remove wet garments
• Protect against heat loss and wind chill (use blankets and insulating equipment)
• Avoid rough movement and excess activity, but do not delay necessary interventions
• Monitor core temperature
• Monitor cardiac rhythm[1]
Assess responsiveness, breathing, and pulse
Pulse and breathing present
Pulse or breathing absent
What is core temperature?
>34°C (>93.2°F)
Mild hypothermia
• Passive rewarming
• Consider active rewarming[2,3]
30°C to 34°C (86°F to 93.2°F)
Moderate hypothermia
• Passive rewarming
• Active external rewarming[2,3]
<30°C (86°F)
Severe hypothermia
• Active internal rewarming sequence (see below)
• Begin CPR without delay (if victim is not breathing, start rescue breathing immediately)
• If VF/VT present, attempt defibrillation; if VF/VT persists after 1 shock, may give additional shocks according to Cardiac Arrest Algorithm
– Biphasic: Manufacturer recommendation (120-200 J); if unknown, use maximum available. Second and subsequent doses should be equivalent, and higher doses may be considered.
– Monophasic: 360 J
– AED: device specific
• Resume CPR immediately
• Secure airway; consider advanced airway
• Establish IV/IO access
• May give vasopressor according to Cardiac Arrest Algorithm
• Look for and treat underlying conditions
• If feasible, rewarm concurrently
Active internal rewarming[2]
• Cardiopulmonary bypass/extracorporeal rewarming
• Warm-water lavage of the thoracic cavity
• Warm IV or IO fluids (43°C [109°F])
• Warm, humidified oxygen (42°C to 46°C [108°F to 115°F])
• Esophageal rewarming tubes[4]
Continue internal rewarming
• To a goal temperature of 32°C to 34°C (89.6°F to 93.2°F) if ROSC is achieved and induced hypothermia is appropriate to patient; maintain according to standard post–cardiac arrest care guidelines, or
• To normal temperatures if ROSC is achieved and there are contraindications to induced hypothermia, or
• Until resuscitative efforts cease
Notes:
1. This may require needle electrodes through the skin.
2. Many experts think these interventions should be done only in-hospital, though practice varies.
3. Methods include electric or charcoal warming devices, hot water bottles, heating pads, radiant heat sources, and warming beds and blankets.
4. Esophageal rewarming tubes are widely used internationally and are expected to become available in the United States.

Figure 119. The Hypothermia Algorithm.

Monitor Core Body Temperature and Cardiac Rhythm

The patient's core body temperature will help determine subsequent treatment decisions. The core temperature is measured using a rectal or tympanic membrane thermometer. Monitor the cardiac rhythm. If the patient's skin is extremely cold, it may be impossible to record the cardiac rhythm using adhesive electrodes. In such cases you may use a sterile needle (1.5 inch, 22 gauge works well) to attach the electrodes to the skin.

Specific Interventions to Consider

- Prevent additional evaporative heat loss by removing wet garments and insulating the victim from further environmental exposures. Passive rewarming is generally adequate for patients with mild hypothermia (temperature greater than 34°C [93.2°F]).
- For patients with moderate (30°C to 34°C [86°F to 93.2°F]) hypothermia and a perfusing rhythm, external warming techniques are appropriate.[27] Passive rewarming alone will be inadequate for these patients.[24]
- For patients with severe hypothermia (<30°C [86°F]) with a perfusing rhythm, core rewarming is often used, although some have reported successful rewarming with active external warming techniques.[28,29] Active external warming techniques include forced air or other efficient surface warming devices.
- Patients with severe hypothermia and cardiac arrest can be rewarmed most rapidly with cardiopulmonary bypass.[2,27,30-34] Alternative effective core rewarming techniques include warm-water lavage of the thoracic cavity[33,35-39] and extracorporeal blood warming with partial bypass.[40-42]
- Adjunctive core rewarming techniques include warmed IV or intraosseous (IO) fluids and warm humidified oxygen.[43] Heat transfer with these measures is not rapid and should be considered supplementary to active warming techniques.
- Do not delay urgent procedures such as airway management and insertion of vascular catheters. Although these patients may exhibit cardiac irritability, this concern should not delay necessary interventions. Beyond these critical initial steps, the treatment of severe hypothermia (temperature <30°C [86°F]) in the field remains controversial. Many providers do not have the time or equipment to assess core body temperature or to institute aggressive rewarming techniques, although these methods should be initiated when available.

Rewarming Techniques

Management of the patient with hypothermia and a perfusing rhythm is determined by the core temperature.

Passive Rewarming

As a general rule, passive rewarming is the treatment of choice for hypothermia patients who can shiver (shivering thermogenesis stops at core temperatures below 32°C or 89.6°F). Blankets and reflective metallic-foil wraps are the most common materials for passive rewarming. Passive rewarming occurs through internal heat generation by the patient. Rewarming rates are relatively slow, in the range of only 0.25°C to 0.5°C (0.45°F to 0.9°F) per hour.[44] Providers should also initiate and maintain passive rewarming for patients with moderate or severe hypothermia (see Table 76). But passive rewarming alone will not effectively raise core body temperature for these patients or patients in cardiac arrest with any level of hypothermia.[45]

Active External Rewarming

Active external rewarming of all areas can be accomplished with a variety of heating and heated devices. Examples of heating devices are radiant heat, forced hot air, warm bath water or other efficient surface-warming devices.[29,46] Heating devices include warmed plastic bags of IV solutions, heated blankets, or chemical-reaction warm packs. In general do not place heated devices directly on the patient's skin. Both the patient and the device must be monitored. With all active external rewarming devices, especially chemical warm packs, verify that the temperature of the warming pack does not increase enough to cause skin burns. This is a particular risk for insensate patients with hypothermia. There are reports of chemical heating packs reaching hazardous temperatures.

Most heating devices should be applied first to the groin and axillary regions. Placement at these locations allows healthcare personnel unrestricted access to the patient's chest, neck, and arms for monitoring, diagnostic testing, and IV access. Active external rewarming of truncal areas can rewarm at a rate of approximately 1°C (1.8°F) per hour.[44]

Active Internal Rewarming

The unique treatment for severe hypothermia is the addition of *active internal rewarming* or *core rewarming.* During active internal rewarming, both passive rewarming and active external rewarming should continue (see Table 76), although some have reported successful rewarming with active external warming techniques alone.[28,29]

Healthcare personnel can accomplish active internal rewarming with several techniques. Active internal rewarming should start with simple, inexpensive, and minimally invasive techniques such as warm IV fluids and warm, humid oxygen. Active internal rewarming techniques also include more complex and invasive interventions. These moderately invasive techniques include lavage of the stomach, colon, bladder, pleural cavity, and mediastinum.

During active internal rewarming of hypothermic patients in cardiac arrest, rescuers should remember the following:

- Use as many rewarming techniques simultaneously as possible while continuing CPR and maintaining access to the patient.

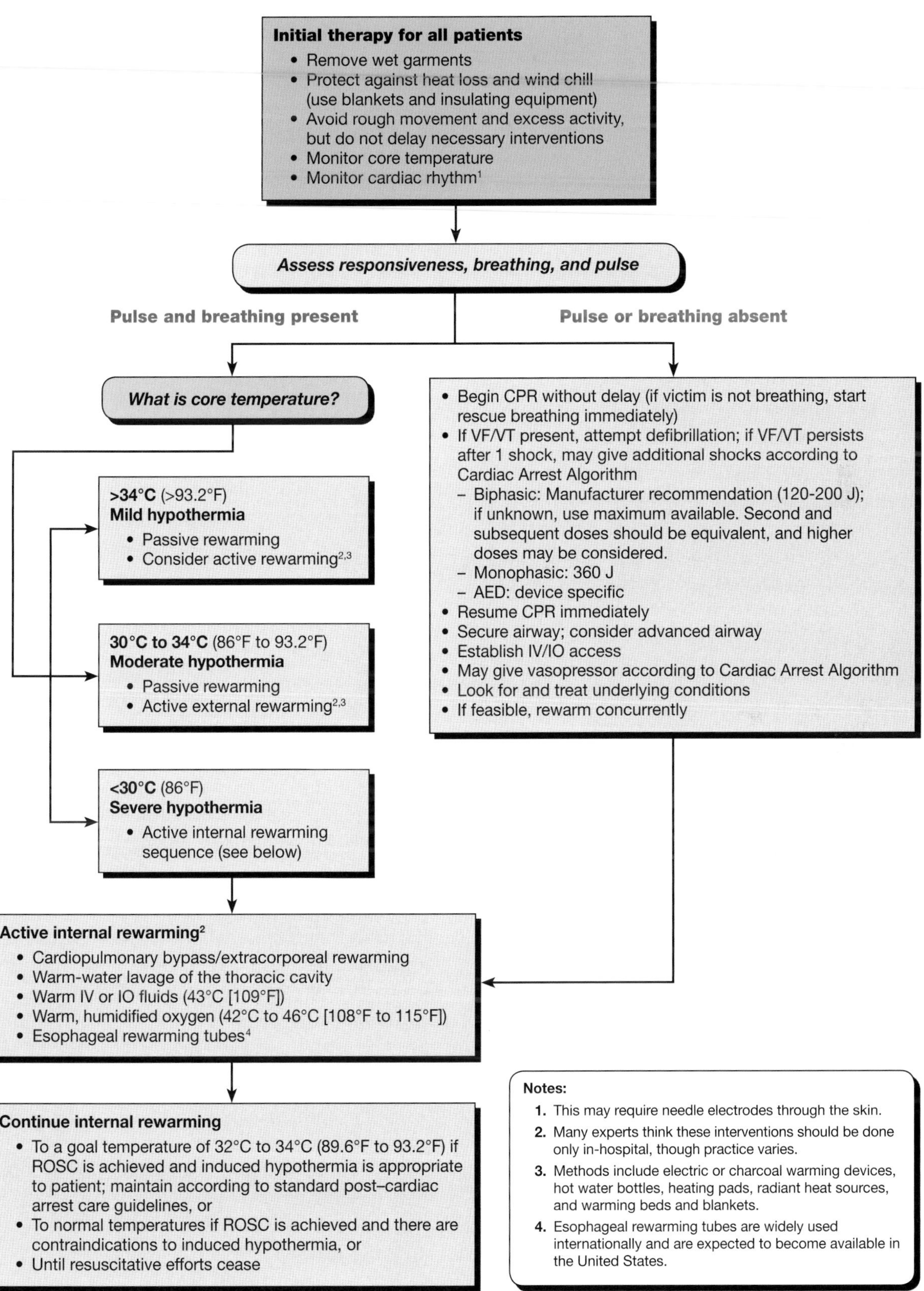
Initial therapy for all patients
• Remove wet garments
• Protect against heat loss and wind chill (use blankets and insulating equipment)
• Avoid rough movement and excess activity, but do not delay necessary interventions
• Monitor core temperature
• Monitor cardiac rhythm[1]
Assess responsiveness, breathing, and pulse
Pulse and breathing present
Pulse or breathing absent
What is core temperature?
>34°C (>93.2°F)
Mild hypothermia
• Passive rewarming
• Consider active rewarming[2,3]
30°C to 34°C (86°F to 93.2°F)
Moderate hypothermia
• Passive rewarming
• Active external rewarming[2,3]
<30°C (86°F)
Severe hypothermia
• Active internal rewarming sequence (see below)
• Begin CPR without delay (if victim is not breathing, start rescue breathing immediately)
• If VF/VT present, attempt defibrillation; if VF/VT persists after 1 shock, may give additional shocks according to Cardiac Arrest Algorithm
– Biphasic: Manufacturer recommendation (120-200 J); if unknown, use maximum available. Second and subsequent doses should be equivalent, and higher doses may be considered.
– Monophasic: 360 J
– AED: device specific
• Resume CPR immediately
• Secure airway; consider advanced airway
• Establish IV/IO access
• May give vasopressor according to Cardiac Arrest Algorithm
• Look for and treat underlying conditions
• If feasible, rewarm concurrently
Active internal rewarming[2]
• Cardiopulmonary bypass/extracorporeal rewarming
• Warm-water lavage of the thoracic cavity
• Warm IV or IO fluids (43°C [109°F])
• Warm, humidified oxygen (42°C to 46°C [108°F to 115°F])
• Esophageal rewarming tubes[4]
Continue internal rewarming
• To a goal temperature of 32°C to 34°C (89.6°F to 93.2°F) if ROSC is achieved and induced hypothermia is appropriate to patient; maintain according to standard post–cardiac arrest care guidelines, or
• To normal temperatures if ROSC is achieved and there are contraindications to induced hypothermia, or
• Until resuscitative efforts cease
Notes:
1. This may require needle electrodes through the skin.
2. Many experts think these interventions should be done only in-hospital, though practice varies.
3. Methods include electric or charcoal warming devices, hot water bottles, heating pads, radiant heat sources, and warming beds and blankets.
4. Esophageal rewarming tubes are widely used internationally and are expected to become available in the United States.

Figure 119. The Hypothermia Algorithm.

hypothermic victim, cardioactive medications can accumulate to toxic levels in the peripheral circulation if given repeatedly. For these reasons, IV drugs are often withheld if the patient's core body temperature is below 30°C (86°F).

In the last decade, a number of animal investigations have been performed evaluating both vasopressors and antiarrhythmic medications that could challenge some of this conventional wisdom.[62 63] In a meta-analysis of these studies, it was found that vasopressor medications (ie, vasopressin or epinephrine) increased rates of return of spontaneous circulation (ROSC) when compared with placebo (62% versus 17%).[64] In addition, coronary perfusion pressures were increased in groups that received vasopressors compared with placebo. However, groups given antiarrhythmics showed no improvement in ROSC compared with control groups (n=34 and n=40, respectively), although sample sizes were relatively small.

One small-animal study found that the application of standard normothermic ACLS algorithms using both drugs (ie, epinephrine and amiodarone) and defibrillation improved ROSC compared with a placebo arm of defibrillation only (91% versus 30%; $P<0.01$; n=21). Human trials of medication use in accidental hypothermia do not exist, although case reports of survival with use of intra-arrest medication have been reported.[34,37,65]

Given the lack of human evidence and relatively small number of animal investigations, the recommendation for administration or withholding of medications is not clear. It may be reasonable to consider administration of a vasopressor during cardiac arrest according to the standard ACLS algorithm concurrent with rewarming strategies (Class IIb, LOE C).

As noted previously, defibrillation attempts (concurrent with rewarming strategies) are appropriate if VF or pulseless VT is present. Sinus bradycardia may be physiologic in severe hypothermia, and cardiac pacing is usually not indicated.

Techniques for in-hospital controlled rewarming include administration of warm, humid oxygen (42°C to 46°C [108°F to 115°F]), warm IV fluids (normal saline) at 42°C to 46°C (109°F), peritoneal lavage with warm fluids, pleural lavage with warm saline through chest tubes, extracorporeal blood warming with partial bypass,[66-69] and cardiopulmonary bypass.[70] A vasopressor may be considered during cardiac arrest according to the standard ACLS algorithm concurrent with rewarming techniques (Class IIb, LOE C).

After ROSC

After ROSC, patients should continue to be warmed to a target temperature of approximately 32°C to 34°C; this can be maintained according to standard postarrest guidelines for mild to moderate hypothermia in patients for whom induced hypothermia is appropriate. For those who have contraindications to induced hypothermia, rewarming can continue to normal temperatures.

Patients who have been hypothermic for more than 45 to 60 minutes are likely to require volume administration during rewarming because their vascular space will expand with vasodilation. Healthcare providers must closely monitor heart rate, perfusion, and hemodynamics at this time. Routine administration of steroids, barbiturates, or antibiotics has not been documented to help increase survival or decrease postresuscitation damage.[71,72]

There may be significant hyperkalemia during rewarming. In fact, the severity of hyperkalemia has been linked with mortality. Management of hyperkalemia should follow the current ACLS guidelines.

Because severe hypothermia is frequently preceded by problems such as drug overdose, alcohol intoxication, or trauma, the clinician must look for and address these underlying conditions while treating the hypothermia. If the patient appears malnourished or has chronic alcoholism, administer thiamine (100 mg IV) early during rewarming.

Termination of Resuscitative Efforts

Prehospital providers should transport the hypothermic patient in persistent cardiac arrest to the nearest appropriate emergency facility. In-hospital personnel can initiate or continue active internal rewarming as clinically indicated. Hypothermia may exert a protective effect on the brain and organs if the hypothermia develops rapidly in cardiac arrest. If submersion with asphyxiation preceded the patient's hypothermia, successful resuscitation is unlikely.

When it is clinically impossible to know whether the arrest or the hypothermia occurred first, providers should try to stabilize the patient with CPR. Basic maneuvers to limit heat loss and begin rewarming should be started. Complete rewarming is not indicated for all patients.

Previous reports have demonstrated survival from accidental hypothermia even with prolonged CPR and downtimes.[4,41] Thus, patients with severe accidental hypothermia and cardiac arrest can benefit from resuscitation even in cases of prolonged downtime and prolonged CPR. Low serum potassium may indicate hypothermia, and not hypoxia, as the primary cause of the arrest.[73] Patients should not be considered dead before warming has been provided. Once in the hospital, physicians should use their clinical judgment to decide when resuscitative efforts should cease in a patient of hypothermic arrest.

Differentiating Cardiac Arrest Due to Hypothermia From Normothermic Cardiac Arrest in a Cold Environment

Hypothermia may exert a protective effect on the brain and organs if core body temperature drops rapidly while the patient is still breathing and has a pulse. If the patient cools rapidly before arrest, a decrease in oxygen consumption and metabolism can precede the arrest and reduce organ ischemia. If the arrest occurs while the patient is normothermic and then the patient later develops hypothermia, the hypothermia cannot exert any protective effect.

The hypothermic patient also may have sustained additional organ insults before the arrest, such as asphyxiation from submersion. In cold-water immersion, for example, significant hypothermia occurs rapidly. But it may be hypothermia-induced exhaustion followed by submersion, aspiration, and hypoxia with eventual cardiac arrest. Successful resuscitation will be very unlikely in such circumstances. The recommended "default decision" is for providers to utilize the systematic approach and initiate full BLS and ACLS interventions when it is clinically impossible to determine whether the arrest or the hypothermia occurred first. Emergency care providers should modify these interventions as described in this chapter if significant hypothermia is documented.

Hypothermia Summary

Unintentional hypothermia is a special resuscitation situation in which prolonged and special resuscitative efforts can be beneficial and improve outcome. Careful management of the patient in the prearrest phase can prevent circulatory arrest and life-threatening arrhythmias. These patients require transport to specialized facilities with equipment and personnel knowledgeable in hypothermia care and rewarming. Many patients will also need integration of care with critical care specialists because multisystem complications are frequent. Table 76 defines the various degrees of hypothermia and correlates core temperature with symptoms and recommended therapy.

Cardiac Arrest in Avalanche Victims

Avalanche-related deaths are on the rise in North America because of winter recreational activities, including backcountry skiing and snowboarding, helicopter and snowcat skiing, snowmobiling, out-of-bounds skiing, ice climbing, mountaineering, and snowshoeing. The most common causes of avalanche-related death are asphyxia, trauma, and hypothermia, or combinations of the 3. Rescue and resuscitation strategies focus on management of asphyxia and hypothermia, because most field research has been done on these 2 conditions.

Avalanches occur in areas that are difficult to access by rescuers in a timely manner, and burials frequently involve multiple victims. The decision to initiate full resuscitative measures should be determined by the number of victims, resources available, and likelihood of survival. Studies of avalanche victims demonstrate a progressive nonlinear reduction in survival as the time of avalanche burial lengthens.[74-77] The likelihood of survival is minimal when avalanche victims are buried more than 35 minutes with an obstructed airway and in cardiac arrest on extrication[40,75,76,78-83] or are buried for any length of time and in cardiac arrest on extrication with an obstructed airway and an initial core temperature of lower than 32°C.[40,76-78,84]

It may be difficult to know with any certainty how long an avalanche victim has been buried. The core temperature at time of extrication provides a proxy for duration of burial. A case series[84] of buried avalanche victims showed a maximum cooling rate of 8°C per hour, whereas a case report[40] described a maximum cooling rate of 9°C per hour. These cooling rates suggest that at 35 minutes of burial, the core temperature may drop as low as 32°C.

If information on the duration of burial or the state of the airway on extrication is not available to the receiving physician, a serum potassium level lower than 8 mmol/L on hospital admission is a prognostic marker for ROSC[79] and survival to hospital discharge.[78,84] High potassium values are associated with asphyxia,[2,78,84,85] and there is an inverse correlation between admission K^+ and survival to discharge in all-cause hypothermic patients.[78,86-89] In a series of 32 avalanche survivors, the highest serum K^+ was 6.4 mmol/L,[84] but there is a single case report of a 31-month-old child with a K^+ of 11.8 mmol/L presenting with hypothermia from exposure unrelated to an avalanche who survived.[34] This suggests that the upper survivable limit of potassium is unknown for children who are hypothermic and victims of avalanche.

Full resuscitative measures, including extracorporeal rewarming when available, are recommended for all avalanche victims without the characteristics outlined above that deem them unlikely to survive or with any obvious lethal traumatic injury (Class I, LOE C).

References

1. Holzer M, Behringer W, Schorkhuber W, Zeiner A, Sterz F, Laggner AN, Frass M, Siostrozonek P, Ratheiser K, Kaff A. Mild hypothermia and outcome after CPR. Hypothermia for Cardiac Arrest (HACA) Study Group. *Acta Anaesthesiol Scand Suppl*. 1997;111:55-58.
2. Farstad M, Andersen KS, Koller ME, Grong K, Segadal L, Husby P. Rewarming from accidental hypothermia by extracorporeal circulation. A retrospective study. *Eur J Cardiothorac Surg*. 2001;20:58-64.
3. Schneider SM. Hypothermia: from recognition to rewarming. *Emerg Med Rep*. 1992;13:1-20.

4. Gilbert M, Busund R, Skagseth A, Nilsen PÅ, Solbø JP. Resuscitation from accidental hypothermia of 13.7°C with circulatory arrest. *Lancet*. 2000;355:375-376.

5. Exposure-related hypothermia deaths—District of Columbia, 1972-1982. *MMWR Morb Mortal Wkly Rep*. 1982;31:669-671.

6. Hypothermia-related deaths—Alaska, October 1998-April 1999, and trends in the United States, 1979-1996. *MMWR Morb Mortal Wkly Rep*. 2000;49:11-14.

7. Hypothermia-related deaths—Cook County, Illinois, November 1992-March 1993. *MMWR Morb Mortal Wkly Rep*. 1993;42:917-919.

8. Hypothermia-related deaths—Georgia, January 1996-December 1997, and United States, 1979-1995. *MMWR Morb Mortal Wkly Rep*. 1998;47:1037-1040.

9. Hypothermia-related deaths—New Mexico, October 1993-March 1994. *MMWR Morb Mortal Wkly Rep*. 1995;44:933-935.

10. Hypothermia-related deaths—North Carolina, November 1993-March 1994. *MMWR Morb Mortal Wkly Rep*. 1994;43:849, 855-856.

11. Hypothermia-related deaths—Suffolk County, New York, January 1999-March 2000, and United States, 1979-1998. *MMWR Morb Mortal Wkly Rep*. 2001;50:53-57.

12. Hypothermia-related deaths—Utah, 2000, and United States, 1979-1998. *MMWR Morb Mortal Wkly Rep*. 2002;51:76-78.

13. Hypothermia-related deaths—Vermont, October 1994-February 1996. *MMWR Morb Mortal Wkly Rep*. 1996;45:1093-1095.

14. Hypothermia-related deaths—Virginia, November 1996-April 1997. *MMWR Morb Mortal Wkly Rep*. 1997;46:1157-1159.

15. Hypothermia-associated deaths—United States, 1968-1980. *MMWR Morb Mortal Wkly Rep*. 1985;34:753-754.

16. Steinman AM, Giesbrecht G. Immersion into cold water. In: Auerbach PS, ed. *Wilderness Medicine*. St Louis, MO: Mosby; 2001:197-225.

17. Tipton M, Eglin C, Gennser M, Golden F. Immersion deaths and deterioration in swimming performance in cold water. *Lancet*. 1999;354:626-629.

18. Ryan JM. Immersion deaths and swim failure—implications for resuscitation and prevention. *Lancet*. 1999;354:613.

19. Teramoto S, Ouchi Y. Swimming in cold water. *Lancet*. 1999;354:1733.

20. Delaney K. Hypothermic sudden death. In: Paradis NA, Halperin HR, Nowak R, eds. *Cardiac Arrest: The Science and Practice of Resuscitation Medicine*. Baltimore, MD: Williams & Wilkins; 1996:745-760.

21. Danzl DF. Accidental hypothermia. In: Rosen P, Barkin R, eds. *Emergency Medicine: Concepts and Clinical Practice*. St Louis, MO: Mosby; 1998:963-986.

22. Danzl DF. Accidental hypothermia. In: Auerbach PS, ed. *Wilderness Medicine*. St Louis, MO: Mosby; 2001:135-177.

23. Sterz F, Behringer W, Berzanovich A. Active compression-decompression of thorax and abdomen (Lifestick CPR) in patients with cardiac arrest. *Circulation*. 1996;94(suppl 1):1-9. Abstract.

24. Larach MG. Accidental hypothermia. *Lancet*. 1995;345:493-498.

25. Bernard SA, Gray TW, Buist MD, Jones BM, Silvester W, Gutteridge G, Smith K. Treatment of comatose survivors of out-of-hospital cardiac arrest with induced hypothermia. *N Engl J Med*. 2002;346:557-563.

26. Hypothermia After Cardiac Arrest Study Group. Mild therapeutic hypothermia to improve the neurologic outcome after cardiac arrest. *N Engl J Med*. 2002;346:549-556.

27. Sheridan RL, Goldstein MA, Stoddard FJ Jr, Walker TG. Case records of the Massachusetts General Hospital. Case 41-2009. A 16-year-old boy with hypothermia and frostbite. *N Engl J Med*. 2009;361:2654-2662.

28. Kornberger E, Schwarz B, Lindner KH, Mair P. Forced air surface rewarming in patients with severe accidental hypothermia. *Resuscitation*. 1999;41:105-111.

29. Roggla M, Frossard M, Wagner A, Holzer M, Bur A, Roggla G. Severe accidental hypothermia with or without hemodynamic instability: rewarming without the use of extracorporeal circulation. *Wien Klin Wochenschr*. 2002;114:315-320.

30. Gilbert M, Busund R, Skagseth A, Nilsen PA, Solbo JP. Resuscitation from accidental hypothermia of 13.7 degrees C with circulatory arrest. *Lancet*. 2000;355:375-376.

31. Coleman E, Doddakula K, Meeke R, Marshall C, Jahangir S, Hinchion J. An atypical case of successful resuscitation of an accidental profound hypothermia patient, occurring in a temperate climate. *Perfusion*. 2010;25:103-106.

32. Walpoth BH, Walpoth-Aslan BN, Mattle HP, Radanov BP, Schroth G, Schaeffler L, Fischer AP, von Segesser L, Althaus U. Outcome of survivors of accidental deep hypothermia and circulatory arrest treated with extracorporeal blood warming. *N Engl J Med*. 1997;337:1500-1505.

33. Althaus U, Aeberhard P, Schupbach P, Nachbur BH, Muhlemann W. Management of profound accidental hypothermia with cardiorespiratory arrest. *Ann Surg*. 1982;195:492-495.

34. Dobson JA, Burgess JJ. Resuscitation of severe hypothermia by extracorporeal rewarming in a child. *J Trauma*. 1996;40:483-485.

35. Kangas E, Niemela H, Kojo N. Treatment of hypothermic circulatory arrest with thoracotomy and pleural lavage. *Ann Chir Gynaecol*. 1994;83:258-260.

36. Plaisier BR. Thoracic lavage in accidental hypothermia with cardiac arrest—report of a case and review of the literature. *Resuscitation*. 2005;66:99-104.

37. Winegard C. Successful treatment of severe hypothermia and prolonged cardiac arrest with closed thoracic cavity lavage. *J Emerg Med*. 1997;15:629-632.

38. Walters DT. Closed thoracic cavity lavage for hypothermia with cardiac arrest. *Ann Emerg Med*. 1991;20:439-440.

39. Hall KN, Syverud SA. Closed thoracic cavity lavage in the treatment of severe hypothermia in human beings. *Ann Emerg Med*. 1990;19:204-206.

40. Oberhammer R, Beikircher W, Hormann C, Lorenz I, Pycha R, Adler-Kastner L, Brugger H. Full recovery of an avalanche victim with profound hypothermia and prolonged cardiac arrest treated by extracorporeal re-warming. *Resuscitation*. 2008;76:474-480.

41. Tiruvoipati R, Balasubramanian SK, Khoshbin E, Hadjinikolaou L, Sosnowski AW, Firmin RK. Successful use of venovenous extracorporeal membrane oxygenation in accidental hypothermic cardiac arrest. *ASAIO J*. 2005;51:474-476.

42. Scaife ER, Connors RC, Morris SE, Nichol PF, Black RE, Matlak ME, Hansen K, Bolte RG. An established extracorporeal membrane oxygenation protocol promotes survival in extreme hypothermia. *J Pediatr Surg*. 2007;42:2012-2016.

43. Weinberg AD. The role of inhalation rewarming in the early management of hypothermia. *Resuscitation*. 1998;36:101-104.
44. Greif R, Rajek A, Laciny S, Bastanmehr H, Sessler DI. Resistive heating is more effective than metallic-foil insulation in an experimental model of accidental hypothermia: a randomized controlled trial. *Ann Emerg Med*. 2000;35:337-345.
45. Larach MG. Accidental hypothermia. *Lancet*. 1995;345:493-498.
46. Kornberger E, Schwarz B, Lindner KH, Mair P. Forced air surface rewarming in patients with severe accidental hypothermia. *Resuscitation*. 1999;41:105-111.
47. Giesbrecht GG, Paton B. Review article on inhalation rewarming. *Resuscitation*. 1998;38:59-60.
48. Weinberg AD. The role of inhalation rewarming in the early management of hypothermia. *Resuscitation*. 1998;36:101-104.
49. Danzl DF, Pozos RS, Auerbach PS, Glazer S, Goetz W, Johnson E, Jui J, Lilja P, Marx JA, Miller J, et al. Multicenter hypothermia survey. *Ann Emerg Med*. 1987;16:1042-1055.
50. Hayward JS. Thermal protection performance of survival suits in ice-water. *Aviat Space Environ Med*. 1984;55:212-215.
51. Miller JW, Danzl DF, Thomas DM. Urban accidental hypothermia: 135 cases. *Ann Emerg Med*. 1980;9:456-461.
52. Brunette DD, McVaney K. Hypothermic cardiac arrest: an 11 year review of ED management and outcome. *Am J Emerg Med*. 2000;18:418-422.
53. Walpoth BH, Walpoth-Aslan BN, Mattle HP, Radanov BP, Schroth G, Schaeffler L, Fischer AP, von Segesser L, Althaus U. Outcome of survivors of accidental deep hypothermia and circulatory arrest treated with extracorporeal blood warming. *N Engl J Med*. 1997;337:1500-1505.
54. Pickering BG, Bristow GK, Craig DB. Case history number 97: core rewarming by peritoneal irrigation in accidental hypothermia with cardiac arrest. *Anesth Analg*. 1977;56:574-577.
55. Lexow K. Severe accidental hypothermia: survival after 6 hours 30 minutes of cardiopulmonary resuscitation. *Arctic Med Res*. 1991;50(suppl 6):112-114.
56. Hall KN, Syverud SA. Closed thoracic cavity lavage in the treatment of severe hypothermia in human beings. *Ann Emerg Med*. 1990;19:204-206.
57. Iversen RJ, Atkin SH, Jaker MA, Quadrel MA, Tortella BJ, Odom JW. Successful CPR in a severely hypothermic patient using continuous thoracostomy lavage. *Ann Emerg Med*. 1990;19:1335-1337.
58. Steinman AM. Cardiopulmonary resuscitation and hypothermia. *Circulation*. 1986;74(pt 2):IV29-IV32.
59. Incagnoli P, Bourgeois B, Teboul A, Laborie JM. Resuscitation from accidental hypothermia of 22 degrees C with circulatory arrest: importance of prehospital management [in French]. *Ann Fr Anesth Reanim*. 2006;25:535-538.
60. Boddicker KA, Zhang Y, Zimmerman MB, Davies LR, Kerber RE. Hypothermia improves defibrillation success and resuscitation outcomes from ventricular fibrillation. *Circulation*. 2005;111:3195-3201.
61. Reuler JB. Hypothermia: pathophysiology, clinical settings, and management. *Ann Intern Med*. 1978;89:519-527.
62. Elenbaas RM, Mattson K, Cole H, Steele M, Ryan J, Robinson W. Bretylium in hypothermia-induced ventricular fibrillation in dogs. *Ann Emerg Med*. 1984;13:994-999.
63. Wira C, Martin G, Stoner J, Margolis K, Donnino M. Application of normothermic cardiac arrest algorithms to hypothermic cardiac arrest in a canine model. *Resuscitation*. 2006;69:509-516.
64. Wira CR, Becker JU, Martin G, Donnino MW. Anti-arrhythmic and vasopressor medications for the treatment of ventricular fibrillation in severe hypothermia: a systematic review of the literature. *Resuscitation*. 2008;78:21-29.
65. Lienhart HG, John W, Wenzel V. Cardiopulmonary resuscitation of a near-drowned child with a combination of epinephrine and vasopressin. *Pediatr Crit Care Med*. 2005;6:486-488.
66. Reuler JB. Hypothermia: pathophysiology, clinical settings, and management. *Ann Intern Med*. 1978;89:519-527.
67. Weinberg AD, Hamlet MP, Paturas JL, White RD, McAninch GW. *Cold Weather Emergencies: Principles of Patient Management*. Branford, CT: American Medical Publishing Co.; 1990.
68. Zell SC, Kurtz KJ. Severe exposure hypothermia: a resuscitation protocol. *Ann Emerg Med*. 1985;14:339-345.
69. Althaus U, Aeberhard P, Schupbach P, Nachbur BH, Muhlemann W. Management of profound accidental hypothermia with cardiorespiratory arrest. *Ann Surg*. 1982;195:492-495.
70. Silfvast T, Pettila V. Outcome from severe accidental hypothermia in Southern Finland—a 10-year review. *Resuscitation*. 2003;59:285-290.
71. Moss J. Accidental severe hypothermia. *Surg Gynecol Obstet*. 1986;162:501-513.
72. Safar P. Cerebral resuscitation after cardiac arrest: research initiatives and future directions [published correction appears in *Ann Emerg Med*. 1993;22:759]. *Ann Emerg Med*. 1993;22:324-349.
73. Kjaergaard B, Jakobsen LK, Nielsen C, Knudsen PJ, Kristensen SR, Larsson A. Low plasma potassium in deep hypothermic cardiac arrest indicates that cardiac arrest is secondary to hypothermia: a porcine study. *Eur J Emerg Med*. 2010;17:131-135.
74. Falk M, Brugger H, Adler-Kastner L. Avalanche survival chances. *Nature*. 1994;368:21.
75. Buser O, Etter HJ, Jaccard C. Probability of dying in an avalanche [in German]. *Z Unfallchir Versicherungsmed*. 1993;Suppl 1:263-271.
76. Brugger H, Falk M. New perspectives of avalanche disasters. Phase classification using pathophysiologic considerations [in German]. *Wien Klin Wochenschr*. 1992;104:167-173.
77. Brugger H, Durrer B, Adler-Kastner L, Falk M, Tschirky F. Field management of avalanche victims. *Resuscitation*. 2001;51:7-15.
78. Locher T, Walpoth B, Pfluger D, Althaus U. Accidental hypothermia in Switzerland (1980-1987)—case reports and prognostic factors [in German]. *Schweiz Med Wochenschr*. 1991;121:1020-1028.
79. Mair P, Kornberger E, Furtwaengler W, Balogh D, Antretter H. Prognostic markers in patients with severe accidental hypothermia and cardiocirculatory arrest. *Resuscitation*. 1994;27:47-54.
80. Grosse AB, Grosse CA, Steinbach LS, Zimmermann H, Anderson S. Imaging findings of avalanche victims. *Skeletal Radiol*. 2007;36:515-521.
81. Stalsberg H, Albretsen C, Gilbert M, Kearney M, Moestue E, Nordrum I, Rostrup M, Orbo A. Mechanism of death in

avalanche victims. *Virchows Arch A Pathol Anat Histopathol*. 1989;414:415-422.

82. Radwin MI, Grissom CK. Technological advances in avalanche survival. *Wilderness Environ Med*. 2002;13:143-152.

83. Paal P, Ellerton J, Sumann G, Demetz F, Mair P, Brugger H. Basic life support ventilation in mountain rescue. Official recommendations of the International Commission for Mountain Emergency Medicine (ICAR MEDCOM). *High Alt Med Biol*. 2007;8:147-154.

84. Locher T, Walpoth BH. Differential diagnosis of circulatory failure in hypothermic avalanche victims: retrospective analysis of 32 avalanche accidents [in German]. *Praxis (Bern 1994)*. 1996;85:1275-1282.

85. Schaller MD, Fischer AP, Perret CH. Hyperkalemia. A prognostic factor during acute severe hypothermia. *JAMA*. 1990;264:1842-1845.

86. Danzl DF, Pozos RS, Auerbach PS, Glazer S, Goetz W, Johnson E, Jui J, Lilja P, Marx JA, Miller J, et al. Multicenter hypothermia survey. *Ann Emerg Med*. 1987;16:1042-1055.

87. Ruttmann E, Weissenbacher A, Ulmer H, Muller L, Hofer D, Kilo J, Rabl W, Schwarz B, Laufer G, Antretter H, Mair P. Prolonged extracorporeal membrane oxygenation-assisted support provides improved survival in hypothermic patients with cardiocirculatory arrest. *J Thorac Cardiovasc Surg*. 2007;134:594-600.

88. Silfvast T, Pettila V. Outcome from severe accidental hypothermia in Southern Finland—a 10-year review. *Resuscitation*. 2003;59:285-290.

89. Hauty MG, Esrig BC, Hill JG, Long WB. Prognostic factors in severe accidental hypothermia: experience from the Mt. Hood tragedy. *J Trauma*. 1987;27:1107-1112.

90. Nozaki R, Ishibashi K, Adachi N, Nishihara S, Adachi S. Accidental profound hypothermia. *N Engl J Med*. 1986;315:1680.

Chapter 22

Cardiac Arrest Associated With Electrical Shock and Lightning Strikes

This Chapter

- Epidemiology of Electrical Shock and Lightning Strike
- Prevention of Electrical Shock and Lightning Strike Injuries
- Major Effects and Pathophysiology of Electrical Shock and Lightning Strike
- Out-of-Hospital and In-Hospital Management
- Critical BLS and ACLS Interventions and Postarrest Management

Introduction

Uncontrolled electrical current can cause severe injuries when it enters the body accidentally. There are 2 major means by which this occurs: technical electrical current (electrical shock) and lightning current. Injuries from electrical shock and lightning strike result from direct effects of current on the heart and brain, cell membranes, and vascular smooth muscle. Additional injuries result from the conversion of electrical energy into heat energy as current passes through body tissues.[1]

Electrical Shock

Technical electrical current or electrical shock can cause massive deep injury and not infrequently death. Loose terminology might refer to any electrical shock as an "electrocution." But this term specifically refers to death from electrical current. Otherwise the victim suffers an "electrical current injury" or "electrical shock injury."

Although fatal electrocutions may occur with household current, high-tension current generally causes the most serious injuries.[2] Contact with alternating current (the type of current commonly present in most North American households and commercial settings) may cause tetanic skeletal muscle contractions, "locking" the victim to the source of the electricity and thereby leading to prolonged exposure. The frequency of alternating current increases the likelihood of current flow through the heart during the relative refractory period, which is the "vulnerable period" of the cardiac cycle. Current impinging on the heart can induce physical injury (such as burning, bruising, and physical disruption) and precipitate arrhythmias, including ventricular fibrillation (VF) and asystole. This is analogous to the R-on-T phenomenon that occurs in nonsynchronized cardioversion.[3] An electrical current may also cause fatal pump impairment and electromechanical dissociation. Even low-voltage sources, such as those involved in bathtub incidents, can cause cardiac arrest.

Lightning Strike

Lightning strike presents a unique injury constellation of its own. Burns are of minimal concern, but cardiovascular, central nervous system, and autonomic nervous system injury can be significant.

Blunt trauma and blunt head injury may occur with both types of current because of muscle contraction or falls, a blast effect from arcing or circuit box explosion, or the concussive effects of being close to a lightning strike point. Long-term neurocognitive damage with chronic pain, sometimes termed *post–electrical shock syndrome,* has been consistently identified.

The ACLS provider who treats cardiac arrest caused by electrical shock or lightning strike must provide cardiopulmonary resuscitation (CPR) and trauma and burn care. In general, more prolonged resuscitative efforts and more aggressive fluid resuscitation are indicated for these patients than for other patients in cardiac arrest.

Epidemiology

Electrical shock injuries cause approximately 500 deaths annually in the United States.[4] The National Weather Service estimates that an average of 54 reported deaths have occurred due to lightning strikes in the United States per year in a 30-year period (1981-2010).[5] Historically, up to 150 to 300 deaths have occurred in a year.[6] Although these are not common causes of traumatic death, they are responsible for an estimated 52 000 trauma admissions per year and 4% to 7% of burn center admissions.[6] Many people who survive electrical shock or lightning strike have permanent sequelae.

Electrical Shock

Various groups are at particular risk for electrical injury. In a comprehensive epidemiological analysis of deaths due to electrical shock, Lindstrom et al[7] identified patterns of injury using data from 285 electricity-related deaths in Sweden from 1975 to 2000. The investigators defined "electrocution" as a *cause of death* that included death from electrical shock, from burns caused by arcs, and from falls from a height. The vast majority of victims were male (94%); 132 incidents (46%) were related to work activities and 151 (53%) to recreational or leisure activities (2 cases unknown). Thirty-six deaths (13%) occurred in adolescents. Approximately 20% of cases involved alcohol. The researchers identified several significantly dangerous activities: performing unauthorized repairs, using alcohol, overlooking overhead power lines, or simply using poor judgment. These findings emphasize the importance of staying clear of fallen lines and of keeping domestic electrical apparatus in good repair.

The most dangerous situation remains accidental contact with aerial power lines, and these deaths are roughly equally distributed between recreational and occupational deaths. Such incidents accounted for 40% of the total.[7]

However, although aerial power lines pose the greatest risk of electrical shock, these injuries can occur in nearly all areas in which people move, including indoor residential properties and even gardens (Table 77). Electrical injuries in the home account for nearly half of the annual deaths from electrical shock.[6] Pediatric electrical shock injuries typically occur around the home—when the child bites an electrical wire, places an object in an electrical socket, contacts an exposed low-voltage wire or appliance, or touches a high-voltage wire outdoors.[8]

Table 77. Common Locations for Electrocution

Location	Occupational	Leisure
Railway site	23/64	41/64
Residential	6/53	49/53
Substation	25/30	5/30
Farmhouse	19/25	6/25
Garden	0/21	21/21
Workshop	15/18	3/18
Construction site	15/16	1/16
Power pole	12/15	3/15
Water area	1/11	10/11
Other	16/32	12/32
TOTAL	**132/285**	**151/285**

Data from Lindström et al.[7] Published by Blackwell. Copyright © 2006 by American Academy of Forensic Sciences.

Lightning Strike

Lightning strike is a leading environmental cause of cardiac arrest. Victims may be injured by a direct strike or through a side flash or splash (Figure 120) or from shock waves created in the surrounding air. Lightning strike injuries can vary widely, even among groups of people struck at the same time. Symptoms are mild in some victims, whereas fatal injuries occur in others.[10,11] Lightning strikes kill hundreds of people internationally every year and injure many times that number. Approximately 30% of victims of lightning strike die, and up to 70% of survivors sustain significant and permanent sequelae.[12-14]

In many cases of apparent direct strike, victims who receive immediate resuscitation can survive because much of the lightning current "flashes over" the victim and only a small amount enters the body. Figure 121 shows the unique

Critical Concept

Disability, Not Death, Is the Issue

Although accidental death is an undoubted tragedy, survivors of electrical injury demonstrate tremendous ongoing disability,[9] which is important both personally and for society.

"ferning" pattern that can be produced on the skin by this flashover phenomenon.

Cloud-to-ground lightning strikes the surface of the US approximately 25 million times per year. The largest number of cloud-to-ground flashes per area is located in central Florida between Tampa and Orlando.[15,16]

Lightning deaths are tracked more carefully than injuries because fatalities are reported more completely.[17] One reason for the difficulty in reporting lightning casualties is that about 90% of all deaths and injuries occur to one person at a time. A ratio of 10 injuries per death is considered to be the most reasonable estimate of injuries over the long term.[18]

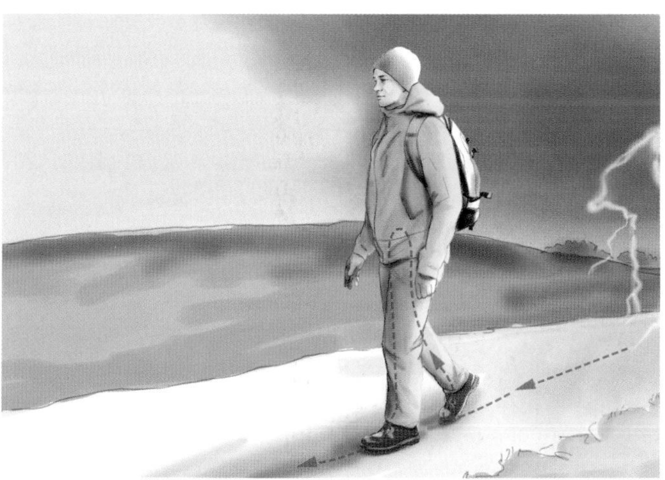

Figure 120. Side flash or splash. Current from a lightning strike is conducted to a nearby victim through the ground. The victim's legs conduct the current through his lower body.

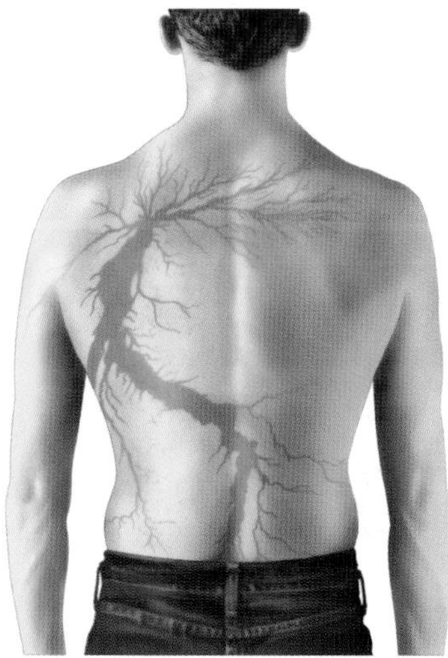

Figure 121. A man struck by lightning. His back displays an erythematous, fern-leaf pattern that was painless. This pattern has been referred to as "Lichtenberg figures."

A century ago, indoor fatalities were the most frequent, but today only 2% of lightning deaths occur inside houses. Outdoor incidents are the most frequent, and victims often are standing under trees.[19] A high percentage of lightning deaths occur during recreation, especially in beach, water, and camping settings. In addition, incidents during sports activities such as soccer, baseball and softball, golf, and hiking have become more common in recent years.[20,21] Rural casualties are now half as frequent as urban cases.

Prevention

Identification of risk groups, the most common settings for electrical shocks and lightning strikes, and epidemiologic trends enables us to introduce measures to prevent many of these injuries and deaths.

Electrical Shock Injury Prevention

Several useful strategies have been developed to help prevent technical electrical injuries. These include building construction techniques and codes to require insulation of conductors in overhead cable swings so that they are insulated where contact might likely occur.

The adoption of standards for safe equipment manufacture has led to the development of circuit breaker closure and reclosure apparatus, semi-insulated cable plugs, and molded integrated plugs and sockets to prevent tampering and unauthorized repair. A significant advance is development of *residual current devices*. These devices compare the current flowing to and from a device, which should be equal. If the device detects an imbalance, it is assumed that the imbalance is caused by diversion of current through a person and the power is disconnected.

Many companies have adopted workplace codes, safe procedures, and specific protocols for responding to accidents. Companies are encouraged to frequently reinforce use of protective devices.

Lightning Strike Injury Prevention

Lightning injury prevention, for the most part, is an individual responsibility unless large venues such as summer camps or sports stadiums are involved.

Prevention requires familiarity with lightning safety guidelines:

1. Know the weather forecast before starting an activity.
2. If bad weather is predicted, make alternative plans.
3. Know the weather patterns in the area where you are planning to be. Be off of mountains, golf courses, and other lightning-prone areas before the time of maximum lightning exposure, which is generally the afternoon hours.

4. Have a "weather eye"—watch the sky for signs of a storm.
5. At the first sound of thunder, which rarely can be heard more than 10 miles away (and often a lot less), you are already in danger and should be in safer shelter, such as a substantial (habitable) building with plumbing and wiring or a fully enclosed metal vehicle with all the windows closed.
6. Do not resume outdoor activities until at least 30 minutes after the last thunder is heard or lightning is seen.

Information about lightning safety for larger venues is available from the National Weather Service (**www.lightningsafety.noaa.gov**).

Major Effects of Electrical Shock and Lightning Strike

Fatal Arrhythmias

The greatest danger for death from electrical shock or lightning strike is the induction of arrhythmias.[7] In the US study by Jones et al,[22] 85% of deaths were due to arrhythmias. The arrhythmias of most importance are those that give rise to cardiac arrest, namely asystole, which is thought to occur more commonly in lightning strike, and VF, thought to occur in "lesser" technical electrical shocks.

Most other arrhythmias, including atrial tachycardia and fibrillation, ventricular tachycardia (VT), and atrial and ventricular ectopia, are inducible with electrical shock. But these arrhythmias do not necessarily lead to immediate death. Some clinicians have observed a delayed induction of arrhythmias within the first few days to 1 to 2 weeks after recovery from electrical shock.

A current of around 20 μA applied directly to the heart is sufficient to induce an asystolic state or VF. Conversely this level of current can act as a defibrillating current when directly applied.

Neural Dysfunction

Common sense assumes that because nervous tissue is by nature electrical in function, it must be susceptible to electrical damage. This view assumes that neural membranes are immediately available to the passage of current. But nerve trunks are enclosed in a protective sheath of highly fatty and relatively resistive tissue, so electrical current may not have the immediately deleterious effects on nerve function as might seem likely at first.

Myocardial Tissue Damage by Burn Injury

Tissue, including myocardial tissue, may be damaged by burns. Burn damage produces a focal area of damaged myocardium not unlike that seen in infarction, and this area can become a site of myocardial rupture. Electrical current most often travels hand to foot, so burn damage usually occurs inferiorly and may be reflected on the electrocardiogram (ECG) in inferior leads II, III, and aVF. Several authors have reported this type of damage and an ECG pattern typical of infarction immediately after electrical injury.[23,24]

The ECG in Electrical Injury

For patients who survive an acute electrical shock, the resolution of ECG changes and abnormal cardiac marker levels are insufficient to indicate recovery of the myocardium. A thorough assessment of the extent and severity of myocardial damage requires additional studies, such as echocardiography and single-photon emission computed tomography (SPECT). Clinicians must also consider the effects of catecholamine excess and hypertension, which can develop from inotropic and vascular changes, on the damaged heart. Chandra et al[25] report that the best clinical predictors of myocardial damage are the extent of surface burns and a pathway of current involving the heart, which they define as one where the entry and exit points are superior and inferior to the heart, respectively. The current-time profile is another parameter to consider.

Critical Concept

Assessing Myocardial Damage in Patients With Electrical Injury

Conventional wisdom has been that once a patient survives an acute electrical shock, the ECG changes and myocardial damage resolve and myocardial function returns. But the clinician should not rely on resolution of ECG changes and abnormal enzyme levels alone to indicate recovery of the myocardium. If clinically indicated, the clinician should also consider

- Findings on additional studies (eg, echocardiography, SPECT)
- Effects of catecholamine excess and hypertension on the damaged heart
- Current-time profile

Perhaps the best clinical predictors of myocardial damage are the extent of surface burns and a pathway of current involving the heart (ie, one where the entry and exit points are superior and inferior to the heart, respectively).[25]

A valuable overview of these issues is given by Fish.[26] The mechanisms of induction of arrhythmias have also been well outlined.[3,27]

Lightning injury seems more straightforward. It is commonly agreed, and appears supported, that even though many different ECG patterns may be seen acutely, full resolution of signs and complete recovery of function is the norm.

Pathophysiology

Electrical Shock Injury

Life-threatening arrhythmias, including VT or ventricular ectopy, may result from either low-intensity or high-intensity electrical current, and cardiopulmonary arrest may result. Low-voltage alternating current typically causes VF, while high-intensity current can cause asystole. In addition to arrhythmias, the current may create a brief but substantial inotropic stimulus, widespread muscle contraction and probable muscle cell rupture, myocardial cell damage, coronary artery spasm, and decreased coronary artery perfusion. These factors can contribute to cardiopulmonary arrest, postshock arrhythmias, and persistent myocardial dysfunction.

Respiratory arrest can be caused by the passage of electrical current through the brain, by contraction of the diaphragm and chest wall muscles, from prolonged paralysis of the respiratory muscles, and by cessation of brain perfusion secondary to cardiac arrest. The respiratory arrest may persist even after circulation is restored.

Metabolic and systemic complications of electrical injury include organ, muscle, and joint injuries and burns. Fractures of long bones and joint dislocations following electrical shock can be caused by severe muscle contractions or falls. Many patients demonstrate hypovolemia and metabolic acidosis from fluid loss through skin damage and tissue destruction. Rhabdomyolysis may result from muscle injury and may lead to renal failure. Vascular complications may compromise perfusion to extremities, and neurologic injuries can range from coma or altered level of consciousness to peripheral nerve damage.

Little is known about how electrical current affects individual cells, but some understanding and data are available based on our knowledge of *electroporation,* a technique used in molecular biology. In this technique electrical current is applied to a cell plasma membrane (or other living surface, such as skin) to increase its electrical conductivity and permeability. With exposure to current, pores will form in the membrane, allowing introduction of a substance such as a drug or coding DNA. If the voltage and duration of exposure are appropriate, these pores will reseal in a short time with no long-term damage to the cell.

Lightning Strike Injury

The most common cause of death in lightning strike is cardiac arrest. The arrest may be associated with primary VF or asystole.[10,11,28,29]

Lightning acts as an instantaneous, massive, direct-current shock that depolarizes the entire myocardium at once.[11,30] In the 70% of lightning strike victims who survive, cardiac automaticity resumes spontaneously. Organized cardiac activity and a perfusing rhythm soon follow.

Victims of lightning strike frequently suffer acute respiratory arrest. Unless ventilatory assistance is provided, a secondary hypoxic (asphyxia) cardiac arrest may occur. This cessation of breathing may be caused by a variety of mechanisms, such as electrical current passing through the brain and stopping further respiratory center activity in the medulla, tetanic contraction of the diaphragm and chest wall musculature during exposure to the current, and prolonged paralysis of respiratory muscles, which may continue for minutes after the electrical shock ends.

A lightning strike has a widespread effect on the cardiovascular system. The strike results in extensive catecholamine release, which stimulates the autonomic nervous system. If cardiac arrest does not occur, the victim may develop hypertension, tachycardia, and nonspecific ECG changes (including prolongation of the QT interval and transient T-wave inversion). Myocardial necrosis with release of MB fraction of creatine kinase (CK-MB) may occur. Right and left ventricular ejection fractions may also be depressed, but this effect appears to be reversible.

Lightning can produce a wide spectrum of neurologic injuries. Injuries may be primary, resulting from effects on the brain, or secondary, developing as complications of cardiac arrest and hypoxia. The current can produce brain hemorrhage, edema, and small-vessel and neuronal injury. Hypoxic encephalopathy can result from cardiac arrest. A lightning strike can also damage myelin of peripheral nerves.

The etiology of respiratory and cardiac arrest following lightning injury has not been well studied, but these events may result from injury to the central nervous system; the autonomic nervous system; or the sinoatrial node, atrioventricular node, or other conducting pathways as current traverses through or around the outside of the body ("flash-over"). Autonomic injury has been reported both clinically and in laboratory studies.[31-34]

Mechanisms of Electrical Current Effects in Lightning Strike

There are 5 mechanisms by which electrical current in a lightning strike may affect a person[35,36]:

- Direct strike—self-explanatory: less than 10% of injuries.
- Side flash or splash—when a person is standing next to a struck object and a portion of current jumps to the person: 25% to 40% of injuries.
- Contact potential—when a person is touching a struck object and a portion of the current is diverted through the person: 3% to 10% of injuries.
- Ground potential (step voltage, stride potential)—when lightning hits an object on the ground at a distance from the person, current is injected into the ground and flows radially from the struck object; injury to a person occurs as the current travels through the ground or as it arcs across an irregular surface through which it is traveling: 30% to 60% of injuries.
- Upward streamer—the electrical field in a thundercloud induces opposite charges and "upward streamers" that may pass through anything in the field, including people. Even when the streamer fails to contact the lightning channel to complete the stroke, the current can be significant enough to cause serious injury or death: 10% to 25% of injuries.

Although it is "common sense" that the direct strike is more likely to cause fatalities, this has never been substantiated by clinical or laboratory studies. The physics of lightning is incredibly complex; lightning is a current phenomenon, not the voltage phenomenon of generated electricity with which we are more familiar.

Out-of-Hospital Management

Electrical Shock

Out-of-hospital management is essentially standard BLS and ACLS management with minor modifications and extra precaution on-site. With electrical shock, the most important consideration is to not convert a situation with one victim into a situation with multiple victims.

The first task is extrication of the victim. It is most important to know—and this is entirely different from lightning-injured persons—that *a victim who remains in contact with electrical current is dangerous to touch.* A rescuer who touches a victim before the source of current is turned off may be shocked. In addition, any material can conduct high-voltage current, and current can flow through the ground surrounding the victim. For these reasons the rescuer should not even approach the victim until the power source is turned off.

The first step is to break the connection between the person and the current source. For incidents involving a utility worker atop a pole, the specific protocols for pole-top rescue must be followed, and all workers should be well trained in these procedures. *Only rescuers specifically trained to break a live connection should attempt this intervention.*

For incidents occurring during recreational activities, the following process can be used:

Safely switch off the power to the apparatus or line that is thought to be the source of the shock, either at the switch or by pulling the plug. This must be done safely—with *no contact with any conductor.* A wise policy is to do this with one hand only and no other environmental body contact. If immediate disconnection is not possible, switch off a circuit breaker or pull the appropriate fuse at the switchboard. Alternatively, turn off the whole installation at the main switch.

Alternative methods of removing a victim from the source have been proposed. These methods include dragging the victim away with insulated hands and using a dry pole as a lever to move the victim. These methods should be used with extreme caution. Once the power supply is off, the victim is safe to touch.

Lightning Strike

As with electrical current injury, the top priority in lightning injury is safety. Victims of lightning strike will not be connected to the source of electricity when rescuers arrive, but if weather conditions are still inclement, the scene is still dangerous. Rescuers should remove the victim from the lightning-prone area to a safe shelter or emergency medical services (EMS) vehicle as soon as possible and provide BLS and ACLS as described below.

Victims are most likely to die of lightning injury if they experience immediate respiratory or cardiac arrest and no treatment is provided. Patients who do not suffer respiratory or cardiac arrest, and those who respond to immediate treatment, have an excellent chance of recovery. Therefore, when multiple victims are struck simultaneously by lightning, rescuers should give the highest priority to patients in respiratory or cardiac arrest.

BLS for Electrical Shock and Lightning Strike Injury

For victims in cardiac arrest, treatment should be early, aggressive, and persistent. If immediate resuscitation is provided, survival from cardiac arrest caused by lightning strike is higher than that reported following cardiac arrest from other non-VF causes. Resuscitative efforts may be effective even when the interval between collapse and the start of resuscitation is prolonged or when cardiac arrest persists despite initial efforts.[37] The goal is to oxygenate the heart and brain adequately until cardiac activity resumes. Victims in respiratory arrest may require only ventilation and oxygenation to avoid secondary hypoxic cardiac arrest.

Once the victim is separated from the source of current and the scene is safe, determine cardiorespiratory status. Immediately after electrocution, respiration or circulation or both may fail. If spontaneous respiration or circulation is absent, immediately initiate BLS, including activation of the EMS system, prompt provision of CPR, and use of an automated external defibrillator (AED) when available. Immediate provision of ventilation and compressions (if needed) is essential. Use the AED to identify and treat VT or VF.

Maintain spinal stabilization throughout extrication and treatment if there is a likelihood of head or neck trauma.[38,39] Both lightning strikes and electrical shock often cause multiple trauma, including injury to the spine,[39] muscular strains, internal injuries from being thrown, and fractures caused by the tetanic response of skeletal muscles.[40] Remove smoldering clothing, shoes, and belts to prevent further thermal damage.

Vigorous resuscitative measures are indicated even for those who appear dead on initial evaluation. Because many victims are young, without preexisting cardiopulmonary disease, they have a good chance of survival if immediate support of cardiopulmonary function is provided.

ACLS for Electrical Shock and Lightning Strike Injury

No modification of standard ACLS care is required for victims of electrical injury or lightning strike, with the exception of paying attention to possible cervical spine injury. Establishing an airway may be difficult for patients with electrical burns of the face, mouth, or anterior neck. Extensive soft-tissue swelling may develop rapidly, complicating airway control measures. Thus, early intubation should be performed for patients with evidence of extensive burns even if the patient has begun to breathe spontaneously.

For victims with significant tissue destruction and in whom a pulse is regained, rapid intravenous fluid administration is indicated to counteract distributive/hypovolemic shock and to correct ongoing fluid losses due to third spacing. Fluid administration should be adequate to maintain diuresis and facilitate excretion of myoglobin, potassium, and other byproducts of tissue destruction (this is particularly true for patients with electrical injury).[30] Regardless of the extent of external injuries following an electrothermal shock, the underlying tissue damage can be far more extensive.

Early Subspecialty Involvement and Transfer

As significant as the external injuries may appear after electrothermal shock, the underlying tissue damage is far more extensive, and survivors may have permanent neurologic and cardiac sequelae. Early consultation with or transfer to a physician and a facility (eg, burn center) familiar with treatment of these injuries is critical.

In-Hospital Management

The Medical Emergency Team

Management of cardiac arrest due to electrical shock or lightning strike generally involves ventilatory support, monitoring, cardiac compression, and standard drugs. However, these patients may have other severe injuries, including trauma from a fall, deep burns, and even injuries due to exposure. A multidisciplinary medical emergency team (MET) with subspecialists from critical care, trauma, neurology, surgery, and cardiology can be very beneficial for these patients and should be activated early.

Differential Diagnoses

Increased capillary permeability will occur in association with tissue injury. Expect the development of local tissue edema at the site of injury. Compartment syndromes can rapidly develop in any extremity, especially if circumferential burns are present. This severe tissue edema can produce local areas of vascular compromise and tissue necrosis.

Electrothermal burns and underlying tissue injury may require surgical attention for debridement or fasciotomies. Seek early consultation with a physician skilled in treatment of electrical injuries.

Postarrest Management

An important question is how long a patient should be monitored after an electrical shock or lightning strike injury. A well person with no signs of cardiac dysfunction, no abnormal cardiac markers, and a normal ECG can generally be discharged within 6 hours of the shock. A middle course is to

Critical Concept **"Reverse Triage" for Multiple Victims of Lightning Strike**	In a multicasualty lightning strike event, the victim who develops immediate cardiac arrest has a high probability of survival and recovery *if BLS is provided without delay.* When multiple victims suffer simultaneous lightning strike, give the highest priority to victims who are in respiratory or cardiac arrest. Victims of lightning strike who do not suffer immediate cardiopulmonary arrest are unlikely to do so. They have an excellent chance of recovery with little additional treatment.

monitor the patient for 24 hours and then, if all remains well, discharge. Any abnormality that develops should be treated as needed before discharge. However, as noted above, many patients with electrical injury will have permanent neurologic, cardiac, or physical sequelae. These patients will require rehabilitation and long-term follow-up care.

References

1. Fish RM, Geddes LA. Conduction of electrical current to and through the human body: a review. *Eplasty*. 2009;9:e44.
2. Budnick LD. Bathtub-related electrocutions in the United States, 1979 to 1982. *JAMA*. 1984;252:918-920.
3. Geddes LA, Bourland JD, Ford G. The mechanism underlying sudden death from electric shock. *Med Instrum*. 1986;20:303-315.
4. National Safety Council. *1999 Injury Facts*. Itasca, IL: National Safety Council; 1999.
5. National Weather Service. Lightning safety. Medical aspects of lightning. http://www.lightningsafety.noaa.gov/medical.htm. Accessed October 10, 2012.
6. Fontanarosa PB. Electrical shock and lightning strike. *Ann Emerg Med*. 1993;22:378-387.
7. Lindstrom R, Bylund PO, Eriksson A. Accidental deaths caused by electricity in Sweden, 1975-2000. *J Forensic Sci*. 2006;51:1383-1388.
8. Kobernick M. Electrical injuries: pathophysiology and emergency management. *Ann Emerg Med*. 1982;11:633-638.
9. Cooper MA, Andrews CJ. Disability, not death, is the issue in lightning injury. Presented at: International Conference on Lightning and Static Electricity; Seattle, WA; 2005.
10. Patten BM. Lightning and electrical injuries. *Neurol Clin*. 1992;10:1047-1058.
11. Browne BJ, Gaasch WR. Electrical injuries and lightning. *Emerg Med Clin North Am*. 1992;10:211-229.
12. Cooper MA. Lightning injuries: prognostic signs for death. *Ann Emerg Med*. 1980;9:134-138.
13. Kleinschmidt-DeMasters BK. Neuropathology of lightning-strike injuries. *Semin Neurol*. 1995;15:323-328.
14. Stewart CE. When lightning strikes. *Emerg Med Serv*. 2000;29:57-67.
15. Huffines GR, Orville RE. Lightning ground flash density and thunderstorm duration in the contiguous United States: 1989-1996. *J Appl Meteorol*. 1999;38:1013.
16. Orville RE, Huffines GR, Burrows WR, Holle RL, Cummins KL. The North American Lightning Detection Network (NALDN)—first results: 1998-2000. *Monthly Weather Rev*. 2002;130:2098.
17. López RE. The underreporting of lightning injuries and deaths in Colorado. *Bull Am Meteorol Soc*. 1993;74:2171.
18. Cherington M, Walker J, Boyson M, Glancy R, Hedegaard H, Clark S. Closing the gap on the actual numbers of lightning casualties and deaths. Presented at: 11th Conference on Applied Climatology; Dallas, TX; January 10-15, 1999.
19. Holle RL, López RE, Navarro BC. Deaths, injuries, and damages from lightning in the United States in the 1890s in comparison with the 1990s. *J Appl Meteorol*. 2005;44:1563-1573.
20. Holle RL. Activities and locations of recreation deaths and injuries from lightning. Presented at: International Conference on Lightning and Static Electricity; Blackpool, UK; September 16-18, 2003.
21. Holle RL. Lightning-caused deaths and injuries during hiking and mountain climbing. Presented at: International Conference on Lightning and Static Electricity; Seattle, WA; September 20-22, 2005.
22. Jones JE, Armstrong CW, Woolard CD, Miller GB Jr. Fatal occupational electrical injuries in Virginia. *J Occup Med*. 1991;33:57-63.
23. Romero B, Candell-Riera J, Gracia RM, Fernandez MA, Aguade S, Peracaula R, Soler-Soler J. Myocardial necrosis by electrocution: evaluation of noninvasive methods. *J Nucl Med*. 1997;38:250-251.
24. Homma S, Gillam LD, Weyman AE. Echocardiographic observations in survivors of acute electrical injury. *Chest*. 1990;97:103-105.
25. Chandra NC, Siu CO, Munster AM. Clinical predictors of myocardial damage after high voltage electrical injury. *Crit Care Med*. 1990;18:293-297.
26. Fish R. Electric shock, part II: nature and mechanisms of injury. *J Emerg Med*. 1993;11:457-462.
27. Bridges JE, Ford CL, Sherman IA, Vainberg M, eds. *Electrical Shock Safety Criteria: Proceedings of the First International Symposium on Electrical Shock Safety Criteria*. New York, NY: Pergamon Press; 1985.
28. Lichtenberg R, Dries D, Ward K, Marshall W, Scanlon P. Cardiovascular effects of lightning strikes. *J Am Coll Cardiol*. 1993;21:531-536.
29. Kleiner JP, Wilkin JH. Cardiac effects of lightning stroke. *JAMA*. 1978;240:2757-2759.
30. Cooper MA. Emergent care of lightning and electrical injuries. *Semin Neurol*. 1995;15:268-278.
31. Grubb BP, Karabin B. New onset postural tachycardia syndrome following lightning injury. *Pacing Clin Electrophysiol*. 2007;30:1036-1038.
32. Weeramanthri TS, Puddey IB, Beilin LJ. Lightning strike and autonomic failure: coincidence or causally related? *J R Soc Med*. 1991;84:687-688.
33. Cooper MA, Kotsos T, Gandhi MV, Neideen T. Acute autonomic and cardiac effects of simulated lightning strike in rodents. Presented at: International Bioengineering Symposium; Chicago, IL; July 2000.
34. Cooper MA. The acute effects of simulated lightning strike on the cardiac and autonomic nervous system in an animal model. Presented at: International Conference in Lightning and Static Electricity; Blackpool, UK; September 15-19, 2003.
35. Cooper MA. A fifth mechanism of lightning injury. *Acad Emerg Med*. 2002;9:172-174.
36. Cooper MA, Andrews CJ, Holle RL. Distribution of lightning injury mechanisms. Presented at: International Lightning Detection Conference; Tucson, AZ; April 24-25, 2006.
37. Milzman DP, Moskowitz L, Hardel M. Lightning strikes at a mass gathering. *South Med J*. 1999;92:708-710.
38. Duclos PJ, Sanderson LM. An epidemiological description of lightning-related deaths in the United States. *Int J Epidemiol*. 1990;19:673-679.
39. Epperly TD, Stewart JR. The physical effects of lightning injury. *J Fam Pract*. 1989;29:267-272.
40. Whitcomb D, Martinez JA, Daberkow D. Lightning injuries. *South Med J*. 2002;95:1331-1334.

Chapter 23

Cardiac Arrest Associated With Cardiac Procedures

This Chapter

- Cardiac Arrest During Percutaneous Coronary Intervention
- Cardiac Arrest After Cardiac Surgery

Cardiac Arrest During Percutaneous Coronary Intervention

During both elective and emergent percutaneous coronary intervention (PCI), there is risk of cardiac arrest. Although high-quality chest compressions improve the chance of successful resuscitation and survival, it is difficult to perform effective, high-quality chest compressions during PCI. Therefore, resuscitation adjuncts have been explored for the treatment of cardiac arrest during PCI. There are no randomized controlled trials evaluating alternative treatment strategies compared with standard care for cardiac arrest during PCI.

Mechanical CPR During PCI

Mechanical chest compression devices have been used successfully in an animal model[1] and adult humans[1-5] to provide maintenance of circulation in cardiac arrest while continuing a percutaneous coronary procedure. It is reasonable to use mechanical cardiopulmonary resuscitation (CPR) during PCI (Class IIa, LOE C).

Emergency Cardiopulmonary Bypass

One case series[6] describes the use of emergency cardiopulmonary bypass to stabilize and facilitate emergency coronary angioplasty in patients with cardiac arrest unresponsive to ACLS during PCI. It is reasonable to use emergency cardiopulmonary bypass during PCI (Class IIb, LOE C).

Cough CPR

Multiple case reports[7-10] describe the use of cough CPR to temporarily maintain adequate blood pressure and level of consciousness in patients who develop ventricular arrhythmias during PCI while definitive therapy for malignant arrhythmias is instituted. It is reasonable to use cough CPR during PCI (Class IIa, LOE C).

Intracoronary Verapamil

One large case series[11] describes the successful use of intracoronary verapamil to terminate reperfusion-induced ventricular tachycardia (VT) following mechanical revascularization therapy. Verapamil was not successful in terminating ventricular fibrillation (VF).

Cardiac Arrest After Cardiac Surgery

The incidence of cardiac arrest after cardiac surgery is in the range of 1% to 3%. Causes include conditions that may be readily reversed, such as VF, hypovolemia, cardiac tamponade, or tension pneumothorax. Pacing wires, if present, may reverse symptomatic bradycardia or asystole. A recent review may be helpful for those seeking additional information.[12]

Resternotomy

Studies of patients with cardiac arrest after cardiac surgery who are treated with resternotomy and internal cardiac compression have reported improved outcome compared with a standard protocol[13-23] when patients are treated by experienced personnel in intensive care units (ICUs). Findings of similar quality studies[24-28] reported no difference in outcomes when resternotomy was compared with standard management of cardiac arrest after cardiac surgery. Resternotomy performed outside an ICU generally has a very poor outcome.[13,20,27]

For patients with cardiac arrest following cardiac surgery, it is reasonable to perform resternotomy in an appropriately staffed and equipped ICU (Class IIa, LOE B). Despite rare case reports describing damage to the heart possibly due to external chest compressions, chest compressions should not be withheld if emergency resternotomy is not immediately available (Class IIa, LOE C).[29,30]

Mechanical Circulatory Support

Nine case series have reported survival of some post–cardiac surgery patients who had cardiac arrest that was refractory to standard resuscitation measures and received extracorporeal membrane oxygenation (ECMO)[31-35] and cardiopulmonary bypass.[23,36-38] In post–cardiac surgery patients who are refractory to standard resuscitation procedures, mechanical circulatory support (eg, ECMO and cardiopulmonary bypass) may be effective in improving outcome (Class IIb, LOE B).

Pharmacologic Intervention

Rebound hypertension following the administration of vasopressors during resuscitation has the potential to induce significant bleeding in this group of patients. Results from a single study of epinephrine[39] and another study evaluating the choice of antiarrhythmics[40] in patients with cardiac arrest following cardiac surgery were neutral. There is insufficient evidence on epinephrine dose, antiarrhythmic use, and other routine pharmacologic interventions to recommend deviating from standard resuscitation guidelines when cardiac arrest occurs after cardiac surgery.

References

1. Grogaard HK, Wik L, Eriksen M, Brekke M, Sunde K. Continuous mechanical chest compressions during cardiac arrest to facilitate restoration of coronary circulation with percutaneous coronary intervention. *J Am Coll Cardiol*. 2007;50:1093-1094.
2. Agostoni P, Cornelis K, Vermeersch P. Successful percutaneous treatment of an intraprocedural left main stent thrombosis with the support of an automatic mechanical chest compression device. *Int J Cardiol*. 2008;124:e19-e21.
3. Steen S, Sjoberg T, Olsson P, Young M. Treatment of out-of-hospital cardiac arrest with LUCAS, a new device for automatic mechanical compression and active decompression resuscitation. *Resuscitation*. 2005;67:25-30.
4. Larsen AI, Hjornevik AS, Ellingsen CL, Nilsen DW. Cardiac arrest with continuous mechanical chest compression during percutaneous coronary intervention. A report on the use of the LUCAS device. *Resuscitation*. 2007;75:454-459.
5. Wagner H, Terkelsen CJ, Friberg H, Harnek J, Kern K, Lassen JF, Olivecrona GK. Cardiac arrest in the catheterisation laboratory: a 5-year experience of using mechanical chest compressions to facilitate PCI during prolonged resuscitation efforts. *Resuscitation*. 2010;81:383-387.
6. Shawl FA, Domanski MJ, Wish MH, Davis M, Punja S, Hernandez TJ. Emergency cardiopulmonary bypass support in patients with cardiac arrest in the catheterization laboratory. *Cathet Cardiovasc Diagn*. 1990;19:8-12.
7. Criley JM, Blaufuss AH, Kissel GL. Cough-induced cardiac compression. Self-administered form of cardiopulmonary resuscitation. *JAMA*. 1976;236:1246-1250.
8. Criley JM, Blaufuss AH, Kissel GL. Self-administered cardiopulmonary resuscitation by cough-induced cardiac compression. *Trans Am Clin Climatol Assoc*. 1976;87:138-146.
9. Keeble W, Tymchak WJ. Triggering of the Bezold Jarisch Reflex by reperfusion during primary PCI with maintenance of consciousness by cough CPR: a case report and review of pathophysiology. *J Invasive Cardiol*. 2008;20:E239-E242.
10. Saba SE, David SW. Sustained consciousness during ventricular fibrillation: case report of cough cardiopulmonary resuscitation. *Cathet Cardiovasc Diagn*. 1996;37:47-48.
11. Kato M, Dote K, Sasaki S, Takemoto H, Habara S, Hasegawa D. Intracoronary verapamil rapidly terminates reperfusion tachyarrhythmias in acute myocardial infarction. *Chest*. 2004;126:702-708.
12. Dunning J, Fabbri A, Kolh PH, Levine A, Lockowandt U, Mackay J, Pavie AJ, Strang T, Versteegh MI, Nashef SA. Guideline for resuscitation in cardiac arrest after cardiac surgery. *Eur J Cardiothorac Surg*. 2009;36:3-28.
13. Mackay JH, Powell SJ, Charman SC, Rozario C. Resuscitation after cardiac surgery: are we ageist? *Eur J Anaesthesiol*. 2004;21:66-71.
14. Raman J, Saldanha RF, Branch JM, Esmore DS, Spratt PM, Farnsworth AE, Harrison GA, Chang VP, Shanahan MX. Open cardiac compression in the postoperative cardiac intensive care unit. *Anaesth Intensive Care*. 1989;17:129-135.
15. Karhunen JP, Sihvo EI, Suojaranta-Ylinen RT, Ramo OJ, Salminen US. Predictive factors of hemodynamic collapse after coronary artery bypass grafting: a case-control study. *J Cardiothorac Vasc Anesth*. 2006;20:143-148.
16. Anthi A, Tzelepis GE, Alivizatos P, Michalis A, Palatianos GM, Geroulanos S. Unexpected cardiac arrest after cardiac surgery: incidence, predisposing causes, and outcome of open chest cardiopulmonary resuscitation. *Chest*. 1998;113:15-19.
17. Dimopoulou I, Anthi A, Michalis A, Tzelepis GE. Functional status and quality of life in long-term survivors of cardiac arrest after cardiac surgery. *Crit Care Med*. 2001;29:1408-1411.
18. el-Banayosy A, Brehm C, Kizner L, Hartmann D, Kortke H, Korner MM, Minami K, Reichelt W, Korfer R. Cardiopulmonary resuscitation after cardiac surgery: a two-year study. *J Cardiothorac Vasc Anesth*. 1998;12:390-392.
19. Fairman RM, Edmunds LH Jr. Emergency thoracotomy in the surgical intensive care unit after open cardiac operation. *Ann Thorac Surg*. 1981;32:386-391.
20. Mackay JH, Powell SJ, Osgathorp J, Rozario CJ. Six-year prospective audit of chest reopening after cardiac arrest. *Eur J Cardiothorac Surg*. 2002;22:421-425.

21. Ngaage DL, Cowen ME. Survival of cardiorespiratory arrest after coronary artery bypass grafting or aortic valve surgery. *Ann Thorac Surg*. 2009;88:64-68.

22. Kriaras I, Anthi A, Michelopoulos A, Karakatsani A, Tzelepis G, Papadimitriou L, Geroulanos S. Antimicrobial protection in cardiac surgery patients undergoing open chest CPR. *Resuscitation*. 1996;31:10-11.

23. Rousou JA, Engelman RM, Flack JE III, Deaton DW, Owen SG. Emergency cardiopulmonary bypass in the cardiac surgical unit can be a lifesaving measure in postoperative cardiac arrest. *Circulation*. 1994;90:II280-II284.

24. Beyersdorf F, Kirsh M, Buckberg GD, Allen BS. Warm glutamate/aspartate-enriched blood cardioplegic solution for perioperative sudden death. *J Thorac Cardiovasc Surg*. 1992;104:1141-1147.

25. Feng WC, Bert AA, Browning RA, Singh AK. Open cardiac massage and periresuscitative cardiopulmonary bypass for cardiac arrest following cardiac surgery. *J Cardiovasc Surg (Torino)*. 1995;36:319-321.

26. Wahba A, Gotz W, Birnbaum DE. Outcome of cardiopulmonary resuscitation following open heart surgery. *Scand Cardiovasc J*. 1997;31:147-149.

27. Pottle A, Bullock I, Thomas J, Scott L. Survival to discharge following open chest cardiac compression (OCCC). A 4-year retrospective audit in a cardiothoracic specialist centre—Royal Brompton and Harefield NHS Trust, United Kingdom. *Resuscitation*. 2002;52:269-272.

28. Kaiser GC, Naunheim KS, Fiore AC, Harris HH, McBride LR, Pennington DG, Barner HB, Willman VL. Reoperation in the intensive care unit. *Ann Thorac Surg*. 1990;49:903-907.

29. Bohrer H, Gust R, Bottiger BW. Cardiopulmonary resuscitation after cardiac surgery. *J Cardiothorac Vasc Anesth*. 1995;9:352.

30. Ricci M, Karamanoukian HL, D'Ancona G, Jajkowski MR, Bergsland J, Salerno TA. Avulsion of an H graft during closed-chest cardiopulmonary resuscitation after minimally invasive coronary artery bypass graft surgery. *J Cardiothorac Vasc Anesth*. 2000;14:586-587.

31. Chen YS, Chao A, Yu HY, Ko WJ, Wu IH, Chen RJ, Huang SC, Lin FY, Wang SS. Analysis and results of prolonged resuscitation in cardiac arrest patients rescued by extracorporeal membrane oxygenation. *J Am Coll Cardiol*. 2003;41:197-203.

32. Dalton HJ, Siewers RD, Fuhrman BP, Del Nido P, Thompson AE, Shaver MG, Dowhy M. Extracorporeal membrane oxygenation for cardiac rescue in children with severe myocardial dysfunction. *Crit Care Med*. 1993;21:1020-1028.

33. Ghez O, Feier H, Ughetto F, Fraisse A, Kreitmann B, Metras D. Postoperative extracorporeal life support in pediatric cardiac surgery: recent results. *ASAIO J*. 2005;51:513-516.

34. del Nido PJ, Dalton HJ, Thompson AE, Siewers RD. Extracorporeal membrane oxygenator rescue in children during cardiac arrest after cardiac surgery. *Circulation*. 1992;86:II300-II304.

35. Duncan BW, Ibrahim AE, Hraska V, del Nido PJ, Laussen PC, Wessel DL, Mayer JE Jr, Bower LK, Jonas RA. Use of rapid-deployment extracorporeal membrane oxygenation for the resuscitation of pediatric patients with heart disease after cardiac arrest. *J Thorac Cardiovasc Surg*. 1998;116:305-311.

36. Newsome LR, Ponganis P, Reichman R, Nakaji N, Jaski B, Hartley M. Portable percutaneous cardiopulmonary bypass: use in supported coronary angioplasty, aortic valvuloplasty, and cardiac arrest. *J Cardiothorac Vasc Anesth*. 1992;6:328-331.

37. Parra DA, Totapally BR, Zahn E, Jacobs J, Aldousany A, Burke RP, Chang AC. Outcome of cardiopulmonary resuscitation in a pediatric cardiac intensive care unit. *Crit Care Med*. 2000;28:3296-3300.

38. Overlie PA. Emergency use of cardiopulmonary bypass. *J Interv Cardiol*. 1995;8:239-247.

39. Cipolotti G, Paccagnella A, Simini G. Successful cardiopulmonary resuscitation using high doses of epinephrine. *Int J Cardiol*. 1991;33:430-431.

40. Kron IL, DiMarco JP, Harman PK, Crosby IK, Mentzer RM Jr, Nolan SP, Wellons HA Jr. Unanticipated postoperative ventricular tachyarrhythmias. *Ann Thorac Surg*. 1984;38:317-322.

Appendix

2010 AHA Guidelines for CPR and ECC *Summary Table*

Topic	2005 Guidelines	2010 Guidelines
Systematic Approach: BLS Survey	• A-B-C-D: Airway, Breathing, Circulation, Defibrillation • "Look, listen, and feel" for breathing and give 2 rescue breaths	• 1-2-3-4 1. **Check responsiveness.** 2. **Activate the emergency response system and get an AED.** 3. **Circulation:** Check the carotid pulse. If you cannot detect a pulse within 10 seconds, start CPR, beginning with chest compressions, immediately. 4. **Defibrillation:** If indicated, deliver a shock with an AED or defibrillator.

Topic	2010 Guidelines
BLS: High-Quality CPR	• A rate of **at least 100** chest compressions per minute • A compression depth of **at least 2 inches** in adults • Allowing complete chest recoil after each compression • Minimizing interruptions in compressions (10 seconds or less) • Switching providers about every 2 minutes to avoid fatigue • Avoiding excessive ventilation
ACLS: Cardiac Arrest and Bradycardia Algorithms	• The *2010 AHA Guidelines for CPR and ECC* simplifies the Cardiac Arrest Algorithm and includes a circular algorithm. • The priority is the 2-minute continuous period of high-quality CPR and defibrillation. • All advanced interventions—including IV access, drug delivery, and advanced airways—should not interrupt chest compressions and shocks. Rather, they should be performed or administered strategically **after** the brief pause for defibrillation. • These actions continue until ROSC, when healthcare providers initiate post–cardiac arrest care protocols. • During cardiac arrest, providers should administer a vasopressor every 3 to 5 minutes. Epinephrine is commonly used, although vasopressin can replace the first or second dose of epinephrine. Regardless of the vasopressor given, one should be administered every 3 to 5 minutes. ACLS providers should administer amiodarone for refractory VF and VT. • The American Heart Association no longer recommends atropine for routine use in managing PEA or asystole. • For treatment of undifferentiated wide-complex tachycardia with regular rhythm, ACLS providers can consider adenosine in the initial treatment. • Atropine remains the first-line treatment for all symptomatic bradycardias, regardless of type. • For symptomatic bradycardia, the American Heart Association now recommends IV infusion of chronotropic agents as an equally effective alternative to external transcutaneous pacing when atropine is ineffective.

(continued)

(continued)

Topic	2010 Guidelines
ACLS: Tachycardia–Synchronized Cardioversion	• The *2010 AHA Guidelines for CPR and ECC* simplifies the Tachycardia Algorithm. • For cardioversion of unstable atrial fibrillation, the *2010 AHA Guidelines for CPR and ECC* recommends that the initial biphasic energy dose be between 120 and 200 J. • For cardioversion of unstable SVT or unstable atrial flutter, the *2010 AHA Guidelines for CPR and ECC* recommends that the initial biphasic energy dose be between 50 to 100 J. • Cardioversion with monophasic waveforms should begin at 200 J and increase in a stepwise fashion if not successful. • The *2010 AHA Guidelines for CPR and ECC* also recommends cardioversion for unstable monomorphic VT, with an initial energy dose of 100 J. • If the initial shock fails, providers should increase the dose in a stepwise fashion.
ACLS: Post–Cardiac Arrest Care	A new section focusing on post–cardiac arrest care was introduced in the *2010 AHA Guidelines for CPR and ECC*. Recommendations aimed at improving survival after ROSC include • Optimizing cardiopulmonary function and vital organ perfusion, especially to the brain and heart • Transporting out-of-hospital cardiac arrest patients to an appropriate facility with post–cardiac arrest care that includes acute coronary interventions, neurologic care, goal-directed critical care, and hypothermia • Transporting in-hospital cardiac arrest patients to a critical care unit capable of providing comprehensive post–cardiac arrest care • Identifying and treating the causes of the arrest and preventing recurrence • Considering therapeutic hypothermia to optimize survival and neurologic recovery in comatose patients • Identifying and treating acute coronary syndromes • Optimizing mechanical ventilation to minimize lung injury • Gathering data for prognosis • Assisting patients and families with rehabilitation services if needed **Critical actions for post–cardiac arrest care:** • Hemodynamic optimization, including a focus on treating hypotension • Acquisition of a 12-lead ECG • Induction of therapeutic hypothermia • Monitoring advanced airway placement and ventilation status with quantitative waveform capnography in intubated patients • Optimizing arterial oxygen saturation
ACLS: Managing the Airway	• The *2010 AHA Guidelines for CPR and ECC* recommends using waveform capnography to monitor the amount of carbon dioxide exhaled by the patient and to verify placement of an endotracheal tube. • Cricoid pressure should not be used routinely during cardiac arrest. This technique is difficult to master and may not be effective for preventing aspiration. It may also delay or prevent placement of an advanced airway. • Agonal gasps are not effective breaths and should not be confused with normal breathing.
High-Quality Patient Care: Systems of Care	• Integrated systems of care should include community members, EMS, physicians, and hospitals.

ACLS Pharmacology Table

Administration Notes	
Peripheral Intravenous (IV)	Resuscitation drugs administered via peripheral IV catheter should be followed by bolus of 20 mL IV fluid to move drug into central circulation. Then elevate extremity for 10 to 20 seconds.
Intraosseous (IO)	ACLS drugs that can be administered by IV route can be administered by IO route.
Endotracheal	IV/IO administration is preferred because it provides more reliable drug delivery and pharmacologic effect. Drugs that can be administered by endotracheal route are noted in the table below. Optimal endotracheal doses have not yet been established. Medication delivered via endotracheal tube should be diluted in sterile water or NS to a volume of 5 to 10 mL. Provide several positive-pressure breaths after medication is instilled.

Drug/Therapy	Indications/Precautions	Adult Dosage
ACE Inhibitors (Angiotensin-Converting Enzyme Inhibitors)	**Indications** • ACE inhibitors reduce mortality and improve LV dysfunction in post-AMI patients. They help prevent adverse LV remodeling, delay progression of heart failure, and decrease sudden death and recurrent MI. • An ACE inhibitor should be administered orally within the first 24 hours after onset of AMI symptoms and continued long term if tolerated. • Clinical heart failure without hypotension in patients not responding to digitalis or diuretics. • Clinical signs of AMI with LV dysfunction. • LV ejection fraction <40%.	**Approach:** ACE inhibitor therapy should start with low-dose oral administration (with possible IV doses for some preparations) and increase steadily to achieve a full dose within 24 to 48 hours. An angiotensin receptor blocker (ARB) should be administered to patients intolerant of ACE inhibitors.
Enalapril Captopril Lisinopril Ramipril	**Precautions/Contraindications for All ACE Inhibitors** • ***Contraindicated*** in pregnancy (may cause fetal injury or death). • Contraindicated in angioedema. • Hypersensitivity to ACE inhibitors. • Reduce dose in renal failure (creatinine >2.5 mg/dL in men, >2 mg/dL in women). Avoid in bilateral renal artery stenosis. • Serum potassium >5 mEq/L. • Do not give if patient is hypotensive (SBP <100 mm Hg or >30 mm Hg below baseline) or volume depleted. • Generally not started in ED; after reperfusion therapy has been completed and blood pressure has stabilized, start within 24 hours.	**Enalapril (IV = Enalaprilat)** • **PO:** Start with a single dose of 2.5 mg. Titrate to 20 mg PO BID. • **IV:** 1.25 mg IV initial dose over 5 minutes, then 1.25 to 5 mg IV every 6 hours. • IV form is contraindicated in STEMI (risk of hypotension). **Captopril, AMI Dose** • Start with a single dose of 6.25 mg PO. • Advance to 25 mg TID and then to 50 mg TID as tolerated. **Lisinopril, AMI Dose** • 5 mg within 24 hours of onset of symptoms, then • 5 mg given after 24 hours, then • 10 mg given after 48 hours, then • 10 mg once daily **Ramipril** • Start with a single dose of 2.5 mg PO. Titrate to 5 mg PO BID as tolerated.
Adenosine	**Indications** • First drug for most forms of stable narrow-complex SVT. Effective in terminating those due to reentry involving AV node or sinus node. • May consider for unstable narrow-complex reentry tachycardia while preparations are made for cardioversion. • Regular and monomorphic wide-complex tachycardia, thought to be or previously defined to be reentry SVT. • Does *not* convert atrial fibrillation, atrial flutter, or VT. • Diagnostic maneuver: stable narrow-complex SVT. **Precautions/Contraindications** • Contraindicated in poison/drug-induced tachycardia or second- or third-degree heart block. • Transient side effects include flushing, chest pain or tightness, brief periods of asystole or bradycardia, ventricular ectopy. • Less effective (larger doses may be required) in patients taking theophylline or caffeine. • Reduce initial dose to 3 mg in patients receiving dipyridamole or carbamazepine, in heart transplant patients, or if given by central venous access. • If administered for irregular, polymorphic wide-complex tachycardia/VT, may cause deterioration (including hypotension). • Transient periods of sinus bradycardia and ventricular ectopy are common after termination of SVT. • Safe and effective in pregnancy.	**IV Rapid Push** • Place patient in mild reverse Trendelenburg position before administration of drug. • Initial bolus of 6 mg given *rapidly* over 1 to 3 seconds followed by NS bolus of 20 mL; then elevate the extremity. • A second dose (12 mg) can be given in 1 to 2 minutes if needed. **Injection Technique** • Record rhythm strip during administration. • Draw up adenosine dose and flush in 2 separate syringes. • Attach both syringes to the IV injection port closest to patient. • Clamp IV tubing above injection port. • Push IV adenosine *as quickly as possible* (1 to 3 seconds). • While maintaining pressure on adenosine plunger, push NS flush *as rapidly as possible* after adenosine. • Unclamp IV tubing.

Drug/Therapy	Indications/Precautions	Adult Dosage
Adenosine Diphosphate (ADP) Antagonists (Thienopyridines)	**Indications** Adjunctive antiplatelet therapy for acute coronary syndrome (ACS) patients. **Precautions/Contraindications** • Do not administer to patients with active pathologic bleeding (eg, peptic ulcer). Use with caution in patients with risk of bleeding. • **Prasugrel is contraindicated in patients with a history of TIA or stroke; use with caution in patients ≥75 years old or <60 kg due to increased risk of fatal and intracranial bleeding and uncertain benefit.** • Use with caution in the presence of hepatic impairment. • **When CABG is planned, withhold ADP antagonists for 5 (for clopidogrel) or 7 (for prasugrel) days before CABG unless need for revascularization outweighs the risk of excess bleeding.**	*Note:* Combinations of loading and maintenance doses of different ADP antagonists (clopidogrel, prasugrel, and ticagrelor) are ***not*** recommended.
Clopidogrel (Plavix) 75 mg and 300 mg tabs available	**Clopidogrel** • For STEMI or moderate- to high-risk non–ST elevation ACS, including patients receiving fibrinolysis. • Limited evidence in patients ≥75 years old. • Substitute for aspirin if patient is unable to take aspirin.	**Clopidogrel** • STEMI or moderate- to high-risk UA/non–ST-segment elevation ACS patient <75 years old: Administer loading dose of 300 to 600 mg orally followed by maintenance dose of 75 mg orally daily; full effects will not develop for several days. • ED patients with suspected ACS unable to take aspirin: loading dose 300 mg.
Prasugrel (Effient) 5 mg and 10 mg tabs available	**Prasugrel** • May be substituted for clopidogrel after angiography in patients with NSTEMI or STEMI who are not at high risk for bleeding. • Not recommended for STEMI patients managed with fibrinolysis or for NSTEMI patients before angiography. • No data to support use in ED or prehospital setting.	**Prasugrel** • STEMI or UA/NSTEMI patient <75 years old managed with PCI: Administer loading dose of 60 mg PO followed by maintenance dose of 10 mg PO daily; full effects will not develop for several days. • Consider dose reduction to 5 mg PO daily in patients weighing <60 kg.
Ticagrelor	**Ticagrelor** • May be administered to patients with NSTEMI or STEMI who are treated with early invasive strategy.	
Amiodarone	Amiodarone is a complex drug with effects on sodium, potassium, and calcium channels as well as α- and β-adrenergic blocking properties. Patients must be hospitalized while the loading doses of amiodarone are administered. Amiodarone should be prescribed only by physicians who are experienced in the treatment of life-threatening arrhythmias, are thoroughly familiar with amiodarone's risks and benefits, and have access to laboratory facilities capable of adequately monitoring the effectiveness and side effects of amiodarone treatment. **Indications** Because its use is associated with toxicity, amiodarone is indicated for use in patients with life-threatening arrhythmias when administered with appropriate monitoring: • VF/pulseless VT unresponsive to shock delivery, CPR, and a vasopressor. • Recurrent, hemodynamically unstable VT. *With expert consultation* amiodarone may be used for treatment of some atrial and ventricular arrhythmias. ***Caution:* Multiple complex drug interactions**	**VF/VT Cardiac Arrest Unresponsive to CPR, Shock, and Vasopressor** First dose: 300 mg IV/IO push. Second dose (if needed): 150 mg IV/IO push. **Life-Threatening Arrhythmias** **Maximum cumulative dose:** 2.2 g IV over 24 hours. May be administered as follows: • **Rapid infusion:** 150 mg IV over first 10 minutes (15 mg per minute). May repeat rapid infusion (150 mg IV) every 10 minutes as needed. • **Slow infusion:** 360 mg IV over 6 hours (1 mg per minute). • **Maintenance infusion:** 540 mg IV over 18 hours (0.5 mg per minute). **Precautions** • Rapid infusion may lead to hypotension. • With multiple dosing, cumulative doses >2.2 g over 24 hours are associated with significant hypotension in clinical trials. • Do not administer with other drugs that prolong QT interval (eg, procainamide). • Terminal elimination is extremely long (half-life lasts up to 40 days).
Amrinone *(See **Inamrinone**)*		
Aspirin	**Indications** • Administer to all patients with ACS, particularly reperfusion candidates, unless hypersensitive to aspirin. • Blocks formation of thromboxane A_2, which causes platelets to aggregate and arteries to constrict. This reduces overall ACS mortality, reinfarction, and nonfatal stroke. • Any person with symptoms ("pressure," "heavy weight," "squeezing," "crushing") suggestive of ischemic pain. **Precautions/Contraindications** • Relatively contraindicated in patients with active ulcer disease or asthma. • Contraindicated in patients with known hypersensitivity to aspirin.	• 160 mg to 325 mg non–enteric-coated tablet as soon as possible (chewing is preferable). • May use rectal suppository (300 mg) for patients who cannot take orally.

Drug/Therapy	Indications/Precautions	Adult Dosage
Atropine Sulfate Can be given via endotracheal tube	**Indications** • First drug for symptomatic sinus bradycardia. • May be beneficial in presence of AV nodal block. **Not likely to be effective for type II second-degree or third-degree AV block or a block in non-nodal tissue.** • Routine use during PEA or asystole is unlikely to have a therapeutic benefit. • Organophosphate (eg, nerve agent) poisoning: extremely large doses may be needed. **Precautions** • Use with caution in presence of myocardial ischemia and hypoxia. Increases myocardial oxygen demand. • Avoid in hypothermic bradycardia. • May not be effective for infranodal (type II) AV block and new third-degree block with wide QRS complexes. (In these patients may cause paradoxical slowing. Be prepared to pace or give catecholamines.) • Doses of atropine <0.5 mg may result in paradoxical slowing of heart rate.	**Bradycardia (With or Without ACS)** • 0.5 mg IV every 3 to 5 minutes as needed, not to exceed total dose of 0.04 mg/kg (total 3 mg). • Use shorter dosing interval (3 minutes) and higher doses in severe clinical conditions. **Organophosphate Poisoning** Extremely large doses (2 to 4 mg or higher) may be needed.
β-Blockers **Metoprolol Tartrate** **Atenolol** **Propranolol** **Esmolol** **Labetalol**	**Indications (Apply to all β-blockers)** • Administer to all patients with suspected myocardial infarction and unstable angina in the absence of contraindication. These are effective antianginal agents and can reduce incidence of VF. • Useful as an adjunctive agent with fibrinolytic therapy. May reduce nonfatal reinfarction and recurrent ischemia. • To convert to normal sinus rhythm or to slow ventricular response (or both) in supraventricular tachyarrhythmias (reentry SVT, atrial fibrillation, or atrial flutter). β-Blockers are second-line agents after adenosine. • To reduce myocardial ischemia and damage in AMI patients with elevated heart rate, blood pressure, or both. • Labetalol recommended for emergency antihypertensive therapy for hemorrhagic and acute ischemic stroke. **Precautions/Contraindications (Apply to all β-blockers unless noted)** • Early aggressive β-blockade may be hazardous in hemodynamically unstable patients. • Do not give to patients with STEMI if any of the following are present: – Signs of heart failure. – Low cardiac output. – Increased risk for cardiogenic shock. • Relative contraindications include PR interval >0.24 second, second- or third-degree heart block, active asthma, reactive airway disease, severe bradycardia, SBP <100 mm Hg. • Concurrent IV administration with IV calcium channel blocking agents like verapamil or diltiazem can cause severe hypotension and bradycardia/heart block. • Monitor cardiac and pulmonary status during administration. • Propranolol is contraindicated and other β-blockers relatively contraindicated in cocaine-induced ACS.	**Metoprolol Tartrate (AMI Regimen)** • Initial IV dose: 5 mg slow IV at 5-minute intervals to a total of 15 mg. • Begin oral regimen to follow IV dose with 50 mg PO; titrate to effect. **Atenolol (AMI Regimen)** • 5 mg IV over 5 minutes. • Wait 10 minutes, then give second dose of 5 mg IV over 5 minutes. • In 10 minutes, if tolerated well, begin oral regimen with 50 mg PO; titrate to effect. **Propranolol (for SVT)** • 0.5 to 1 mg over 1 minute, repeated as needed up to a total dose of 0.1 mg/kg. **Esmolol** • 0.5 mg/kg (500 mcg/kg) over 1 minute, followed by 0.05 mg/kg (50 mcg/kg) per minute infusion; maximum: 0.3 mg/kg (300 mcg/kg) per minute. • If inadequate response after 5 minutes, may repeat 0.5 mg/kg (500 mcg/kg) bolus and then titrate infusion up to 0.2 mg/kg (200 mcg/kg) per minute. Higher doses unlikely to be beneficial. • Has a short half-life (2 to 9 minutes). **Labetalol** • 10 mg IV push over 1 to 2 minutes. • May repeat or double every 10 minutes to a maximum dose of 150 mg, *or* give initial dose as a bolus, then start infusion at 2 to 8 mg per minute.
Calcium Chloride 10% solution is 100 mg/mL	**Indications** • Known or suspected hyperkalemia (eg, renal failure). • Ionized hypocalcemia (eg, after multiple blood transfusions). • As an antidote for toxic effects (hypotension and arrhythmias) from calcium channel blocker overdose or β-blocker overdose. **Precautions** • Do not use routinely in cardiac arrest. • Do not mix with sodium bicarbonate.	**Typical Dose** • 500 mg to 1000 mg (5 to 10 mL of a 10% solution) IV for hyperkalemia and calcium channel blocker overdose. May be repeated as needed. • *Note:* Comparable dose of 10% calcium gluconate is 15 to 30 mL.
Clopidogrel *(See* ***ADP Antagonists****)*		
Digoxin-Specific Antibody Therapy Digibind (38 mg) or DigiFab (40 mg) (each vial binds about 0.5 mg digoxin)	**Indications** Digoxin toxicity with the following: • Life-threatening arrhythmias. • Shock or congestive heart failure. • Hyperkalemia (potassium level >5 mEq/L). • Steady-state serum levels >10 to 15 ng/mL for symptomatic patients. **Precautions** • Serum digoxin levels rise after digoxin antibody therapy and should not be used to guide continuing therapy.	**Chronic Intoxication** 3 to 5 vials may be effective. **Acute Overdose** • IV dose varies according to amount of digoxin ingested. See ACLS Toxicology. • Average dose is 10 vials; may require up to 20 vials. • See package insert for details.

Drug/Therapy	Indications/Precautions	Adult Dosage
Digoxin 0.25 mg/mL or 0.1 mg/mL supplied in 1 or 2 mL ampule (totals = 0.1 to 0.5 mg)	**Indications (may be of limited use)** • To slow ventricular response in atrial fibrillation or atrial flutter. • Alternative drug for reentry SVT. **Precautions** • Toxic effects are common and are frequently associated with serious arrhythmias. • Avoid electrical cardioversion if patient is receiving digoxin unless condition is life-threatening; use lower dose (10 to 20 J).	**IV Administration** • Loading doses: 0.004 to 0.006 mg/kg (4 to 6 mcg/kg) initially over 5 minutes. Second and third boluses of 0.002 to 0.003 mg/kg (2 to 3 mcg/kg) to follow at 4- to 8-hour intervals (total loading dose 8 to 12 mcg/kg divided over 8 to 16 hours). • Check digoxin levels no sooner than 4 hours after IV dose; no sooner than 6 hours after oral dose. • Monitor heart rate and ECG. • Maintenance dose is affected by body mass and renal function. • ***Caution:*** Amiodarone interaction. Reduce digoxin dose by 50% when used with amiodarone.
Diltiazem	**Indications** • To control ventricular rate in atrial fibrillation and atrial flutter. May terminate reentrant arrhythmias that require AV nodal conduction for their continuation. • Use after adenosine to treat refractory reentry SVT in patients with narrow QRS complex and adequate blood pressure. **Precautions** • Do not use calcium channel blockers for wide-QRS tachycardias of uncertain origin or for poison/drug-induced tachycardia. • Avoid calcium channel blockers in patients with Wolff-Parkinson-White syndrome plus rapid atrial fibrillation or flutter, in patients with sick sinus syndrome, or in patients with AV block without a pacemaker. • ***Caution:*** Blood pressure may drop from peripheral vasodilation (greater drop with verapamil than with diltiazem). • Avoid in patients receiving oral β-blockers. • Concurrent IV administration with IV β-blockers can cause severe hypotension and AV block.	**Acute Rate Control** • 15 to 20 mg (0.25 mg/kg) IV over 2 minutes. • May give another IV dose in 15 minutes at 20 to 25 mg (0.35 mg/kg) over 2 minutes. **Maintenance Infusion** 5 to 15 mg per hour, titrated to physiologically appropriate heart rate (can dilute in D_5W or NS).
Dobutamine IV infusion	**Indications** • Consider for pump problems (congestive heart failure, pulmonary congestion) with SBP of 70 to 100 mm Hg and *no* signs of shock. **Precautions/Contraindications** • **Contraindication:** Suspected or known poison/drug-induced shock. • Avoid with SBP <100 mm Hg and signs of shock. • May cause tachyarrhythmias, fluctuations in blood pressure, headache, and nausea. • Do not mix with sodium bicarbonate.	**IV Administration** • Usual infusion rate is 2 to 20 mcg/kg per minute. • Titrate so heart rate does not increase by >10% of baseline. • Hemodynamic monitoring is recommended for optimal use. • Elderly patients may have a significantly decreased response.
Dopamine IV infusion	**Indications** • Second-line drug for symptomatic bradycardia (after atropine). • Use for hypotension (SBP ≤70 to 100 mm Hg) with signs and symptoms of shock. **Precautions** • Correct hypovolemia with volume replacement before initiating dopamine. • Use with caution in cardiogenic shock with accompanying CHF. • May cause tachyarrhythmias, excessive vasoconstriction. • Do not mix with sodium bicarbonate.	**IV Administration** • Usual infusion rate is 2 to 20 mcg/kg per minute. • Titrate to patient response; taper slowly.
Epinephrine Can be given via endotracheal tube Available in 1:10 000 and 1:1000 concentrations	**Indications** • **Cardiac arrest:** VF, pulseless VT, asystole, PEA. • **Symptomatic bradycardia:** Can be considered after atropine as an alternative infusion to dopamine. • **Severe hypotension:** Can be used when pacing and atropine fail, when hypotension accompanies bradycardia, or with phosphodiesterase enzyme inhibitor. • **Anaphylaxis, severe allergic reactions:** Combine with large fluid volume, corticosteroids, antihistamines. **Precautions** • Raising blood pressure and increasing heart rate may cause myocardial ischemia, angina, and increased myocardial oxygen demand. • High doses do not improve survival or neurologic outcome and may contribute to postresuscitation myocardial dysfunction. • Higher doses *may* be required to treat poison/drug-induced shock.	**Cardiac Arrest** • **IV/IO dose:** 1 mg (10 mL of 1:10 000 solution) administered every 3 to 5 minutes during resuscitation. Follow each dose with 20 mL flush, elevate arm for 10 to 20 seconds after dose. • **Higher dose:** Higher doses (up to 0.2 mg/kg) may be used for specific indications (β-blocker or calcium channel blocker overdose). • **Continuous infusion:** Initial rate: 0.1 to 0.5 mcg/kg per minute (for 70-kg patient: 7 to 35 mcg per minute); titrate to response. • **Endotracheal route:** 2 to 2.5 mg diluted in 10 mL NS. **Profound Bradycardia or Hypotension** 2 to 10 mcg per minute infusion; titrate to patient response.

Drug/Therapy	Indications/Precautions	Adult Dosage
Fibrinolytic Agents **Alteplase, Recombinant** (Activase); **Tissue Plasminogen Activator (rtPA)** 50- and 100-mg vials reconstituted with sterile water to 1 mg/mL For all 4 agents, insert 2 peripheral IV lines; use 1 line exclusively for fibrinolytic administration	**Indications** **Cardiac arrest:** Insufficient evidence to recommend routine use. **AMI in adults (see ACS section):** • ST elevation (threshold values: J-point elevation of 2 mm in leads V_2 and V_3* and 1 mm in all other leads) or new or presumably new LBBB. • In context of signs and symptoms of AMI. • Time from onset of symptoms ≤12 hours. • See "Acute Coronary Syndromes: Fibrinolytic Checklist for STEMI" and Fibrinolytic Therapy under "ST-Segment Elevation Therapies: Fibrinolytic Strategy" for guidance on use of fibrinolytics in patients with STEMI. **Acute ischemic stroke (see Stroke section):** (Alteplase is the only fibrinolytic agent approved for acute ischemic stroke.) • Sudden onset of focal neurologic deficits or alterations in consciousness (eg, facial droop, arm drift, abnormal speech). • See "Use of IV rtPA for Acute Ischemic Stroke: Inclusion and Exclusion Characteristics" for guidance on which patients can be treated with rtPA based on time of symptom onset.	**Alteplase, Recombinant (rtPA)** Recommended total dose is based on patient's weight. **STEMI:** • Accelerated infusion (1.5 hours) — Give 15 mg IV bolus. — Then 0.75 mg/kg over next 30 minutes (not to exceed 50 mg). — Then 0.5 mg/kg over 60 minutes (not to exceed 35 mg). — Maximum total dose: 100 mg. **Acute ischemic stroke:** • Give 0.9 mg/kg (maximum 90 mg) IV, infused over 60 minutes. • Give 10% of total dose as an initial IV bolus over 1 minute. • Give remaining 90% of total dose IV over next 60 minutes.
Reteplase, Recombinant (Retavase) 10-unit vials reconstituted with sterile water to 1 unit/mL	**Precautions and Possible Exclusion Criteria for AMI in Adults/Acute Ischemic Stroke** • For AMI in adults, see "Acute Coronary Syndromes: Fibrinolytic Checklist for STEMI" and Fibrinolytic Therapy under "ST-Segment Elevation Therapies: Fibrinolytic Strategy" for indications, precautions, and contraindications. • For acute ischemic stroke, see "Use of IV rtPA for Acute Ischemic Stroke: Inclusion and Exclusion Characteristics" for indications, precautions, and contraindications.	**Reteplase, Recombinant** • Give first 10-unit IV bolus over 2 minutes. • 30 minutes later give second 10-unit IV bolus over 2 minutes. (Give NS flush before and after each bolus.)
Streptokinase (Streptase) Reconstitute to 1 mg/mL		**Streptokinase** 1.5 million units in a 1-hour infusion.
Tenecteplase (TNKase) 50-mg vial reconstituted with sterile water		**Tenecteplase** • Bolus, weight adjusted — <60 kg: Give 30 mg. — 60-69 kg: Give 35 mg. — 70-79 kg: Give 40 mg. — 80-89 kg: Give 45 mg. — ≥90 kg: Give 50 mg. • Administer single IV bolus over 5 seconds. • Incompatible with dextrose solutions.
Flumazenil	**Indications** Reverse respiratory depression and sedative effects from pure benzodiazepine overdose. **Precautions** • Effects may not outlast effect of benzodiazepines. • Monitor for recurrent respiratory depression. • Do not use in suspected tricyclic overdose. • Do not use in seizure-prone patients, chronic benzodiazepine users, or alcoholics. • Do not use in unknown drug overdose or mixed drug overdose with drugs known to cause seizures (tricyclic antidepressants, cocaine, amphetamines, etc).	**First Dose** 0.2 mg IV over 15 seconds. **Second Dose** 0.3 mg IV over 30 seconds. If no adequate response, give third dose. **Third Dose** 0.5 mg IV given over 30 seconds. If no adequate response, repeat once every minute until adequate response or a total of 3 mg is given.
Furosemide	**Indications** • For adjuvant therapy of acute pulmonary edema in patients with SBP >90 to 100 mm Hg (without signs and symptoms of shock). • Hypertensive emergencies. **Precautions** Dehydration, hypovolemia, hypotension, hypokalemia, or other electrolyte imbalance may occur.	**IV Administration** • 0.5 to 1 mg/kg given over 1 to 2 minutes. • If no response, double dose to 2 mg/kg, given slowly over 1 to 2 minutes. • For new-onset pulmonary edema with hypovolemia: <0.5 mg/kg.
Glucagon Powdered in 1-mg vials Reconstitute with provided solution	**Indications** Adjuvant treatment of toxic effects of calcium channel blocker or β-blocker. **Precautions** • May cause vomiting, hyperglycemia.	**IV Infusion** 3 to 10 mg IV slowly over 3 to 5 minutes, followed by infusion of 3 to 5 mg per hour.

*2.5 mm in men <40 years; 1.5 mm in all women.

Drug/Therapy	Indications/Precautions	Adult Dosage
Glycoprotein IIb/IIIa Inhibitors	**Indications** These drugs inhibit the integrin glycoprotein IIb/IIIa receptor in the membrane of platelets, inhibiting platelet aggregation. **Precautions/Contraindications** Active internal bleeding or bleeding disorder in past 30 days, history of intracranial hemorrhage or other bleeding, surgical procedure or trauma within 1 month, platelet count <150 000/mm^3, hypersensitivity and concomitant use of another GP IIb/IIIa inhibitor (also see "ACS: Treatment for UA/NSTEMI").	*Note:* **Check package insert for current indications, doses, and duration of therapy.** Optimal duration of therapy has not been established.
Abciximab (ReoPro)	**Abciximab Indications** FDA approved for patients with NSTEMI or UA with planned PCI within 24 hours. **Abciximab Precautions/Contraindications** Must use with heparin. Binds irreversibly with platelets. Platelet function recovery requires 48 hours (regeneration). Readministration may cause hypersensitivity reaction.	**Abciximab** • **PCI:** 0.25 mg/kg IV bolus (10 to 60 minutes before procedure), then 0.125 mcg/kg per minute (to maximum of 10 mcg per minute) IV infusion for 12 hours. • **ACS with planned PCI within 24 hours:** 0.25 mg/kg IV bolus, then 10 mcg per minute IV infusion for 18 to 24 hours, concluding 1 hour after PCI.
Eptifibatide (Integrilin)	**Eptifibatide Indications** For high-risk UA/NSTEMI and patients undergoing PCI. **Actions/Precautions** Platelet function recovers within 4 to 8 hours after discontinuation.	**Eptifibatide** • **PCI:** 180 mcg/kg IV bolus over 1 to 2 minutes, then begin 2 mcg/kg per minute IV infusion, then repeat bolus in 10 minutes. • Maximum dose (121-kg patient) for PCI: 22.6 mg bolus; 15 mg per hour infusion. • Infusion duration 18 to 24 hours after PCI. • Reduce rate of infusion by 50% if creatinine clearance <50 mL per minute.
Tirofiban (Aggrastat)	**Tirofiban Indications** For high-risk UA/NSTEMI and patients undergoing PCI. **Actions/Precautions** Platelet function recovers within 4 to 8 hours after discontinuation.	**Tirofiban** • **PCI:** 0.4 mcg/kg per minute IV for 30 minutes, then 0.1 mcg/kg per minute IV infusion (for 18 to 24 hours after PCI). • Reduce rate of infusion by 50% if creatinine clearance <30 mL per minute.
Fondaparinux (Arixtra)	**Indications** • For use in ACS. • To inhibit thrombin generation by factor Xa inhibition. • May be used for anticoagulation in patients with history of heparin-induced thrombocytopenia. **Precautions/Contraindications** • Hemorrhage may complicate therapy. • Contraindicated in patients with creatinine clearance <30 mL per minute; use with caution in patients with creatinine clearance 30 to 50 mL per minute. • Increased risk of catheter thrombosis in patients undergoing PCI; coadministration of unfractionated heparin required.	**STEMI Protocol** • Initial dose 2.5 mg IV bolus followed by 2.5 mg subcutaneously every 24 hours for up to 8 days. **UA/NSTEMI Protocol** • 2.5 mg subcutaneously every 24 hours.
Heparin, Unfractionated (UFH) Concentrations range from 1000 to 40 000 units/mL	**Indications** • Adjuvant therapy in AMI. • Begin heparin with fibrin-specific lytics (eg, alteplase, reteplase, tenecteplase). **Precautions/Contraindications** • Same contraindications as for fibrinolytic therapy: active bleeding; recent intracranial, intraspinal, or eye surgery; severe hypertension; bleeding disorders; gastrointestinal bleeding. • Doses and laboratory targets appropriate when used with fibrinolytic therapy. • Do not use if platelet count is or falls below <100 000 or with history of heparin-induced thrombocytopenia. For these patients consider direct antithrombins. See bivalirudin on the next page as part of LMWH.	**UFH IV Infusion—STEMI** • Initial bolus 60 units/kg (maximum bolus: 4000 units). • Continue 12 units/kg per hour, round to the nearest 50 units (maximum initial rate: 1000 units per hour). • Adjust to maintain aPTT 1.5 to 2 times the control values (50 to 70 seconds) for 48 hours or until angiography. • Check initial aPTT at 3 hours, then every 6 hours until stable, then daily. • Follow institutional heparin protocol. • Platelet count daily. **UFH IV Infusion—UA/NSTEMI** • Initial bolus 60 units/kg. Maximum: 4000 units. • 12 units/kg per hour. Maximum initial rate: 1000 units per hour. • Follow institutional protocol (see Heparin in ACS section).

Drug/Therapy	Indications/Precautions	Adult Dosage
Heparin, Low Molecular Weight (LMWH)	**Indications** For use in ACS, specifically patients with UA/NSTEMI. These drugs inhibit thrombin generation by factor Xa inhibition and also inhibit thrombin indirectly by formation of a complex with antithrombin III. These drugs are **not** neutralized by heparin-binding proteins. **Precautions** • Hemorrhage may complicate any therapy with LMWH. Contraindicated in presence of hypersensitivity to heparin or pork products or history of sensitivity to drug. Use **enoxaparin** with extreme caution in patients with type II heparin-induced thrombocytopenia. • Adjust dose for renal insufficiency. • Contraindicated if platelet count <100 000. For these patients consider direct antithrombins. **Heparin Reversal** ICH or life-threatening bleed: Administer protamine; refer to package insert.	**STEMI Protocol** • Enoxaparin — Age <75 years, normal creatinine clearance: initial bolus 30 mg IV with second bolus 15 minutes later of 1 mg/kg subcutaneously, repeat every 12 hours (maximum 100 mg/dose for first 2 doses). — Age ≥75 years: Eliminate initial IV bolus, give 0.75 mg/kg subcutaneously every 12 hours (maximum 75 mg/dose for first 2 doses). — If creatinine clearance <30 mL per minute, give 1 mg/kg subcutaneously every 24 hours. **UA/NSTEMI Protocol** • Enoxaparin: Loading dose 30 mg IV bolus. Maintenance dose 1 mg/kg subcutaneously every 12 hours. If creatinine clearance <30 mL per minute, give every 24 hours. • Bivalirudin: Bolus with 0.1 mg/kg IV; then begin infusion of 0.25 mg/kg per hour.
Ibutilide Intervention of choice is DC cardioversion	**Indications** Treatment of supraventricular arrhythmias, including atrial fibrillation and atrial flutter when duration ≤48 hours. Short duration of action. Effective for the conversion of atrial fibrillation or flutter of relatively brief duration. **Precautions/Contraindications** Contraindication: Do not give to patients with QT_C >440 milliseconds. Ventricular arrhythmias develop in approximately 2% to 5% of patients (polymorphic VT, including torsades de pointes). *Monitor ECG continuously for arrhythmias during administration and for 4 to 6 hours after administration with defibrillator nearby.* Patients with significantly impaired LV function are at highest risk for arrhythmias.	**Dose for Adults ≥60 kg** 1 mg (10 mL) administered IV (diluted or undiluted) over 10 minutes. A second dose may be administered at the same rate 10 minutes later. **Dose for Adults <60 kg** 0.01 mg/kg initial IV dose administered over 10 minutes.
Inamrinone Phosphodiesterase enzyme inhibitor	**Indications** Severe congestive heart failure refractory to diuretics, vasodilators, and conventional inotropic agents. **Precautions** • Do not mix with dextrose solutions or other drugs. • May cause tachyarrhythmias, hypotension, or thrombocytopenia. • Can increase myocardial ischemia.	**IV Loading Dose and Infusion** • 0.75 mg/kg (not to exceed 1 mg/kg) given over 2 to 3 minutes. Give loading dose over 10 to 15 minutes with LV dysfunction (eg, postresuscitation). • Follow with infusion of 5 to 15 mcg/kg per minute titrated to clinical effect. • Additional bolus may be given in 30 minutes. • Requires hemodynamic monitoring. • Creatinine clearance <10 mL per minute: reduce dose 25% to 50%.
Isoproterenol IV infusion	**Indications** • *Use cautiously as temporizing measure if external pacer is not available* for treatment of symptomatic bradycardia. • Refractory torsades de pointes unresponsive to magnesium sulfate. • *Temporary* control of bradycardia in heart transplant patients (denervated heart unresponsive to atropine). • Poisoning from β-blockers. **Precautions** • Do not use for treatment of cardiac arrest. • Increases myocardial oxygen requirements, which may increase myocardial ischemia. • Do not give with epinephrine; can cause VF/VT. • Do not give to patients with poison/drug-induced shock (except for β-blocker poisoning). • May use higher doses for β-blocker poisoning.	**IV Administration** • Infuse at 2 to 10 mcg per minute. • Titrate to adequate heart rate. • In torsades de pointes titrate to increase heart rate until VT is suppressed.
Lidocaine Can be given via endotracheal tube	**Indications** • Alternative to amiodarone in cardiac arrest from VF/VT. • Stable monomorphic VT with preserved ventricular function. • Stable polymorphic VT with normal baseline QT interval and preserved LV function when ischemia is treated and electrolyte balance is corrected. • Can be used for stable polymorphic VT with baseline QT-interval prolongation if torsades suspected. **Precautions/Contraindications** • **Contraindication:** *Prophylactic* use in AMI is contraindicated. • Reduce maintenance dose (not loading dose) in presence of impaired liver function or LV dysfunction. • Discontinue infusion immediately if signs of toxicity develop.	**Cardiac Arrest From VF/VT** • Initial dose: 1 to 1.5 mg/kg IV/IO. • For refractory VF may give additional 0.5 to 0.75 mg/kg IV push, repeat in 5 to 10 minutes; maximum 3 doses or total of 3 mg/kg. **Perfusing Arrhythmia** For stable VT, wide-complex tachycardia of uncertain type, significant ectopy: • Doses ranging from 0.5 to 0.75 mg/kg and up to 1 to 1.5 mg/kg may be used. • Repeat 0.5 to 0.75 mg/kg every 5 to 10 minutes; maximum total dose: 3 mg/kg. **Maintenance Infusion** 1 to 4 mg per minute (30 to 50 mcg/kg per minute).

Drug/Therapy	Indications/Precautions	Adult Dosage
Magnesium Sulfate	**Indications** • Recommended for use in cardiac arrest only if torsades de pointes or suspected hypomagnesemia is present. • Life-threatening ventricular arrhythmias due to digitalis toxicity. • Routine administration in hospitalized patients with AMI is **not** recommended. **Precautions** • Occasional fall in blood pressure with rapid administration. • Use with caution if renal failure is present.	**Cardiac Arrest** **(Due to Hypomagnesemia or Torsades de Pointes)** 1 to 2 g (2 to 4 mL of a 50% solution) diluted in 10 mL of D_5W IV/IO. **Torsades de Pointes With a Pulse or AMI With Hypomagnesemia** • Loading dose of 1 to 2 g mixed in 50 to 100 mL of D_5W, over 5 to 60 minutes IV. • Follow with 0.5 to 1 g per hour IV (titrate to control torsades).
Mannitol Strengths: 5%, 10%, 15%, 20%, and 25%	**Indications** Increased intracranial pressure in management of neurologic emergencies. **Precautions** • Monitor fluid status and serum osmolality (not to exceed 310 mOsm/kg). • Caution in renal failure because fluid overload may result.	**IV Administration** • Administer 0.5 to 1 g/kg over 5 to 10 minutes through in-line filter. • Additional doses of 0.25 to 2 g/kg can be given every 4 to 6 hours as needed. • Use with support of oxygenation and ventilation.
Milrinone Shorter half-life than inamrinone	**Indications** Myocardial dysfunction and increased systemic or pulmonary vascular resistance, including • Congestive heart failure in postoperative cardiovascular surgical patients. • Shock with high systemic vascular resistance. **Precautions** May produce nausea, vomiting, hypotension, particularly in volume-depleted patients. Shorter half-life and less effect on platelets but more risk for ventricular arrhythmia than inamrinone. Drug may accumulate in renal failure and in patients with low cardiac output; reduce dose in renal failure.	**Loading Dose** 50 mcg/kg over 10 minutes IV loading dose. **IV Infusion** • 0.375 to 0.75 mcg/kg per minute. • Hemodynamic monitoring required. • Reduce dose in renal impairment.
Morphine Sulfate	**Indications** • Chest pain with ACS unresponsive to nitrates. • Acute cardiogenic pulmonary edema (if blood pressure is adequate). **Precautions** • Administer slowly and titrate to effect. • May cause respiratory depression. • Causes hypotension in volume-depleted patients. • Use with caution in RV infarction. • May reverse with naloxone (0.04 to 2 mg IV).	**IV Administration** • STEMI: Give 2 to 4 mg IV. May give additional doses of 2 to 8 mg IV at 5- to 15-minute intervals. Analgesic of choice. • UA/NSTEMI: Give 1 to 5 mg IV only if symptoms not relieved by nitrates or if symptoms recur. Use with caution.
Naloxone Hydrochloride Can be given via entotracheal tube	**Indications** Respiratory and neurologic depression due to opiate intoxication unresponsive to oxygen and support of ventilation. **Precautions** • May cause severe opiate withdrawal, including hypertensive crisis and pulmonary edema when given in large doses (titration of small doses recommended). • Half-life shorter than narcotics, repeat dosing may be needed. • Monitor for recurrent respiratory depression. • Rare anaphylactic reactions have been reported. • Assist ventilation before naloxone administration, avoid sympathetic stimulation. • Avoid in meperidine-induced seizures.	**Administration** • Typical IV dose 0.04 to 0.4 mg, titrate until ventilation adequate. • Use higher doses for complete narcotic reversal. • Can administer up to 6 to 10 mg over short period (<10 minutes). • If total reversal is not required (eg, respiratory depression from sedation), smaller doses of 0.04 mg repeated every 2 to 3 minutes may be used. • IM/subcutaneously: 0.4 to 0.8 mg. • For chronic opioid-addicted patients, use smaller dose and titrate slowly.
Nicardipine (Cardene) Calcium channel blocker	**Indications** • Hypertensive emergencies. • Decrease blood pressure to ≤185/110 mm Hg before administration of fibrinolytic therapy. **Precautions/Contraindications** • Avoid rapid decrease in blood pressure. • Reflex tachycardia or increased angina may occur in patients with extensive coronary disease. • Avoid use in patients with severe aortic stenosis. • Do not mix with sodium bicarbonate or Ringer's lactate solution.	**Acute Hypertension Emergencies** • Initial infusion rate 5 mg per hour; may increase by 2.5 mg per hour every 5 to 15 minutes to maximum of 15 mg per hour. • Decrease infusion rate to 3 mg per hour once desired blood pressure reached.

Drug/Therapy	Indications/Precautions	Adult Dosage
Nitroglycerin Available in IV form, sublingual tablets, and aerosol spray	**Indications** • Initial antianginal for suspected ischemic pain. • For initial 24 to 48 hours in patients with *AMI and CHF*, large anterior wall infarction, persistent or recurrent ischemia, or hypertension. • Continued use (beyond 48 hours) for patients with recurrent angina or persistent pulmonary congestion (nitrate-free interval recommended). • Hypertensive urgency with ACS. **Contraindications** • Hypotension (SBP <90 mm Hg or ≥30 mm Hg below baseline). • Severe bradycardia (<50 per minute) or tachycardia (>100 per minute). • RV infarction. • Use of phosphodiesterase inhibitors for erectile dysfunction (eg, sildenafil and vardenafil within 24 hours; tadalafil within 48 hours). **Precautions** • Generally, with evidence of AMI and normotension, do not reduce SBP to <110 mm Hg. If patient is hypertensive, do not decrease mean arterial pressure (MAP) by >25% (from initial MAP). • Do not mix with other drugs. • Patient should sit or lie down when receiving this medication. • Do not shake aerosol spray because this affects metered dose.	**IV Administration** • **IV bolus:** 12.5 to 25 mcg (if no SL or spray given). • **Infusion:** Begin at 10 mcg per minute. Titrate to effect, increase by 10 mcg per minute every 3 to 5 minutes until desired effect. Ceiling dose of 200 mcg per minute commonly used. — Route of choice for emergencies. **Sublingual Route** • 1 tablet (0.3 to 0.4 mg), repeated for total of 3 doses at 5-minute intervals. • 1 to 2 sprays for 0.5 to 1 second at 5-minute intervals (provides 0.4 mg per dose). Maximum 3 sprays within 15 minutes. • *Note:* Patients should be instructed to contact EMS if pain is unrelieved or increasing after 1 tablet or sublingual spray.
Nitroprusside (Sodium Nitroprusside)	**Indications** • Hypertensive crisis. • To reduce afterload in heart failure and acute pulmonary edema. • To reduce afterload in acute mitral or aortic valve regurgitation. **Precautions** • May cause hypotension and cyanide toxicity. • May reverse hypoxic pulmonary vasoconstriction in patients with pulmonary disease, exacerbating intrapulmonary shunting, resulting in hypoxemia. • Other side effects include headaches, nausea, vomiting, and abdominal cramps. • Contraindicated in patients who have recently taken phosphodiesterase inhibitors for erectile dysfunction (eg, sildenafil).	**IV Administration** • Add 50 or 100 mg to 250 mL D_5W. (Refer to your institutional pharmacy policy.) • Begin at 0.1 mcg/kg per minute and titrate upward every 3 to 5 minutes to desired effect (usually up to 5 mcg/kg per minute, but higher doses up to 10 mcg/kg may be needed). • Use with an infusion pump; use hemodynamic monitoring for optimal safety. • Action occurs within 1 to 2 minutes. • Light sensitive; cover drug reservoir and tubing with opaque material.
Norepinephrine	**Indications** • Severe cardiogenic shock and hemodynamically significant hypotension (SBP <70 mm Hg) with low total peripheral resistance. • Agent of last resort for management of ischemic heart disease and shock. **Precautions** • Increases myocardial oxygen requirements; raises blood pressure and heart rate. • May induce arrhythmias. Use with caution in patients with acute ischemia; monitor cardiac output. • Extravasation causes tissue necrosis. • If extravasation occurs, administer phentolamine 5 to 10 mg in 10 to 15 mL saline solution; infiltrate into area. • Relatively contraindicated in patients with hypovolemia.	**IV Administration (Only Route)** • Initial rate: 0.1 to 0.5 mcg/kg per minute (for 70-kg patient: 7 to 35 mcg per minute); titrate to response. • Do not administer in same IV line as alkaline solutions. • Poison/drug-induced hypotension may require higher doses to achieve adequate perfusion.

<table>
<tr><th>Drug/Therapy</th><th>Indications/Precautions</th><th>Adult Dosage</th></tr>
<tr>
<td>Oxygen
Delivered from portable tanks or installed, wall-mounted sources through delivery devices</td>
<td>Indications
• Any suspected cardiopulmonary emergency.
• Complaints of shortness of breath and suspected ischemic pain.
• For ACS: May administer to all patients until stable. Continue if pulmonary congestion, ongoing ischemia, or oxygen saturation <94%.
• For patients with suspected stroke and hypoxemia, arterial oxygen desaturation (oxyhemoglobin saturation <94%), or unknown oxyhemoglobin saturation. May consider administration to patients who are not hypoxemic.
• After ROSC following resuscitation: Use the minimum inspired oxygen concentration to achieve oxyhemoglobin saturation ≥94%. If equipment available, to avoid hyperoxia, wean inspired oxygen when oxyhemoglobin saturation is 100% but maintain ≥94%.
Precautions
• Observe closely when using with pulmonary patients known to be dependent on hypoxic respiratory drive (very rare).
• Pulse oximetry may be inaccurate in low cardiac output states, with vasoconstriction, or with exposure to carbon monoxide.</td>
<td><table>
<tr><th>Device</th><th>Flow Rate</th><th>O_2 (%)</th></tr>
<tr><td>Nasal cannula</td><td>1-6 L per minute</td><td>21-44</td></tr>
<tr><td>Venturi mask</td><td>4-12 L per minute</td><td>24-50</td></tr>
<tr><td>Partial rebreathing mask</td><td>6-10 L per minute</td><td>35-60</td></tr>
<tr><td>Nonrebreathing oxygen mask with reservoir</td><td>6-15 L per minute</td><td>60-100</td></tr>
<tr><td>Bag-mask with nonrebreathing "tail"</td><td>15 L per minute</td><td>95-100</td></tr>
</table>
Note: Pulse oximetry provides a useful method of titrating oxygen administration to maintain physiologic oxygen saturation (see Precautions).</td>
</tr>
<tr>
<td>Procainamide</td>
<td>Indications
• Useful for treatment of a wide variety of arrhythmias, including stable monomorphic VT with normal QT interval and preserved LV function.
• May use for treatment of reentry SVT uncontrolled by adenosine and vagal maneuvers if blood pressure stable.
• Stable wide-complex tachycardia of unknown origin.
• Atrial fibrillation with rapid rate in Wolff-Parkinson-White syndrome.
Precautions
• If cardiac or renal dysfunction is present, reduce maximum total dose to 12 mg/kg and maintenance infusion to 1 to 2 mg per minute.
• Proarrhythmic, especially in setting of AMI, hypokalemia, or hypomagnesemia.
• May induce hypotension in patients with impaired LV function.
• Use with caution with other drugs that prolong QT interval (eg, amiodarone). Expert consultation advised.</td>
<td>Recurrent VF/VT
• 20 mg per minute IV infusion (maximum total dose: 17 mg/kg).
• In urgent situations, up to 50 mg per minute may be administered to total dose of 17 mg/kg.
Other Indications
• 20 mg per minute IV infusion until one of the following occurs:
— Arrhythmia suppression.
— Hypotension.
— QRS widens by >50%.
— Total dose of 17 mg/kg is given.
• Use in cardiac arrest limited by need for slow infusion and uncertain efficacy.
Maintenance Infusion
1 to 4 mg per minute (dilute in D_5W or NS). Reduce dose in presence of renal insufficiency.</td>
</tr>
<tr>
<td>Sodium Bicarbonate</td>
<td>Indications
• Known preexisting hyperkalemia.
• Known preexisting bicarbonate-responsive acidosis; eg, diabetic ketoacidosis or overdose of tricyclic antidepressant, aspirin, cocaine, or diphenhydramine.
• Prolonged resuscitation with effective ventilation; on return of spontaneous circulation after long arrest interval.
• Not useful or effective in hypercarbic acidosis (eg, cardiac arrest and CPR without intubation).
Precautions
• Adequate ventilation and CPR, not bicarbonate, are the major "buffer agents" in cardiac arrest.
• Not recommended for routine use in cardiac arrest patients.</td>
<td>IV Administration
• 1 mEq/kg IV bolus.
• If rapidly available, use arterial blood gas analysis to guide bicarbonate therapy (calculated base deficits or bicarbonate concentration). During cardiac arrest, ABG results are not reliable indicators of acidosis.</td>
</tr>
<tr>
<td>Sotalol
Seek expert consultation</td>
<td>Indications
Treatment of supraventricular arrhythmias and ventricular arrhythmias in patients without structural heart disease.
Precautions/Contraindications
• Should be avoided in patients with poor perfusion because of significant negative inotropic effects.
• Adverse effects include bradycardia, hypotension, and arrhythmias (torsades de pointes).
• Use with caution with other drugs that prolong QT interval (eg, procainamide, amiodarone).
• May become toxic in patients with renal impairment; contraindicated if creatinine clearance <40 mL per minute.</td>
<td>IV Administration
• 1 to 1.5 mg/kg.
• Check hospital protocol for infusion rate. Package insert recommends slow infusion, but literature supports more rapid infusion of 1.5 mg/kg over 5 minutes or less.</td>
</tr>
<tr>
<td>Thienopyridines
(see ADP Antagonists)</td>
<td colspan="2"></td>
</tr>
<tr>
<td>Thrombolytic Agents
(see Fibrinolytic Agents)</td>
<td colspan="2"></td>
</tr>
</table>

Drug/Therapy	Indications/Precautions	Adult Dosage
Vasopressin Can be given via endotracheal tube	**Indications** • May be used as alternative pressor to epinephrine in treatment of adult shock-refractory VF. • May be useful alternative to epinephrine in asystole, PEA. • May be useful for hemodynamic support in vasodilatory shock (eg, septic shock). **Precautions/Contraindications** • Potent peripheral vasoconstrictor. Increased peripheral vascular resistance may provoke cardiac ischemia and angina. • Not recommended for responsive patients with coronary artery disease.	**IV Administration** **Cardiac arrest:** One dose of 40 units IV/IO push may replace either first or second dose of epinephrine. Epinephrine can be administered every 3 to 5 minutes during cardiac arrest. **Vasodilatory shock:** Continuous infusion of 0.02 to 0.04 units per minute.
Verapamil	**Indications** • Alternative drug (after adenosine) to terminate re-entry SVT with narrow QRS complex and adequate blood pressure and *preserved LV function.* • May control ventricular response in patients with atrial fibrillation, flutter, or multifocal atrial tachycardia. **Precautions** • Give *only* to patients with narrow-complex reentry SVT or known supraventricular arrhythmias. • Do not use for wide-QRS tachycardias of uncertain origin, and avoid use for Wolff-Parkinson-White syndrome and atrial fibrillation, sick sinus syndrome, or second- or third-degree AV block without pacemaker. • May decrease myocardial contractility and can produce peripheral vasodilation and hypotension. IV calcium may restore blood pressure in toxic cases. • Concurrent IV administration with IV β-blockers may produce severe hypotension. Use with extreme caution in patients receiving oral β-blockers.	**IV Administration** • **First dose:** 2.5 to 5 mg IV bolus over 2 minutes (over 3 minutes in older patients). • **Second dose:** 5 to 10 mg, if needed, every 15 to 30 minutes. Maximum total dose: 20 mg. • **Alternative:** 5 mg bolus every 15 minutes to total dose of 30 mg.

Appendix

Index

- Start with the simple and minimally invasive techniques. Initiate more complex approaches as more resources and personnel become available.
- Do not delay urgent procedures such as airway management and insertion of vascular catheters. Although these patients may exhibit cardiac irritability, this concern should not delay necessary interventions.

Warm, Humid Oxygen (Administration Temperature: 42°C to 46°C or 108°F to 115°F)

Most experts recommend administration of warm, humid oxygen as a mainstay of active internal rewarming for patients with severe hypothermia but no cardiac arrest.[20-22,47,48] With the aerosol heated to 40°C (104°F), this technique rewarms at a rate of 1°C to 1.5°C (1.8°F to 2.7°F) per hour. Heated to 45°C (113°F), the rewarming rate increases to 1.5°C to 2°C (2.7°F to 3.6°F) per hour.[49-51]

Warm IV Fluids (42°C to 44°C or 108°F to 111°F)

Warm IV fluid is also infused centrally at a rate of approximately 150 to 200 mL/h IV. Avoid excessive fluid administration and provide sufficient fluid to maintain urinary output of 0.5 to 1 mL/kg per hour.[43]

Warm-Water Lavage (KCl-Free Fluid, Warmed to 43°C or 109°F)

Many experienced clinicians consider peritoneal lavage the preferred run-in/run-out heated lavage technique.[49] Other anatomic sites may be used for heated lavage, including the stomach, colon, bladder, chest (closed thoracic cavity lavage),[49,51] and heart (direct cardiac lavage can be performed after open thoracotomy and cardiac massage).[33,35-39,52]

Extracorporeal Rewarming (Cardiac Bypass)

Extracorporeal rewarming is the most effective technique for core rewarming of hypothermic patients in cardiac arrest.[53] Extracorporeal rewarming techniques have considerable advantages. They provide adequate support of oxygenation, ventilation, and perfusion, and they enable rapid core rewarming (up to 1°C or 1.8°F every 5 minutes).[32,40-42]

Other Active Internal Warming Techniques

Several other active internal rewarming techniques have resulted in neurologically intact survival from hypothermic cardiac arrest. These techniques include peritoneal lavage[54]; peritoneal lavage combined with warm water bags, warm IV fluids, and continuous CPR[55]; and continuous, closed thoracostomy lavage using 2 chest tubes.[56,57]

Cardiac Arrest Interventions

Patients in ***hypothermic cardiac arrest*** will require CPR with some modifications from conventional BLS and ACLS care and will require active internal rewarming.

Modifications to BLS for Hypothermia

For patients in cardiac arrest, the general approach to BLS management should still target breathing and circulation but with some modifications in approach. When the patient is hypothermic, pulse and respiratory rates may be slow or difficult to detect.[49,58]

If the hypothermic victim has no signs of life or if there is any doubt about whether a pulse is present, begin CPR without delay. If the victim is not breathing, start rescue breathing immediately. Do not wait to check the victim's temperature to initiate CPR. If possible, administer warm (42°C to 46°C [108°F to 115°F]), humid oxygen during bag-mask ventilation.

The temperature at which defibrillation should first be attempted in the severely hypothermic patient and the number of defibrillation attempts that should be made have not been established. There are case reports of refractory ventricular arrhythmias with severe hypothermia; however, in a recent animal model it was found that an animal with a temperature of as low as 30°C had a better response to defibrillation than did normothermic animals in arrest.[59,60]

In general, providers should attempt defibrillation (1 shock) without regard to core body temperature. It is unacceptable to delay defibrillation attempts to assess core temperature. If VT or VF is present, defibrillation should be attempted. Automated external defibrillators may be used for these patients. If VF is detected, it should be treated with 1 shock, immediately followed by resumption of CPR. If VT or VF persists after a single shock, the value of deferring subsequent defibrillations until a target temperature is achieved is uncertain. It may be reasonable to perform further defibrillation attempts according to the standard BLS algorithm concurrent with rewarming techniques (Class IIb, LOE C).

Modifications to ACLS for Hypothermia

For unresponsive patients or those in arrest, advanced airway insertion is appropriate as recommended in the standard ACLS guidelines. Advanced airway management serves 2 purposes in the management of hypothermia: it enables provision of effective ventilation with warm, humidified oxygen, and it can isolate the airway to reduce the likelihood of aspiration for patients in peri-arrest.

ACLS management of cardiac arrest due to hypothermia focuses on more aggressive active core rewarming techniques as the primary therapeutic modality. Conventional wisdom indicates that the hypothermic heart may be unresponsive to cardiovascular drugs, pacemaker stimulation, and defibrillation; however, the data to support this are essentially theoretical.[61] In addition, drug metabolism is reduced. There is theoretical concern that in the severely